Taphonomy of Human Remains

Forensic Analysis of the Dead and the Depositional Environment

Edited by

Eline M.J. Schotsmans
PACEA De La Préhistoire à l'Actuel: Culture, Environnement et Anthropologie, UMR 5199, CNRS-Université de Bordeaux, Pessac, France

Nicholas Márquez-Grant
Cranfield Forensic Institute, Defence Academy of the United Kingdom, Cranfield University, Shrivenham, UK

Shari L. Forbes
Centre for Forensic Science, University of Technology Sydney, Sydney, Australia

université de BORDEAUX

WILEY

This edition first published 2017

Registered Office: John Wiley & Sons Ltd, The Atrium, Southern Gate, Chichester, West Sussex, PO19 8SQ, UK

Editorial offices: 9600 Garsington Road, Oxford, OX4 2DQ, UK
The Atrium, Southern Gate, Chichester, West Sussex, PO19 8SQ, UK
111 River Street, Hoboken, NJ 07030-5774, USA

For details of our global editorial offices, for customer services and for information about how to apply for permission to reuse the copyright material in this book please see our website at www.wiley.com/wiley-blackwell.

Library of Congress Cataloging-in-Publication Data

Names: Schotsmans, Eline M.J., 1981– editor. | Márquez-Grant, Nicholas, 1976– editor. | Forbes, Shari L., 1977– editor.
Title: Taphonomy of human remains : forensic analysis of the dead and the depositional environment / edited by Eline M. Schotsmans, Nicholas Márquez-Grant, Shari L. Forbes.
Description: Chichester, West Sussex ; Hoboken, NJ : John Wiley & Sons, Inc., 2017. | Includes bibliographical references and index.
Identifiers: LCCN 2016036072 (print) | LCCN 2016037394 (ebook) | ISBN 9781118953327 (cloth) | ISBN 9781118953334 (pdf) | ISBN 9781118953341 (epub)
Subjects: | MESH: Forensic Anthropology | Fossils | Postmortem Changes | Environment
Classification: LCC RA1055 (print) | LCC RA1055 (ebook) | NLM W 750 | DDC 614/.17–dc23
LC record available at https://lccn.loc.gov/2016036072

A catalogue record for this book is available from the British Library.

Wiley also publishes its books in a variety of electronic formats. Some content that appears in print may not be available in electronic books.

Cover image:
Front Cover: Human remains from a mass grave at Kozluk - Courtesy of T. Loveless
Back Cover: The hand from a body recovered from water - Courtesy of S.J. Hamilton & M.A. Green
Eroded teeth from an acid experiment - Courtesy of Rep EX/98-44.
Preserved human remains from a crypt in Italy - Courtesy of R.G. Beckett
Preserved brain from a Spanish Civil War mass grave - Courtesy of F. Serrulla

Set in 10/12pt Warnock by SPi Global, Chennai, India

Contents

List of Contributors

Maurice C.G. Aalders
Academic Medical Center
Amsterdam
The Netherlands

Esma Alicehajic
European Union Rule of Law Mission (EULEX)
Kosovo

Ruggero D'Anastasio
Museo Universitario
Università 'G. d'Annunzio'
Chieti e Pescara
Italy

Caroline Barker
Independent Forensic Anthropologist and Archaeologist

Ronald G. Beckett
Quinnipiac University
Hamden
Connecticut
USA

Bram Bekaert
KU Leuven - University of Leuven
Department of Imaging & Pathology
Forensic Biomedical Sciences
Leuven
Belgium

University Hospitals Leuven
Department of Forensic Medicine
Laboratory of Forensic Genetics and Molecular Archaeology
Leuven
Belgium

Jelena J. Bekvalac
Centre for Human Bioarchaeology
Museum of London
UK

Charles E.H. Berger
Netherlands Forensic Institute (NFI)
The Hague
The Netherlands

Institute for Criminal Law and Criminology
Faculty of Law
Leiden University
Leiden
The Netherlands

Frédérique Blaizot
Inrap
Centre Archéologique Rhône-Alpes-Auvergne
Lyon
France

PACEA De la Préhistoire à l'Actuel: Culture, Environnement et Anthropologie, UMR 5199
CNRS-Université de Bordeaux
Pessac
France

Soren Blau
Victorian Institute of Forensic Medicine
Southbank
Australia

Department of Forensic Medicine
School of Public Health and Preventive Medicine
Monash University
Australia

Martin Brown
The Plugstreet Project
Belgium

David O. Carter
Forensic Sciences Unit
Division of Natural Sciences and Mathematics
Chaminade University of Honolulu
Hawaii

Annalisa Cappella
LABANOF (Laboratorio di antropologia e odontologia forense)
Sezione di Medicina Legale e delle Assicurazioni
Dipartimento di Scienze Biomediche per la Salute
Università degli Studi di Milano
Italy

José Luis Cascallana
Instituto de Medicina Legal de Galicia
Unidad de Antropología Forense
Hospital de Verin
Ourense
Spain

Dominique Castex
PACEA De la Préhistoire à l'Actuel: Culture, Environnement et Anthropologie, UMR 5199
CNRS-Université de Bordeaux
Pessac
France

Cristina Cattaneo
LABANOF (Laboratorio di antropologia e odontologia forense)
Sezione di Medicina Legale e delle Assicurazioni
Dipartimento di Scienze Biomediche per la Salute
Università degli Studi di Milano
Italy

Emily Cline
Cranfield Forensic Institute
Defence Academy of the United Kingdom
Cranfield University
Shrivenham
UK

Jenna L. Comstock
Faculty of Science
University of Ontario Institute of Technology
Ontario
Canada

Anne Coulombeix
Institut de Recherche Criminelle de la Gendarmerie Nationale (IRCGN)
Pontoise
France

Eva Cuypers
KU Leuven - University of Leuven
Toxicology and Pharmacology
Campus Gasthuisberg
Leuven
Belgium

Franklin E. Damann
Defense POW/MIA Accounting Agency
Central Identification Laboratory
Offutt Air Force Base
Nebraska
USA

Ronny Decorte
KU Leuven - University of Leuven
Department of Imaging & Pathology
Forensic Biomedical Sciences
Leuven
Belgium

University Hospitals Leuven
Department of Forensic Medicine
Laboratory of Forensic Genetics and Molecular Archaeology
Leuven
Belgium

Roosje de Leeuwe
Netherlands Forensic Institute (NFI)
The Hague
The Netherlands

Julio Del Olmo
Asociación para la Recuperación de la Memoria Histórica de Valladolid
Spain

Maria Cristina de Mendonça
Instituto Nacional de Medicina Legal e Ciências Forenses
Coimbra
Portugal

Joanne B. Devlin
Forensic Anthropology Center
Department of Anthropology
University of Tennessee Knoxville
Tennessee
USA

Marie Christine Dussault
Department of Anatomy
Faculty of Health Sciences
University of Pretoria
South Africa

Faculty of Science and Technology
Bournemouth University
UK

Gerda J. Edelman
Netherlands Forensic Institute (NFI)
The Hague
The Netherlands

Francisco Etxeberría
Sociedad de Ciencias Aranzadi
Spain

Universidad del Pais Vasco
Spain

Julie Evans
ROAR Forensics
Malvern Hills Science Park
Malvern
Worcestershire
UK

Elissa Fleak
Los Angeles County Department of Medical Examiner-Coroner
Los Angeles
California
USA

Leonardo R. Flores Pérez
Universidad Autónoma Chapingo
Texcoco
México

Jean-François Focant
CART, Organic and Biological Analytical Chemistry Group
Chemistry Department
University of Liège
Belgium

Shari L. Forbes
Centre for Forensic Science
University of Technology Sydney
Sydney
Australia

Heather Gill-Frerking
NTK Services
Concord
New Hampshire
USA

David Gonçalves
Research Centre for Anthropology and Health (CIAS)
University of Coimbra
Coimbra
Portugal

Laboratório de Arqueociências
Direção Geral do Património Cultural and LARC/CIBIO/InBIO
Lisboa
Portugal

Laboratory of Forensic Anthropology
Department of Life Sciences
University of Coimbra
Coimbra
Portugal

Michael A. Green
Department of Forensic Pathology
University of Sheffield
Sheffield
UK

W.J. Mike Groen
Netherlands Forensic Institute (NFI)
The Hague
The Netherlands

Department of Archaeological Sciences
Faculty of Archaeology
Leiden University
Leiden
The Netherlands

Stuart J. Hamilton
East Midlands Forensic Pathology Unit
Leicester Royal Infirmary
Leicester
UK

Karl Harrison
Cranfield Forensic Institute
Defence Academy of the United Kingdom
Cranfield University
Shrivenham
UK

Lourdes Herrasti
Sociedad de Ciencias Aranzadi
Spain

Jean-Bernard Huchet
Archéozoologie, Archéobotanique: Sociétés, Pratiques et Environnements, UMR 7209
Muséum National d'Histoire Naturelle
Paris
France

Institut de Systématique, Évolution, Biodiversité (ISYEB), UMR 7205
Département Systématique et Evolution (Entomologie)
Muséum National d'Histoire Naturelle
Paris
France

PACEA De la Préhistoire à l'Actuel: Culture, Environnement et Anthropologie, UMR 5199
CNRS-Université de Bordeaux
Pessac
France

Rob C. Janaway
School of Archaeological Sciences
University of Bradford
Bradford
UK

Lee Meadows Jantz
Forensic Anthropology Center
Department of Anthropology
University of Tennessee
Knoxville
Tennessee
USA

Emily N. Junkins
Department of Microbiology and Plant Biology
University of Oklahoma
Norman
Oklahoma
USA

Richard Lloyd
Cranfield Forensic Institute
Defence Academy of the United Kingdom
Cranfield University
Shrivenham
UK

Nicholas Márquez-Grant
Cranfield Forensic Institute
Defence Academy of the United Kingdom
Cranfield University
Shrivenham
UK

Institute of Human Sciences
School of Anthropology and Museum Ethnography
University of Oxford
Oxford
UK

Jennifer Miller
School of Science and Technology
Nottingham Trent University
Clifton Campus
Nottingham
UK

Humberto Molina Chávez
Procuraduría General de Justicia del Distrito Federal – Faculty of Medicine
Universidad Nacional Autónoma de México
México

Javier Naranjo Santana
Independent Forensic Archaeologist

Manuel Nava Hernández
Procuraduría General de Justicia del Distrito Federal – Faculty of Medicine
Universidad Nacional Autónoma de México
México

Richard Osgood
The Plugstreet Project
Belgium

Claudio Ottoni
University of Oslo
Department of Biosciences
Centre for Ecological and Evolutionary Synthesis (CEES)
Oslo
Norway

KU Leuven - University of Leuven
Department of Earth and Environmental Sciences
Center for Archaeological Sciences
Leuven
Belgium

KU Leuven - University of Leuven
Department of Imaging and Pathology
Forensic Biomedical Sciences
Leuven
Belgium

Chelsea Parham
Cranfield Forensic Institute
Defence Academy of the United Kingdom
Cranfield University
Shrivenham
UK

Fray M. Pérez Villegas
Servicio Médico Forense
Pachuca de Soto
Estado de Hidalgo
México

Katelynn A. Perrault
Centre for Forensic Science
University of Technology Sydney
Sydney
Australia

Dario Piombino-Mascali
Department of Cultural Heritage and of Sicilian Identity
Palermo
Italy

Robin Quataert
Department of Anthropology
University of Indianapolis
Indiana
USA

Rebecca C. Redfern
Centre for Human Bioarchaeology
Museum of London
UK

Elien Rosier
KU Leuven - University of Leuven
Toxicology and Pharmacology
Campus Gasthuisberg
Leuven
Belgium

Christopher W. Schmidt
Department of Anthropology
University of Indianapolis
Indiana
USA

Eline M.J. Schotsmans
PACEA De la Préhistoire à l'Actuel: Culture, Environnement et Anthropologie, UMR 5199
CNRS-Université de Bordeaux
Pessac
France

School of Archaeological Sciences
University of Bradford
Bradford
UK

Yves Schuliar
Institut de Recherche Criminelle de la Gendarmerie Nationale (IRCGN)
Pontoise
France

Fernando Serrulla
Sociedad de Ciencias Aranzadi
Spain

Instituto de Medicina Legal de Galicia
Unidad de Antropología Forense
Hospital de Verin
Ourense
Spain

Tal Simmons
Department of Forensic Science
Virginia Commonwealth University
Richmond
Virginia
USA

Dawnie W. Steadman
Forensic Anthropology Center
Department of Anthropology
University of Tennessee Knoxville
Tennessee
USA

Pierre-Hugues Stefanuto
CART, Organic and Biological Analytical Chemistry Group
Chemistry Department
University of Liège
Belgium

Barbara H. Stuart
Centre for Forensic Science
University of Technology Sydney
Sydney
Australia

Kirsty Squires
Department of Forensic and Crime Science
Faculty of Computing, Engineering and Sciences
Staffordshire University
Stoke-on-Trent
UK

Tim J.U. Thompson
School of Science & Engineering
Teesside University
Middlesbrough
UK

Jan Tytgat
KU Leuven - University of Leuven
Toxicology and Pharmacology
Campus Gasthuisberg
Leuven
Belgium

Maiken Ueland
Centre for Forensic Science
University of Technology Sydney
Sydney
Australia

Stefano Vanin
School of Applied Sciences
University of Huddersfield
Huddersfield
UK

Wim Van de Voorde
KU Leuven - University of Leuven
Department of Imaging & Pathology
Forensic Biomedical Sciences
Leuven
Belgium

University Hospitals Leuven
Department of Forensic Medicine
Leuven
Belgium

Arpad A. Vass
Nebulytics Inc.
Oak Ridge
Tennessee
USA

Giovanna M. Vidoli
Forensic Anthropology Center
Department of Anthropology
University of Tennessee Knoxville
Tennessee
USA

Priscilla Ulguim
School of Science & Engineering
Teesside University
Middlesbrough
UK

Andrew S. Wilson
School of Archaeological Sciences
University of Bradford
Bradford
UK

Alexandria Young
Independent Forensic Anthropologist and Archaeologist

Fatma Zalzala
Department of Anthropology
University of Indianapolis
Indiana
USA

Notes on Contributors

Eline M.J. Schotsmans is a researcher at the University of Bordeaux in France and an honorary research fellow at the University of Bradford, UK, specialising in taphonomy and forensic archaeology. Her research is focused on inorganic materials in burials and lies at the interface between archaeo-anthropology and forensic sciences. Originally from Belgium, she completed a PhD at the University of Bradford on a taphonomy topic, more specifically the effects of lime on the decay of human remains by studying forensic and archaeological lime burials. Eline is regularly consulted on forensic casework and has a wide range of forensic experience gained through continuous professional collaboration with the Belgian DVI, different police forces in the UK and Kenyon International Emergency Services. Her field forensic experience includes the response to five aircraft accidents and one terrorist attack. She also travelled to Burundi to join a team of forensic experts from the University of Leuven (KUL) and DVI Belgium, to search for the remains of the last Burundian King assassinated in 1972. Eline publishes regularly in forensic journals, acts as guest lecturer in France and the UK, and delivers forensic training courses and exercises.

Nicholas Márquez-Grant is a Lecturer in Forensic Anthropology and Course Director of the MSc Forensic Archaeology and Anthropology at Cranfield Forensic Institute, Cranfield University, UK. Previously, he worked for several years as a Specialist Forensic Practitioner and a Reporting Scientist in Anthropology and Archaeology for two of the largest independent forensic science providers in the UK. Having worked for over 15 years as a specialist in human skeletal remains from archaeological sites, both on a freelance basis and for a number of commercial archaeological companies, he has considerable experience in the excavation and the study of cremated and unburnt bones from sites dating from Prehistory to the present day, and from a variety of geographical areas, in particular Britain and Spain. In addition, he is often consulted and deployed to other European countries to assist in the identification of WWI and WWII casualties. He has worked on more than 70 forensic cases for over 20 different police forces, in addition to many bone identification enquiries, and he continues to consult in forensic cases today. Nicholas has acted as an expert witness and he is an accredited Level 1 Forensic Anthropologist by the Royal Anthropological Institute in the UK. He is also a Research Associate of the School of Anthropology and Museum Ethnography at the University of Oxford, where he has taught biological anthropology since 2001 and where he obtained his doctoral degree in 2006. Nicholas is co-editor of the *Routledge Handbook of Archaeological Human Remains and Legislation* (Routledge, 2011), *Forensic Ecology Handbook* (Wiley-Blackwell, 2012) and *Forensic Archaeology: A Global Perspective* (Wiley-Blackwell, 2015).

Shari L. Forbes is a Professor at the University of Technology Sydney (UTS) in Australia. She completed a Bachelor of Science (Hons) in Applied Chemistry and Forensic Science and a PhD (Forensic Chemistry) at UTS. She spent two years as a Postdoctoral Fellow at the Centre for Forensic Science, University of Western Australia. In 2005, she moved to Canada as the founding Director of the Forensic Science programme at the University of Ontario Institute of Technology (UOIT). Shari spent seven applications of forensic taphonomy, and illustrating how to proceed in specific situations, such as a body in concrete, a saponified brain, interpretation of textile degradation, or various types of burials.

We congratulate the editors on compiling such a wide range of topics and perspectives from Europe, Australia and North America. We are especially pleased to see the editors' incorporation of a broad purview that integrates forensic and strictly archaeological time frames. The relatively fine-grained, actualistic knowledge about death events in forensic taphonomy has potentially much to teach more traditional taphonomic efforts. The breadth of experience represented here, and the comprehensive coverage of the most important topics in forensic taphonomy, is a real contribution to the field.

Marcella H. Sorg
Research Professor, Department of Anthropology, University of Maine, Orono, Maine, USA

William D. Haglund
Senior Forensic Consultant, Shoreline, Washington, USA

Acknowledgements

Our heartfelt gratitude goes to numerous people. We would like to thank all 77 authors for their excellent contributions and for their patience during the progress of this volume. We also offer our gratitude to Marcella Sorg and William Haglund who provided the foreword to this volume and triggered our interest in forensic taphonomy many years ago.

We are much obliged to our colleagues and friends for their support, helpful comments and chapter reviews, in particular Dominique Castex, Christopher Knüsel, Jean-Bernard Huchet, Kris Vleeschouwer, Sébastien Villotte, Jacqueline Towers, Rémy Chapoulie, Priscilla Bayle, Marie-Paule De Brabander and Tatyana Shvedchikova. We are also very grateful to Tim Loveless for providing some of his touching photographs for us to select an image for the cover of this book.

Grateful thanks goes to all our family members, friends and colleagues for their encouragement, support and advice during the progress of this book. We are truly indebted to them.

The editors would like to thank Denny Collie, Jennifer Grant and Lucy Douglas from ELES Editing (UK) for diligently proofreading the entire manuscript. Likewise, a special thanks goes to the entire Wiley team.

Finally, we are very grateful to the Excellence Initiative of the University of Bordeaux (FR) for funding this project (IdEx Bordeaux ANR-10-IDEX-03-02). This would not have been possible without the help of Cathérine Morel-Chevillet, Jean-François Caro, Carlos Mendoza-Palomares and Maison des Sciences de l'Homme d'Aquitaine.

We also thank our institutions for supporting this project: Université de Bordeaux (FR), University of Bradford (UK), Cranfield University (UK) and University of Technology Sydney (AU).

Introduction

Eline M.J. Schotsmans, Nicholas Márquez-Grant and Shari L. Forbes

Over the last 35 years, taphonomy has gained increased importance in several disciplines such as palaeontology, archaeology, anthropology, zoology and geology. As a result of this focus on taphonomy, the depositional environment has also become more important for the contextual information that it can provide. Without studying the depositional environment, carrying out a thorough death investigation becomes more difficult.

This used to be different in the past. Many remains, whether forensic evidence, human remains, animal remains or even stone tools, were (and are) often studied outside their depositional context. Although there is some overlap, the division between archaeology and anthropology in most European countries is an interesting example of this separation between the field and the laboratory: the archaeologist attends the search and recovers the remains in the field, whilst the anthropologist studies skeletal remains, often in the laboratory or in a morgue setting[1]. Fortunately, this approach is changing and understanding the context, in which human remains have been found, is gaining increased importance. One example of the value of this can be found in the work of Henri Duday on archaeothantology, which emphasises the importance of analysis in the field (Duday 2006, 2009) (Chapter 19).

The same is noticed in forensic science. Far too often, evidence is processed in the laboratory, by scientists who did not attend the (crime) scene, and sometimes communication is limited between the crime scene investigator who collected the evidence and the forensic scientists who analyse the evidence. The forensic taphonomy volumes written by Haglund and Sorg (1997a, 2002), which still have a large influence today, helped to increase the awareness of the environmental context and prompted an improvement in death investigations. Over the years, research in this area has grown and much more experimental work is now undertaken.

This book aims to provide an update of current research in forensic taphonomy, including all stages of a decaying body from soft tissue to skeletal remains. It demonstrates the close association between human remains, and the need for analysis and interpretation by an interdisciplinary team to better understand the science of taphonomy.

I.1 Efremov: from Taphonomy to Science Fiction

The term 'taphonomy' (from Greek *taphos* meaning burial and *nomos* meaning law) was introduced to palaeontology in 1935 by the Russian scientist Ivan Antonovich Yefremov (often spelled as Efremov).

1 For more information about the disciplines of forensic archaeology and anthropology in different parts of the world: see Groen *et al.* 2015.

Taphonomy of Human Remains: Forensic Analysis of the Dead and the Depositional Environment, First Edition.
Edited by Eline M.J. Schotsmans, Nicholas Márquez-Grant and Shari L. Forbes.

In palaeontology, Efremov introduced taphonomy to indicate the study of the transition of organisms from the biosphere to the lithosphere or geological record (Efremov 1940; Lyman 1994; Turner *et al.* 2013). Outside Russia, the term 'taphonomy' is directly associated with Efremov and palaeontology. Inside Russia, however, Efremov is only known as a famous science fiction author.

Efremov was born in 1908 near St Petersburg. He served and engaged in military action with the Red Army from 1919 to 1921. After taking courses in biology, in 1925 he became the assistant of a professor in Leningrad. He defended his doctorate in biology in 1941. Efremov spent several years working on Mongolian fossil reptile deposits, making taphonomic interpretations in the overlap area between biology and geology. His basic ideas of taphonomy were described in a paper from 1935 entitled 'Falling out of transitional forms in the conditions of burial of the oldest quadruped' (Turner *et al.* 2013). While he was awarded several scientific prizes within Russia (e.g. the State prize in 1952), he was accused of serving as a spy and had to leave on early retirement in 1957. Restrained from science, he started to write science fiction novels. He died in Moscow in 1972 under suspicious circumstances (Shvedchikova 2013; Turner *et al.* 2013). It is very difficult to find primary sources relating to his retirement, his 'alleged' acting as a spy and the circumstances surrounding his death. Therefore it is almost ironic that Ivan Efremov became well known in the world of forensic science.

1.2 The Meaning of Taphonomy

The definition of taphonomy is slightly different in every discipline. Amongst many proposed definitions, we chose the following three examples. In archaeology, Renfrew and Bahn (1991) described taphonomy as 'the assessment of what has happened to an object or organism between its deposition and its recovery'. In palaeobiology, taphonomy is seen as 'the study of processes of preservation and how they affect information' (Behrensmeyer and Kidwell 1985). The forensic definition provided by Haglund and Sorg (1997a) states that forensic taphonomy is the use of taphonomic models, approaches and analyses in forensic contexts to estimate the time since death, reconstruct the circumstances before and after decomposition, and discriminate the products of human behaviour from those created by the earth's biological, physical, chemical and geological subsystems.

In this volume, we suggest combining those definitions into a broad spectrum one: forensic taphonomy as the interdisciplinary study of what has happened to an organism between death and its recovery. However, some may want to include taphonomic factors that affect human remains after recovery (e.g. modifications due to transportation, storage, destructive sampling, etc.) (Chapter 24). Taphonomy assesses the depositional environment and examines peri- and post-mortem processes, which affect the preservation and degradation, in order to discriminate human behaviour from natural processes. As such, the original conditions could be reconstructed and event sequences recreated. An important aim of forensic taphonomy is to serve the justice system and the law. The main goals of applying taphonomy to forensic investigations are to identify the remains, estimate post-mortem interval (PMI), investigate the circumstances surrounding death, including cause and manner of death and, if applicable, identify clues that can lead to the person who executed a criminal act. Therefore, it is a key in distinguishing natural processes from human-induced actions, considering all factors that could affect the rate of decomposition and the conditions in which the remains have been found.

It is the combination of intrinsic and extrinsic factors, which make every deposition unique, a division that was originally proposed by Henderson (1987). Intrinsic factors depend on the nature of the body itself and the complexity of its structure such as age, sex, body mass and physical state at the time of death. Extrinsic factors can be divided into two main categories: the depositional context and human behaviour including cultural aspects. Amongst the environmental factors that affect decomposition are water, soil, temperature, oxygen and local fauna and flora. Human behaviour could be the cause of death and includes when, how and where a body is deposited. Moreover, the latter includes treatment of the body, such as dismemberment or the application of certain chemicals to the body.

Often, taphonomic questions are being asked when decomposed or skeletal remains are on the mortuary table. This leads to a misunderstanding that (forensic) taphonomy starts when human remains are skeletonised. It is important to highlight that forensic taphonomy is more than the study of skeletal remains and that it includes the study of remains with soft tissue.

This introduction does not aim to rewrite the theory behind forensic taphonomy and will not propose models. For a concise and thorough theoretical overview, the chapters by Haglund and Sorg (1997b,1997c), Sorg and Haglund (2002) and Nordby (2002) are recommended literature. Further modelling and the application of the archaeological paradigm to crime scene investigation are provided by Groen and Berger in Chapter 36.

I.3 The Rationale Behind this Volume

During the past three decades, the field of forensic taphonomy has grown intensely with ground-breaking research and experiments in many sub-disciplines. Forensic taphonomy is applied to various criminal, medico-legal and civil law contexts by scientists of a number of disciplines. Up-to-date research is presented in journals such as *Forensic Science International* or *Journal of Forensic Sciences*. Despite this, there are few publications that provide a holistic overview, bringing together diverse approaches from a variety of disciplines, including case studies and the most recent research and developments.

The first volume in the field of forensic taphonomy, entitled *Forensic Taphonomy, the Postmortem Fate of Human Remains*, was published in 1997 and edited by William D. Haglund and Marcella H. Sorg. As a result of its international success as a world reference, the editors published a second edition in 2002, titled *Advances in Forensic Taphonomy; Method, Theory, and Archaeological Perspectives*. It was not until 2010 that another book on forensic taphonomy was published, edited by Mark Tibbett and David O. Carter with a focus on soils, called *Soil Analysis in Forensic Taphonomy: Chemical and Biological Effects of Buried Human Remains*. In 2013, a fourth volume on forensic taphonomy was published, edited by James T. Pokines and Steven A. Symes, focusing on skeletal remains and entitled *Manual of Forensic Taphonomy*.

All the above texts have provided valuable new data to the study of forensic taphonomy. However, the field has continued to grow and has encompassed an even broader range of scientific disciplines over the past two decades. While there are many volumes on forensic anthropology and forensic pathology, there appears to be a lack of literature that is focused on the chemical and biological processes of soft tissue decomposition of human remains, and the degradation of associated artefacts or textiles, particularly in the depositional environment. Moreover, there is a need for more comparative case studies.

Thus, this volume aims to provide a comprehensive representation of the disciplines now studied within forensic taphonomy and to fill any gaps in the literature. Chapters and case studies have been written by international colleagues whose expertise is invaluable. The authors consist of a combination of young and senior researchers worldwide: upcoming scholars in the field and forensic practitioners, working within different jurisdictions and frameworks, and exposed to a variety of scenarios and contexts. It is written by and for specialists of different forensic disciplines, such as pathology, anthropology, archaeology, entomology, botany, chemistry, microbiology and soil science.

I.4 Challenges in Forensic Taphonomy

While working on this volume, the editors compiled a list of future considerations in forensic taphonomy. Surprisingly, almost 20 years after Haglund and Sorg's (1997b) publications, the list appeared to be very similar to their recommendations in 'suggestions for the future of forensic taphonomy'. Haglund and Sorg (1997b) based their description on five hindrances described by Marshall (1989) regarding bone modification and taphonomy. The issues included:

1) lack of standard nomenclature
2) lack of comparative case studies
3) unsynthesised and scattered data sets
4) limited data sets
5) researchers who lack a broad knowledge base appropriate for this multidisciplinary field

While some progress has been made on all five points in the field of forensic anthropology, in the field of forensic taphonomy, less progress has been documented.

One of the main issues is that forensic taphonomy is seen as a multidisciplinary field instead of an interdisciplinary one. The difference and the implications between those two terms are large. Multidisciplinary means that many disciplines work next to each other, while interdisciplinary means that they work collaboratively with each other. What is the place of forensic taphonomy in these various disciplines? Many volumes describe forensic taphonomy as a sub-discipline of forensic anthropology (e.g. Haglund and Sorg 1997a; Pokines and Symes 2013). However, should we consider forensic taphonomy as an umbrella that covers several sub-disciplines? After all, forensic taphonomy encompasses other sciences such as forensic pathology, anthropology, archaeology, entomology, botany, chemistry, microbiology and soil science to name just a few.

The difference between multidisciplinary and interdisciplinary is also noticed in forensic taphonomy as part of law enforcement investigations. Unfortunately, as Groen and Berger state in Chapter 36:

> Most forensic scientists tend to work within a narrow forensic discipline and generally do not (or are not allowed to) correlate their results with the results obtained from other forensic disciplines. This is, generally speaking, the prosecution's job, or that of the police. Scenes of Crime Officers and forensic scientists rarely receive feedback from magistrates concerning the consequences of their reports.

Clearly, a good collaboration, updates and feedback are vital between law enforcement and scientists.

If forensic taphonomy becomes an interdisciplinary study, as our broad-spectrum definition suggests, we might be able to solve a second problem: the lack of a standard terminology. Terms tend to vary with different languages, in different parts of the world and between different disciplines. A confusing example of the language difference is the word 'cranium'. In English, the term 'cranium' refers only to that structure which houses the brain (neurocranium) and accommodates the sense organs of the face (viscerocranium), while the term 'skull' refers to both the cranium and the mandible (Knüsel 2014). Contrastingly, in French, 'crâne' refers to the skull (cranium with mandible) and 'bloc craniofacial' is utilised for the cranium without mandible (Boulestin 2015). Literal translations from non-English languages to English lead to a potpourri of terms and thus often to wrongly compared data. Additionally, and even more confusing, are the different meanings of a word across disciplines. For example, in forensic medicine, the term 'peri-mortem' refers literally to the period at or near the time of death. In anthropology, peri-mortem refers to a longer period after death, when the bone is still green (Chapter 23). Another example is the use of the terms multiple and collective burial. In France, a collective burial is a burial with human remains deposited over a longer time period, often following a natural pattern of death, whereas a multiple burial is considered as a simultaneous deposit of several cadavers (Castex *et al.* 2014). This subtle word difference has huge implications on the interpretation, and a distinction can only be made based on thorough archaeological analysis. Confusingly, in many other countries, multiple and collective burials are used as synonyms. And what is the definition of the term 'mass burial'? An interesting discussion on this subject is provided by Barker *et al.* in Chapter 18. A final example is the word 'mummification'. Does this term only apply to artificial mummified bodies or does it also include preservation by natural processes. Originally, the word mummification is derived from the Persian word *mumiya* (or *mûm* in Arabic) meaning bitumen. Technically, it could be argued that the term should be reserved for cases of artificial preservation of soft tissue. As Aufderheide (2003) states in *The Scientific Study of Mummies*, the word 'mummification' can be interpreted by its strict definition of desiccation, or by the broader common usage of the word; survival of soft tissue by any mechanism. Even in the making of this volume, we had discussions about the meaning of this word. Clearly, the development of a standard vocabulary is important work for the near future and, as long as there is no accepted standardised lexicon, terms should be described when employed in reports and articles.

A third issue is the lack of comparative case studies. This is not only due to different environmental circumstances that makes every case unique, it is also caused by the aforementioned separation between forensic field work and post-field analysis in the laboratory. Simply put, people who are based in law enforcement do not have the time and means to write articles about case studies. Even if it is finally decided to publish a case, the authors are not allowed to mention details and are instructed to make it as anonymous as possible. As such, much information is lost, which makes any form of comparison difficult. Additionally, not every author of a case study works in the same legislative framework, and scientists may have different formations. This means that not every forensic process is the same, implying that observations and interpretations might be different too. We cannot deny that the case study part was the hardest part of this volume.

A further issue relates back to points 3 and 4 from Marshall (1989) and Haglund and Sorg (1997b), and is also discussed by Groen and Berger in Chapter 36: a lack of synthesised data sets and interpretative framework. This could be related to the fact that forensic science concentrates on single cases and does not try to reconstruct a population and past (human) activity, as in traditional archaeology and anthropology. Another cause might be the lack of interdisciplinary collaborations, hindering the creation of concise databases. As Pokines and Symes (2013) state in their introduction: 'forensic taphonomy is the least quantified field'. Although research in forensic taphonomy has increased and more experimental work on human remains has recently been undertaken in several research facilities across the USA (Chapter 35) and in Australia, experimental work is still faced with the same problem as the case studies. There are so many extrinsic and intrinsic variables that make comparison difficult.

Despite all these issues, it is timely that forensic taphonomic data are being compiled, so that they can lead to the development of a digitally shared taphonomic database that will be linked to a map, in order to create an interpretative framework. Centralisation of taphonomic data will provide an invaluable resource for investigations. After all, the forensic community aims to increase efficiency by improving the quality of forensic investigations, including better search procedures and more accurate PMI estimations.

I.5 Organisation of the Volume

This volume is divided into five main parts. A clear understanding of the natural processes of decay is necessary in order to recognise the influence of environmental and human factors. This is covered in the first part, which includes macroscopic post-mortem changes (Chapter 1), microscopic post-mortem changes (Chapter 2), the study of volatile organic compounds that are released during decomposition (Chapter 3), the degradation of blood (Chapter 4), the degradation of DNA (Chapter 5), the decay of hair and nail (Chapter 6) and teeth (Chapter 7). This is followed by cases of natural preservation (Chapter 8), the degradation of clothing (Chapter 9) and an overview of techniques to estimate PMI (Chapter 10).

The second part of this book concentrates on the depositional environment, consisting of a description of the environmental factors that influence decomposition (Chapter 11), including bacterial symbionts as taphonomic agents (Chapter 12), entomology (Chapter 13), botany and the emerging area of stomach contents analysis (Chapter 14), the processes of weathering on bone (Chapter 15) and animal scavenging (Chapter 16). Furthermore, it discusses decomposition in an aquatic environment (Chapter 17) and differential preservation in mass burials (Chapter 18). This part concludes with a chapter on archaeothanatology in order to illustrate this analytical approach and demonstrate its potential to forensic cases (Chapter 19).

The third part concentrates on factors that might complicate forensic analysis and could lead to misinterpretations, including the presence of drugs in the body (Chapter 20), the exposure of human remains to fire (Chapter 21) and the effects of chemicals on human tissues (Chapter 22). Chapter 23 describes how to distinguish peri- from post-mortem trauma. The final chapter of this part deals with taphonomy beyond recovery (Chapter 24).

The fourth part of the volume focuses on case studies, which are not always present in the forensic literature. Ten case studies are presented, which can be related back to the theory chapters of the other parts. They are derived from different geographical and chronological contexts and a good illustration of different types of depositional environments. The first case study uses volatile fatty acid biomarkers to estimate PMI (Chapter 25). Next, an overview of Dutch taphonomic observations is given (Chapter 26) followed by different cemetery burials (Chapter 27). Mexican case studies are presented, focused on entomological analysis (Chapter 28), along with a case study on textile degradation (Chapter 29) and brain preservation in mass graves from Spain (Chapter 30). Burned human remains are described in Chapter 31, whilst Chapter 32 contains a blast injury example. This part ends with two case studies of bodies in concrete (Chapter 33 and 34). As mentioned above, some case studies have limited details because of forensic restrictions.

The final part of this volume covers past and future considerations in forensic taphonomy. The first chapter describes the first anthropology research facility in Tennessee and other decomposition and/or experimental facilities (Chapter 35). The second chapter discusses the lack of a scientific framework in forensic science, and explores the applicability of the archaeological paradigm in crime scene investigation (Chapter 36).

In summary, this book aims to fill a gap between different forensic taphonomy disciplines. Only by knowledge of the natural processes and by studying the depositional context, can we make more accurate interpretations of suspicious circumstances, and death investigations can be improved. We believe that the information presented in this volume will be useful to scientists and non-scientists from different fields, so that they become aware of the wide array of factors that play a part in forensic taphonomy, including the challenges and limitations. Our hope is that this book will spark interest and future research, which will lead to better forensic investigations.

References

Aufderheide, A.C. (2003) *The Scientific Study of Mummies.* Cambridge University Press: Cambridge.

Behrensmeyer, A.K. and Kidwell, S.M. (1985) Taphonomy's contriubitions to paleobiology. *Paleobiology*, **11**: 105–119.

Boulestin, B. (2015) Conservation du crâne et terminologie: pour en finir avec quelques mots de tête. *Bulletins et Mémoires de la Société d'Anthropologie de Paris*, **27**: 16–25.

Castex, D., Kacki, S., Réveillas, H., Souquet-Leroy, Y., Sachau-Carcel, G. *et al.* (2014) Revealing of archaeological features linked to mortality increases. *Anthropologie: International Journal of the Science of Man*, **3**: 299–318.

Duday, H. (2006) L'archéothanatologie ou l'archeologie de la mort (Archeothanatology of the Archaeology of Death). In: Gowland, R. and Knüsel, C. (eds), *Social Archaeology of Funerary Remains.* Oxbow Books: Oxford, pp. 30–56.

Duday, H. (2009) *The Archaeology of the Death: Lectures in archaeothanatology.* Oxbow Books: Oxford.

Efremov, I.A. (1940) Taphonomy, a new branch of paleontology. *Pan-American Geologist*, **74**: 81–93.

Groen, W.J.M., Marquez-Grant, N. and Janaway, R.C. (2015) *Forensic Archaeology: A global perspective.* Wiley-Blackwell: Chichester.

Haglund, W.D. and Sorg, M.H. (1997a) *Forensic Taphonomy. The Postmortem Fate of Human Remains.* CRC Press: Boca Raton.

Haglund, W.D. and Sorg, M.H. (1997b) Introduction to forensic taphonomy. In: Haglund, W.D. and Sorg, M.H. (eds), *Forensic Taphonomy. The Postmortem Fate of Human Remains.* CRC Press: Boca Raton, pp. 1–9.

Haglund, W.D. and Sorg, M.H. (1997c) Method and theory of forensic taphonomy research. In: Haglund, W.D. and Sorg, M.H. (eds), *Forensic Taphonomy. The Postmortem Fate Of Human Remains.* CRC Press: Boca Raton, pp. 13–26.

Haglund, W.D. and Sorg, M.H. (2002) *Advances in Forensic Taphonomy. Method, Theory and Archaeological Perspectives.* CRC Press: Boca Raton.

Henderson, J. (1987) Factors determining the state of preservation of human remains. In: Boddington, A., Garland, A.N. and Janaway, R.C. (eds), *Death, Decay and Reconstruction.* Manchester University Press: Manchester, pp. 43–54.

Knüsel, C.J. (2014) Crouching in fear: terms of engagement for furnerary remains. *Journal of Social Archaeology*, **14**: 26–58.

Lyman, R.L. (1994) *Vertebrate Taphonomy.* Cambridge University Press: Cambridge.

Marshall, L.G. (1989) Bone modification and 'the laws of burial'. In: Bonnichsen, R. and Sorg, M.H. (eds), *Bone Modification.* Center for the Study of the First Americans: Orono: pp. 7–24.

Nordby, J.J. (2002) Is forensic taphonomy scientific? In: Haglund, W.D. and Sorg, M.H. (eds), *Advances in Forensic Taphonomy. Method, Theory and Archaeological Perspectives.* CRC Press: Boca Raton, pp. 31–42.

Pokines, J. and Symes, S.A. (2013) *Manual of Forensic Taphonomy.* CRC Press: Boca Raton.

Renfrew, C. and Bahn, P. (1991) *Archaeology. Theories, Methods and Practice.* Thames & Hudson: London.

Shvedchikova, T. (2013) Taphonomic studies in Russia: past and future. *Second European Meeting on Forensic Archaeology.* The Hague: Netherlands Forensic Institute.

Sorg, M.H. and Haglund, W.D. (2002) Advancing forensic taphonomy: purpose, theory and process. In: Haglund, W.D. and Sorg, M.H. (eds), *Advances in Forensic Taphonomy. Method, Theory and Archaeological Perspectives*. CRC Press: Boca Raton, 3–29.

Tibbett, M. and Carter, D.O. (2008) *Soil Analysis in Forensic Taphonomy*. CRC Press: Boca Raton.

Turner, C.G.I., Ovodov, N.D. and Pavlova, O.V. (2013) *Animal Teeth and Human Tools. A Taphonomic Odyssey in Ice Age Siberia*. Cambridge University Press: Cambridge.

Part I

General Post-Mortem Processes: Degradation of Soft Tissue, Bone and Associated Materials

1

Gross Post-Mortem Changes in the Human Body

Stuart J. Hamilton and Michael A. Green

1.1 Introduction

All organisms die and the natural consequence of this is decomposition. The rate of decomposition is determined by numerous factors, both intrinsic to the body such as body habitus, and environmental factors such as predators, ambient temperature and humidity. Decomposition may broadly be divided into putrefaction and arrested decay, although these processes are not mutually exclusive and may be seen in the same body.

Post-mortem changes produce both artefacts that may mislead the unwary and obscure findings that point to the events immediately before, and indeed leading directly to, the death of the person. Recommended literature regarding forensic pathology is DiMaio and DiMaio (2001) and Knight and Saukko (2004). In this chapter the processes that occur in the body after death are discussed, along with the ways in which human and other environmental factors can affect these processes. The potential pitfalls faced in examination of the deceased are highlighted. In particular, some post-mortem changes may be mistaken for injuries sustained shortly before death.

1.2 The Immediate Post-Mortem Period

While most people know what death is, it is remarkably difficult to define scientifically and is best considered a process during which the cells and tissues that make up an organism cease to function. This is not the same as the 'time of death' recorded on the death certification, which is usually the time at which life is pronounced extinct by a suitably qualified person. In the UK, to diagnose brain death, a series of appropriate tests are performed twice at different times and the time of death is considered to be the time of the first set of tests. The tests include shining a torch into both eyes to see if they react to the light, stroking the cornea, pinching the nose, inserting ice-cold water in each ear, trying to provoke gagging or coughing by placing a plastic tube down the trachea, amongst other tests (National Health Service 2015).

One of the first notable features is that thermoregulation stops and the body temperature will naturally move towards ambient temperature. In most cases, this means the body will cool, but in particularly warm climates the body may actually increase in temperature.

The cooling of the body has long been of interest to the forensic community, particularly with respect to estimating the post-mortem interval (PMI). A historical review on the early work of estimating time since death is described by Knight and Madea (2016). A common 'rule of thumb' is that

Taphonomy of Human Remains: Forensic Analysis of the Dead and the Depositional Environment, First Edition.
Edited by Eline M.J. Schotsmans, Nicholas Márquez-Grant and Shari L. Forbes.

a body tends to cool at a rate of one degree Celsius per hour. A slightly more refined version takes into account the sigmoid nature of the cooling curve and assumes that the body does not begin to cool for around three hours after death, but cools at around one degree Celsius per hour thereafter, called the 'initial temperature plateau' (Al-Alousi *et al.* 2002). The authors politely submit that such calculations are so 'rough and ready' as to be of no real value in criminal investigations. By way of example, the case of *R v Lattimore and Leighton* (1974) involved a body recovered from a fire scene. Because of the possibility of sexual activity, a rectal temperature was not taken at the scene and later excessive reliance on post-mortem phenomena to estimate the time of death (particularly given that the body had been exposed to an unusually high ambient temperature) became an important aspect of the case with respect to the defendants' alibis. This ultimately led to a successful appeal and the case initiated research funded by the UK Home Office. Unfortunately, this extensive and expensive study only confirmed the unreliabilities, which had been known for years.

A more refined calculation is the Henssge equation and nomogram that take into account numerous factors including body weight, gender, body coverings, whether the body is wet or dry and ambient temperature (Henssge and Madea 2004; Henssge *et al.* 2002; Madea and Henssge 2016). The nomogram is useful, but as with any hand-drawn graphical method there is potential for user error. While the equation may appear daunting, there are now apps available for smartphones that can perform the calculation with relative ease. It should also be noted that any estimate of the PMI is based on a 'normal' initial body temperature, but particularly in cases of overwhelming infection or strenuous exercise, the initial temperature may be higher, and indeed in cases of sepsis, a transient post-mortem rise in temperature may be seen. Equally, hypothermia will cause a low core body temperature in life, also affecting estimates of the PMI. Even without such extreme changes, it is known that the human core temperature may vary under normal circumstances (the changes associated with the menstrual cycle are so well recognised that they can be used for family planning) and so one must bear in mind that there is an inherent potential error of up to two hours in any PMI calculation, and even the Henssge calculation includes a range of ±2.8 hours as a minimum range, rising to as much as ±7 hours.

Furthermore, the so-called 'normal temperature' in any individual may vary by as much as 1°C from the assumed 37.4, so all calculations start with a built-in potential error of up to 2 hours. It is also the case that the ambient temperature is based on a single measurement, and as this temperature can fluctuate over time, both outdoors and indoors with automatic central heating, its measurement may not accurately reflect the average temperature to which the body has been exposed throughout the post-mortem period.

Concurrently with cooling, rigor mortis (post-mortem stiffening) will develop as the muscles become depleted of adenosine triphosphate (ATP) and the muscle fibres permanently cross-link. As the reader may recall from his or her studies of basic physiology, muscle fibres are composed of actin and myosin, with the myosin heads binding to actin during muscle contraction and hydrolysing ATP to adenosine diphosphate (ADP) to allow the myosin to release the actin. Once ATP is depleted then cross-linking of the actin/myosin becomes permanent until decomposition causes breakdown of the molecules, or mechanical force is applied as discussed below. A logical corollary of this is that individuals who die shortly after exercise may have already depleted their stores of energy and ATP and therefore may develop rigor mortis more rapidly than an identical person who died at rest.

Rigor mortis is first observed in the small muscle groups such as the fingers, eyelids and lower jaw, which has produced the age-old practices of 'pennies on the eyelids', and the timely application of a jaw bandage or prop. The appearance of a slack-jawed, half-staring body can be highly distressing to relatives. Furthermore, if the eyes remain open, a dark discoloration occurs in the exposed conjunctiva, the so-called *tâche noire de la sclérotique* (Figure 1.1). In the early stages of its development, this may be mistaken for petechial haemorrhage (pinpoint haemorrhages resulting from

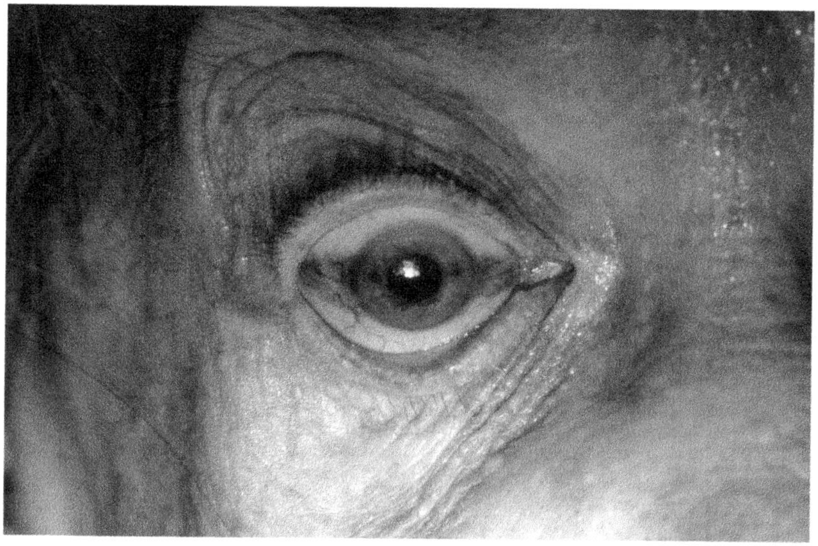

Figure 1.1 The *tâche noire de la sclérotique*, a post-mortem artefact.

ruptured venules, a common finding in strangulation), which the inexperienced may interpret as a sign of asphyxial death.

Rigor mortis then gradually becomes apparent in larger muscle groups until the body is essentially stiff. As the muscle decomposes, rigor mortis will pass. The rate at which rigor appears and disappears is extremely variable, as is its intensity. Individuals with large muscle bulk can develop very strong degrees of rigor, while particularly cachexic elderly people with very low muscle mass may show only weak rigor, or in extreme cases no recognisable rigor mortis at all. The 'strength' of rigor mortis is not a matter of forensic relevance. However, there are two aspects of rigor mortis that are worthy of consideration by the forensic pathologist. First, rigor in the heart can make it appear contracted and hypertrophic; therefore any assessment of cardiac hypertrophy should also include weight as well as wall thickness. Second, rigor developing in the muscles of the iris may cause dilation or contraction after death and therefore clinically useful signs such as the pinpoint pupils of the opiate overdose may be compromised. The pupils will react to mydriatic and meiotic drugs such as atropine or pilocarpine for a few hours after death. This phenomenon was extensively studied in the 1960s and 1970s as a method of estimating time of recent death, but proved to be totally unreliable (Madea 1994, 2016; Prasad 2003).

Some authors argue that rigor mortis can occur instantaneously (cadaveric spasm) (Figures 1.2 and 1.3), although this is by no means universally accepted (Pirch *et al.* 2013).

Rigor mortis can be 'broken' by physical force. If a body has been lying in an unusual position, this may occur when the body is manipulated during transfer to the mortuary and so any assessment of the degree of rigor mortis in the mortuary should take this into account. It has also been shown that it is possible for rigor mortis to become re-established after being mechanically broken, albeit more weakly than the original (Krompecher *et al.* 2008). Although it is rare that this phenomenon is likely to have forensic relevance, one of the authors (MAG) has seen such a case where a weapon was placed in the hand of a decedent in order to stage a scene of a suicidal shooting.

Similarly, once active circulation of blood ceases, blood will tend to gravitate to the most dependant parts of the body, producing a dark discoloration known as hypostasis, livor mortis or lividity, alternating with pallid areas of 'contact flattening' (Figure 1.4). This usually relates to where the body

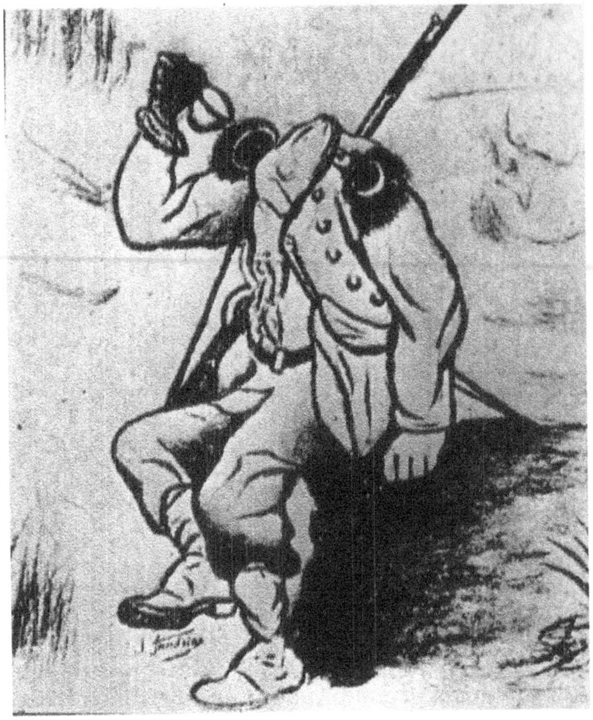

Figure 1.2 A sketch of a case of cadaveric spasm from a 19th-century pathology textbook showing a soldier who is enjoying a beverage while his head has been blown off by a shell explosion.

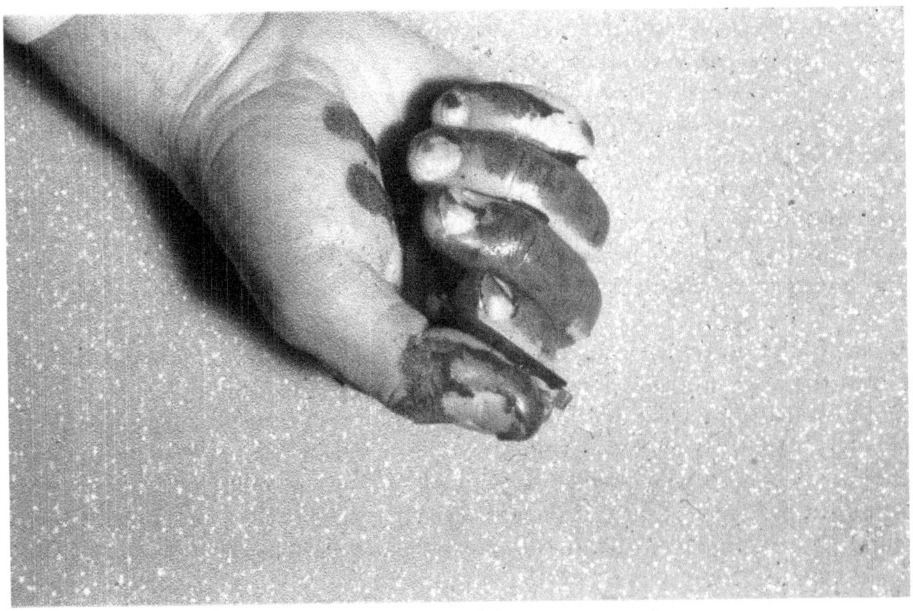

Figure 1.3 A razor blade clutched in the hand, an apparent example of cadaveric spasm.

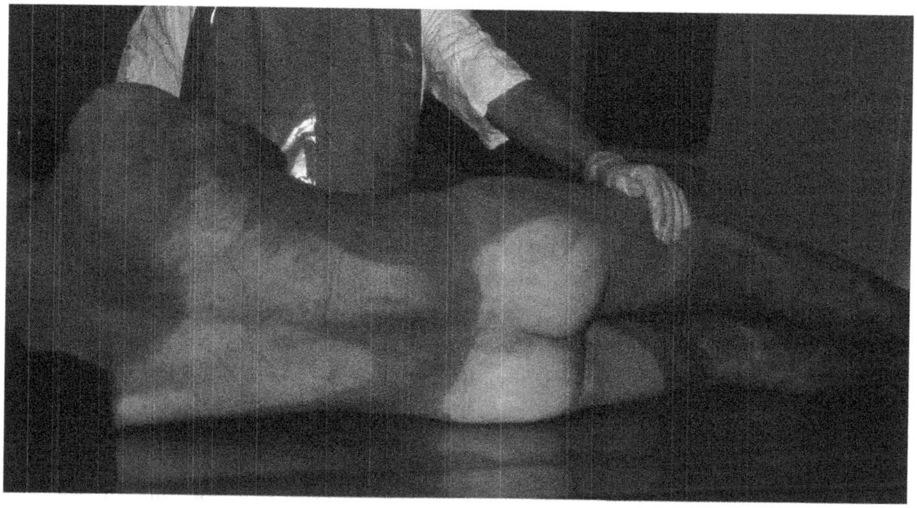

Figure 1.4 Clear sparing in hypostasis from the body lying on a hard surface and the small blood vessels being compressed, preventing hypostasis developing in these areas.

is in contact with the surface on which it lies, although pressure from clothing can also lead to regions of pallor. This can sometimes be so well defined as to allow the embossed brand name in the elasticated waistband of some brands of underwear to be read upon the surface of the underlying discoloured skin.

Hypostasis also occurs within the internal organs, and there also it can cause pitfalls for the unwary. In particular, hypostasis in the left ventricle of the heart may mimic a posterior myocardial infarct (death of cardiac muscle resulting from inadequate blood flow) and hypostasis in the intestines can be mistaken for ischaemia (injury from lack of oxygen) or infarction (tissue death from lack of oxygen). Artefactual post-mortem haemorrhage in the neck muscles (the Prinsloo Gordon artefact) should not be mistaken for evidence of strangulation and it is recommended that the head is opened before the neck is dissected to minimise the risk of this developing. Over time haemolysis occurs and the hypostasis becomes 'fixed', that is to say if the body is moved the hypostasis will not move to the new position. Again, the rate at which hypostasis develops and becomes fixed is highly variable, and not of value in estimating the PMI. Some factors alter the colour of hypostasis, in particular carbon monoxide poisoning causes cherry red hypostasis and cyanide poisoning causes brick red hypostasis. Blue/brown hypostasis is seen in cases where methaemoglobin is produced, such as poisoning with chlorate weed killers. Extreme cold may cause pink discoloration. While under no circumstances should such observations replace adequate toxicological analysis, they may assist in directing the observer towards a possible cause of death.

Overall, rigor mortis and hypostasis cannot give an accurate estimate of the time of death. However, if the pattern of these phenomena does not match the position in which the body is found, this may be of value in indicating that the body has been moved sufficiently long after death for these features to be present, which may in itself be of value to the investigation of the cause of death.

It is also relevant that non-forensically trained persons may make observations regarding bodies feeling cold or rigor mortis being present. Given that direct observation of such features by an experienced practitioner cannot offer a precise time of death, using such second-hand observations to make pronouncements would be unwise. So-called 'undertaker's bruises' seen over the shoulders should not be mistaken for evidence of intravital trauma.

1.3 Subsequent Weeks

Even as the very early post-mortem changes become apparent, the processes that produce the features of decomposition are developing. Autolysis refers to the chemical breakdown of tissue, and tends to be first observed in the pancreas where escape of the proteolytic enzymes causes digestion of the organ itself. This will rapidly become apparent on histological examination, although naked eye appearances are less clear and if necessary, microscopic examination may be needed to differentiate between a haemorrhagic, autolytic pancreas and one that was truly inflamed in life. Simultaneously, the active processes that prevent bacteria escaping the bowel fail and the microorganisms that colonise the gut will migrate through the intestinal wall and begin to break down tissue (Finley *et al.* 2014). Haemolysis and the associated degradation of haemoglobin causes the classic green coloration associated with decomposition, and the high bacterial load in the caecum means that the first sign of decomposition that is usually noticed is green discoloration of the abdominal wall in the right lower quadrant of the abdomen, spreading to the rest of the abdominal wall. As bacteria propagate along blood vessels, they can cause haemolysis that stains the course of the vessels, known as 'marbling'. Marbling of the veins of the forearms and groins has sometimes been misinterpreted as evidence of intravenous drug use. Bacterial activity can also generate ethanol (alcohol) that may be a confounding factor in toxicological analysis. For this reason alcohol levels in the vitreous humour (eye fluid) are more reliable in cases where decomposition is beginning to occur (Kugelberg and Jones 2007).

At this stage, the skin will also begin to blister and slough, and fluid may begin to purge from bodily orifices. Sloughing may begin to obscure injuries, but loss of the epidermis may cause tattoos and old scars to be more clearly discernible. Purge fluid should not be confused with bleeding and considered evidence of, for example, sexual assault. Putrefaction gas will also begin to generate, which is usually most apparent in the abdomen and scrotum.

At the same time as the external aspects of the body decay, similar processes will be occurring internally. Changes in the pancreas are noted above, and the changes of decomposition manifest in different organs at different rates and in different ways. The brain, lacking a fibrous supporting structure, develops the well-recognised 'Swiss cheese' artefact before liquefying. In buried or encoffined bodies, or when adipocere has formed, the brain's putrefaction may arrest at the Swiss Cheese stage, and be found in this condition hundreds of years later (Fiedler *et al.* 2015). More fibrous organs such as the heart and uterus tend to retain their appearance for longer, and calcified structures (including calcified atheromatous vessels) may be readily identified for prolonged periods. The spleen may soften and this should not be confused with the diffluent spleen of systemic sepsis. Fat will often liquefy, coating the viscera in a slippery translucent yellow film. The blood, while initially remaining liquid, will begin to form post-mortem clots. This tends to be an admixture of red and white jelly-like material (sometimes described as having a 'turkey fat and cranberry jelly' appearance) that should be readily distinguished from the firmer, more organised and granular thrombus that occurs in life.

While such changes do hamper the examination of the body, this should never preclude a full autopsy examination when required, as macroscopic and microscopic features are often surprisingly well preserved compared to what may be expected based on external examination. As with the features discussed in the early post-mortem period, the rate at which such changes develop is extremely variable and therefore even greater ranges of PMI exist.

1.4 Other Post-Mortem Modifications

1.4.1 Scavenging

The dead organism is a source of nutrition for any number of predators: insects may deposit eggs very early in the peri-mortem period. Beloved, but hungry family pets will bite the hand and face that no longer feeds them (Colard *et al.* 2015; Tsokos and Schulz 1999). In the wild, carnivores can cause extensive and rapid tissue destruction, the extent and nature of which is very much dependent upon the local fauna, and knowledge of what animals may have access to a body should be obtained when assessing the appearance of that body (Dabbs and Martin 2013; O'Brien *et al.* 2010; Young *et al.* 2015). The role of entomology is well established in forensic investigation; detailed discussion is extensively covered elsewhere in this work and is beyond the scope of this chapter (Chapter 13). Suffice to say, a case with insect activity and infestation warrants the involvement of an experienced forensic entomologist, therefore such advice should be obtained, and the appropriate samples taken, before the body is moved. The site of each sample should be carefully recorded. In the case of *R v Sutcliffe* (1981), the well-documented 'Yorkshire Ripper' case, one of the victims had been partially moved from shade to sunlight and different fauna were present in shaded and exposed parts of the body (Bilton 2003).

The body of another of Sutcliffe's victims, found in a city centre, was colonised by the larvae of a fly found more commonly in the vicinity of cows and cowsheds. This led to the assumption that the woman had been transported from a rural setting, and led to the fruitless redirection of the inquiry for many weeks. The significance of such evidence may not be apparent immediately and the authors are of the view that retention of material that does not result in significant evidence is vastly preferable to the loss of material that may, at a later date, become important.

Post-mortem predation produces its own challenges for assessment of the body. On the one hand, any tissue loss may alter or efface injuries or stigmata of disease, but on the other hand, predation can mimic injuries, for example maggots burrowing through the skin may give the appearance of a shotgun wound on cursory examination or ant bites may give the appearance of abrasions (Byard and Heath 2014; Campobasso *et al.* 2009).

1.4.2 Arrested Decay

Bodies that lie in very dry environments may become naturally desiccated, also called natural mummification (Chapter 8). In contrast to putrefactive decomposition, which commonly obscures or destroys injuries and external marks, mummification has a tendency to preserve tissue and features may be readily identifiable for many years, even centuries. Putrefaction and mummification may be seen in a single cadaver. Mummification is most commonly seen in the extremities in such circumstances, with putrefaction of the torso.

1.4.3 Adipocere

This is a relatively uncommon phenomenon, sometimes referred to as 'grave wax' characterised by hydrolysis and hydrogenation of body fat by bacteria (Chapter 2). Bacteria in an anaerobic environment produce a waxy cast of tissue containing palmitic, oleic and stearic fatty acids. Although this is often seen externally, it is a process that can affect any body fat that is exposed to the appropriate conditions, and therefore can also be seen, for example, in association with hepatic steatosis (fatty liver) and mesenteric fat.

In the so-called 'Moors Murders' (*R v Brady and Hindley* 1963), the saponification of the fatty tissues led to extremely good preservation of the first two bodies recovered. Likewise, when a third body was recovered in 1985, rehydration in a solution of polyethylene glycol restored the facial features to a degree of normality.

A gruesome example of artificial and deliberate creation of adipocere was the 'hand of glory'. This was a candle created from the severed hand of a hanged murderer, ideally with the deceased's hair for the wick, preserved and said to render people motionless or unlock doors, and was therefore considered a highly desirable item for burglars and other persons with nefarious intent. The authors are not aware of any peer-reviewed literature detailing the efficacy of this item, but those interested may wish to read the poem 'The Hand of Glory' in the Ingoldsby Legends published by Richard Barham between 1840 and 1847 (Ingoldsby 1870).

Sleep all who sleep, wake all who wake
But be as the dead for the dead man's sake

1.4.4 Maceration

Maceration is a very particular form of post-mortem change that is typically only encountered in intrauterine death (IUD). As the normal uterine cavity is sterile (unless infection is present), then putrefaction does not occur and decomposition results entirely from autolysis. Skin slip begins to appear within 48 hours of IUD. The skin becomes progressively more dried out and friable, concomitant changes occur in the internal organs, and the whole body undergoes progressive shrinkage. Eventually, if amniotic fluid has been completely lost or re-absorbed, the end product is the shrunken brittle *foetus papyraceus* (Keeling 1978). In a long buried body, the general changes throughout the maternal cadaver will mask these changes.

Maceration from a pathology point of view should not be confused with maceration as a bone preparing technique used in forensic anthropology. Sometimes forensic bones have adhering soft tissues, which make direct observation of the bone difficult. The process of removing soft tissue can be done by different maceration techniques such as submerging in heated water (Lee *et al.* 2010; White *et al.* 2012).

1.4.5 Bodies Recovered from Water

Bodies recovered from water present their own particular challenges (Chapter 9). The first is to determine whether the cause of death is drowning, natural disease or injury sustained prior to immersion or while the body is in the water. If a body is recovered quickly, classic features such as the *champignon de mousse* (literally a mushroom of foam) and overlapping, crepitant, hyperinflated lungs (*emphysema aequosum*) may point to drowning as a cause of death, which may be altered by resuscitation attempts. The *champignon de mousse* is a very transient finding at the best of times, and has often disappeared by the time of autopsy if there is any delay between recovery of the body and examination. Sometimes the *champignon* is copious, and reappears as fast as it is wiped away; this can be very distressing when a body has been prepared for viewing by the relatives only a few minutes before. In the initial phase, bodies will tend to float if the water is sufficiently deep. Simple physics will usually cause the body to float face down with the limbs dependent. Far be it for the authors to disagree with literary genius, but forensic pathology would not appear to support the following contention by Aldous Huxley (Huxley 1933):

Second Philosopher's Song

If, O my Lesbia, I should commit,
Not fornication, dear, but suicide,
My Thames-blown body (Pliny vouches it)
Would drift face upwards on the oily tide
With the other garbage, till it putrefied.

But you, if all your lovers' frozen hearts
Conspired to send you, desperate, to drown –

Your maiden modesty would float face down,
And men would weep upon your hinder parts.

'Tis the Lord's doing. Marvellous is the plan
By which this best of worlds is wisely planned.
One law he made for women, one for man:
We bow the head and do not understand.

In shallower bodies of water, the knuckles and lower limbs may brush against rough surfaces and cause abrasion that may be misinterpreted by the unwary as evidence that the deceased had been beaten, or had made attempts at self-defence. Even with true, ante-mortem injuries, water will tend to wash away blood patterns associated with injuries. Post-mortem artefacts may occur if the body strikes solid objects causing fractures, and most pathologists who work near a body of water large enough for boating will be familiar with the regular, parallel incised wounds caused by the passage of a propeller across the body (Figure 1.5).

With time, bodies that are not recovered will sink. The thicker skin of the palms and soles will become waterlogged, giving a pale, wrinkled appearance such as may be observed in one who has overindulged in bathing or has undertaken household chores, giving rise to the description of washerwoman change (Figure 1.6). The skin of the hands and feet can slough in totality. Fingerprint impressions may often be recovered from the under-surfaces of these degloved digits.

In most cases the water in which the body sinks will be relatively cold and therefore acts to retard decomposition (De Donno *et al.* 2014; Mateus and Vieira 2014). However, this will also increase the time that the body is exposed to aquatic predators. Such creatures tend to focus on exposed areas

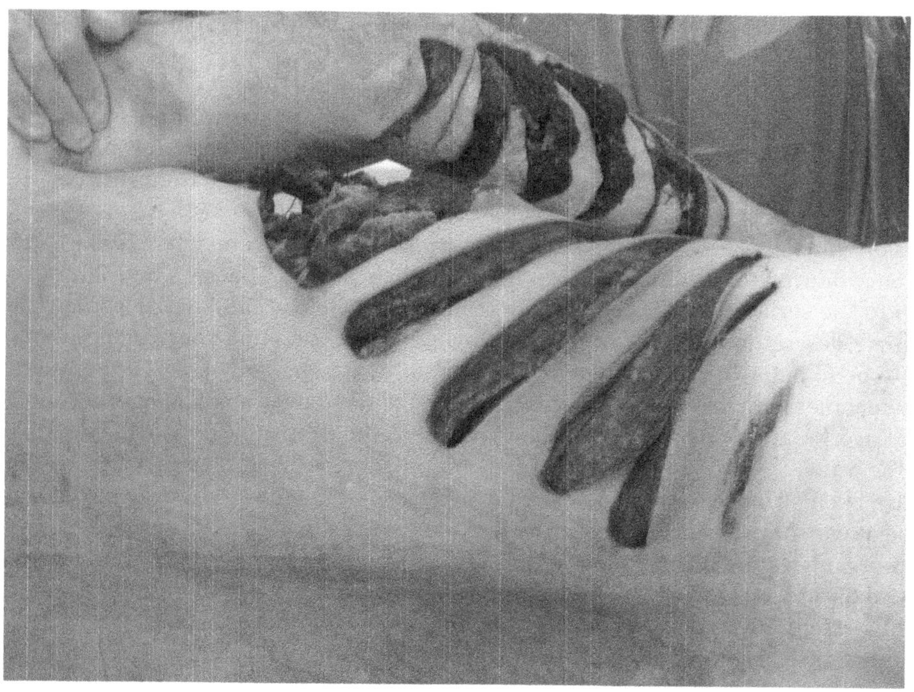

Figure 1.5 Propeller injuries. The regular, parallel-incised wounds are the result of the propeller passing over the body as the boat moves through the water.

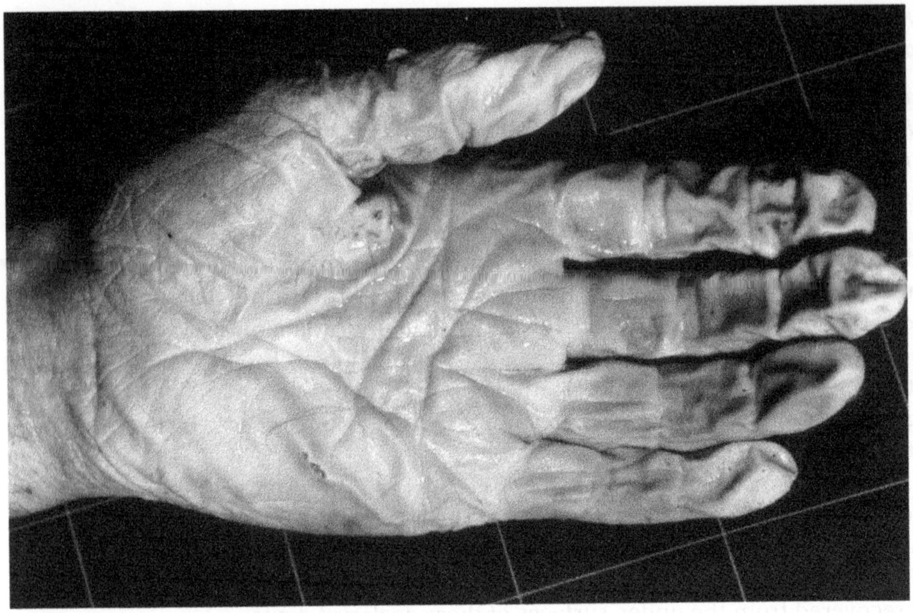

Figure 1.6 So-called 'washerwoman change'. The waterlogged skin becomes wrinkled and may slough off. The sloughed skin can still be used to obtain fingerprints.

(often the hands and face), which causes significant difficulties in using the face for identification, and will obscure or erase injuries to the soft tissues of the face that are all too common in interpersonal violence.

A common finding in bodies that have undergone prolonged immersion or even burial is 'pink teeth'. In the case of *R v Christie* (1953), the pathologist insisted that this phenomenon was the result of poisoning with coal gas, but in reality the presence of such a change is of limited, if any, pathological significance. Middle ear haemorrhage is also common, but most likely results from hydrostatic pressure rather than drowning *per se*.

Although immersion in cold water will retard decomposition, it will not completely halt it, and eventually gas will be produced (as discussed above) that causes the body to become buoyant once again and to return to the surface. This is colloquially referred to as 'bloat and float', a somewhat distasteful but accurate description of what occurs. In flowing water, there may be specific places where bodies tend to be found, which may be many miles from where the body entered the water. Equally, a body may become entangled close to the place where it entered the water and may be found there. Bodies in tidal rivers may travel back and forth with the tide, but ultimately remain close to the point of entry into the water.

Many findings have been proposed as 'diagnostic' of drowning. In the authors' opinion most are, at best, spurious and at worst misleading. Probably the best-known test is to seek diatoms. Diatoms are silicaceous microorganisms and different species exist in different proportions in different bodies of water. Testing is predicated upon the principle that if an unbreathing body is deposited in water then the water, and by extension the diatoms in it, enters the lungs, but in the absence of an active circulation are not transported to distant organs. If, however, the person is alive, then diatoms enter the lungs, cross into the circulation and are deposited elsewhere in the body. This is said to confirm drowning, and the species and proportions of diatoms would, in theory, suggest in which body of water the person drowned. While there may be some merit in this, the question of whether a body entering water is 'diatom free' prior to the incident, the shortage of experts who can perform detailed analysis of diatom species, and the presence of such organisms in soil and even some toothpaste, to some extent undermine the utility of the test.

More recently, molecular biological methods utilising polymerase chain reaction (PCR) to identify bacterioplankton (Kakizaki *et al.* 2008; Rutty *et al.* 2015) have been developed and at least one trial has shown them to be useful in clinical practice. This method has the advantage of requiring less tissue retention and does not require organs to be dissolved in hot acid, a process that has implications in the era of Work Health and Safety (WH&S) rules.

1.4.6 Artificial Preservation, Burial and Cremation

Human beings interact with the dead, and these interactions have their own impact upon the dead. While a detailed discussion of cultural and religious practices is beyond the scope of this chapter, the changes caused by deliberate human actions are worthy of consideration and may have a bearing on the interpretation of findings (Green 2006).

These matters are extensively covered in 'Dealing with Death' (Green and Green 2006) and in 'Essentials of Autopsy Practice' (Rutty 2001, 2004), to which those interested should refer. The attitude to the dead is very much culturally determined, and it is self-evident that the mummified bodies in the ornate tombs of pharaohs in the Valley of the Kings in Egypt will produce post-mortem appearances that differ greatly from the findings in a cremated body or a body from a Zoroastrian 'Tower of Silence', where vultures cleaned corpses as part of a burial rite (Boyce 1979). This practice of disposal by exposure to aerial predators is fast dying out. The Indian vulture population has been decimated by the practice of treating cattle with non-steroidal anti-inflammatory drugs (NSAIDS). The birds, lacking the necessary liver enzymes, die shortly after feasting on the corpses of cattle so treated (Taggart *et al.* 2009).

In general, funerary practices tend to either hasten the breakdown of the body or retard it. The most destructive practice is probably cremation where, with a modern efficient crematorium, a body can be reduced to calcined bone fragments and ash in a matter of hours and leave next to nothing for an investigator to examine (Bohnert *et al.* 1998; Eckert *et al.* 1988; Ubelaker 2009) (Chapter 21).

On the other hand, preservation can allow relatively easy interpretation of findings. The most relevant practice with respect to deaths in the late 20th and early 21st centuries is the increasing prevalence of embalming. Introduction of chemicals can preserve bodies to a high standard for many years (such as the body of Vladimir Lenin in Moscow) (Aufderheide 2003), although in the authors' experience there is a considerable degree of variation in the quality of the embalming process. Although embalming tends to render bodies more firm and difficult to manipulate, the preservation of the surface of the body and internal organs can greatly assist in the assessment of injuries and disease even many months or years after death. However the embalming process may produce lesions that are important to recognise. Cannulae are often inserted into the carotid vessels or the axillae and groins to instil embalming fluid and therefore stitched incised wounds may be apparent at these sites. Similarly, a plastic 'button' may be present, particularly on the abdomen as the result of the injection of cavity fluid in the embalming process. Some embalming involves the introduction of a sharp cutting ended trocar that can leave large puncture wounds in underlying organs, particularly the liver or heart, and should not be misinterpreted as ante-mortem stab wounds. It should be borne in mind, that while embalming fluids vary in their composition, many contain not only formalin, but also ethanol and glycerine that will interfere with some post-mortem toxicological analysis (Chapter 20).

1.5 Skeletonisation

Eventually, many bodies are reduced to skeletal remains and at this point examination and interpretation moves towards the expertise of the (forensic) anthropologist. The time for this to occur varies greatly. The recovery of partial or complete skeletal remains is far from uncommon. For the forensic practitioner there are two questions of immediate significance, specifically whether the remains are human or non-human and whether they are recent enough to warrant a criminal investigation. The former issue is usually relatively simple, although the latter may be less so. As the PMI increases, bones tend to become lighter in weight and drier.

While it is self-evident that the loss of internal and external soft tissue will reduce the evidence available, skeletal features will be useful in determining features such as age class, sex and stature of the deceased. The presence of skeletal trauma may assist in determining a likely cause and manner of death, and other features including medical interventions following fractures, prostheses, and cosmetic or reconstructive dental work, may assist in identifying the individual. Isotope analysis can point to where in the world a person may have lived in his childhood. In the 'Torso in the Thames' case, when a young boy's torso was discovered in the River Thames (UK) in 2001, such analysis allowed investigators to identify an area in Africa where the deceased had lived, which is clearly of value in investigations involving decedents whose identity is unknown (Hoskins 2012; Sanders 2003).

A recent and well-publicised example of the information available from skeletal remains is the discovery of the body of Richard III (1483–1485), the last English king to die in The Battle of Bosworth, in Leicester (UK) in 2012. A range of forensic examinations has not only confirmed his identity but also provided a wealth of information regarding his appearance, life and ultimate death (Buckley *et al.* 2013).

As this chapter is being written, a new method for determining the PMI based on degradation of skeletal muscle has been published. Whether this is to become a vital weapon in the forensic armoury or another false dawn remains to be seen (Pittner *et al.* 2015) (Chapter 10).

1.6 Conclusion and Future Research

As alluded to earlier, there have been many efforts to utilise the changes affecting the body after death to elicit a PMI, but mostly these have met with limited success. It is generally agreed that many of the features that result from post-mortem changes are not sufficiently uniform or accurate to provide precise information regarding the PMI, and any estimates made on, for example, body temperature should be regarded as just that and include appropriately wide possible ranges. To the frustration of many forensic pathologists, examination of the body may ultimately lead them to express the opinion that the person died at some point between the last time that he or she was reliably known to be alive and the point where they are declared legally dead. More recently, taphonomic processes have been studied at facilities known as 'body farms', research facilities where relatively specific conditions can be recreated and used as experimental models. The first such facility was set up at the University of Tennessee in 1981, with additional facilities opening across the USA since then (Chapter 35). A similar establishment has been recently set up at the University of Technology Sydney in Australia called AFTER, Australian Facility for Taphonomic Experimental Research.

In the last few years, the 'virtopsy' approach, using radiological techniques to examine the internal structures of the body, has been the subject of considerable research in forensic medicine. Such an approach has some advantages, particularly for faith groups for whom an invasive autopsy contradicts their belief systems. The authors' view is that at present such an approach may be useful in some cases, but in homicidal deaths, while radiology often provides a useful adjunct, a traditional autopsy is still the most appropriate method of examination.

References

Al-Alousi, L.M., Anderson, R.A., Worster, D.M. and Land, D.V. (2002) Factors influencing the precision of estimating the postmortem interval using the triple-exponential formulae (TEF). Part II: A study of the effect of body temperature at the moment of death on the postmortem brain, liver and rectal cooling in 117 forensic cases. *Forensic Science International*, **125**: 231–236.

Aufderheide, A.C. (2003) *The Scientific Study of Mummie*. Cambridge University Press: Cambridge.

Bilton, M. (2003) *Wicked Beyond Belief*. Harper Collins: London.

Bohnert, M., Rost, T. and Pollak, S. (1998) The degree of destruction of human bodies in relation to the duration of the fire. *Forensic Science International*, **95**: 11–21.

Boyce, M. (1979) *Zoroastrians: Their religious beliefs and practices*. Routledge: London.

Buckley, R., Morris, M., Appleby, J., King, T.L., O'Sullivan, D. and Foxhall, L. (2013) The king in the car park: new light on the death and burial of Richard III in the Grey Friars church, Leicester, in 1485. *Antiquity*, **87**: 519–538.

Byard, R.W. and Heath, K.J. (2014) Patterned postmortem ant abrasions outlining clothing and body position after death. *Journal of Forensic and Legal Medicine*, **26**: 10–13.

Campobasso, C.P., Marchetti, D., Introna, F. and Colonna, M.F. (2009) Postmortem artifacts made by ants and the effect of ant activity on decompositional rates. *American Journal of Forensic Medicine and Pathology*, **30**: 84–87.

Colard, T., Delannoy, Y., Naji, S., Gosset, D., Hartnett, K. and Bécart, A. (2015) Specific patterns of canine scavenging in indoor settings. *Journal of Forensic Sciences*, **60**: 495–500.

Dabbs, G.R. and Martin, D.C. (2013) Geographic variation in the taphonomic effect of vulture scavenging: the case for Southern Illinois. *Journal of Forensic Sciences*, **58**: S20–25

De Donno, A., Campobasso, C.P., Santoro, V., Leonardi, S., Tafuri, S. and Introna, F. (2014) Bodies in sequestered and non-sequestered aquatic environments: a comparative taphonomic study using decompositional scoring system. *Science and Justice*, **54**: 439–46

DiMaio, V. and DiMaio, D. (2001) *Forensic Pathology*, 2nd edition. (Practical aspects of criminal and forensic investigations). CRC Press: Boca Raton.

Eckert, W.G., James, S. and Katchis, S. (1988) Investigation of cremations and severely burned bodies. *American Journal of Forensic Medicine and Pathology*, **9**: 188–200.

Fiedler, S., Berns, A.E., Schwark, L., Woelk, A.T. and Graw, M. (2015) The chemistry of death – Adipocere degradation in modern graveyards. *Forensic Science International*, **257**: 320–328.

Finley, S.J., Benbow, M.E. and Javan, G.T. (2014) Microbial communities associated with human decomposition and their potential use as postmortem clocks. *International Journal of Legal Medicine*, **129**: 623–632.

Green, M.A. (2006) The examination of 83 vault-interred bodies. *Journal of Forensic Medicine and Pathology*, **2**: 19–24.

Green, M.A. and Green, J.B (2006) *Dealing with Death*. Jessica Kingsley: London.

Henssge, C., Knight, B., Krompecher, T., Madea, B. and Nokes, L. (2002) *The Estimation of the Time since Death in the Early Postmortem Period*. London: Arnold Publishing.

Henssge, C. and Madea, B. (2004) Estimation of the time since death in the early post-mortem period. *Forensic Science International*, **144**: 167–175.

Hoskins, R. (2012) *The Boy in the River*. Pan Macmillan: London.

Huxley, A. (1933) *Retrospect: An Omnibus of Aldous Huxley's books.* Doubleday Doran and Co.: New York.

Ingoldsby, T. (1870) *The Ingoldsby Legends or Mirth and Marvels.* Richard Bentley: London

Kakizaki, E., Takahama, K., Seo, Y., Kozawa, S., Sakai, M. and Yukawa, N. (2008) Marine bacteria comprise a possible indicator of drowning in seawater. *Forensic Science International,* **176**: 236–247.

Keeling, J.W. (1978) Macerated stillbirth. In: Keeling, J.W. (ed.), *Fetal and Neonatal Pathology.* Springer-Verlag: Berlin, pp. 167–178.

Knight, B. and Saukko, P. (2004) *Knight's Forensic Pathology.* Arnold: New York.

Knight, B. and Madea, B. (2016) Historical review on early work on estimating the time since death. In: Madea, B. (ed.), *Estimation of the Time since Death.* CRC Press: Boca Raton, pp. 7–16.

Krompecher, T., Gilles, A., Brandt-Casadevall, C. and Mangin, P. (2008) Experimental evaluation of rigor mortis. IX: The influence of the breaking (mechanical solution) on the development of rigor mortis. *Forensic Science International,* **176**: 157–162.

Kugelberg, F.C. and Jones, A.W. (2007) Interpreting results of ethanol analysis in postmortem specimens: a review of the literature. *Forensic Science International,* **165**: 10–29.

Lee, E.J., Luedtke, J.G., Allison, J.L., Arber, C.E., Merriwether, D.A. and Steadman, D.W. (2010) The effects of different maceration techniques on nuclear DNA amplification using human bone. *Journal of Forensic Science,* **55**: 1032–1038.

Madea, B. (1994) Importance of supravitality in forensic medicine. *Forensic Science International,* **69**: 221–241.

Madea, B. (2016) Supravitality in tissues. In: Madea, B. (ed.), *Estimation of the Time since Death.* CRC Press: Boca Raton, pp. 17–40.

Madea, B. and Henssge, C. (2016) General remarks on estimating the time since death. In: Madea, B. (ed.), *Estimation of the Time since Death.* CRC Press: Boca Raton, pp. 1–6.

Mateus, M. and Vieira, V. (2014) Study on the postmortem submersion interval and accumulated degree days for a multiple drowning accident. *Forensic Science International,* **238**: e15–e19.

National Health Service, www.nhs.uk/Conditions/Brain-death/Pages/diagnosis.aspx (Accessed 15 November 2015).

O'Brien, R.C., Forbes, S.L., Meyer, J. and Dadour, I. (2010) Forensically significant scavenging guilds in the southwest of Western Australia. *Forensic Science International,* **198**: 85–91.

Pirch, J., Schulz, Y. and Klintschar, M. (2013) A case of instantaneous rigor? *International Journal of Legal Medicine,* **127**: 971–974.

Pittner, S., Monticelli, F.C., Pfisterer, A., Zissler, A., Sänger, A.M. *et al.* (2015) Postmortem degradation of skeletal muscle proteins: a novel approach to determine the time since death. *International Journal of Legal Medicine,* **PMID**: 26041514.

Prasad, B.K. (2003) Post-mortem ocular changes: a study on autopsy cases in Bharatpur Hospital. *Kathmandu University Medical Journal,* **1**: 276–277.

Rutty, G.N., Bradley, C.J., Biggs, M.J., Hollingbury, F.E., Hamilton, S.J. *et al.* (2015) Detection of bacterioplankton using PCR probes as a diagnostic indicator for drowning; the Leicester experience. *Legal Medicine (Tokyo),* **pii**: S1344-6223(15)00071-1.

Rutty, J. (2001) Religious attitudes to death: What every pathologist needs to know. In: Rutty, G. (ed.), *Essentials of Autopsy Practice,* vol. **1**. Springer Verlag: London.

Rutty, J. (2004) Religious attitudes to death: What every pathologist needs to know. Part 2. In: Rutty, G. (ed.), *Essentials of Autopsy Practice,* vol. **2**. Springer Verlag: London.

Sanders, T. (2003) Imagining the dark continent: the met, the media and the Thames torso. *The Cambridge Journal of Anthropology,* **23**: 53–66.

Taggart, M.A., Senacha, K.R., Green, R.E., Cuthbert, R., Jhala, Y.V. *et al.* (2009) Analysis of nine NSAIDs in ungulate tissues available to critically endangered vultures in India. *Environmental Science and Technology*, **43**: 4561–4566

Tsokos, M. and Schulz, F. (1999) Indoor postmortem animal interference by carnivores and rodents: report of two cases and review of the literature. *International Journal of Legal Medicine*, **112**: 115–119.

Ubelaker, D. (2009) The forensic evaluation of burned skeletal remains: a synthesis. *Forensic Science International*, **183**: 1–5.

White, T.D., Black, M.T. and Folkens, P.A. (2012) *Human Osteology*. Elsevier: London.

Young, A., Stillman, R., Smith, M.J. and Korstjens, A.H. (2015) Applying knowledge of species-typical scavenging behaviour to the search and recovery of mammalian skeletal remains. *Journal of Forensic Sciences*, doi: 10.1111/1556-4029.12974.

Cited court cases

R v Brady and Hindley (1963)
R v Christie (1953)
R v Lattimore and Leighton (1974)
R v Sutcliffe (1981)

2

Microscopic Post-Mortem Changes: the Chemistry of Decomposition

Shari L. Forbes, Katelynn A. Perrault and Jenna L. Comstock

2.1 Introduction

Death is often referred to as a process rather than an event, and there are typically two types of death that can be described: somatic death and cellular death. Somatic death results when a person becomes unconscious, being unable to initiate voluntary movement or respond to sensory stimuli, and being unaware of their surrounding environment. While somatic death is often equated with brain death, circulatory and respiratory functions will continue, either naturally or with artificial support, ensuring that tissues and cells in the body remain alive and functioning (Knight 2004). When a person's cardiorespiratory functions fail, then cellular death results, where the tissues and cells are no longer functioning and have no metabolic activity. This is often referred to as the 'irreversible cessation of blood circulation' (Tsokos 2004). Cellular death is the process typically used to describe post-mortem changes and the chemistry of decomposition.

The physical, chemical and biological processes that a body undergoes after death are highly complex, with a broad range of variables influencing the subsequent post-mortem changes to the body's composition (Tsokos 2004). Body composition can be described by molecular structure, which includes water, proteins, lipids, carbohydrates, DNA and apatite (in bone). Alternatively, it can be described by elemental composition including oxygen, carbon, hydrogen, nitrogen, calcium, phosphorous, potassium, sulphur, sodium, chlorine and magnesium, as well as other trace elements. In forensic taphonomy, the body's composition is typically referred to by tissue type (e.g. fat, muscle, connective tissue and bone), but for the purposes of discussing microscopic post-mortem changes, it is also necessary to discuss changes at a cellular level.

Strictly speaking, the entire post-mortem process is a continuum; however, it can be divided into several stages that demonstrate relatively predictable patterns (Prahlow 2010). The stages most relevant to this discussion include early post-mortem changes (i.e. physical processes such as *livor* and *algor mortis*, physiochemical processes, such as *rigor mortis*, and metabolic processes, such as supravital reactions (Zapico *et al.* 2014), autolysis, putrefaction and skeletonisation. This chapter will only focus on the autolytic and putrefactive processes, as the microscopic post-mortem changes that occur throughout the chemical degradation of soft tissue predominantly result from autolysis and putrefaction. Early post-mortem changes and skeletonisation are addressed in detail in Chapters 1 and 23, respectively. The major biochemical reactions, particularly those that result from macromolecule degradation, are discussed here in detail. Factors that commonly affect autolysis and putrefaction are also discussed, along with the impact of these biochemical processes on the surrounding environment.

Taphonomy of Human Remains: Forensic Analysis of the Dead and the Depositional Environment, First Edition.
Edited by Eline M.J. Schotsmans, Nicholas Márquez-Grant and Shari L. Forbes.

2.2 Autolysis

The processes of autolysis and putrefaction are collectively referred to as decomposition, although the term decomposition should more accurately be used to describe the entire post-mortem continuum. Autolysis is defined as the post-mortem self-digestion and degradation of the cells and organs by intracellular enzymes (Di Maio and Di Maio 2001). The lack of oxygen supply after death, combined with a decrease in cytoplasmic pH, results in the loss of cell membrane integrity (Tsokos 2004). Loss of cellular structure leads to the release of lysosomes, membrane-bound cell organelles that contain hydrolytic enzymes. The destructive hydrolytic enzymes are released into the cytoplasm where they denature molecules and the remaining membrane (Gill-King 1997). These enzymes have the capacity to break down almost all macromolecules in the body, including proteins, lipids, carbohydrates, nucleic acids and cellular debris.

Organs rich in lysosomes, and thus enzymes, will undergo autolysis faster than those with reduced enzyme concentrations. The pancreas, stomach and liver undergo rapid deterioration due to the large number of hydrolytic enzymes present, including gastric and pancreatic lipases, carbohydrate-digesting amylases and a variety of peptidases and nucleotidases (Gill-King 1997). The lungs and airways will also deteriorate rapidly due to the high number of macrophages, which contain lysosomes and hydrolytic enzymes that are activated at low cytoplasmic pH. Kidneys, bladder, brain and nervous tissue may also be among the first tissues to autolyse (Gill-King 1997). Autolysis can begin in some tissue cells while other cells are still alive. Connective tissue and muscle can take several hours – and in some environments – days, before cellular death and degradation is evidenced (Knight 2004). Tissues such as collagen may last indefinitely, due to their triple-helical structure and strong inter- and intra-molecular forces. Like all chemical processes, autolysis is impacted by environmental variables, particularly temperature.

True autolytic changes are typically only visible using microscopy to confirm the loss or fading of cellular structure (Tsokos 2004). For example, the release of hydrolytic enzymes into intercellular regions leads to tissue necrosis, evidenced microscopically by the absence of cell nuclei (Gill-King 1997). However, some macroscopic changes that result from autolytic self-digestion may be visible to the naked eye, as evidenced in necrotic tissue, which is typically paler and more friable. Additionally, the cornea may demonstrate a cloudy appearance and liquefaction of the splenic pulp may be evident. Haemolysis of the blood serum results from degradation of erythrocyte membranes causing a red-brown discolouration of the larger and smaller arteries. Skin slippage may also result as the outer layers of the skin slip off the body (Dix and Graham 2000). Additionally, hair will loosen and be removed with the skin. Skin slippage is sometimes considered to result from autolysis, and other times to result from putrefaction. The distinction is not clear, since the processes of autolysis and putrefaction can occur in parallel. By definition, autolytic changes result only from endogenous enzyme activity, whereas putrefactive changes are a result of microbial activity. Considering that both processes can occur concomitantly within a body, many of the macroscopic and microscopic changes cannot be attributed specifically to autolysis or putrefaction and are simply described as part of the decomposition process.

2.3 Putrefaction

The process of putrefaction is typically described sequentially following the end-stage of autolysis; however, the two processes can occur simultaneously within different regions of a body. Putrefaction is a microbial-driven process, predominantly governed by anaerobic bacteria, that degrades and liquefies tissues (Campobasso *et al.* 2001; Gill-King 1997; Janaway *et al.* 2009; Vass *et al.* 2002). The first signs of putrefaction are visible as a green/purple discolouration of the skin on the abdominal region, caused by the conversion of haemoglobin to sulf-haemoglobin (Janaway *et al.* 2009; Swann *et al.* 2010; Vass *et al* 2002). Other indicators of putrefaction include bloating, due to the accumulation of fermentative gases, and foul odours released by the action of bacteria (Gill-King 1997; Swann *et al.* 2010; Vass *et al.* 2002).

2.3.1 Liquefaction and Properties of Liquefaction Products

The liquefaction of soft tissues commences shortly after death, initiated by the processes of putrefaction (Janaway 1997). Bacterial enzymes originating in the gastrointestinal tract are responsible for the widespread decomposition of tissues in the body (Janaway 1997; Janaway *et al.* 2009), which become increasingly more liquid. These liquefied products, mixed with other bodily fluids, will enter the surrounding environment via natural orifices and post-mortem skin ruptures.

Liquefied remains have been shown to exhibit changes in their properties throughout the decay process, as influenced by extrinsic organisms. The pH of purged fluid has been measured and reported as being initially neutral, but increases in alkalinity when insects are present on the remains (Comstock 2014). Maggots release ammonia (NH_3) as they feed, which is subsequently converted into ammonium (NH_4^+) (Turner 2005), thus leading to increased alkalinity (Hopkins *et al.* 2000). Following the insect activity stages, however, the pH decreases to levels above those initially detected (Comstock 2014). Conductivity, the measure of the total amount of dissolved ionic compounds, of liquefied tissue has also been measured, and displays a general increase during the early decay stages (Comstock 2014). This is caused by the concerted release of ions, such as NH_4^+, K^+, Cl^- and SO_4^{2-} during these early stages (Vass *et al.* 1992). During the insect activity stages, however, the conductivity of purged fluids decreases (Comstock 2014). It is likely that the liquefied products, rich in ions, are utilised by the bacteria brought to the carcasses by insects for metabolism (Vass *et al.* 1992).

The human body is predominantly composed of water (approximately 64%) and approximately 20% protein, 10% fat, 1% carbohydrate and 5% minerals (Janaway *et al.* 2009). The degradation of soft tissue involves the breakdown of these macromolecules and the breakdown products should therefore reflect the proportion of compounds initially present within the body (Dent *et al.* 2004; Swann *et al.* 2010). In addition to the aforementioned properties, purged liquefied remains have been shown to contain high levels of lipids and their degradation products (Comstock 2014). It is hypothesised that they also contain degradation products of the other macromolecules, but this has not been investigated in the same level of detail.

2.3.2 Protein Degradation

Proteins within the body are degraded by bacterial enzymes via proteolysis (Evans 1963). The process takes place at variable rates and is dependent on the action of bacteria, the amount of moisture, and the temperature of the surrounding environment (Forbes 2008; Janaway *et al.* 2009). Proteolysis first takes place in soft tissues, such as the neuronal and epithelial tissues (Forbes 2008; Janaway *et al.* 2009), and occurs during the early stages of decomposition in the brain, liver and kidneys (Forbes 2008; Janaway *et al.* 2009). Connective tissues and integuments (tissues containing the collagen protein), including the epidermis, reticulin and muscle protein, are more resistant to proteolysis (Dent *et al.* 2004; Forbes 2008; Gill-King 1997), but will eventually succumb to degradation. Collagen and keratin, as noted previously, will survive for longer post-mortem periods, as they are highly resistant to both hydrolytic enzymes and microbial degradation (Forbes 2008).

Type I collagen proteins are found in hard tissues, such as bone and tooth enamel (Collins *et al.* 2002). The breakdown of collagen in bone is largely restricted due to its physical exclusion from microbial extracellular enzymes (Collins *et al.* 2002). However, the rate of collagen degradation is dependent upon time, temperature and environmental pH (Collins *et al.* 2002). Nonetheless, these hard tissues are largely protected from proteolysis as a result of their association with biological apatite, and thus persist into the archaeological record (Collins *et al.* 2002).

Similarly, hair, skin and nails, which contain keratin (an insoluble fibrous protein) (Gupta and Ramnani 2006; Janaway *et al.* 2009), also have the potential to remain intact into the archaeological record (Forbes 2008; Linch and Prahlow 2001; Macko *et al.* 1999; Wilson *et al.* 2007). Keratin is a secondary protein with a rigid structure created by extensive disulphide bonds and cross-linkages (Gupta and Ramnani 2006). Its structure prevents its degradation by common proteolytic enzymes (Macko *et al.* 1999) and is only used as a nutrient source by specialised keratinolytic microorganisms (Gupta and Ramnani 2006; Janaway *et al.* 2009), which influence the rate at which these structures are broken down (Wilson *et al.* 2007).

In general, proteolysis breaks down proteins into proteoses, peptones and polypeptides (Forbes 2008; Janaway 1997; Janaway *et al.* 2009). Bacterial exoenzymes denature proteins and eventually release their constituent amino acids (Gill-King 1997). Amino acids subsequently undergo deamination (removal of amine groups) or decarboxylation (removal of carboxyl groups) (Gill-King 1997). Amino acids containing sulphur (i.e. cysteine, cystine and methionine) undergo desulfhydralation, which produces hydrogen sulphide gas, sulphides, ammonia, thiols and pyruvic acid (Forbes 2008; Gill-King 1997; Janaway *et al.* 2009).

Two decarboxylation products have been frequently reported as resulting from protein degradation, and are aptly named putrescine (derived from ornithine) and cadaverine (derived from lysine) (Gill-King 1997; Forbes 2008; Pessione *et al.* 2005; Vass 2001). However, these diamines have been consistently absent from volatile organic compound (VOC) profiles of pig and human remains (Dekeirsschieter *et al.* 2009; Hoffman *et al.* 2009; Stadler *et al.* 2013; Statheropoulos *et al.* 2005; Vass *et al.* 2004). Their significance as protein degradation products is therefore unclear.

2.3.3 Lipid Degradation

Adipose tissue occupies 15% of the body (Kagawa *et al.* 1996) and consists of approximately 5–30% water, 2–3% protein and 60–85% lipids, 90–99% of which are triglycerides (Reynold and Cahill 1965). Triglycerides are composed of a glycerol molecule containing three hydroxyl groups that form ester linkages with fatty acids (Campbell and Farrell 2006). Six fatty acids in particular account for over 90% of the fatty acids detected in adipose tissue: monounsaturated oleic and palmitoleic acids, saturated palmitic, myristic and stearic acids, and polyunsaturated linoleic acid (Calder *et al.* 1992; Hirsch *et al.* 1960; Insull and Bartsch 1967; Krut and Bronte-Stewart 1964).

Neutral lipids are the dominant lipid forms within adipose tissue and collectively refer to di- and tri-glycerides and cholesterol esters (Kramer and Hulan 1978). Hydrolysis of these neutral lipids is the first step in the lipid degradation process (Forbes 2008). Intrinsic lipases act upon the lipids to free the fatty acids from their glycerol backbone, creating a mixture of free saturated and unsaturated fatty acids (Evans 1963; Forbes *et al.* 2005; Janaway 1997; Janaway *et al.* 2009; Notter *et al.* 2009) (Figure 2.1). Following hydrolysis, the fatty acids can undergo one of two routes of degradation, depending on the availability of oxygen.

Anaerobic microorganisms dominate within a body following death because the redox potential of tissues falls, which limits the number of aerobes that can survive (Gill-King 1997). As a result, anaerobic microorganisms will invade surrounding tissues and promote the anaerobic degradation of fatty acids via hydrogenation (Gill-King 1997; Janaway *et al.* 2009). Unsaturated fatty acids, such as palmitoleic and oleic acids, will undergo hydrogenation, which is the process by which hydrogen atoms are added to the double bonds in the fatty acids to convert them into their saturated

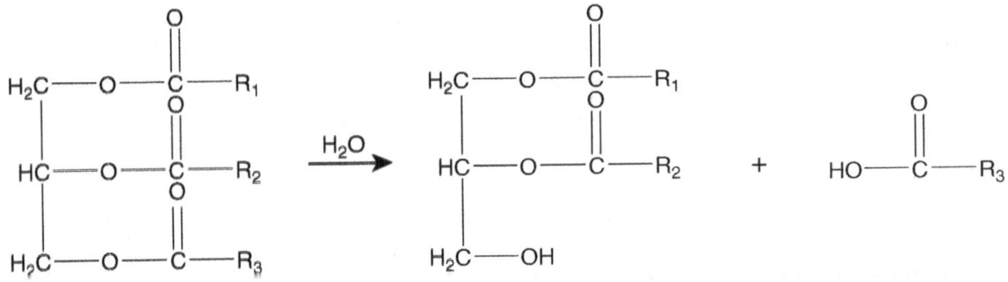

Figure 2.1 Example of a hydrolysis reaction.

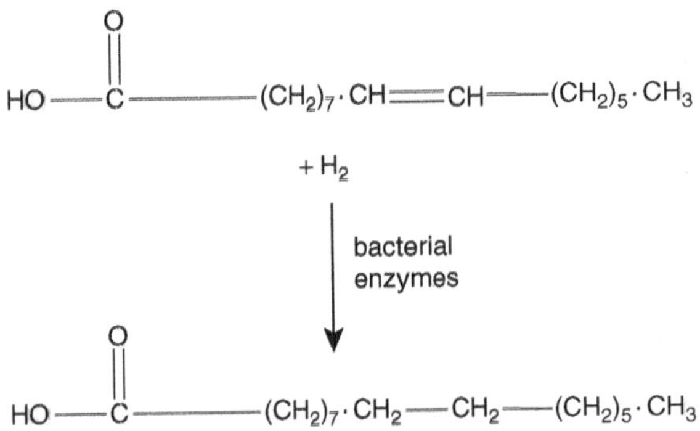

Figure 2.2 Example of a hydrogenation reaction.

counterparts (Figure 2.2) (Fiedler and Graw, 2003; Forbes 2008; Forbes *et al.* 2005; Jones 2005; Notter *et al.* 2009).

Hydrogenation increases the amount of saturated fatty acids, while decreasing the amount of unsaturated fatty acids, and therefore hydrogenation of palmitoleic and oleic acids should yield palmitic and stearic acids, respectively (Evans 1963; Notter *et al.* 2009). Evidence of hydrogenation in soft tissue has been observed to take place during the later stages of decay (Comstock 2014).

Under aerobic conditions, fatty acids undergo oxidation, which is aided by bacteria, fungi and oxygen (Forbes 2008). Oxidation produces peroxide linkages, initiated by oxygen attacking the double bonds in unsaturated fatty acids (Gray 1978), and eventually leads to the production of aldehydes and ketones (Evans 1963; Forbes 2008; Janaway 1997; Janaway *et al.* 2009).

2.3.4 Adipocere Formation

One of the most common by-products of lipid degradation is the formation of adipocere, a greyish-white substance that can become solid and resistant to further putrefactive changes (Cotton *et al.* 1987; Forbes *et al.* 2005; Gill-King 1997; Notter *et al.* 2009). When sufficient water and bacterial enzymes are present, hydrolysis will continue until neutral lipids are completely reduced to free fatty acids (Forbes 2008), which subsequently liquefy and penetrate surrounding tissues (Fiedler andGraw 2003). These free fatty acids can be converted into hydroxyl fatty acids by the action of bacterial enzymes (Forbes 2008; Janaway *et al.* 2009), which will remain as adipocere if no further chemical changes take place (Gill-King 1997; Notter *et al.* 2009; Pfeiffer *et al.* 1998). Alternatively, fatty acids can react with sodium and potassium ions in tissue to produce fatty acid salts (Forbes 2008; Notter *et al.* 2009). When located in a soil environment, the sodium and potassium ions can be replaced by calcium and magnesium ions to form fatty acid soaps (Gill-King 1997; Forbes 2008).

2.3.5 Carbohydrate Degradation

The degradation of carbohydrates in soft tissue occurs early in the decomposition process (Evans 1963; Janaway *et al.* 2009), because hexoses, such as glucose, are the preferred carbon and energy source for many endogenous bacteria (Boumba *et al.* 2008). Glucose monomers are produced from the microorganism-induced degradation of the glycogen polysaccharide (Corry 1978). The complete oxidation of glucose leads to the production of carbon dioxide and water, while the incomplete degradation of sugars results in a variety of organic acids and alcohols (Ellis and Wilson 2002; Paczkowski and Schütz 2011; Ueno *et al.* 2001).

A variety of products can be formed through carbohydrate degradation, which is dependent on the initiating organism. Glucose degradation by yeast yields pyruvate, which is decarboxylated to acetaldehyde and is subsequently reduced to ethanol (Boumba *et al.* 2008; Ziavrou *et al.* 2014). Enterobacteria ferment glucose to produce a mixture of acids, including lactic, acetic, succinic, formic, butanoic and propanoic (Boumba *et al.* 2008; Paczkowski and Schütz 2011). Additionally, aerobic degradation by fungi results in the production of organic acids, such as glucuronic, citric and oxalic (Paczkowski and Schütz 2011), which are responsible for the acidic environment created around carcasses during the early stages of decomposition (Gill-King 1997). Additional fermentative products include alcohols, such as ethanol, methanol and isomers of propanol and butanol (Boumba *et al.* 2008; Paczkowski and Schütz 2011; Ziavrou *et al.* 2014), acetone, acetate (Boumba *et al.* 2008; Paczkowski and Schütz 2011; Ziavrou *et al.* 2014), lactate, formate, propionate, *n*-butyrate (Ueno *et al.* 2001), and gases, including hydrogen, methane and hydrogen sulphide (Ueno *et al.* 2001).

2.3.6 Nucleic Acid Degradation

Nucleic acids are macromolecules comprising DNA. DNA molecules will be attacked by nucleases, which are enzymes that specifically target nucleic acids (Perry *et al.* 1988). The degradation of nucleic acids results in the formation of nucleotides and nucleosides, which will subsequently decay into sugars, phosphate and nitrogenous purine and pyrimidine bases (Hodgson 1962; Dekeirsschieter *et al.* 2009; Statheropoulos *et al.* 2005; Vass *et al.* 2002). The resulting sugars, such as pentose and ribose, will be degraded via the same pathways as those originating from carbohydrates.

The phosphorus released does not follow simple degradation pathways and can be found in many different forms in the surrounding environment (Dent *et al.* 2004). Oxidised forms of phosphorus are the most thermodynamically stable and mobile; however they are favoured in slightly acidic soils (Hem 1989). Outside a pH range of 6–7, the phosphorus will exist in its insoluble inorganic forms, which may be associated with iron, calcium, magnesium and aluminium (Dent *et al.* 2004).

The purine bases (adenine and guanine) compose both DNA and RNA and will be released in greater amounts than pyridine bases (Hodgson 1962). Degradation of the purine bases will lead to the formation of xanthine and hypoxanthine, which are commonly collected from the vitreous humour to estimate the post-mortem interval (PMI) (Donaldson and Lamont 2014). Detection of pyridine bases has been limited due to their lower abundance within the body (Hodgson 1962). Nitrogen may be released from the bases and enter the surrounding soil, where it will enter the nutrient cycle.

2.4 Factors Affecting Autolysis and Putrefaction

As a general rule, changes in environmental variables may impact the rate, but do not change the underlying chemical and biological mechanisms of decomposition (Tsokos 2004). Temperature, both physiologically and environmentally, has the greatest impact on the decomposition process (Gill-King 1997). With respect to the chemical processes of autolysis and putrefaction, it is generally reported that heat increases the decomposition rate and cold impedes it (Carter *et al.* 2007; Dent 2004; Dix and Graham 2000; Forbes 2008; Gill-King 1977; Janaway 1997; Knight 2004; Prahlow 2001; Vass 2002). A high ambient temperature will also accelerate decomposition through the activation of other biological activity such as vertebrate and invertebrate scavenging (Di Maio and Di Maio 2001). Freezing will typically inhibit decomposition due to the inactivation of enzymes and bacteria and the absence of invertebrate scavengers at temperatures below zero (Di Maio and Di Maio 2001; Micozzi 1997).

The physical location and/or deposition of the body will influence the rate of decomposition and dictate whether or not the process occurs. In addition to temperature, other climatic conditions such as humidity, rainfall, solar radiation and air movement can influence the decomposition rate. A body discovered in a forested area may have been exposed to varying amounts of sun and shade from surrounding vegetation, which can change the exposure to solar radiation and increase the internal temperature of the body. A body discovered inside a home or other structure may have been exposed to heating or cooling in a relatively dry environment, depending on the time of year and whether an air conditioner was on at the time of death (Di Maio and Di Maio 2001).

Buried remains are known to decompose at a slower rate than remains left on the surface in the same environment (Dix and Graham 2000). A body buried in a deep (cemetery-like) grave will be better preserved than a body buried in a shallow (forensic-like) grave. The presence of a coffin will also slow decomposition and aid preservation in some soil environments, which can be particularly important during archaeological recoveries (Knight 2004). Bodies in water also decompose at a slower rate but typically faster than those buried in soil (Prahlow 2010). The reduced rate of decomposition in both soil and water is mostly due to cooler temperatures and a reduction (or absence) of small mammal and invertebrate scavenging (Knight 2004). The variation even within soil and water can be large and it is important to remember that differences in soil type (e.g. sand versus clay), different types of water (e.g. fresh, brackish, salt) and even differences in air (e.g. dry versus humid) will vary the rate of decomposition (Prahlow 2010). Bodies buried in soil, submerged in water, or found in a cool basement, will all appear very different after the same post-mortem period (Dix and Graham 2000). Decomposition can also vary within a body, with one region of the body appearing leathery and mummified while another region is still in a state of putrefaction and liquefaction (Knight 2004; Schotsmans *et al.* 2011). Particularly, hot/dry or cold/dry environments can lead to the inhibition of decomposition through tissue desiccation resulting in mummification (Di Maio and Di Maio 2001).

2.5 Impact of the Decomposition Process on the Surrounding Environment

The chemistry of decomposition is not an isolated process and extends beyond the body's internal microenvironment. In forensic and archaeological contexts, it is common to encounter remains deposited on or below the soil surface in outdoor terrestrial settings. Decomposing remains can have a profound effect on the surrounding environment due to the release of nutrients and energy into the immediate vicinity. In outdoor environments, this may include physical and chemical changes to soil, vegetation, microorganisms and associated evidence (e.g. textiles, documents, etc.) surrounding the remains. The degree of change in soil and vegetation around decomposing remains is likely to be high during the initial purging of liquefactive fluid and will decrease as the time since deposition or burial of the remains increases (Watson and Forbes 2008). Characterisation of these physical disturbances has assisted forensic experts in improving visual search procedures (Caccianiga *et al.* 2012; France *et al.* 1992; Watson and Forbes 2008). New research in this area is attempting to identify chemical biomarkers of decomposition within the surrounding environment that could assist with post-burial interval estimation (Benninger *et al.* 2008; Donaldson and Lamont 2013, 2014, 2015; Larizza and Forbes 2013; Van Belle *et al.* 2009; Vass *et al.* 1992).

Physical changes to the immediate surroundings can vary depending on many variables (e.g. vegetation species assemblage, geographical location, biomass of remains, season, etc.) but can give a visual indication that remains are or were present. Few visual changes to the environment are observed during the early stages of decomposition as cadaveric materials are contained within the cadaver until the skin ruptures or fluids purge from body orifices. For surface-deposited remains, once the body deflates, fluids leach into the surrounding soil and a cadaver decomposition island (CDI) forms (Carter *et al.* 2007). The CDI is a darkened area of moistened soil, as seen in Figure 2.3. The vegetation within the CDI may die and disintegrate depending on the soil nutrient status (Bornemissza 1952; Towne 2000; Watson and Forbes 2008). Vegetation located further from the remains is less likely to be affected by these disturbances. As the PMI increases, the vegetation will regenerate, often healthier than it was originally, which can cause a clear delineation of the site in some cases (Watson and Forbes 2008). Species assemblage of vegetation may become altered, especially where the vegetation cover is completely destroyed upon burial (Caccianiga *et al.* 2012). This is often the response of opportunistic plants colonising areas of increased nutrient availability (France *et al.* 1992) (Figure 2.4) and some species may therefore act as grave indicators (Watson and Forbes 2008). These physical changes may originate from a variety of causes existing at a microscopic level.

Decomposition produces a localised pulse of nutrients into the soil, whereby dispersal depends largely on biomass and season (Danell *et al.* 2002). The human body is comprised of a variety of elements, which are housed in different reservoirs (i.e. bone, soft tissue, etc.) and become released during decomposition. Carbon, nitrogen, phosphorus and other elements enter the area surrounding a decomposing cadaver and become available to enter ecological nutrient cycles. The availability and

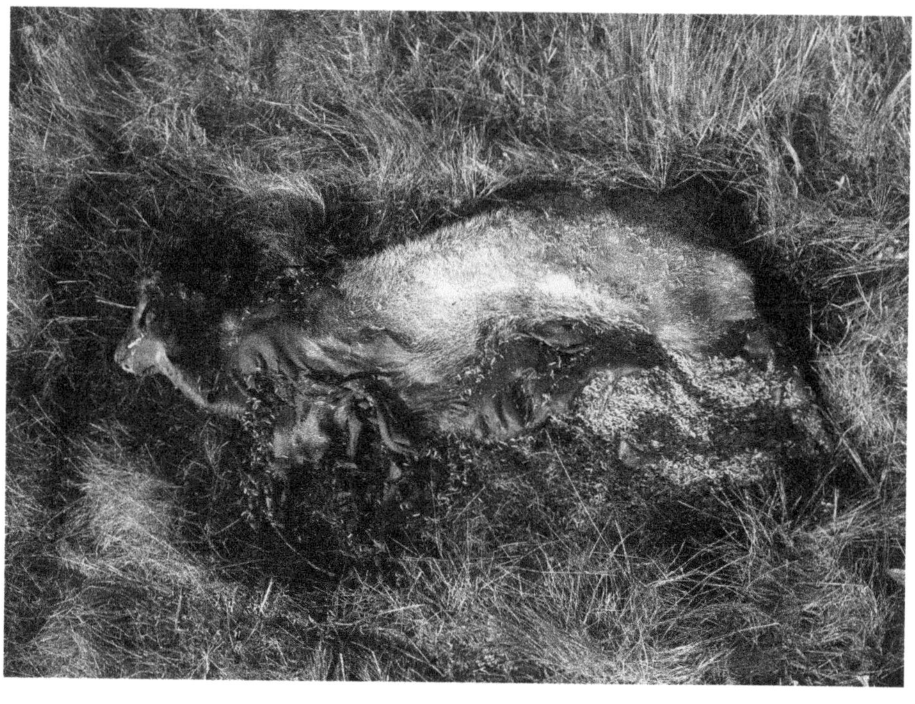

Figure 2.3 Carcass decomposition depicting a cadaver decomposition island (CDI) surrounding a decomposing pig carcass.

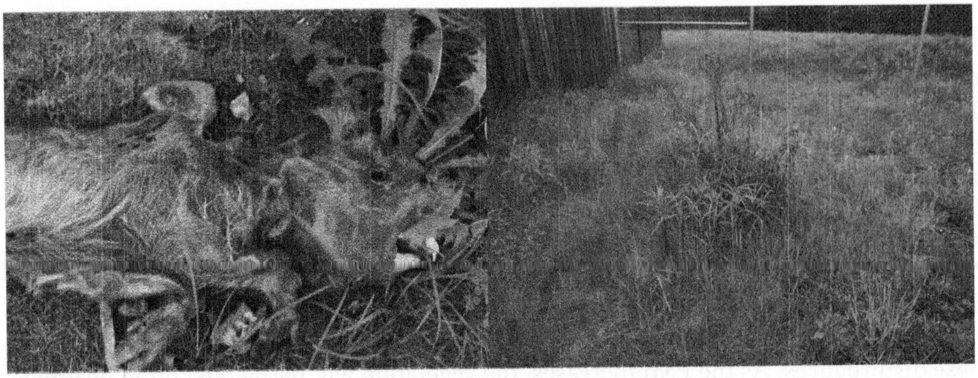

Figure 2.4 Opportunistic plants colonise areas of ideal nutrient availability.

transformation of nutrients in the soil after this influx will impact macroscopic changes. The mobility of introduced nutrients through soil particles is largely dependent on the physicochemical properties of the soil in the immediate area. Since many nutrients are solubilised and transported in groundwater, the soil texture, porosity and moisture content can largely impact nutrient mobility. For example, soils with high compaction or high clay content will impede the transportation of cadaveric nutrients through soil, whereas soils with larger particles (i.e. higher porosity) will promote nutrient transport. In clandestine burials, the soil exhibits decreased compaction compared with the surrounding soil that has been undisturbed, which can promote the mobility of nutrients within the grave (Dent *et al.* 2004). The pulse of nutrients into the environment, in addition to the increased nutrient availability to plant roots, is associated with flourishing vegetation that may be seen on grave sites. High moisture in soils with adequate porosity will be conducive to the transport of introduced nutrients through the soil. Soil pH can also affect the form and solubility of the nutrients entering the soil and may also impact the health of living organisms (i.e. plants, bacteria, fungi) that play a role in their transformation.

The nutritional status of the soil preceding the influx of cadaveric material can also impact the soil chemistry during cadaver decomposition. For example, if a lacking nutrient is augmented by liquefactive by-products, it may increase the health of the soil system thereby improving nutrient availability for soil bacteria, fungi and plants (Watson and Forbes 2008). Decomposition by-products entering the soil may not be immediately present in plant-usable forms and therefore may undergo processing by bacteria or fungi, causing a lag in nutrient availability or a cycling to occur. However, some organisms may be highly sensitive to fluctuations in particular elements, and surplus nutrients can overload the soil thereby causing toxicity symptoms in living organisms. If a nutrient deficiency was experienced prior to the introduction of cadaveric material, new plant growth often occurs rather than necrotic symptoms.

Leachate from a decomposing body can provide valuable commodities to the surrounding plants and soil microbial community. The flow of cadaveric nutrients to soil, plants, bacteria and fungi as well as the symbiotic nature of living organisms in this system is complex to define. Minor fluctuations in extrinsic factors (e.g. precipitation, temperature, pH, etc.) can have a major effect on these interactions. For example, alterations in soil pH can alter the soil microbial community, thereby affecting soft tissue decay in direct contact with the soil. Changes in soil pH can also impact the solubility of nutrients reaching plants and fungi. The temperature is also known to impact the pH of the soil surrounding decomposing remains (Carter *et al.* 2008). The interactions of these events can be challenging to interpret as they are interrelated in nature and do not exist independently in a soil environment (Carter *et al.* 2007; Hopkins *et al.* 2000).

2.6 Conclusion

The microscopic post-mortem changes that occur during decomposition involve a range of complex chemical and biological reactions. These are initiated soon after death and during the early post-mortem period, but are predominantly observed during autolysis and putrefaction. The loss of cellular structure, as a result of autolysis, releases hydrolytic enzymes that break down the body's macromolecules including proteins, lipids, carbohydrates, nucleic acids and cellular debris. The microbial-driven process of putrefaction further degrades and liquefies the tissues, resulting in the release of smaller molecules as liquids and gases to the surrounding environment. Environmental and physiological factors will impact the rate of decomposition including the weather conditions (e.g. temperature, humidity, rainfall and solar radiation), microorganisms in and around the body, invertebrate and vertebrate scavengers, and whether the body is buried in soil or concealed in other environments such as water. The decomposition of soft tissue releases nutrients to the environment causing physical and chemical changes to soil, vegetation, microorganisms and associated evidence (e.g. textiles, documents, etc.). The flow of nutrients to soil, plants, bacteria and fungi produces a highly complex system around the body. While research has been ongoing in this field for decades, much still needs to be done in order to better understand the symbiotic relationship between decomposition and the environment in which it occurs.

References

Benninger, L.A., Carter, D.O. and Forbes, S.L. (2008) The biochemical alteration of soil beneath a decomposing carcass. *Forensic Science International*, **180**: 70–75.

Bornemissza, G.F. (1952) An analysis of arthropod succession in carrion and the effect of its decomposition on the soil fauna. *Australian Journal of Zoology*, **5**: 1–12.

Boumba, V.A., Ziavrou, K.S. and Vougiouklakis, T. (2008) Biochemical pathways generating post-mortem volatile compounds co-detected during forensic ethanol analyses. *Forensic Science International*, **174**: 133–151.

Caccianiga, M., Bottacin, S. and Cattaneo, C. (2012) Vegetation dynamics as a tool for detecting clandestine graves. *Journal of Forensic Sciences*, **57**: 983–988.

Calder, P.C., Harvey, D.J., Pond, C.M. and Newsholme, E.A. (1992) Site-specific differences in the fatty acid composition of human adipose tissue. *Lipids*, **27**: 716–720.

Campbell, M.K. and Farrell, S.O. (2006) *Biochemistry*. Thomson Learning Inc.: Toronto.

Campobasso, C.P., Di Vella, G. and Introna, F. (2001) Factors affecting decomposition and Diptera colonization. *Forensic Science International*, **120**: 18–27.

Carter, D.O., Yellowlees, D. and Tibbett, M. (2007) Cadaver decomposition in terrestrial ecosystems. *Naturwissenschaften*, **94**: 12–24.

Carter, D.O., Yellowlees, D. and Tibbett, M. (2008) Temperature affects microbial decomposition of cadavers (*Rattus rattus*) in contrasting soils. *Applied Soil Ecology*, **40**: 129–137.

Collins, M., Nielsen-Marsh, C. and Hiller, J. (2002) The survival of organic matter in bone: a review. *Archaeometry*, **44**: 383–394.

Comstock, J. (2014) Elucidation of the lipid degradation process in soft tissue and fluid during decomposition, in the presence and absence of insects. Unpublished PhD thesis, University of Ontario Institute of Technology.

Corry, J.E. (1978) A review. Possible sources of ethanol ante- and post-mortem: its relationship to the biochemistry and microbiology of decomposition. *The Journal of Applied Bacteriology*, **44**: 1–56.

Cotton, G., Aufderheide, A. and Goldschmidt, V. (1987) Preservation of human tissue immersed for five years in fresh water of known temperature. *Journal of Forensic Sciences*, **32**: 1125–1130.

Danell, K., Berteaux, D. and Bråthen, K.A. (2002) Effect of musk ox carcasses on nitrogen concentration in tundra vegetation. *Arctic*, **55**: 389–392.

Dekeirsschieter, J., Verheggen, F.J., Gohy, M., Hubrecht, F., Bourguignon, L. *et al.* (2009) Cadaveric volatile organic compounds released by decaying pig carcasses (*Sus domesticus* L.) in different biotopes. *Forensic Science International*, **189**: 46–53.

Dent, B.B., Forbes, S.L. and Stuart, B.H. (2004) Review of human decomposition processes in soil. *Environmental Geology*, **45**: 576–585.

Di Maio, V.J.M. and Di Maio, D.J. (2001) *Forensic Pathology*. CRC Press: Boca Raton.

Dix, J. and Graham, M. (2000) *Time of Death, Decomposition and Identification: An atlas*. CRC Press: Boca Raton.

Donaldson, A.E. and Lamont, I.L. (2013) Biochemistry changes that occur after death: potential markers for determining post-mortem interval. *PLoS One*, **8**: e82011

Donaldson, A.E. and Lamont, I.L. (2014) Estimation of post-mortem interval using biochemical markers. *Australian Journal of Forensic Sciences*, **46**: 8–26.

Donaldson, A.E. and Lamont, I.L. (2015) Metabolomics of post-mortem blood: identifying potential markers of post-mortem interval. *Metabolomics*, **11**: 237–245.

Ellis, A.V. and Wilson, M.A. (2002) Carbon exchange in hot alkaline degradation of glucose. *The Journal of Organic Chemistry*, **67**: 8469–8474.

Evans, W.E.D. (1963) *The Chemistry of Death*. Thomas: Springfield.

Fiedler, S. and Graw, M. (2003) Decomposition of buried corpses, with special reference to the formation of adipocere. *Naturwissenschaften*, **90**: 291–300.

Forbes, S.L. (2008) Decomposition chemistry in a burial environment. In: Tibbett, M. and Carter, D.O. (eds), *Soil Analysis in Forensic Taphonomy. Chemical and Biological Effects of Buried Human Remains. CRC Press*: Boca Raton, pp. 203–223.

Forbes, S.L., Stuart, B.H. and Dent, B.B. (2005) The effect of the burial environment on adipocere formation. *Forensic Science International*, **154**: 24–34.

France, D.L., Griffin, T.J., Swanburg, J.G., Lindemann, J.W., Davenport, G.C. *et al.* (1992) A multidisciplinary approach to the detection of clandestine graves. *Journal of Forensic Sciences*, **37**: 1445–1458.

Gill-King, H. (1997) Chemical and ultrastructural aspects of decomposition. In: Haglund, W.D. and Sorg, M.H. (eds), *Forensic Taphonomy. The Postmortem Fate Of Human Remains*. CRC Press: Boca Raton, pp. 93–105.

Gray, J. (1978) Measurement of lipid oxidation: a review. *Journal of the American Oil Chemists' Society*, **55**: 539–546.

Gupta, R. and Ramnani, P. (2006) Microbial keratinases and their prospective applications: an overview. *Applied Microbiology and Biotechnology*, **70**: 21–33.

Hem JD (1989) *Study and Interpretation of the Chemical Characteristics of Natural Water*, 3rd edition. US Geological Survey: Alexandria.

Hirsch, J., Farquhar, J. and Ahrens, E. (1960) Studies of adipose tissue in man. A microtechnic for sampling and analysis. *The American Journal of Clinical Nutrition*, **8**: 499–511.

Hodgson, C. (1962) Nucleic acids and their decomposition products in normal and pathological horny layers. *Journal of Investigative Dermatology*, **39**: 69–79.

Hoffman, E.M., Curran, A.M., Dulgerian, N., Stockham, R.A. and Eckenrode, B.A. (2009) Characterization of the volatile organic compounds present in the headspace of decomposing human remains. *Forensic Science International*, **186**: 6–13.

Hopkins, D., Wiltshire, P.E.J. and Turner, B.D. (2000) Microbial characteristics of soils from graves: an investigation at the interface of soil microbiology and forensic science. *Applied Soil Ecology*, **14**: 283–288.

Insull, W. and Bartsch, G. (1967) Fatty acid composition of human adipose tissue related to age, sex, and race. *The American Journal of Clinical Nutrition*, **20**: 13–23.

Janaway, R.C. (1997) The decay of buried human remains and their associated materials. In: Hunter, J., Roberts, C. and Martin, A. (eds), *Studies in Crime: An introduction to forensic archaeology*. Routledge: London, pp. 58–85.

Janaway, R.C., Percival, S.L. and Wilson, A.S. (2009) Decomposition of human remains. In: Percival, S.L. (ed.), *Microbiology and Aging*. Humana Press: Totowa, pp. 313–334.

Jones, M. (2005) *Organic Chemistry*, 3rd edition. Norton & Company Inc.: New York.

Kagawa, M., Matsubara, K. and Kimura, K. (1996) Species identification by the positional analysis of fatty acid composition in triacylglyceride of adipose and bone tissues. *Forensic Science International*, **79**: 215–226.

Knight, B. (2004) *Knight's Forensic Pathology*, 3rd edition. CRC Press: Boca Raton.

Kramer, J.M. and Hulan, H.W. (1978) A comparison of procedures to determine free fatty acids in rat heart. *Journal of Lipid Research*, **19**: 103–106.

Krut, L.H. and Bronte-Stewart, B. (1964) The fatty acids of human depot fat. *Journal of Lipid Research*, **5**: 343–351.

Larizza, M. and Forbes, S.L. (2013) Detection of fatty acids in the lateral extent of the cadaver decomposition island. *Geological Society London, Special Publications*, **384**: 209–219.

Linch, C.A. and Prahlow, J.A. (2001) Postmortem microscopic changes observed at the human head hair proximal end. *Journal of Forensic Sciences*, **46**: 15–20.

Macko, S.A., Lubec, G., Teschler-Nicola, M., Andrusevich, V. and Engel, M.H. (1999) The Ice Man's diet as reflected by the stable nitrogen and carbon isotopic composition of his hair. *FASEB Journal: Official Publication of the Federation of American Societies for Experimental Biology*, **13**: 559–562.

Micozzi, M.Z. (1997) Frozen environments and soft tissue preservation. In: Haglund, W.D. and Sorg, M.H. (eds), *Forensic Taphonomy. The postmortem fate of human remains*. CRC Press: Boca Raton, pp. 93–105.

Notter, S.J., Stuart, B.H., Rowe, R. and Langlois, N. (2009) The initial changes of fat deposits during the decomposition of human and pig remains. *Journal of Forensic Sciences*, **54**: 195–201.

Paczkowski, S. and Schütz, S. (2011) Post-mortem volatiles of vertebrate tissue. *Applied Microbiology and Biotechnology*, **91**: 917–935.

Perry, W.L., Bass, W.M., Riggsby, W.S. and Sirotkin, K. (1988) The autodegradation of deoxyribonucleic acid (DNA) in human rib bone and its relationship to the time interval since death. *Journal of Forensic Sciences*, **33**: 144–153.

Pessione, E., Mazzoli, R., Giuffrida, M.G., Lamberti, C., Garcia-Moruno, E. *et al.* (2005) A proteomic approach to studying biogenic amine producing lactic acid bacteria. *Proteomics*, **5**: 687–698.

Pfeiffer, S., Milne, S. and Stevenson, R.M. (1998) The natural decomposition of adipocere. *Journal of Forensic Sciences*, **43**: 368–370.

Prahlow, J. (2010) *Forensic Pathology for Police, Death Investigators, Attorneys and Forensic Scientists*. Springer: New York.

Reynold, A. and Cahill, G. (1965) *Handbook of Physiology: Adipose tissue*. American Physiological Society: Washington.

Schotsmans, E.M.J., Van de Voorde, W., De Winne, J. and Wilson, A.S. (2011) The impact of shallow burial on differential decomposition to the body: a temperate case study. *Forensic Science International*, **206**: e43–e48.

Stadler, S. (2013) Analysis of the volatile organic compounds produced by the decomposition of pig carcasses and human remains. Unpublished PhD thesis, University of Ontario Institute of Technology.

Statheropoulos, M., Spiliopoulou, C. and Agapiou, A. (2005) A study of volatile organic compounds evolved from the decaying human body. *Forensic Science International*, **153**: 147–155.

Swann, L.M., Forbes, S.L. and Lewis, S.W. (2010) Analytical separations of mammalian decomposition products for forensic science: A review. *Analytica Chimica Acta*, **682**: 9–22.

Towne, E.G. (2000) Prairie vegetation and soil nutrient responses to ungulate carcasses. *Oecologia*, **122**: 232–239.

Tsokos, M. (2004) Postmortem changes and artifacts occurring during the early postmortem interval. In: Tsokos, M. (ed.), *Forensic Pathology Reviews*, vol. **3**. Humana Press: Totowa, pp. 183–237.

Turner, B. (2005) Blowfly maggots: the good, the bad and the ugly. *Comparative Clinical Pathology*, **14**: 81–85.

Ueno, Y., Haruta, S., Ishii, M. and Igarashik, Y. (2001) Changes in product formation and bacterial community by dilution rate on carbohydrate fermentation by methanogenic microflora in continuous flow stirred tank reactor. *Applied Microbiology and Biotechnology*, **57**: 65–73.

Van Belle, L.E., Carter, D.O. and Forbes, S.L. (2009) Measurement of ninhydrin reactive nitrogen influx into grave soil during aboveground and belowground carcass (*Sus domesticus*) decomposition. *Forensic Science International*, **193**: 37–41.

Vass, A.A. (2001) Beyond the grave-understanding human decomposition. *Microbiology Today*, **28**: 190–193.

Vass, A.A., Barshick, S,-A., Sega, G., Caton, J., Skeen, J.T. *et al.* (2002) Decomposition chemistry of human remains: a new methodology for determining the postmortem interval. *Journal of Forensic Sciences*, **47**: 542–553.

Vass, A.A., Bass, W.M., Wolt, J.D., Foss, J.E. and Ammonsk, J.T (1992) Time since death determinations of human cadavers using soil solution. *Journal of Forensic Sciences*, **37**: 1236–53.

Vass, A.A., Smith, R.R., Thompson, C.V., Burnett, M.N., Wolf, D.A. *et al.* (2004) Decompositional odor analysis database. *Journal of Forensic Sciences*, **49**: 760–769.

Watson, C.J. and Forbes, S.L. (2008) An investigation of the vegetation associated with grave sites in Southern Ontario. *Journal of the Canadian Society of Forensic Science*, **41**: 199–207.

Wilson, A.S., Dodson, H.I., Janaway, R.C., Pollard, A.M. and Tobin, D.J. (2007) Selective biodegradation in hair shafts derived from archaeological, forensic and experimental contexts. *The British Journal of Dermatology*, **157**: 450–457.

Zapico, S.C., Menendez, S.T. and Nunez, P. (2014) Cell death proteins as markers of early postmortem interval. *Cellular and Molecular Life Sciences*, **71**: 2957–2962.

Ziavrou, K., Boumba, V.A. and Vougiouklakis, T.G. (2014) Insights into the origin of postmortem ethanol. *International Journal of Toxicology*, **24**: 69–77.

3

Profiling Volatile Organic Compounds of Decomposition

Pierre-Hugues Stefanuto, Elien Rosier*, Jan Tytgat, Jean-François Focant and Eva Cuypers*

3.1 Introduction

During the decomposition of human or animal remains, a wide spectrum of volatile organic compounds (VOCs) are emitted into the environment, resulting in what is commonly known as 'the smell of death'. Due to the VOC's specific chemical profile and a canine's excellent olfactory capacity, human remains detection (HRD) canines (more commonly called 'cadaver dogs') can be trained to locate (buried) corpses. As these dogs can differentiate between odours produced by human and animal remains, it is believed that the decomposition of human remains generates a unique scent (Vass *et al.* 2004). HRD canines can even make a distinction between the odour of living persons and recently deceased individuals (DeGreeff *et al.* 2011). Training and cultivating such a selective sense of detection in HRD canines consequently requires a high level of understanding of cadaveric decomposition chemistry. Therefore, the physicochemical identification of specific VOCs generated by the complex and dynamic human decomposition process could contribute to increase the efficiency of HRD canine training. Additionally, HRD canines have a short working life and variable performances (depending on the dog) (Statheropoulos *et al.* 2007). The development of a portable device that could efficiently detect specific markers would be complementary to the work of HRD canines and enhance the power of forensic research in the discovery of buried bodies. However, for now, these detectors are not as sensitive as the HRD dogs.

In forensic entomology, insects that inhabit decomposing remains are used to aid forensic investigations. Although it can take days, weeks or longer to find a body, insects are typically attracted to the odour of decomposed bodies within minutes. Depending on the decomposition stage and the released VOCs, different insects will be attracted. The distribution, biology and behaviour of insects found on a decomposing body can provide information in an investigation (Amendt *et al.* 2006, 2011; Farinha *et al.* 2014). Since different insect activities are associated with each stage in the decomposition process, the most important application of forensic entomology is the estimation of the minimum post-mortem interval (PMI). Despite the fact that the exact mechanisms that attract insects are still not completely understood, it is believed that the nature of released VOCs plays a major role (Statheropoulos *et al.* 2011). The field of entomology would thus also benefit from the physicochemical identification of stage-specific VOCs to provide better insights in forensic investigations.

---

* Equal contribution

Taphonomy of Human Remains: Forensic Analysis of the Dead and the Depositional Environment, First Edition.
Edited by Eline M.J. Schotsmans, Nicholas Márquez-Grant and Shari L. Forbes.

To date, it is known that a wide variety of VOCs are formed during the decomposition process arising from degraded proteins, carbohydrates and fat in the human body. Several research groups have studied these post-mortem dynamic VOC mixtures and different chemical classes such as alkanes, alcohols, acids, esters, ketones, aldehydes, cyclic hydrocarbons, aromatic compounds, sulphur- and nitrogen-containing compounds have already been identified. Nevertheless, it is important to further study the VOC signature of the 'smell of death' and to determine whether the identified compounds are specific to human decomposition (Brasseur *et al.* 2012; Cablk *et al.* 2012; DeGreeff and Furton 2011; Dekeirsschieter *et al.* 2009, 2012; Forbes and Perrault 2014; Hoffman *et al.* 2009; Perrault *et al.* 2014; Rosier *et al.* 2014; Stadler *et al.* 2013; Statheropoulos *et al.* 2005, 2007; Stefanuto *et al.* 2014; Vass 2012; Vass *et al.* 2004, 2008).

3.2 Matrices and Sampling Methods

3.2.1 Matrices

The materials on which studies are carried out are defined as matrices. These can be divided into primary and secondary matrices. The decomposing body or tissue that is used in the study is considered a primary matrix. During decomposition investigations, different materials such as soil, water or air can also be used to determine the VOC signature. These matrices are considered to be secondary matrices.

3.2.1.1 Primary Matrices

The preferred matrix to use in human decomposition studies is human cadavers. Nevertheless, due to ethical restrictions and limited availability this is not always possible (Statheropoulos *et al.* 2011). Therefore, organs or tissues from humans such as muscle, fat tissue, bones, liver, intestines and blood can be used in studies. Domestic pigs (*Sus scrofa domesticus* L.) are also considered to be acceptable analogues for human decomposition studies due to the similarities including comparable internal organs/anatomy and fat distribution across the torso, similar hair coverage and comparable gut fauna. Pigs are therefore widely used in studies of decomposition (Brasseur *et al.* 2012; Dekeirsschieter *et al.* 2009, 2012; Forbes and Perraut 2014; Perrault *et al.* 2014; Stadler *et al.* 2013; Statheropoulos *et al.* 2011).

3.2.1.2 Secondary Matrices

When human or animal remains are decomposing in a specific environment, secondary matrices can also be analysed. Compounds produced during the decomposition process are released and migrate into different sub-media. Depending on their physicochemical properties (molecular weight, vapour pressure, boiling point, etc.), these compounds can be found predominantly in specific secondary matrices such as air (above the corpse or the grave), soil (above and below for buried corpses or below for corpses deposited on the surface), and water (moisture or immersion) (Brasseur *et al.* 2012; Forbes and Perrault 2014).

3.2.2 Sampling Methods

Since the composition of the air (i.e. headspace) above the body seems the most relevant in finding decomposition VOC signatures, most research groups focus on the secondary matrix. To study this matrix, air-sampling methods are required. Although the odour of decomposition might be very strong, the concentration of VOCs in the air is in most cases relatively low. A concentration step is therefore required in order to be able to detect trace VOCs. Concentrated air sampling can be carried out using two distinct methods.

3.2.2.1 Headspace Solid-Phase Microextraction

In this solvent-free sample preparation technique, a fused silica fibre is immersed for a certain time in the headspace/air collected above the remains. During this time, the VOCs that are released can be adsorbed in a *passive* way on the fibre coating. The fibre coating can be made of a single or multiple adsorbents. Selecting the more suitable coating will allow different types of molecules to be adsorbed. Trapped VOCs are then thermally desorbed from the fibre into the injection port of the gas chromatograph (GC) (see below). The advantage of headspace solid-phase microextraction (HS-SPME) is that no solvent is used, allowing solvent-independent VOC transfer (no solvent peak and no solubility issues), and preventing VOC dilution. Major disadvantages are:

1) thermally unstable compounds can be degraded when the fibre is heated;
2) this method can only be used in a passive way that requires the equilibrium stage to be reached; and
3) the trapping efficiency is dependent on the fibre coating (Ramírez *et al.* 2010; Ras *et al.* 2009; Woolfenden 2010).

3.2.2.2 Sorbent Tube

Sorbent tubes can collect the VOCs in a *dynamic way*, by drawing air through the tube, or in a *passive way*, by placing the tubes in the headspace so that the VOCs are passively adsorbed onto the sorbent. Sorbent tubes can be packed with one or multiple adsorbents. The adsorbent bed will influence the trapping efficiency. The collected and concentrated VOCs on the sorbent tube must be desorbed before chromatographic analysis.

Compared to HS-SPME, sorbent tubes have a higher loading capacity due to the larger amount of sorbent present. Another advantage of using sorbent tubes is the possibility of dynamic sampling, providing a higher volume of airflow through the tube. As a consequence, a higher number and abundance of VOCs can be collected and thus the sensitivity is greater compared to passive sampling. Two desorption techniques can be used with sorbent tubes: 1) solvent extraction (SE) and 2) thermal desorption (TD).

3.2.2.2.1 Solvent Extraction The VOCs that are adsorbed on the tubes can be eluted using *organic solvents* (e.g. carbon disulphide, ether). This is a simple method where VOCs with high molecular masses or thermally unstable compounds can be collected and analysed. However, there are also several drawbacks:

1) After concentration on the tubes, there is a dilution of the VOCs in the organic solvent.
2) When the VOCs are collected passively, the sampling period is longer.
3) More polar and reactive compounds often have poor desorption efficiencies.
4) The chemical nature of compounds collected depends on the type of organic solvent used.
5) Long-term storing is highly dependent on the solvent volatility and stability (Ramírez *et al.* 2010; Ras *et al.* 2009).

3.2.2.2.2 Thermal Desorption Thermal desorption (TD) is a *solvent-free* sampling technique in which sorbent tubes are used. Desorption is carried out by heating the tube to high temperatures. In TD, another concentration step can be introduced as there is a possibility of placing a cold trap between the sorbent tubes and the GC column. Using this cold trap, a focusing effect takes place to compress signals and increase the sensitivity.

Enhanced sensitivity of TD compared to SE is introduced due to the focusing step in the cold trap. However, thermally unstable compounds and compounds with high boiling points (>300°C) are not adequately analysed using TD because of their poor desorption efficiency (Ramírez *et al.* 2010; Ras *et al.* 2009; Woolfenden 2010).

3.2.3 Analytical Methods

Decrypting the composition of the volatile mixtures released by decaying mammalian bodies represents an analytical challenge. During the decomposition, complex reactions are taking place, leading to the chemical degradation of the body's constituents (Swann *et al.* 2010). The resulting by-products require a high-resolution separation for a complete analysis. Decomposition VOC mixtures are characterised by a high variability in chemical composition and a large dynamic range (Dekeirsschieter *et al.* 2012; Stadler *et al.* 2013). Nowadays, several analytical methods are commonly used for analyses of volatile matrices.

3.2.3.1 Gas Chromatography

The most common methods of VOC analysis are based on gas chromatography (GC) techniques. Chromatographic methods separate different components of a complex mixture based on particular affinities of the compounds between a stationary phase and a mobile phase. Compounds with a higher affinity for the mobile phase will elute faster than those more strongly retained on the stationary phase. Following separation, a detector is able to detect and identify the successive compounds eluting from the chromatographic system (Dekeirsschieter *et al.* 2009; Forbes and Perrault 2014; Hoffman *et al.* 2009; Perrault *et al.* 2014; Rosier *et al.* 2014; Statheropoulos *et al.* 2005, 2007, 2011; Vass 2012; Vass *et al.* 2004, 2008).

3.2.3.2 Comprehensive Two-Dimensional Gas Chromatography

The matrix complexity of decomposition odour has led to challenges in separation using classical GC (1DGC) techniques. To overpass these limitations, a higher peak capacity is required. To increase the separation power, the use of comprehensive two-dimensional gas chromatography (GC×GC) has been proposed (Brasseur *et al.* 2012; Dekeirsschieter *et al.* 2012; Stadler *et al.* 2013). GC×GC uses two separation dimensions (two GC columns) connected together. The stationary phase of each dimension is different to offer different separation mechanisms. These columns are serially connected and a special device called a modulator is placed between the two dimensions. The modulator allows the transfer of compounds eluting from the first dimension (^{1}D) to the second dimension (^{2}D), while maintaining the separation achieved in ^{1}D. Moreover, the two stationary phases should be different to ensure a maximum separation. The chemistry of separation taking place in ^{1}D (e.g. volatility) has to be different in the ^{2}D (e.g. polarity). This requirement is called the orthogonality of the two dimensions.

The modulator of choice for decomposition headspace analysis is a liquid nitrogen-based cryogenic system that allows efficient trapping-releasing of volatile analytes. It ensures a high sampling rate and a quantitative transfer between the two dimensions. In practice, the modulator continuously samples the eluent of ^{1}D into several slices that correspond to fast repeated injections of ^{1}D material into ^{2}D for further separation. This occurs based on a specific interval called the modulation period (P_M). Each P_M corresponds to a fast secondary separation. The modulator is the heart of the GC×GC system and allows both the conservation and the orthogonality rules to be fulfilled. Based on this 'sliced chromatogram', specific software can be used to create a multidimensional plot used to visualise the entire separation (Figure 3.1). Such an image can be used and considered as the fingerprint of the VOC profile. By fine tuning of the GC phase combinations in ^{1}D and ^{2}D, compounds potentially still co-eluting after ^{1}D elution can be resolved based on different separation mechanisms in ^{2}D. When properly selected, column combinations can also generate structured chromatograms that allow chemical similarities to be used during the identification process. The enhanced separation power is additionally completed by a global sensitivity enhancement as the modulation process

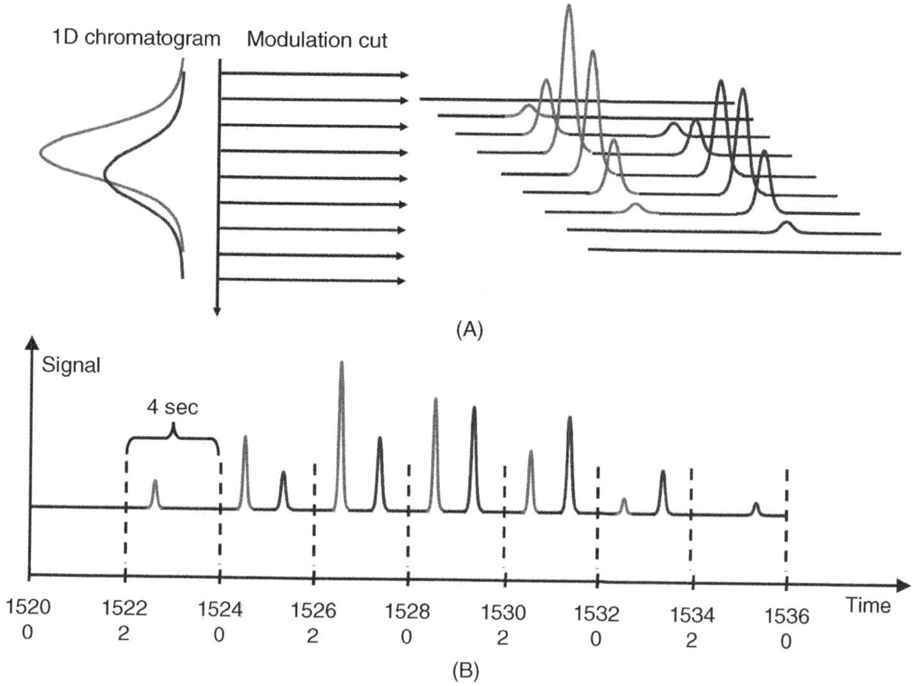

Figure 3.1 (A) In classical GC the two peaks are co-eluting. The modulator cuts this peak to generate a 2D (GC × GC) plot where the two peaks are resolved. (B) The 1D traces of a GC × GC analysis is a succession of fast GC separations that are software transformed to obtain the 2D plot.

also results in zone compression of the chromatographic signals while mass conservation is present (Patterson *et al.* 2011).

The decision of the use of either a 1DGC or a GC×GC system should be based on the application of interest. For the targeting of the main compounds produced in the decomposition headspace, the 1DGC approach provides adequate separation resolution. However, for a complete screening of the complex volatile mixture above decomposed remains, GC×GC is required.

3.2.3.3 Chromatography Detectors

For both chromatographic methods, mass spectrometry (MS) has been used to study the decomposition headspace. MS is used to ionise GC eluents and separate produced ions based on their respective masses. Resulting mass spectra are specific to each analyte by combining both fragment and parent ion information. They are compared to MS libraries for identification purposes. For classical 1DGC-MS, simple scanning quadrupole systems are commonly used as they offer good sensitivity and good dynamic range (Cablk *et al.* 2012; DeGreeff and Furton 2011; Dekeirsschieter *et al.* 2009; Forbes and Perrailt 2014; Hoffman *et al.* 2009; Perrault *et al.* 2014; Rosier *et al.* 2014; Statheropoulos *et al.* 2005, 2007, 2011; Vass 2012; Vass *et al.* 2004, 2008). For GC×GC, time-of-flight mass spectrometers (TOFMS) are typically used as they offer the fast acquisition rate required to characterise very narrow (<200 ms wide) ^{2}D peaks. Moreover, because TOFMS are non-scanning instruments, mass spectra are free from mass skewing, and signals of possibly co-eluting analytes can be deconvoluted to extract analyte-specific information and identification. Regardless of the type of MS used, electron impact (EI) ionisation sources are used to ensure appropriate production of reproducible mass spectra, representing the fingerprint of chemical compounds, which can be compared with databases (e.g. NIST and Wiley). Retention indices can also be used to improve the identification for both 1DGC and GC×GC, at least in ^{1}D.

1DGC and GC×GC methods are powerful for describing the content of a complex mixture. However, the disadvantage to these techniques is the complexity of the data set generated. For each peak detected, several identification points are available: a retention time, intensity and a mass spectral identification. This becomes more complex when GC×GC is used as a ^{2}D retention time value and a chromatographic pattern description is obtained. Despite the added value of collecting more information, the decrypting of this information requires powerful statistical tools to be used. Principal component analysis (PCA) is the most commonly used multivariate method in decomposition studies (Brasseur *et al.* 2012; Dekeirsschieter *et al.* 2009, 2012; Forbes and Perrault 2014; Perrault *et al.* 2014; Stadler *et al.* 2013). PCA allows the combination of multiple variables to obtain a usable visualisation of the information present in a massive data set. More recently, Stefanuto *et al.* (2014) developed supervised filtration approaches to improve the PCA visualisation power. The establishment of a specific decomposition biomarkers database will only happen via specific statistical method development, in order to sort out compounds of interest from the hundreds of signals that are typically recorded during such analyses. The difficulty in replicating putrefaction experiments, and the potentially large biological variability, further make data treatment an analytical challenge.

3.2.3.4 Data Treatment and Validation

When such complex data are considered, the quality of the data treatment is as important as the quality of the analytical method itself. Indeed, the ethical and logistical limitations linked to decomposition studies require a powerful tool to obtain the maximum information from a limited number of replicates. Thus, the data handling requires the application of robust statistics. Statheropoulos *et al.* (2006) were the first to use strong univariant and multivariant statistics in the decomposition field. They applied various clustering methods to compare VOC mixtures from different origins. Dekeirsschieter *et al.* (2009) used PCA to study the link between differences in decomposition stage profiles and the environment. Based on these papers, the subsequent studies in decomposition also contained strong data handling methods.

For GC×GC-TOFMS, the larger amount of data increases the need for robust data handling methods. Indeed, behind each chromatographic peak, there are two retention times, full mass spectra and intensity information. Stadler *et al.* (2013) used a strong data alignment technique to monitor the decomposition headspace of pig decomposition samples. This method was based on peak table alignment to obtain an accurate day-to-day comparison. However, dealing with large tables of data is not user-friendly and requires grouping in chemical family prior to the statistical treatment. Based on the same approach, but shifting from family profiling to individual biomarker identification, Stefanuto *et al.* (2014) developed an image analysis approach to decrypt the decomposition volatile signature. This approach gives good preliminary results but more work is needed to produce a comprehensive decomposition VOC biomarkers list. All these studies used multivariate statistic methods to reduce the data dimensionality. The data filtration process in these kinds of mathematical methods allows conversion from chemical family comparison to individual compound comparison. This represents a major step in the methods of biomarker validation (Figure 3.2) (Stefanuto *et al.* 2014).

The combination of comprehensive hyphenated methods and statistics provides a powerful tool for decomposition investigation. However, this approach still requires a validation process for the

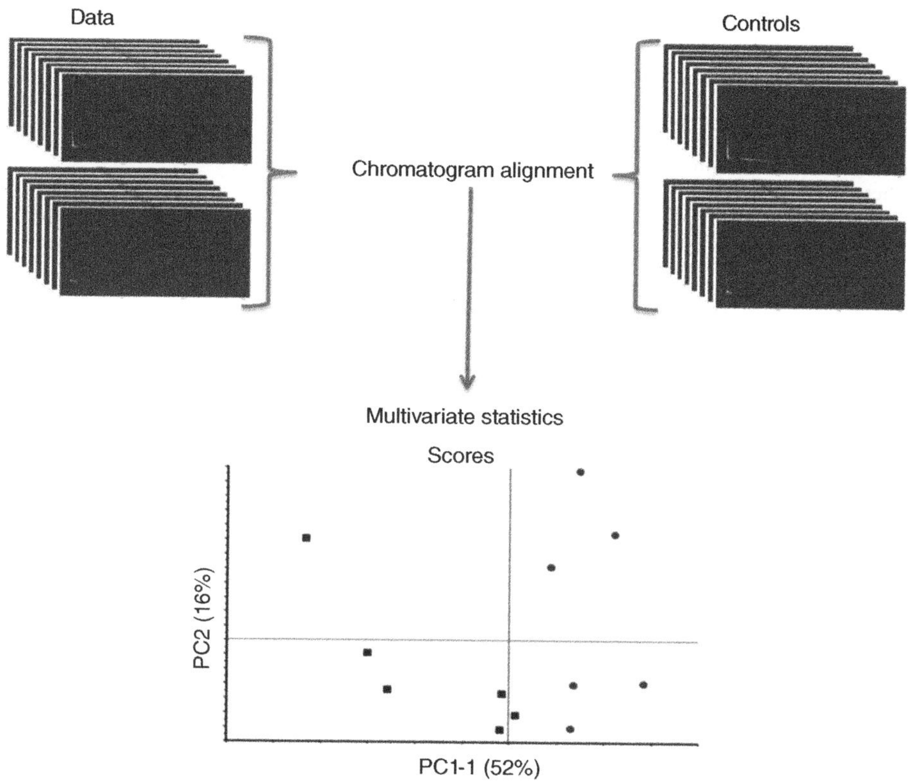

Figure 3.2 Illustration of the data processing method to analyse data from decomposition headspace compared to control samples.

chemical identification confirmation. Moreover, the quantification aspects need to be investigated and validated to obtain a full description of the decaying body headspaces. High-resolution mass spectrometry could provide such information. Accurate mass data would aid in confirming compound identities by reducing the range of possible attributions from a more accurate molecular formula. Tandem MS data could also give access to supplementary structural information to help in biomarker identification.

For all methods described, the validation process is a major step in decomposition headspace profiling. Indeed, several studies have already demonstrated the meaningful information that can be obtained from decomposition odour (DeGreeff and Furton *et al.* 2011; Stadler *et al.* 2012). However, to date there is no validated method for decomposition VOC biomarker identification that can be used to produce a list of specific compounds. The major reason for this lack of validation is directly linked to the limitation of decomposition studies. Indeed, it is almost impossible to obtain a true biological replicate. In classical biological study, this limitation is overcome by increasing the number of replicates. Nevertheless, for decomposition, access to bodies is limited for ethical and logistical reasons. Rosier *et al.* (2014) were the first group to focus on the validation of some decomposition markers and to establish a validation process. They developed a repeatable TD-GC-MS method. For the future, some effort will have to be directed towards the validation of decomposition monitoring methods.

Table 3.1 VOCs and their possible origin (Dekeirsschieter *et al.* 2012; Paczkowski and Schütz 2011; Stadler *et al.* 2013; Statheropoulos *et al.* 2011).

VOCs	Possible origin
Oxygenated compounds (acids, alcohols, ketones, aldehydes, esters and ethers)	Lipids (triglycerides) Sugars (carbohydrates)
Sulphur-containing compounds	Sulphur-containing amino acids (cysteine and methionine)
Nitrogen-containing compounds	Nucleic acids Amino acids
Aromatic compounds (phenol, indole, skatole, benzonitrile, benzaldehyde)	Amino acids (tyrosine, tryptophan, phenylalanine)

3.3 Results and Discussion

3.3.1 Identified Decomposition VOCs

Decomposition is initiated by endogenous enzymes, but during the active and the advanced stages of decay, microorganisms originating endogenously from for example the gut and mucous membrane of the respiratory system, but also from the environment, play the most important role. Lipids, proteins and carbohydrates will break down to amino acids, fatty acids and glucose (Paczkowski and Schütz 2011). An overview of VOCs and their possible origins can be found in Table 3.1. A wide variety of compounds that are released during the decomposition process have already been identified. VOCs from different chemical classes include alkanes, alkenes, aromatic and cyclic compounds, acids, esters, ketones, aldehydes, alcohols, ethers, halogen compounds, sulphur- and nitrogen-containing compounds (Brasseur *et al.* 2012; Cablk *et al.* 2012; DeGreeff and Furton 2011; Dekeirsschieter *et al.* 2009, 2012; Forbes and Perrault 2014; Hoffman *et al.* 2009; Perrault *et al.* 2014; Rosier *et al.* 2014; Stadler *et al.* 2012; Statheropoulos *et al.* 2005, 2007, 2011; Vass 2012; Vass *et al.* 2004, 2008).

The first investigation of decomposition headspace was conducted by Vass *et al.* (2004). The authors used a TD-GC-MS method to study the VOC emission from buried human bodies. The aim of this study was to create a 'decompositional odour analysis database'. This research reports hundreds of compounds that were grouped by chemical family for the data interpretation. Grouping compounds by chemical family or decomposition stage allows for the identification of the main contributors of decomposition odour. Dimethyl disulphide (DMDS) and other sulphides are typically the compounds with the highest concentration. They are produced by the degradation of amino acids (cysteine and methionine) that are the building block sulphide bridges in protein. A large number of amine and hydrocarbon compounds are also usually detected. However, these compounds do not seem to be specific to one species. They are typically detected in the headspace of animal as well as human decomposition. These compounds probably come from amino acid degradation and are the by-products of deamination and decarboxylation. The volatile fatty acids (e.g. butyric acid) and their derivatives (ester) are mainly produced via the degradation of sugars. Tracking the origin of VOCs is not straightforward. The chemicals produced from biomolecule degradation generally undergo secondary reactions (e.g. oxidation, reduction, esterification). Until now, there is no specific validated list for human decomposition VOCs. Nevertheless, almost all the articles published contain a compound list from the decomposition headspace. The aim of decomposition odour profiling is to advance the biomarkers list to improve HRD dog-training methods or to develop target detectors.

Remarkably, during all described decomposition studies, cadaverine and putrescine have never been reported. They are both produced from the decarboxylation of specific amino acids. Cadaverine is produced from lysine and putrescine from ornithine (resulting from arginine) (Statheropoulos *et al.* 2005). These two diamine compounds were previously associated with human decomposition and were assumed to be essential for HRD canines to find human remains. Hence, these two compounds were used in training formulations for dogs (Stadler *et al.* 2012; Tipple *et al.* 2014; Vass *et al.* 2004). Several hypotheses to explain the lack of cadaverine and putrescine detection have been described, including their fast metabolism by bacteria, or that they are thermally labile and therefore destroyed in GC and not detected, hence liquid chromatography is therefore more suitable to detect cadaverine and putrescine. Dekeirsschieter *et al.* (2009, 2012) detected piperidin-2-one and reported that this could be a metabolite of cadaverine. Another hypothesis is that cadaverine and putrescine are not produced in partial-pressure oxygen atmospheres (Dekeirsschieter *et al.* 2009, 2012; Statheropoulos *et al.* 2005; Vass *et al.* 2004).

3.3.2 Differences in Decomposition VOCs Between Primary Matrices

Since cadaver dogs can differentiate between odours emitted by human and animal remains, differences between species are likely (Vass *et al.* 2004). Several research groups have therefore tried to identify differences between human and animal specific markers from the headspace of the remains (Cablk *et al.* 2012; DeGreeff and Furton 2011; Rosier *et al.* 2014).

DeGreeff *et al.* (2011) used the STU-100 to collect samples and analysed the samples with SPME-GC-MS. The air was sampled above human remains in a morgue and above animal remains in a laboratory (canine, tuna, chicken, beef, hamburger, lamb and pork chops). They found many similarities between the profiles, but styrene and benzoic acid methyl ester were only detected in the human remains samples (DeGreeff and Furton 2011). However, styrene was also detected in pig remains by Statheropoulos *et al.* (2011) and Forbes and Perrault (2014).

Cablk *et al.* (2012) sampled the air above bone, fat, muscle and skin samples of cow, pig and chicken and compared their VOC profile with a study by Hoffman *et al.* (2009) who sampled the air above human remains. They found 11 'human specific' compounds (Cablk *et al.* 2012), but of these 11 compounds only 4 compounds were not detected in pig remains in other decomposition studies: (1) hexanoic acid, hexyl ester, (2) 2-octene-3-ol, (3) 2-hexenal and (4) tetrachloroethylene. Notably, these compounds were also never detected in other human sample studies.

Rosier *et al.* (2015) compared the released VOCs of 6 decomposing human and 26 decomposing animal remains in a lab-controlled environment using a validated TD-GC-MS-method. They found a combination of eight compounds that separated human and pig remains from the other animal remains using PCA-analyses: ethyl propionate, propyl propionate, propyl butyrate, ethyl pentanoate, pyridine, diethyl disulphide, methyl(methylthio)ethyl disulphide and 3-methylthio-1-propanol. Further research in the field using full bodies has to corroborate these results.

Stefanuto *et al.* (2015) analysed the VOCs emitted by human bodies and pig carcasses during the first days of decomposition. This study was conducted to demonstrate the differences between species, since pigs are commonly used as a human analogue. Different factors were compared in order to demonstrate their impacts on the decomposition process of both species. Two trials were conducted (summer and winter) on two humans and one pig. One human was protected from insect colonisation. This study was conducted in an open environment.

3.3.3 Differences in Decomposition VOCs Between Secondary Matrices

The secondary matrix will also impact the decomposition VOCs detected. In 2014, Forbes and Perrault (2014) placed domestic pig carcasses on the soil surface and compared the VOC profile obtained from the air above the pig remains with the profile obtained from the soil below the remains. In order to accumulate the VOCs in the headspace, they placed a stainless steel hood over the carcasses prior to sampling. To facilitate the sampling in soil, they used VOC-Mole™ Soil Probes. Both samples were analysed with TD-GC-MS. When they compared the results they found 207 compounds in soil compared to 100 compounds in air samples. Only 23% of all described VOCs were found in both air and soil. This demonstrates that sampling in soil and air are complementary techniques. An explanation for the increased number in soil samples could be:

1) the microorganisms in the soil, hence more VOCs can be produced and detected;
2) adsorption of VOCs on soil particle causing a longer retention; and
3) rapid dispersion of VOCs in air due to wind and evaporation.

They also noted that the majority of the compounds identified in the air samples were detected during bloat, active decay, advanced decay stages and skeletonisation, while in soil samples the majority of VOCs were detected starting from the active decay stage. Since the liquefaction of the soft tissue starts during active decay, and there is a release and leaching of the compounds into the surrounding soil, this could explain why VOCs were not detected earlier. When VOC profiles of the air and the soil samples were compared, a comparable profile was reported (Forbes and Perrault 2014).

The majority of other published decomposition studies focused on air samples only. In the studies where soil samples were collected, VOCs were dominated by ketones, alcohols and esters. This was comparable with the results of the Forbes and Perrault (2014) study, where the soil samples mainly consisted of aromatics, esters, ketones, alcohols and hydrocarbons. In air samples, Forbes and Perrault (2014) found mainly sulphides, nitrogen-containing compounds, aromatics and alcohols. In other studies, air samples were dominated by sulphur and nitrogen-containing compounds, ketones, alcohols, acids and aromatics. Acids were mainly found in air samples, also described by Forbes and Perrault (2014). The corresponding esters were also detected in soil (Forbes and Perrault 2014), but this result was not reported in other decomposition studies.

3.3.4 Differences in Decomposition VOCs Based on Sampling Methods

TD is the most commonly used method for sampling VOCs from various decomposition matrices. However, other sampling techniques are available for VOC profiling, for example HS-SPME and SE. Based on non-forensic VOC studies, it may be presumed that TD is the most suitable method for sample collection and introduction into the GC (Agelopoulos and Pickett 1998; Brokl *et al.* 2013). Indeed, the HS-SPME technique is a static equilibrium procedure. The time required to reach this equilibrium state is different for every compound based on their physicochemical properties.

In 2014, Perrault *et al.* compared the efficiency of TD and HS-SPME to monitor the VOCs in soil beneath decomposing pig remains. They illustrated the differences between TD and HS-SPME sampling for decomposition matrices. Depending on the chemical property of the compound, differences in trapping efficiency were reported between different methods. All polar compounds (sulphur, nitrogen) were more efficiently trapped on the sorbent tubes, while carbonyl compounds (aldehydes, ketones, carboxylic acids) were more efficiently trapped using HS-SPME. The authors also demonstrated that the VOC profile obtained by TD is more discriminatory for the analysis of the decomposition process. HS-SPME appears to be more suitable when specific target compounds are monitored. In the latter case, a good choice of the fibre coating is required in order to obtain good results.

The SE approach has not been widely used for decomposition studies. Indeed, several disadvantages are linked to SE application (see Section 3.2.2 above). However, this method was applied with GC×GC-TOFMS producing interesting results (Brasseur *et al.* 2012; Dekeirsschieter *et al.* 2009, 2012). Dekeirsschieter *et al.* (2009, 2012) demonstrated the time evolution in the headspace above pig remains. The consistency of these results was confirmed by Stadler *et al.* (2013), who also studied pig carcasses on the soil surface using TD-GC×GC-TOFMS. In both studies, the same main chemical families were detected: alcohols, carboxylic acids, aromatics, and sulphides and along with ketones and aldehydes, were the major contributors to the overall VOC profile. Moreover, the main compounds of each family were the same. Although these two studies were conducted in different geographical areas (i.e. Belgium and Canada) with different meteorological parameters, the general profile was consistent.

3.3.5 Differences in Decomposition VOCs Based on Analytical Methods

Most research groups studying decomposition have used GC-MS methods. It was only very recently that GC×GC-TOFMS was implemented into the study of decomposition VOCs (Dekeirsschieter *et al.* 2012). An overview of research groups and their developed methods can be found in the supplementary information.

Dekeirsschieter *et al.* (2012) conducted the first study using GC×GC that monitored the headspace of pig remains in 2012. The authors applied the same data treatment previously used with classical 1DGC, but demonstrated an enhancement for the number of compounds detected due to the separation capacity and the deconvolution of the TOFMS. This research presented the main compounds detected through the first 40 days of decomposition. Around 830 compounds were detected. This number represented a vast increase from the first database previously reported (Vass *et al.* 2004). Studying the occurrence of these compounds, the 1H-indole, DMDS, dimethyl trisulphide (DMTS) and other well-known compounds of the decomposition signature were identified as the most detected compounds. The time evolution of the number of compounds also displayed the parallel that can be drawn between the decomposition activities and the number of VOCs detected in the corpse headspace. Moreover, the evolution of the occurrence of different chemical classes in the headspace was monitored and appeared to be dependent on the decomposition stage. For example, the carbonyl families (aldehydes, carboxylic acid) were the major compounds detected during active decay. Stadler *et al.* (2013) confirmed this time evolution during another study on pig carcasses.

3.3.6 Factors that Influence the Detection of Decomposition VOCs

Differences in detected compounds can be explained by the use of different soil (sample) types. Indeed, differences in physical, chemical and microbial properties of the soil can influence the speed and/or type of compounds formed and released. When the soil is dry, water will compete with the VOCs on the soil surface, but when the soil is wet, water can act as a solvent for VOCs. Temperature can also influence the detection of VOCs, the number of detected compounds can increase and different types can be identified when other microorganisms are involved in the decomposition process (Forbes and Perrault 2014). Therefore, the comparison of results obtained from decomposition profiling studies represents a challenging task. Indeed, each group applies its own analytical approach limiting the comparison possibilities.

3.4 Conclusion and Future Research

The study of 'the smell of death' has increased considerably since robust analytical methods appeared in the field, for the results to date have assisted in better understanding of canine olfaction processes and entomological colonisation. Although several research groups are exploring this field and hundreds of compounds have already been described, it remains challenging to compare these studies in order to find 'specific human markers'. This is because different matrices are typically studied, different analysis techniques are often used and even different data analysis tools are introduced.

Fortunately, increasing attention is being given to the validation of methods and data analysis. This standardisation of methods will certainly lead to a better comparison of analysis results and ultimately an increased understanding of animal and human decomposition odour.

References

Agelopoulos, N.G. and Pickett, J.A. (1998) Headspace analysis in chemical ecology: effects of sampling methods on ratios of volatile compounds present in headspace samples. *Journal of Chemical Ecology*, **24**: 1–12.

Amendt, J., Campobasso, C.P., Gaudry, E., Reiter, C., LeBlanc, H.N. and Hall, M.J. (2006) Best practice in forensic entomology – standards and guidelines. *International Journal of Legal Medicine*, **121**: 90–104.

Amendt, J., Richards, C.S., Campobasso, C.P., Zehner, R. and Hall, M.J.R. (2011) Forensic entomology: applications and limitations. *Forensic Science, Medicine, and Pathology*, **7**: 379–392.

Brasseur, C., Dekeirsschieter, J., Schotsmans, E.M.J., de Koning, S., Wilson, A.S. *et al.* (2012) Comprehensive two-dimensional gas chromatography-time-of-flight mass spectrometry for the forensic study of cadaveric volatile organic compounds released in soil by buried decaying pig carcasses. *Journal of Chromatography A*, **1255**: 163–170.

Brokl, M., Bishop, L., Wright, C.G., Liu, C., McAdam, K. and Focant, J.-F. (2013) Analysis of mainstream tobacco smoke particulate phase using comprehensive two-dimensional gas chromatography-time-of-flight mass spectrometry. *Journal of Separation Science*, **36**: 1037–1044.

Cablk, M.E., Szelagowski, E.E. and Sagebiel, J.C. (2012) Characterization of the volatile organic compounds present in the headspace of decomposing animal remains, and compared with human remains. *Forensic Science International*, **220**: 118–125.

DeGreeff, L.E. and Furton, K.G. (2011) Collection and identification of human remains volatiles by non-contact, dynamic airflow sampling and SPME-GC/MS using various sorbent matrials. *Analytical and Bioanalytical Chemistry*, **401**: 1295–1307.

DeGreeff, L.E., Weakley-Jones, B. and Furton, K.G. (2011) Creation of training aids for human remains detection canines utilizing a non-contact, dynamic airflow volatile concentration technique. *Forensic Science International*, **209**: 133–142.

Dekeirsschieter, J., Verheggen, F.J., Gohy, M., Hubrecht, F., Bourguignon, L. *et al.* (2009) Cadaveric volatile organic compounds released by decaying pig carcasses (*Sus domesticus* L.) in different biotopes *Forensic Science International*, **189**: 46–53.

Dekeirsschieter, J., Stefanuto, P.-H., Brasseur, C., Haubruge, E. and Focant, J.-F. (2012) Enhanced characterization of the smell of death by Comprehensive Two-Dimensional Gas Chromatography-Time-of-Flight Mass Spectrometry (GCxGC-TOFMS). *PLoS ONE*, **7**: e39005.

Farinha, A., Dourado, C.G., Centeio, N., Oliveira, A.R., Dias, D. and Rebelo, M.T. (2014) Small bait traps as accurate predictors of dipteran early colonizers in forensic studies. *Journal of Insect Science*, **14**: 1–16.

Forbes, S.L. and Perrault, K.A. (2014) Decomposition odour profiling in the air and soil surrounding vertebrate carrion. *PLoS ONE*, **9**: e95107.

Hoffman, E., Curran, A. and Dulgerian, N. (2009) Characterization of the volatile organic compounds present in the headspace of decomposing human remains. *Forensic Science*, **186**: 6–13.

Paczkowski, S. and Schütz, S. (2011) Post-mortem volatiles of vertebrate tissue. *Applied Microbiology and Biotechnology*, **91**: 917–935.

Patterson, D.G. Jr., Welch, S.M., Turner, W.E., Sjödin, A. and Focant, J.-F. (2011) Cryogenic zone compression for the measurement of dioxins in human serum by isotope dilution at the attogram level using modulated gas chromatography coupled to high resolution magnetic sector mass spectrometry. *Journal of Chromatography A*, **1218**: 3274–3281.

Perrault, K., Stuart, B. and Forbes, S. (2014) A longitudinal study of decomposition odour in soil using sorbent tubes and solid phase micro-extraction. *Chromatography*, **1**: 120–140.

Ramírez, N., Cuadras, A., Rovira, E., Borrull, F. and Marcé, R.M. (2010) Comparative study of solvent extraction and thermal desorption methods for determining a wide range of volatile organic compounds in ambient air. *Talanta*, **82**: 719–727.

Ras, M.R., Borrull, F. and Marcé, R.M. (2009) Sampling and pre-concentration techniques for determination of volatile organic compounds in air samples. *Trends in Analytical Chemistry*, **28**: 347–361.

Rosier, E., Cuypers, E., Dekens, M., Verplaetse, R., Develter, W. *et al.* (2014) Development and validation of a new TD-GC/MS method and its applicability in the search for human and animal decomposition products. *Analytical and Bioanalytical Chemistry*, **406**: 3611–3619.

Rosier, E., Loix, S., Develter, W., Van de Voorde, W., Tytgat, J. and Cuypers, E. (2015) The search for a volatile human specific marker in the decomposition process. *PLoS ONE*, **10**: e0137341

Stadler, S., Stefanuto, P.-H., Byer, J.D., Brokl, M., Forbes, S. and Focant, J.-F. (2012) Analysis of synthetic canine training aids by comprehensive two-dimensional gas chromatography-time of flight mass spectrometry. *Journal of Chromatography A*, **1255**: 202–206.

Stadler, S., Stefanuto, P.-H., Brokl, M., Forbes, S.L. and Focant, J.-F. (2013) Characterization of Volatile Organic Compounds from human analogue decomposition using thermal desorption coupled to comprehensive two-dimensional Gas Chromatography-Time-of-Flight Mass Spectrometry. *Analytical Chemistry*, **85**: 998–1005.

Statheropoulos, M., Spiliopoulou, C. and Agapiou, A. (2005) A study of volatile organic compounds evolved from the decaying human body. *Forensic Science International*, **153**: 147–155.

Statheropoulos, M., Mikedi, K., Agapiou, A., Georgiadou, A. and Karma, S. (2006) Discriminant Analysis of Volatile Organic Compounds data related to a new location method of entrapped people in collapsed buildings of an earthquake. *Analytica Chimica Acta*, **566**: 207–216.

Statheropoulos, M., Agapiou, A., Spiliopoulou, C., Pallis, G.C. and Sianos, E. (2007) Environmental aspects of VOCs evolved in the early stages of human decomposition. *The Science of the Total Environment*, **385**: 221–227.

Statheropoulos, M., Agapiou, A., Zorba, E., Mikedi, K., Karma, S, *et al.* (2011) Combined chemical and optical methods for monitoring the early decay stages of surrogate human models. *Forensic Science International*, **210**: 154–163.

Stefanuto, P.-H., Perrault, K., Stadler, S., Pesesse, R., Brokl, M. *et al.* (2014) Reading cadaveric decomposition chemistry with a new pair of glasses. *ChemPlusChem*, **79**: 786–789.

Stefanuto, P.-H., Perrault, K., Stadler, S., Pesesse, R., LeBlanc, H. *et al.* (2015) GC × GC – TOFMS and supervised multivariate approaches to study human cadaveric decomposition olfactive signatures. *Analytical Bioanalytical Chemistry*, **407**: 4767–4778.

Swann, L.M., Forbes, S.L. and Lewis, S.W. (2010) Analytical separations of mammalian decomposition products for forensic science: a review. *Analytica Chimica Acta*, **682**: 9–22.

Tipple, C.A., Caldwell, P.T., Kile, B.M., Beussman, D.J., Rushing, B. *et al.* (2014) Comprehensive characterization of commercially available canine training aids. *Forensic Science International*, **242**: 242–254.

Vass, A.A. (2012) Odor mortis. *Forensic Science International*, **222**: 234–241.
Vass, A.A., Smith, R.R., Thompson, C.V., Burnett, M.N., Wolf, D.A. *et al.* (2004) Decompositional odor analysis database. *Journal of Forensic Science,* **49**: 760–769.
Vass, A.A., Smith, R.R., Thompson, C.V., Burnett, M.N., Dulgerian, N. and Eckenrode, B.A. (2008) Odor analysis of decomposing buried human remains. *Journal of Forensic Science,* **53**: 384–391.
Woolfenden, E. (2010) Sorbent-based sampling methods for volatile and semi-volatile organic compounds in air. Part 1: Sorbent-based air monitoring options. *Journal of Chromatography A*, **1217**: 2674–2684.

4

Blood Degradation and Bloodstain Age Estimation

Gerda J. Edelman and Maurice C.G. Aalders

4.1 Introduction: Forensic relevance of bloodstains

Blood, the major biological fluid of the human body, is one of the most common traces encountered at a crime scene. Bloodstains can be of great value in forensic investigations, as they provide information at the source level, useful for the identification of the donor, and at the activity level, to enable the reconstruction of events at the crime scene (Cook *et al.* 1998). Historically, blood typing was used to gain information about the bloodstain donor, a classification technique limited by the low variation of blood groups. Following the advances in forensic genetics, DNA analysis nowadays enables the identification of victims, perpetrators or witnesses with high accuracy and reliability. Current developments in 'DNA intelligence' are expected to help police investigations concentrate towards finding unknown individuals, by predicting the donor's physical characteristics, such as eye and hair colour, skin pigmentation, bio-ancestry and facial features (Walsh *et al.* 2011).

Apart from source level information, bloodstain pattern analysis (BPA) may also provide information on the activity level. The analysis of the size, shape and distribution of bloodstains enables forensic investigators to reconstruct a crime, to verify statements, or to identify bloodstains which are likely to be donated by an offender (Peschel *et al.* 2008). By calculating the area of origin of a bloodstain pattern, information can be provided about the position of the victim (e.g. standing, sitting, lying) at the moment of the bloodshed. Sometimes the sequence of events can also be determined using BPA, for example a bloodied shoeprint overlaid by an impact pattern indicates that the impact happened after the shoeprint was created (Laber *et al.* 2014). Likewise, altered bloodstain patterns, for example a bloodstain wiped prior to drying, provides evidence of movement after creation of the stain. This information can be used to generate a relative timeline of events.

To gain even more information, several techniques have been explored for the age estimation of bloodstains. Knowledge of the absolute time of bleeding can be highly relevant in forensic investigations. The age of bloodstains of a victim may give an indication of the moment the person was injured. When bloodstains of a suspect are found, estimation of the age can indicate their presence at the scene in a certain timeframe. Some bloodstains may not be related to the crime, but may be caused during an earlier or later incident. This is relevant information that crime scene investigators can use in their selection of traces for further analysis.

Driven by the forensic relevance, scientists have explored techniques to determine the age of bloodstains for more than a century. An overview of these techniques, mainly developed and tested under laboratory conditions, is given below. During the last decade the main focus was on optical, non-destructive techniques. Current developments in optical methods are described in

Taphonomy of Human Remains: Forensic Analysis of the Dead and the Depositional Environment, First Edition.
Edited by Eline M.J. Schotsmans, Nicholas Márquez-Grant and Shari L. Forbes.

more detail, after which a case example is given. To conclude, expected future developments and recommendations for future work are described.

4.2 Blood Degradation

Various techniques have been proposed for measuring the process of blood degradation, with the ultimate goal being to develop a method for age determination of blood (Bremmer *et al.* 2012b). Such a method must be based on a changing property with predictable kinetics, preferably with low inter-donor variability, and with known influences of environmental factors such as temperature and humidity. The degradation of blood causes chemical, morphological and mechanical changes of the blood cells, all potential predictive processes, which have been under investigation for designing a method for age determination of blood.

4.2.1 Chemical Changes

The most obvious chemical change is the conversion of haemoglobin into various haemoglobin derivatives. Because haemoglobin is the main chromophore (pigment) of blood, causing its red colour, this process is visible to the human eye. Optical techniques have been explored for more than a century, as described in the next section. Other techniques for monitoring the degradation of haemoglobin are summarised below. The degradation of plasma proteins and hormones can also be used to determine the time interval since deposition. Techniques described in the literature cover a broad range of analytical chemistry techniques, such as Electron Paramagnetic Resonance (EPR), High Performance Liquid Chromatography (HPLC), oxygen electrodes and many other analytical chemistry techniques.

4.2.1.1 Oxidation and Breakdown of Haemoglobin Derivatives

Fujita *et al.* (2005) published on the use of EPR for estimating the age of human bloodstains, based on the hypothesis that the spin rate of the iron in the haemoglobin molecule will change over time. By plotting double logarithms of the EPR intensity ratio of ferric low spin and ferric non-haem versus the time after bleeding, a linear correlation of up to 432 days, with an error range within 25% of the actual number of days, was found. These results were obtained under controlled conditions. The researchers stated that environmental factors such as differences of light exposure and fluctuations of storage temperature did have an influence on the changes of the EPR-active compounds. However, these factors were not further investigated.

In 1997, Andrasko investigated the feasibility of using HPLC for estimating the age of bloodstains deposited on clothing. Degradation products of haemoglobin were studied quantitatively, and found suitable for age estimation of the stains. By relating peak areas of these products to each other, ages of bloodstains could be estimated. Moreover, the ratio between the different peaks formed by ageing was practically independent of temperatures between 0°C and 37°C.

Matsuoka *et al.* (1995) studied the temporal ratio of oxyhaemoglobin versus total haemoglobin (fractional oxyhaemoglobin) in the bloodstain using oxygen electrodes and conventional colorimetry. The decay of HbO_2 was attributed to the conversion to methaemoglobin, at several temperatures. The results of the measurements were used to build a data table relating the fractional oxyhaemoglobin and the ambient temperature to the time of deposition.

4.2.1.2 Changes in Plasma Proteins

Guo *et al.* (2012) published an animal study by investigating the fluorescence lifetime of blood for bloodstain ageing. Fluorescence lifetime is an intrinsic property of the fluorophore and refers to the average time the molecule can exist in the excited state prior to emitting a photon. The method uses the structural changes of the tryptophan-containing proteins, such as albumin and γ-globulin, which constitute more than 95% of the protein mass in blood. The authors showed a steady decrease of the lifetime of up to 400 hours and speculated that in addition to the proposed change in protein conformation, the release of a variety of organic and inorganic quenchers, such as free amines or unbound Fe ions, might also contribute to the change of fluorescence lifetime. A disadvantage of the technique is that it is destructive, as the blood has to be dissolved in a phosphate buffered saline.

The use of the aspartic acid racemisation (AAR) rate for the age estimation of bloodstains was also studied (Arany and Ohtani 2011). AAR is a common method for age determination in chronological age in tooth, bone, cartilage and elastin. The method is based on the estimation of the AAR. In a preliminary report, the authors showed that the time lapse after the creation of a bloodstain could be determined *ex vivo* by measuring the extent of aspartic acid racemisation although, as noted by the authors, further stepwise refinement and corrections regarding post-mortem conditions were clearly required.

Odriozola *et al.* (2014) showed proof-of-concept, using microRNA (miRNA) markers for time of death determination. The markers – miRNA-142-5p and miRNA-541 – were reported to show considerable expression differences in vitreous humour between individuals who died during the day or at night. Lech *et al.* (2014) also investigated whether these miRNA markers showed the same diurnal expression pattern in blood, which would make them useful for estimating bloodstain deposition time to allow molecular alibi testing for forensic casework (Lech *et al.* 2014). However, they concluded that the two miRNA markers previously suggested for time of death determination in vitreous humour were not suitable for estimating the deposition time of forensic bloodstains. No statistically significant expression differences between blood samples collected during day time and night time were found, nor was a statistically significant rhythmicity found during the 24-hour day/night period.

4.3 Mechanical and Morphological Changes

In 2007, Strasser *et al.* proposed the use of atomic force spectroscopy, a high-resolution technique, to measure the elasticity changes of the erythrocytes in a blood sample on a nanometre scale. The analytical procedure was applied to an ageing blood spot on a glass slide and the elasticity pattern was shown to decrease over time, an effect that was most probably influenced by the alteration of the blood spot during the drying and coagulation process. The presented preliminary data demonstrated the capacity of this method to be used for the development of calibration curves, which could be subsequently used for estimation of bloodstain age during forensic investigations. In 2012, this method was applied to study the elasticity of red blood cells, which had been preserved in the Iceman tissue samples for more than 5,000 years (Janko *et al.* 2012). Young's modulus, the measure of elasticity, was significantly lower in the ancient red blood cells compared to Young's modulus for the recent red blood cells.

4.4 Optical Methods

Haemoglobin accounts for approximately 97% of dry blood content and is the main chromophore in blood; the red appearance of blood is due to the absorption properties of oxygenated haemoglobin. After blood leaves the body's circulation, it changes colour from bright red to dark brown. The human observation of this colour change motivated researchers to find a chemical explanation and to find a quantitative way to measure the colour and use it for age estimations.

4.4.1 Chemical Explanation

In 1903, Leers was the first to study the chemical reactions underlying the colour change of blood stains, and attributed it to the oxidation of the iron atoms present in the haemoglobin molecules, resulting in a transition of oxyhaemoglobin (HbO_2) to methaemoglobin (MetHb) (Leers 1910). This is a well-known reaction, which also takes place within the human body. HbO_2 is a haemoglobin derivative saturated with oxygen, which can be released to form deoxyhaemoglobin (Hb). This cycle is responsible for the oxygen transport from the lungs to the rest of the body. MetHb is incapable of binding oxygen and is therefore useless in the human body, and will be reduced back to Hb by the reductase protein cytochrome b5. Outside the body, haemoglobin in bloodstains will completely saturate to HbO_2 when exposed to the air, with part of it oxidising to MetHb. Once oxidised however, MetHb molecules will not be reduced back to Hb by proteins. Instead, the molecules lose their original structure and will denature in time to form haemichrome (HC). Although no consensus can be derived from the literature, this is the most probable mechanism occurring in an ageing bloodstain. Thus, a combination of HbO_2, MetHb and HC is expected to be present within each bloodstain (Bremmer *et al.* 2011).

4.4.2 Spectral Changes

All haemoglobin derivatives present in a bloodstain have specific absorption properties. The visible absorption spectrum of HbO_2 shows peaks at 540 and 576 nm, MetHb has an absorption peak at 630 nm and HC shows less pronounced peaks (Figure 4.1a). Reflectance spectra of bloodstains show the inverse of these characteristics. Figure 4.1b clearly shows two dips in the reflectance spectrum of a fresh bloodstain, which reduce over time. Contrary to this, the dip caused by the presence of MetHb becomes more prominent while ageing.

Several approaches have been proposed to relate the spectral changes to the age of the bloodstain. In 1972, Kind *et al.* calculated the ratio of the reflectance at 540 and 576 nm – the location of the HbO_2 absorption peaks – and found a time dependence, which enabled age estimation; the ratio decreased on timescales from 1 hour to 8 years (Bremmer *et al.* 2012a). More recently, Li *et al.* (2011) proposed the use of spectral measurements of a broad spectral region (442–585 nm) combined with

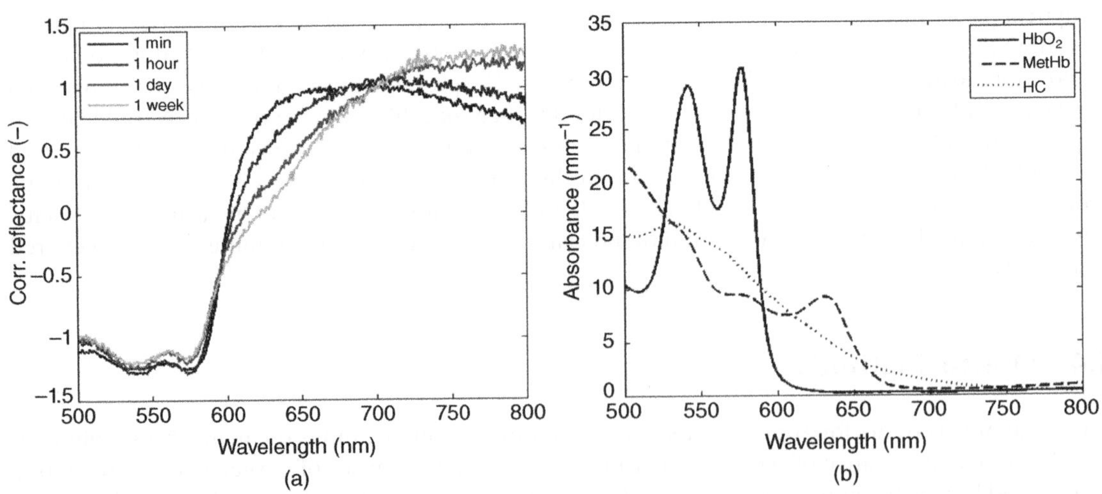

Figure 4.1 Reflectance spectra of bloodstains of different ages, and absorption spectra of the haemoglobin derivatives oxyhaemoglobin (HbO_2), methaemoglobin (MetHb) and haemichrome (HC).

Linear Discriminant Analysis (LDA). LDA is a multivariate statistical classification technique used to visualise trends in data sets. Using this method, the age of unknown bloodstains is predicted, using a statistical model based on a training set with spectra of bloodstains of known ages. Another approach, proposed by Bremmer *et al.* (2011), made use of a physical light transport model to calculate the relative contribution of HbO_2, MetHb and HC to the measured reflectance spectrum. They demonstrated that the amount of HbO_2 decreases with time, while the amount of HC increases with time, and the amount of MetHb starts with an increase followed by a decrease.

Apart from the visible wavelength range, reflectance spectra measured in the ultraviolet wavelength range also show typical characteristics changing over time. Hanson *et al.* (2011) described a change in the absorption band at 414 nm, the so-called Soret band (Hanson and Ballantyne 2010). The maximal absorption shifts to a shorter wavelength, and this blue-shift correlates with the age of the bloodstain. On the other side of the spectrum, the near infrared (NIR) region also provides functional information dependent on the molecules present in a bloodstain. Edelman *et al.* (2012a,b) demonstrated spectral features in the NIR range, which could be used for age estimation of bloodstains (Figure 4.2). A complicating factor in this wavelength range however, is the contribution of other constituents present in blood. Spectral characteristics not only originate from haemoglobin molecules, but other constituents, for example albumin, globulin and water also contribute to the spectra.

4.4.3 Equipment

The first efforts to address the challenge of bloodstain age estimation date back to the early 1900s. In 1907, Tomellini described the colour changes of a bloodstain up to one year after deposition,

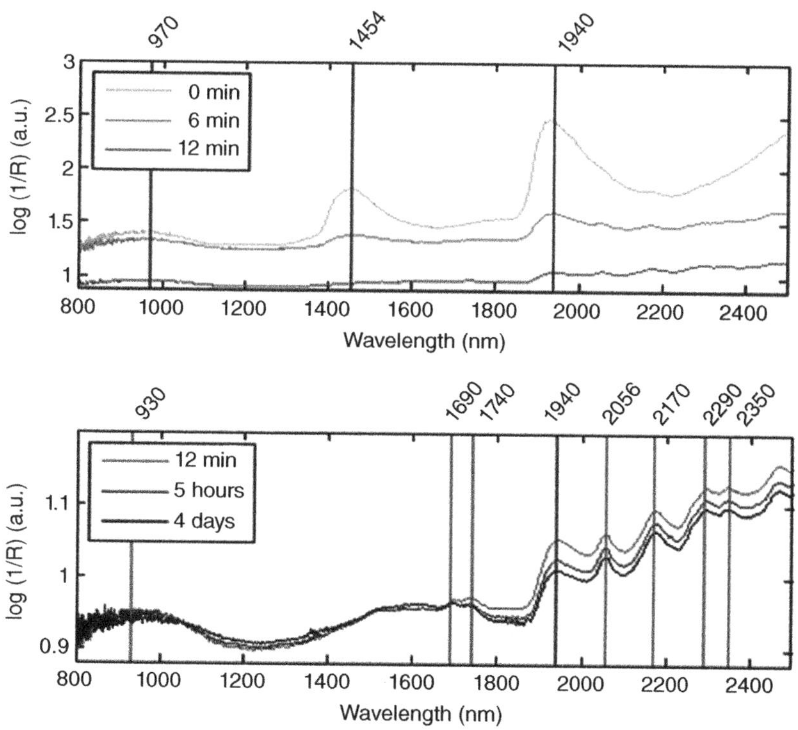

Figure 4.2 Near infrared absorbance spectra of bloodstains of different ages (Source : Edelman 2012. Reproduced with permission of Elsevier.).

and developed a chart illustrating that changes in the colour of blood correlated with the age (Bremmer *et al.* 2012a, 2012b). A drawback of this method was the objectivity of the visual observations, and the dependence on human visual performance. In 1960, Patterson *et al.* used a colorimeter to measure the reflectance of bloodstains quantitatively (Bremmer *et al.* 2012a, 2012b). Currently, an established method for colour measurements is reflectance spectroscopy, which uses a white light source and a spectrometer, both guided to the sample by an optical fibre probe. When measuring bloodstains however, a drawback of this equipment is that measurements have to be performed from a short distance, which makes some bloodstains difficult to reach, and may increase the risk of contamination. The procedure is also labour-intensive, because only one bloodstain can be measured at a time. The development of spectral imaging systems solves these problems. Spectral imaging combines spectroscopy with digital imaging and can be performed from a distance. A spectral camera records reflectance spectra of millions of pixels in an image at the same time, which makes this method very time-efficient. Additionally, images for each specific wavelength can be extracted from the dataset, showing the measured bloodstain within the original context.

Recently, it was shown that spectral imaging enables the age estimation of bloodstains under controlled circumstances (Edelman *et al.* 2012b; Janchaysang *et al.* 2012; Li *et al.* 2013). When moving a laboratory technique to the crime scene, the measurement set-up is typically less controlled, for example the distance from different samples to the detector may vary. Edelman *et al.* (2012a) were able to correct for spectral differences, which were due to physical variability, such as illumination intensity differences rather than chemical variability, and demonstrated that spectral imaging can be used for the age estimation of bloodstains at a simulated crime scene (Edelman *et al.* 2012b). They scanned the entire scene and were able to distinguish bloodstain groups of different ages, by extracting the relative amount of haemoglobin derivatives from the spectra.

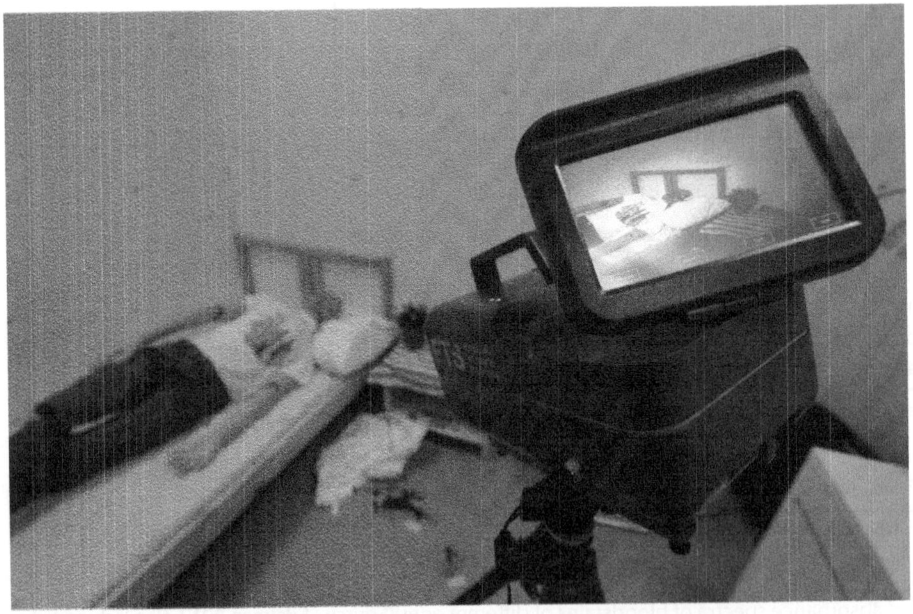

Figure 4.3 Forensic spectral camera at a simulated crime scene.

Apart from data analysis, equipment used by investigators at the crime scene has different requirements, for example ideally it is portable, wireless, waterproof, easily decontaminated and user-friendly. Recent technological advances enabled the development of fast, wireless, high resolution spectral imaging systems, facilitating the transfer from the laboratory to the crime scene. The development of portable equipment enables the analysis of an unknown stain at the crime scene without waiting for results from the laboratory (Figure 4.3).

Due to current developments, spectral imaging systems become smaller, more sensitive, user-friendly and cost-effective (Edelman *et al.* 2012a). A next generation of snapshot systems is expected in the near future, which would filter specific wavelengths simultaneously. Another technology expected in the future is the use of adapted smart phones with additional filters, which can be used for the analysis of bloodstains at the crime scene. Thanakiatkrai *et al.* (2013) recently proposed to use smart phone cameras for the age estimation of bloodstains. Using an optimally controlled light box, they successfully classified bloodstains in broad age intervals. However, the described technique is expected to be highly sensitive to minimal changes in this set-up, such as the camera used, the background colour, the intensity of the light source, or the distance to the bloodstain. Nevertheless, it is worthwhile to explore these new technologies for forensic analysis.

4.5 Practical Implementation

4.5.1 Hypothetical Case Description

To demonstrate the possible benefits of estimating the age of bloodstains in forensic casework, a crime scene was simulated. At the hypothetical scene of a presumed homicide, Mr Jenkins was found dead in the bedroom (Figure 4.3). The time of death was unknown. In the bedroom, multiple bloodstain patterns could be observed. DNA analysis of selected samples indicated that the bloodstains were a match to Mr Jenkins. In the bathroom, a handkerchief was found stained with blood from his wife, who was also living in the residence. When interrogated by a police officer, Mrs Jenkins stated that she had cut her finger two days earlier, which could explain her bloodstains at the scene. To verify this scenario, the age of the bloodstains was estimated.

4.5.2 Method

All bloodstains were scanned using a wireless hyperspectral imaging system (Figure 4.3) and a halogen white light source. The hyperspectral camera recorded the reflected light of all wavelengths between 400 and 1,000 nm separately, using a line spectrograph. By moving the lens systematically, the room was scanned, reflectance spectra were depicted on a chip and were automatically recorded on an internal hard disk.

Reflectance spectra of all pixels were normalised and compared to the theoretical spectra of oxyhaemoglobin, methaemoglobin and haemichrome, to see whether the spectra correlated with blood (Bremmer *et al.* 2011). For pixels with a high correlation, the relative contributions of these molecules to the overall spectrum was calculated (Edelman *et al.* 2012b). Comparison with a reference data set of bloodstains up to 2 years old then revealed the estimated age of the bloodstains.

4.5.3 Results

Figure 4.4 shows the results for the bloodstains found on the cloth in the bathroom. First, a colour image was created from the hyperspectral image (Figure 4.4a) showing the visual appearance of the

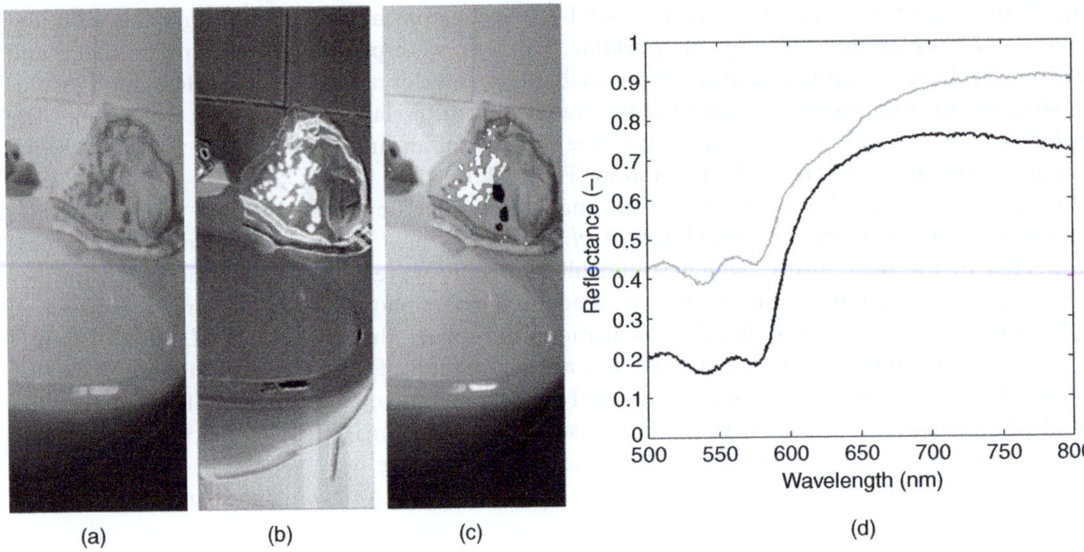

Figure 4.4 (a) Grey scale image created from the hyperspectral image of the blood on the handkerchief. (b) Image showing pixels highly correlating with blood based on the reflectance spectra in white, low correlations are shown in black. (c) Grey scale image of the scene overlaid with white (Mrs Jenkins' blood) and black (unknown source) pixels showing bloodstains of different ages. (d) Reflectance spectra of the selected bloodstains.

stains. Next, pixels showing bloodstains were identified using the correlation with theoretical blood spectra (Figure 4.4b). Finally, the ages were calculated for pixels identified as blood, based on the reflectance spectra (Figures 4.4c, d).

The results of the age estimation task indicated that the bloodstains donated by Mrs Jenkins were created approximately two days earlier. Between Mrs Jenkins' bloodstains however, three stains could be observed to be much fresher and were indicated to be created eight hours before the moment Mr Jenkins was bleeding too (Figure 4.4). Additional DNA analysis of these stains may lead to a suspect.

4.5.4 Discussion

This hypothetical case demonstrates the possible value of age estimations of bloodstains in forensic casework. Knowledge of the time of bleeding can primarily help to reconstruct the timeline of events. When bloodstains of a victim are analysed, a maximum post-mortem time interval can be determined. Furthermore, knowledge of the time of events can help by verifying statements and possible scenarios. Being able to distinguish bloodstains with different ages also helps investigators in their selection of stains for DNA analysis. When searching for bloodstains donated by a suspect amongst blood from the victim, bloodstain pattern experts normally analyse which stains differ from the patterns. Bloodstain age estimation can be an extra aid to finding deviant bloodstains based on age differences, as illustrated by the example.

4.6 Crime Scene Challenges of Bloodstain Age Estimation

For more than a century, much research has been devoted to the development of techniques for age estimation of bloodstains, because the results would be highly relevant in forensic casework.

However, to our knowledge, none of the techniques have yet been implemented in standard forensic practice, but the spectroscopic techniques are on the eve of implementation. Current research focuses on parameters, which potentially affect the results, and can vary extremely between crime scenes, for example human variability, environmental influences and substrate properties. The effect of these parameters on the spectroscopic measurements and potential limitations of the method for age estimation of bloodstains are described below.

4.6.1 Human Variability

An important factor to be studied is the biological variability between and within persons. The visible spectroscopic techniques described above are all based on the colour change of blood, which is influenced by the haemoglobin molecules within blood. In a study by Bremmer *et al.* (2011), no significant differences were found between or within healthy non-smoking volunteers. Possible sources of human variability are the initial amounts of carboxyhaemoglobin and methaemoglobin in a bloodstain. Bloodstains of non-smoking volunteers usually contain a small percentage (<4%) of carboxyhaemoglobin (Woebkenberg *et al.* 2011). The increased level of carboxyhaemoglobin expected for smokers, fire victims or in cases of fatal carbon monoxide poisoning, may influence the results in forensic practice (Sears *et al.* 2001; Teige *et al.* 1977; Wald *et al.* 1981). Diseases influencing the haemoglobin molecules, for example sickle cell disease, may also cause unexpected results.

4.6.2 Environmental Influences

Already in the 1960s, Patterson reported that the changing colour of the bloodstain depends on environmental conditions, including temperature and humidity (Bremmer *et al.* 2012b). Bremmer *et al.* (2012a) studied the influence of temperature and humidity on the kinetics of the haemoglobin derivatives. Measurements performed under several known environmental circumstances indicated that a higher temperature increases the speed of the chemical reactions in a bloodstain, whereas humidity only influences the denaturation of methaemoglobin into haemichrome. The influence of environmental factors at the crime scene will make precise estimation of the absolute age of bloodstains challenging. If the environmental factors can be reconstructed, we will be able to study the kinetics of the haemoglobin derivatives, which can then be used to estimate the absolute ages of bloodstains. In unknown circumstances, relative ages of bloodstains can be estimated to determine the order of formation of different bloodstains, under the assumption that they were exposed to similar environmental conditions.

4.6.3 Substrate Interference

One of the main challenges when performing spectral measurements at the crime scene is how to correct for substrate interferences. These interferences are a general problem encountered in forensic applications, where traces are typically not found on the ideal neutrally reflecting substrates used in laboratories; instead, all possible substrates can be encountered (e.g. with varying texture, roughness, porosity, colour, reflectance, etc.). The way bloodstains interact with porous and non-porous substrates is physically different; blood is absorbed by porous substrates, while it sits on top of non-porous substrates, which influences the interaction with light and thus the measured reflectance spectrum. Likewise, coloured substrates influence the measured reflectance spectrum, because they absorb specific wavelengths, which should be corrected for. Currently, experiments are being performed to find the limitations of the technique. Although all spectroscopic techniques are hampered by certain substrates, different techniques can be complementary. For example, where visible reflectance spectroscopy is difficult on black backgrounds, near infrared spectroscopy can be successful. Therefore, next to the development of adequate correction methods, a multidisciplinary approach is advised in which several techniques are combined to optimise the results for each specific substrate.

4.6.4 Evidential Value

Apart from detector noise, the factors described above contribute to spectral differences, which lead to measurement uncertainty. It is important to calculate confidence intervals in forensic practice. The accuracy of the estimated age will depend on the actual age of the bloodstain and knowledge of the environmental conditions. The chemical reactions taking place in the bloodstains are rapid in the beginning, but slower in a later stage (Bremmer *et al.* 2012a). As a result, the accuracy of age estimations decreases with the age of the bloodstain. How this influences the evidential value depends on the hypotheses relevant to the case. Confidence intervals in casework are generally expected to be larger than intervals resulting from measurements performed in a laboratory set-up. To culminate small age intervals, we recommend performing spectroscopic measurements as soon as possible.

4.7 Conclusion

To be able to implement techniques for age estimation of bloodstains in practice, and to apply them to more decomposed remains in taphonomic research, key steps in the research process are refining and validating the data to meet the needs of the legal and scientific communities. It is important to explore the boundaries of the technique and to describe the limitations, for example minimal bloodstain size, minimal and maximum bloodstain thickness and requirements of the background colour, porosity, etc. Testing the technique at real crime scenes, on bloodstains of which the age is known, can help when exploring these boundaries and limitations. Meanwhile, additional experiments in the laboratory and advanced data analysis may help to increase the applicability in forensic practice.

References

Andrasko, J. (1997) The estimation of age of bloodstains by HPLC analysis. *Journal of Forensic Science*, **42**: 601–607.

Arany, S. and Ohtani, S. (2011) Age estimation of bloodstains: a preliminary report based on aspartic acid racemization rate. *Forensic Science International*, **212**: e36–e39.

Bremmer, R.H., Nadort, A., van Leeuwen, T.G., van Gemert, M.J. and Aalders, M.C. (2011) Age estimation of blood stains by hemoglobin derivative determination using reflectance spectroscopy. *Forensic Science International*, **206**: 166–171.

Bremmer, R.H., de Bruin, D.M., de Joode, M., Buma, W.J., van Leeuwen, T.G. and Aalders, M.C.G. (2012a) Biphasic oxidation of oxy-hemoglobin in bloodstains. *PLoS One*, **6**: e21845.

Bremmer, R.H., de Bruin, K.G., van Gemert, M.J.C., van Leeuwen, T.G. and Aalders, M.C.G. (2012b) Forensic quest for age determination of bloodstains. *Forensic Science International*, **216**: 1–11.

Cook, R., Evett, I.W., Jackson, G., Jones, P.J. and Lambert, J.A. (1998) A hierarchy of propositions: deciding which level to address in casework. *Science and Justice*, **38**: 231–239.

Edelman, G.J., Gaston, E., van Leeuwen, C.P.J. and Aalders, M.C. (2012a) Hyperspectral imaging for non-contact analysis of forensic traces. *Forensic Science International*, **223**: 28–39.

Edelman, G.J., van Leeuwen, T.G. and Aalders, M.C.G. (2012b) Hyperspectral imaging for the age estimation of blood stains at the crime scene. *Forensic Science International*, **223**: 72–77.

Fujita, Y., Tsuchiya, K., Abe, S., Takiguchi, Y., Kubo, S. and Sakurai, H. (2005) Estimation of the age of human bloodstains by electron paramagnetic resonance spectroscopy: long-term controlled experiment on the effects of environmental factors. *Forensic Science International*, **152**: 39–43.

Guo, K., Achilefu, S. and Berezin, M.Y. (2012) Dating bloodstains with fluorescence lifetime measurements. *Chemistry*, **18**: 1303–1305.

Hanson, E.K. and Ballantyne, J. (2010) A blue spectral shift of the hemoglobin Soret band correlates with the age (time since deposition) of dried bloodstains. *PLoS One*, e12830.

Hanson, E., Albornoz, A. and Ballantyne, J. (2011) Validation of the hemoglobin (Hb) hypsochromic shift assay for determination of the time since deposition (TSD) of dried bloodstains. *Forensic Science International Genetics Supplement Series*, **3**: e307–e308.

Janchaysang, S., Sumriddetchkajorn, S. and Buranasiri, P. (2012) Tunable filter-based multispectral imaging for detection of blood stains on construction material substrates. Part 1: Developing blood stain discrimination criteria. *Applied Optics*, **51**: 6984–6996.

Janko, M., Stark, R.W. and Zink, A. (2012) Preservation of 5,300-year-old red blood cells in the Iceman. *Jounal of the Royal Society Interface*, **9**: 2581–2590.

Laber, T.L., Taylor, M.C. and Kish, P.E. (2014) The reliability of current methods of sequencing bloodstain patterns. *Journal of Bloodstain Pattern Analysis*, **30**: 3–10.

Lech, K., Ackermann, K., Wollstein, A., Revell, V.L., Skene, D.J. and Kayser, M. (2014) Assessing the suitability of miRNA-142-5p and miRNA-541 for bloodstain deposition timing. *Forensic Science International Genetics*, **12**: 181–184.

Leers, O. (1910) *Die forensische Blutuntersuchung*. Springer: Berlin.

Li, B., Beveridge, P., O'Hare, W.T. and Islam, M. (2011) The estimation of the age of a blood stain using reflectance spectroscopy with a microspectrophotometer, spectral pre-processing and linear discriminant analysis. *Forensic Science International*, **212**: 198–204.

Li, B., Beveridge, P., O'Hare, W.T. and Islam, M. (2013) The age estimation of blood stains up to 30 days old using visible wavelength hyperspectral image analysis and linear discriminant analysis. *Science and Justice*, **53**: 270–277.

Matsuoka, T., Taguchi, T. and Okuda, J. (1995) Estimation of bloodstain age by rapid determinations of oxyhemoglobin by use of oxygen electrode and total hemoglobin. *Biological and Pharmaceutical Bulletin*, **18**: 1031–1035.

Odriozola, A., Riancho, J.A., de la Vega, R., Agudo, G., Garcia-Blanco, A. and de Cos, E. (2014) MiRNA analysis in vitreous humor to determine the time of death: a proof-of-concept pilot study. *Forensic Science International Genetics*, **12**: 181–184.

Peschel, O., Muetzel, E. and Rothschild, M.A. (2008) Blood stain pattern analysis. *Rechtsmedizin*, **18**: 131–145.

Sears, D.A., Udden, M.M. and Thomas, J. (2001) Carboxyhemoglobin levels in patients with sickle-cell anemia: relationship to hemolytic and vasoocclusive severity. *American Journal of the Medical Sciences*, **322**: 345–348.

Strasser, S., Zink, A., Kada, G., Hinterdorfer, P., Peschel, O. *et al.* (2007) Age determination of blood spots in forensic medicine by force spectroscopy. *Forensic Science International*, **170**: 8–14.

Teige, B., Lundevall, J. and Fleischer, E. (1977) Carboxyhemoglobin concentrations in fire victims and in cases of fatal carbon-monoxide poisoning. *Zeitschrift fur Rechtsmedizin-Journal of Legal Medicine*, **80**: 17–21.

Thanakiatkrai, P., Yaodam, A. and Kitpipit, T. (2013) Age estimation of bloodstains using smartphones and digital image analysis. *Forensic Science International*, **233**: 288–297.

Wald, N.J., Idle, M., Boreham, J. and Bailey, A. (1981) Carbon monoxide in breath in relation to smoking and carboxyhaemoglobin levels. *Thorax*, **36**: 366–369.

Walsh, S., Liu, F., Ballantyne, K.N., van Oven, M., Lao, O. and Kayser, M. (2011) IrisPlex: a sensitive DNA tool for accurate prediction of blue and brown eye colour in the absence of ancestry information. *Forensic Science International Genetics*, **5**: 170–180.

Woebkenberg, N.R., Mostardi, R.A., Ely, D.L. and Worstell, D. (2011) Carboxyhemoglobin and methemoglobin levels in residents living in industrial and non-industrial communities. *Environmental Research*, **26**: 347–352.

5

DNA Degradation: Current Knowledge and Progress in DNA Analysis

Claudio Ottoni, Bram Bekaert and Ronny Decorte

5.1 Introduction

Our knowledge about the biochemical and physical processes that lead to DNA degradation has been increased considerably over the past decade. In particular, the field of palaeogenetics has not only contributed to our understanding of DNA degradation, but also to the development of sensitive methodologies to analyse genetic variation in degraded DNA. The latter is of extreme importance in forensic genetics, not only in the context of identification of the donors of biological stains in criminal cases, but especially in the identification of human remains in criminal cases and mass fatality incidents. Therefore, this review will be focused on the processes involved in the degradation of DNA, but will also highlight the methodological advances that have taken place or might be promising in the future for the analysis of degraded DNA. For an introduction to DNA profiling and identification, we refer the reader to the books of Butler (2009) and Goodwin *et al.* (2010).

5.2 Mechanisms of DNA Degradation

5.2.1 Short-Term Effects of Body Decomposition on DNA

Within the body, approximately 20,000 lesions occur in each cell's DNA on a daily basis, caused by either cell-specific processes such as reactive oxygen/nitrogen species production or by external agents like UV-radiation, chemical damage, etc. (Derheimer *et al.* 2007). The cell has a number of internal controls prior to cell replication to prevent the exponential multiplication of DNA sequence errors in a tissue. Damages are repaired by DNA repair enzymes in living cells. This enzymatic process stops when the body dies or when biological material is deposited (e.g. blood stains; Alaeddini *et al.* 2010). Soon after biological material is depleted of oxygen and nutrients because of blood flow cessation, cellular death is initiated through either programmed energy dependent (ATP) apoptosis or less orderly energy independent necrosis. Apoptosis is a well-studied phenomenon and is characterised by cytoplasm condensation, chromosomal fragmentation into 180–200 bp fragments by caspase-activated nucleases, cellular collapse and apoptotic body formation (Wyllie *et al.* 1984). In living organisms, this type of cell death is responsible for physiological cell turnover.

Necrosism, on the other hand, is caused by external factors such as inflammation, trauma or environmental insults to the body such as toxins; however, it also occurs during normal processes like tissue renewal (Mayhew *et al.* 1999). During necrosis, lysosomes undergo membrane permeabilisation causing the contents to spill out into the intracellular matrix and start the process of autolysis.

Taphonomy of Human Remains: Forensic Analysis of the Dead and the Depositional Environment, First Edition.
Edited by Eline M.J. Schotsmans, Nicholas Márquez-Grant and Shari L. Forbes.

Lysosomes are small cellular organelles packed with hydrolysis enzymes that digest all types of biological polymers, proteins, nucleic acids, carbohydrates and lipids. During autolysis, the digestion enzymes break down the cellular and nuclear membranes (Proskuryakov *et al.* 2003) and release the cell's contents into the extracellular matrix. One category of digestion enzymes released by the lysosome is nucleases. When these nucleases are released into the cellular environment, they can cause severe DNA damage. Endonucleases recognise unique palindromic sequences called restriction sites and cleave the double-stranded DNA sequence by hydrolysing the phosphodiester bond resulting in either 'sticky' ends (with single-stranded overhang) or 'blunt' ends (no overhangs). Exonucleases, on the other hand, chew off the ends of a DNA strand, also by a hydrolysing reaction, resulting in randomly-sized DNA fragments. In the meantime, colonisation by bacteria and fungi leads to further release of bacteria and fungi-specific nucleases, causing further enzymatic breakdown of DNA strands. DNA degradation starts almost immediately after death but is cell type and organ dependent. Morphological changes can be observed in heart tissue 20 minutes post-mortem (Jennings *et al.* 1975). It takes about 1 hour to occur in liver tissue and about 24 hours to occur in skeletal muscle (Tomita *et al.* 2004). What remains of the DNA structure depends on how long and at what temperature the autolysis process is allowed to proceed, but will always result in the individual nucleotides being released into the environment for recycling.

5.2.2 Long-Term Effects of the Depositional Environment on DNA Degradation

Following the early mechanisms of decomposition, slower but relentless processes intervene in the long term. The degradation of DNA in post-depositional contexts, also known as DNA diagenesis, is a complex and multifaceted process that accounts for multiple factors. External microbial activity in the form of extracellular nuclease secretion has a strong impact in DNA degradation pathways across geological time. A key role is also played by chemical and physical factors, which in turn are linked to large- (latitude and geographic location) and small-scale (specific depositional context of a body) environmental conditions. Long-term chemical modifications to which the DNA is subject are mostly ascribable to hydrolytic and oxidative reactions, key players of which are respectively water and oxygen. Hydrolytic reactions are responsible for the fragmentation of the polynucleotide strands, the most obvious type of damage encountered in DNA extracted from ancient biological samples. Water attacks the glycosidic bond between the nitrogenous bases and the sugar backbone, thus creating abasic sites. This occurs 20 times more often in purines than in pyrimidines, hence the so-called depurination rate (Lindahl and Karlstrom 1973; Lindahl and Nyberg 1972; Shapiro 1981). Abasic sites undergo a chemical rearrangement that leads to the cleavage of the polynucleotide strand, consequently a series of nicks appear in either strands of the DNA and inexorably lead to its fragmentation when they occur in contiguous regions. Similarly, accumulation of single-stranded nicks and consequent progressive fragmentation of the DNA is determined by direct hydrolytic cleavage of phosphodiester bonds in the phosphate-sugar backbone. As a result of fragmentation mechanisms, short DNA molecules harbouring single-stranded overhangs originate.

Hydrolytic reactions are also responsible for the deamination of nitrogenous bases. Such modifications accumulate mainly in the single-stranded overhangs of DNA fragments (Briggs *et al.* 2007) and give rise to the so-called miscoding lesions, which cause incorrect bases to be inserted (i.e. misincorporations) during PCR amplification (Hansen *et al.* 2001). The most common miscoding lesion is cytosine deamination, the product of which is uracil that leads during the first PCR cycle to the incorporation of an A and eventually to an artefactual C to T transition in the final sequences, or a G to A when the other strand of the PCR product is sequenced. Oxidation reactions are responsible for the occurrence of blocking lesions, which hinder the elongation of DNA strands by *Taq* polymerase during PCR reactions. Oxidation of DNA may also affect purine and pyrimidine bases, determining a ring-saturation, or the sugar, which breaks down due to the opening of the ribose ring.

Another type of diagenetic DNA damage is represented by intermolecular cross-links resulting from Maillard reactions, which occur between sugars and amino acids, thus linking DNA and peptides. Cross-links hinder PCR amplification of template molecules and have mostly been observed in ancient faecal remains (i.e. coprolite; Poinar *et al.* 1998) and in the presence of soluble soil organics like humic acids (Hedges 2002). Cosmic, ultraviolet and geological radiations must also be taken into account with regard to the integrity of DNA and biomolecules in general (Brown and Brown 2011). Ultraviolet radiation in particular can form links between purines on the same strand, thus acting as a blocking agent of PCR. It is clear that by influencing the kinetics of the chemical decay reactions described above, physical factors like temperature, pH, ionic strength and the availability of water and oxygen, become decisive in DNA diagenesis.

Finally, a large part of DNA degradation is linked to human activity, either between death and deposition (e.g. artificial mummification or cremation practices, cooking of animal bones) or during recovery and post-recovery procedures (*in-situ* sample collection, storage conditions, treatments of fossil bones in museum collections). With regards to pre-deposition practices, the high temperature reached during cremation leaves slim chances of DNA survival, which might be possible in cooked bones. In particular, a recent study showed that 128 bp-long DNA fragments could be amplified by standard PCR in mid-shaft femur samples of a modern bovine that were experimentally heated for 1 hour at 140°C, whereas raising the temperature to 170°C determined the almost total loss of even shorter (i.e. 62 bp) DNA fragments (Ottoni *et al.* 2009). Notwithstanding general belief, artificial mummification processes are not necessarily a treasure trove of ancient biomolecules. In fact, DNA preservation in soft tissues might not be better than in bones and, in particular, the organic compounds and embalming fluids used in mummification practices (e.g. in Egyptian mummies but also in modern activities of body preservation) may interfere with molecular analyses and reduce the efficiency of DNA retrieval (Brown and Brown 2011). Concerning recovery, freshly excavated and untreated (unwashed) bones were demonstrated to be the preferred material for ancient DNA (aDNA) analyses (Pruvost *et al.* 2007).

Genetic studies conducted more than 30 years ago on an extinct 140-year-old equid specimen (Higuchi *et al.* 1984) and a 2,400-year-old Egyptian mummy (Pääbo 1985) represents the pioneering studies of aDNA research, which is defined broadly as 'the retrieval of DNA sequences from museum specimens, archaeological finds, fossil remains and other unusual sources of DNA' (Pääbo *et al.* 2004), including ancient sediments, ice and faeces, even in the absence of visible macrofossils (so-called 'dirt' DNA; Willerslev *et al.* 2007).

5.2.3 Survival of DNA in Geological Times

Understanding the mechanisms responsible for DNA decay is key to predicting the degree of DNA preservation in biological samples, thus avoiding destructive sampling of valuable material and saves time and cost-consuming analyses of extremely degraded samples. Several efforts have been addressed to study *in vitro* chemical processes responsible for DNA degradation in order to model diagenetic trajectories. A seminal theoretical study of 1972 by Lindahl and Nyberg estimated the rate of depurination of DNA in physiological solution at 15°C and neutral pH, which would account for the total degradation of 10^{12} chloroplast DNA molecules to less than 800 bp-long DNA fragments in 5,000 years (Pääbo and Wilson 1991). By speeding up chemical decay, heat is clearly detrimental to DNA survival and later studies highlighted the key role played by temperature, revealing that the thermal history of a fossil, more than its geological age, is decisive for DNA survival. This has led to the definition of thermal age (Smith *et al.* 2003), which by assuming depurination as the main driver of DNA fragmentation and following Lindahl and Nyberg's kinetics, accounts for the thermal history of a biological sample (including factors like altitude and palaeoclimatic curves), in order to predict the likely survival of DNA in a sample.

Though indicative of DNA preservation, such theoretical models rely on assumptions that inevitably overlook the complexity of DNA degradation processes, and empirical studies have demonstrated that in specific depositional contexts the rate of DNA fragmentation is up to 400 times slower than predicted *in vitro* (Allentoft *et al.* 2012). Empirical methods have been developed aimed at directly screening for the preservation of biomolecules in ancient samples prior to DNA analysis, amongst which, at least for bones, the presence of collagen is a good indicator. Nevertheless, DNA and collagen seem to follow different diagenetic trajectories, and whereas the absence of collagen may be useful for ruling out ancient samples for DNA analysis, its presence does not necessarily indicate adequate DNA preservation. Aspartic acid racemisation (AAR) has been widely adopted as a DNA survival screening method due to the very low amount of bone material needed (<10 mg) and to its comparable kinetics with DNA depurination in solution (Poinar *et al.* 1996). Nevertheless, such similarity may not hold true in bone, as demonstrated by a recent study in which no correlation was found between the extent of AAR and DNA amplification success in a wide range of bone samples (Collins *et al.* 2009). Although not widely adopted, other screening methods indicative of DNA preservation have been proposed (Scorrano *et al.* 2015) including: degree of histological degradation (Colson *et al.* 1997; Jans *et al.* 2004); X-ray diffraction to assess mineral alteration (Götherström *et al.* 2002); mass spectrometry (Poinar and Stankiewicz 1999); collagen alteration (Koon *et al.* 2003); and mercury-intrusion porosimetry (Nielsen-Marsh and Hedges 1999).

The multifaceted nature of DNA preservation makes it hard to accurately predict when DNA is degraded to a level where it is no longer suitable for genetic analysis. Much remains to be learnt about how and where DNA is preserved microscopically inside bone, with particular regards to potential 'protective' interactions with the organic (binding to collagen) and inorganic (adsorption to hydroxyapatite) components of the bone (Campos *et al.* 2012). For example, in conditions of rapid desiccation of body tissues after death, DNA may be adsorbed in the mineral matrix and may escape the initial enzymatic and microbial degradation (Pääbo *et al.* 2004). Given the key role played by temperature in the longevity of aDNA molecules, the overall success of DNA retrieval from archaeological samples seems to follow a latitudinal trend, with yields decreasing from arctic to temperate regions. Not surprisingly, most of the recent ancient genomic data have been retrieved in samples from high latitudes (e.g. Prufer *et al.* 2014; Raghavan *et al.* 2014). Nevertheless, this is not always the case and the success rate of DNA recovery may vary strikingly even in the same site. It is still not clear what the limits are for survival of DNA, at least to an extent that makes it feasible for analysis. Claims of antediluvian DNA (120 million years ago) retrieval in the early 1990s have been widely discredited as results of contamination (Lindahl 1993); however, the recent technological advances achieved by high-throughput sequencing (HTS) technologies, also called next-generation sequencing (NGS), has remarkably stretched the timescale up to which DNA can be analysed, thus reaching thresholds that were barely imaginable before. To date of writing, the oldest DNA sequenced belongs to a horse bone recovered from Siberian permafrost dated to 560–780 kyr BP (Orlando *et al.* 2013), whereas the oldest hominin DNA (mtDNA) has been sequenced in bone samples of a 400-kyr-old specimen from Spain (Meyer *et al.* 2014). This result proves that authentic aDNA data can be retrieved from samples hundreds of thousands years old outside of permafrost.

5.3 Preservation of DNA: Recommendations Concerning Sampling and Storage

The choice of samples to be used for DNA analyses and their storage may be decisive in obtaining optimal results. After the 2004 Tsunami disaster in Southeast Asia, the International Society for Forensic Genetics (ISFG) proposed recommendations (Table 5.1) for collecting and storing post-mortem samples suitable for DNA analysis as part of the Disaster Victim Identification

Table 5.1 Recommendations of the International Society for Forensic Genetics (Prinz *et al.* 2007) concerning post-mortem sampling of human remains for genetic identification.

Condition of body	Sample to be collected
Not decomposed, whole body	Blood and buccal swab
Not decomposed, fragmented	If available, blood and deep red muscle tissue
Decomposed, whole bodies and fragmented remains	Long compact bones (e.g. femur, humerus) and/or healthy teeth without fillings (molars preferable) and/or any bone available (dense cortical bone)
Severely burnt bodies	Any of the above samples (if available)

Source: Prinz 2007. Reproduced with permission of Elsevier.

procedure (Prinz *et al.* 2007). Sample collection at the site should follow forensic collection principles ('chain-of-custody'), including preventive measures to avoid contamination, documentation of the sampling, proper conservation and labelling of the samples. Depending on the preservation of the body, different samples should be collected including bone and teeth, which are the most reliable sources of DNA when collection activities span several weeks or take place in adverse environmental conditions.

Experience with the identification of the skeletal remains in the mass graves in former Yugoslavia has revealed that apart from teeth, bone samples from the lower part (femur, fibula and tibia) of the skeleton provides the highest success rate for DNA analysis (Milos *et al.* 2007). It has also been demonstrated that finger or toenails are attractive DNA sources for genetic identification of decomposed or desiccated remains (Allouche *et al.* 2008; Bengtsson *et al.* 2012), even after 32 months of presence in flooding water (Decorte, personal information). Fragmented remains must be collected separately and receive unique traceable identification labels without any presumption of association. Multiple samples (at least 2) per body (part) assure that sufficient samples are available for DNA analysis, even if one of them shows insufficient DNA for analysis. These samples should be stored in a sealed and uniquely labelled container, preferably frozen at $-20°C$ or lower, in order to prevent any further DNA degradation. Preservative solutions such as DMSO, ethanol, DNA lysis buffer (Kilpatrick *et al.* 2002) or commercial solutions such as GenoFix (Fregeau *et al.* 2001) can be used to store soft tissue samples at room temperature; however, formalin is not recommended as it leads to DNA degradation. In the long term, skeletal tissues are those with the highest chance of survival, therefore compact bone samples and teeth have represented the preferred material for aDNA analyses for years. Nevertheless, in recent times and with the advent of HTS technologies, a variety of ancient tissues have been used in human and animal archaeological remains and museum specimens (Bengtsson *et al.* 2012; Olsen *et al.* 2012).

Several sources of contamination threaten the analysis of 'trace' DNA, both modern and ancient. The most acknowledged and feared one is the handling of specimens at every stage, from recovery to the laboratory, which can transfer modern human DNA from skin, sweat and saliva (Gilbert *et al.* 2005; Pilli *et al.* 2013). Personal protective equipment (e.g. gloves, cover all and face mask) is therefore essential and should be worn at all times when collecting biological material. The 'double-gloving' technique can be used to quickly and easily change gloves between collecting samples from different remains. Pre-recovery activities such as handling of the bones in the past (e.g. in secondary burials or burial disturbing due to tomb raiding), exposure to urine and faeces or DNA leaching through sediments due to vertical percolation of liquids, may also be a source of contamination (Haile *et al.* 2007). No effective solution can be taken to reduce this kind of contamination, though a study of the soil and the depositional context may help to account for it. Collection and storage of samples for DNA analyses already *in situ* without further post-excavation treatment (e.g. washing, consolidation) might also reduce significantly the risk of external contamination (Brown and Brown 2011; Pruvost *et al.* 2007).

5.4 Methodologies to Analyse Degraded DNA

5.4.1 Challenges to the Study of aDNA and Precautions

The retrieval of DNA from archaeological and palaeontological remains can provide significant contributions to the study of the past, both at the ecological and the evolutionary side. During the past three decades, the success of aDNA studies has run parallel to technological advances, from the initial use of bacterial cloning (e.g. Higuchi *et al.* 1984; Pääbo 1985), through to the ground-breaking invention of DNA amplification by means of PCR, up to the recent HTS technologies (Margulies *et al.* 2005), which has paved the way to palaeogenomics. Nevertheless, diagenetic changes that affect the DNA post-mortem make it fraught with pitfalls and technical challenges that have to be routinely faced. A large part of these pitfalls is certainly represented by contamination: in fact, the extreme sensitivity of PCR and the fragmented nature of aDNA increase the risk of preferentially amplifying modern contaminant DNA and obtaining false-positive results. An additional source of contamination during molecular analyses is represented by amplicons from previous PCR experiments (carry-over contamination), which remain airborne for long periods and can be transferred and introduced through personnel or equipment into PCR reactions during their preparation. Contamination can also arise from trace DNA molecules, both animal and human, present in commercial plastic ware and reagents used during analytical processes (Leonard *et al.* 2007).

After a first decade of aDNA studies highlighting their successes but even more strikingly their pitfalls (Lindahl 1993), and once DNA amplification through standard PCR became commonly used, nine key criteria were compiled as technical guidelines for conducting aDNA studies and minimise the risk of contamination (Cooper and Poinar 2000). The criteria included the use of dedicated laboratories with isolated work areas in order to separate archaeological samples and DNA extracts from amplified products (pre- and post-PCR facilities), the analysis of a large number of negative controls, appropriate analytical approach (e.g. amplification of short fragments) and the reproducibility and independent replication of data. Across the years, further precautions and authentication methods have been introduced, for example, the adoption of enzymatic decontamination procedures based upon dUTPs and Uracyl-N Glycosilase to reduce the risk of carry-over contamination (Pruvost *et al.* 2005), or strategies to directly decontaminate PCR reagents (Champlot *et al.* 2010). Nevertheless, even a slavish compliance to these rules may not necessarily imply the success of an aDNA study and in some instances a critical evaluation of how the data were produced and a self-questioning approach might be decisive to circumvent the potential flaws (Gilbert *et al.* 2005).

5.4.2 Progress in Methodologies for the Analysis of Degraded DNA

5.4.2.1 Forensic Genetic Identification

Since 1995, forensic genetic identification has relied on the use of DNA amplification and the analysis of mainly Short Tandem Repeat (STR) loci on the human genome. This procedure works well when the DNA is of sufficient quantity and quality, with typically one or two balanced peaks (alleles) per STR (Figure 5.1a), in proportion to the amount of DNA input in the PCR reaction. However, as DNA degradation fragments the DNA sequence into smaller pieces, STR regions might become broken up, resulting in a reduced efficiency of the PCR process and loss of the correlation between the height of

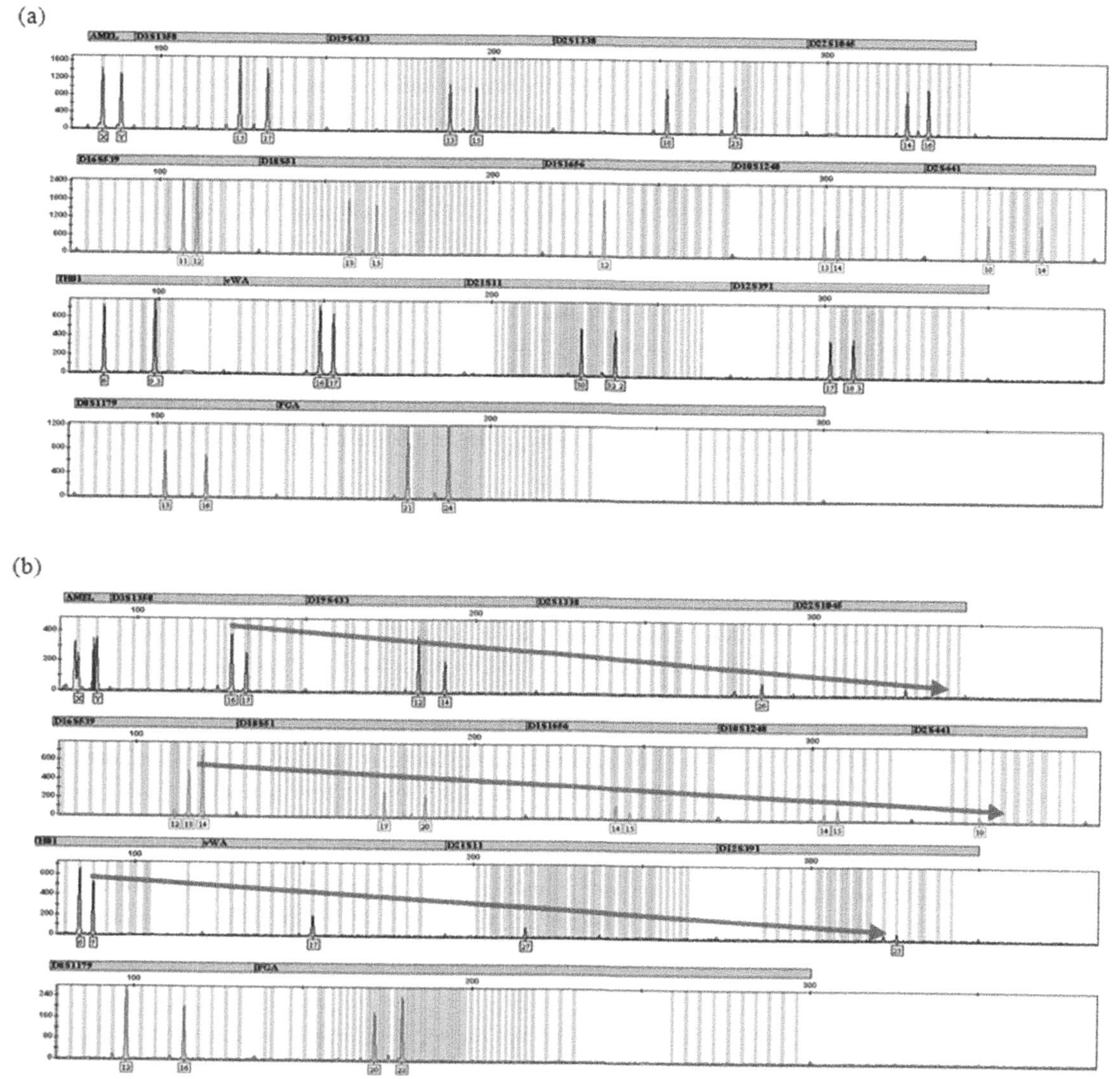

Figure 5.1 Electropherograms produced using the Powerplex® ESI 16 system (Promega). (a) DNA profile from a pristine sample. All loci and alleles are well balanced. (b) DNA profile from a degraded sample. A decrease in peak height with increasing molecular weight of the loci is observed in the first, second and third channel.

the alleles and input DNA amount. Lower PCR efficiency due to degraded DNA will cause lower peak heights and perhaps even cause some of them to 'dropout' of the DNA profile, leaving a partial profile with limited power of discrimination to include or exclude a potential contributor to the sample or to establish biological relationships. The profile of a degraded DNA sample is therefore characterised by a downward slope of the peak heights with increasing allele and marker lengths (Figure 5.1b).

DNA degradation became a major topic within forensic research with the mass identification of the victims of the 9/11 disaster. Many of the biological samples recovered from the disaster area could not be analysed with traditional methods, even with enhancing techniques such as increasing the number of PCR cycles, purification and concentration of PCR products or higher capillary electrophoresis injection settings. It became clear that novel methodologies or the use of alternative genetic markers had to be used in order to identify the remains. By decreasing the length of the DNA sequence necessary to amplify the STR region due to relocating the primers closer to the actual repeat region compared to the traditional STR assays, the sensitivity for degraded DNA increased and resulted in more complete DNA profiles (Butler *et al.* 2003). This mini-STR design shortens the DNA sequence to less than 200 bp in comparison to up to 400 bp of the conventional STR assays. Mini-STR multiplex assays are now routinely used to analyse samples with limited or low-quality DNA.

Single nucleotide polymorphisms or SNPs are single base changes in the DNA sequence that are commonly observed in a population. Forensically relevant SNPs can be categorised into four different classes: identity-testing SNPs, lineage-informative SNPs (Y chromosome and mitochondrial DNA), ancestry-informative SNPs and phenotype-informative (e.g. iris colour) SNPs (Budowle and van Daal 2008). As the region to be analysed is only a single base pair, the length of the DNA sequence required for PCR amplification can be kept to a minimum, making it suitable for the analysis of degraded DNA. An international group of researchers known as the SNP *for* ID consortium have published a 52 SNP-multiplex for human identification, which is suitable for degraded DNA analysis (Sanchez *et al.* 2006).

Degradation of DNA or the absence of sufficient nuclear DNA makes conventional STR or even mini-STR and SNP analysis sometimes difficult or perhaps impossible. Mitochondrial DNA (mtDNA) is an alternative as it is more abundantly present in a cell: several hundred to thousands of copies compared to two copies of the nuclear DNA. The chances are therefore much greater that sufficient mtDNA is present in degraded DNA samples and can be used for identification of remains. Nevertheless, maternal inheritance of mtDNA strongly limits its applicability in genetic identification of remains. Most mtDNA genetic variation is localised in the non-coding or control (d-loop) region concentrated into two hotspots. Similarly to the STRs, revised methodologies have been developed for analysing mtDNA in degraded samples in forensic identifications or in aDNA research (Berger and Parson 2009; Jehaes *et al.* 2001; Kim *et al.* 2013). Within the forensic community, efforts are underway to extend the mitochondrial target sequence from the currently analysed mutation hotspot region to the entire mitochondrial genome, most of which is coding DNA. This would increase the discrimination power of mtDNA and provide more conclusive results. However, analysing the coding region might also reveal mutations with clinical phenotypes and therefore strict ethical and legal rules should be established before mitochondrial genome analysis can be applied in a forensic context.

5.4.2.2 High-Throughput Sequencing (HTS) Technologies in Forensic Genetics and Ancient DNA Research

Recent advances in sequencing technology are starting to replace current techniques, such as capillary sequencing, in molecular research studies and in clinical diagnostic tests (Tucker *et al.* 2009). HTS technology is based on simultaneous parallel sequencing of large numbers of DNA fragments. The sheer volume and speed at which terabytes of data can be produced using HTS platforms have only recently been explored by the forensic community. Published forensic HTS protocols have focused mostly on either the mitochondrial genome (or part thereof; e.g. Bekaert *et al.* 2013; Mikkelsen *et al.* 2014; Parson *et al.* 2013), autosomal STR profiling (e.g. Rockenbauer *et al.* 2014; Van Neste *et al.* 2012; Zeng *et al.* 2014) or SNP markers (Seo *et al.* 2014). Recently, the company Illumina released details of the first commercially available forensic NGS kit. This kit is able to analyse 233 individual markers for human identification, phenotyping and biogeographic ancestry estimation and allows simultaneous analysis of up to 32 stain samples or 96 reference samples. However, several challenges remain to be overcome before HTS methodologies can be incorporated into routine forensic practice. Limitations such as the required sample input amounts, longer hands-on time in the laboratory and a high price/sample ratio still need to be surmounted.

Methodological improvements in HTS in the forensic field will mainly come from palaeogenetics, where HTS technologies have dramatically boosted the field by marking the entrance of the new era of palaeogenomics. In tune with the fragmented nature of aDNA, HTS methodologies are designed to sequence short DNA molecules. Apart from the massive output of sequencing data returned by HTS platforms, the key methodological change introduced in this new technology is represented by ligation to both ends of DNA fragments of universal oligonucleotide sequences (i.e. adapters) containing primer-binding and sequencing sites, the so-called genomic libraries. This makes it possible to amplify and sequence a wide range of DNA molecules (endogenous but also exogenous) present in a DNA extract and more importantly to target even the short-size molecules previously escaping standard PCR techniques. Sequencing of genomic libraries revealed empirically the extremely fragmented nature of aDNA, with average fragment lengths as low as 30–40 bp (Meyer *et al.* 2012; Prufer *et al.* 2014). Moreover, the population of longer molecules targeted by standard PCR methods, when still accessible, represents only a small fraction of all DNA molecules extracted from an ancient biological sample.

HTS methods are not exempt from challenges inherent to aDNA analyses, and the nature of the damage of DNA molecules (degree of fragmentation, cytosine deamination) and the method adopted for library preparation (blunt- versus sticky-end ligation, purification steps) may significantly affect the efficiency of the analysis in poorly preserved samples (e.g. see Heyn *et al.* 2010). More importantly, contamination issues may arise, particularly during library preparation, when contamination from previously amplified libraries may occur (Green *et al.* 2009). In the computational data processing step, authentication and discrimination of endogenous from exogenous sequences, particularly in human samples, may be challenging and a number of criteria have been described to unravel it (Krause *et al.* 2010; Sawyer *et al.* 2012).

Increased efforts in the study of ancient genomes have recently led to significant changes in the preparation of genomic libraries, from the single-stranded method (Gansauge and Meyer 2013) that has been used to sequence extinct hominin genomes at high coverage (Meyer *et al.* 2012; Prufer *et al.* 2014) and in a range of samples of different age and geographic provenance (Bennett *et al.* 2014), up to the more recent U-enrichment (Gansauge and Meyer 2014), which specifically selects and captures deaminated (and most likely ancient) DNA molecules. HTS strategies may change according to the sample material and the specific objective of a study. The simplest one is the 'shotgun' sequencing, which consists of direct sequencing of genomic libraries without any previous targeted enrichment. This technique provides key information about the quality of extracted DNA by returning the relative amount of endogenous sequences versus exogenous contaminants, the majority of which is represented by 'environmental' sequences of fungi and bacteria. Shotgun sequencing has been used to produce draft and high-coverage complete genomes of ancient animals (Orlando *et al.* 2013), humans (e.g. Lazaridis *et al.* 2014) amongst the most recent ones and hominins (Meyer *et al.* 2012; Prufer *et al.* 2014), the quality of which varied from 0.1–10% of endogenous DNA in samples from temperate conditions up to (exceptionally) 84% in permafrost hair samples (Rasmussen *et al.* 2010; Shapiro and Hofreiter 2014).

More recently, enrichment methods have been developed in order to target specific genomic regions through PCR amplification or hybridisation capture. Whereas the former clearly suffers from the limitations of standard PCR, the latter makes use of oligonucleotide probes that hybridise and immobilise target DNA molecules, either on glass substrates (on-array), or by recovery in solution with magnetic beads (Gnirke *et al.* 2009). Target enrichment methods have been successfully used in ancient specimens for sequencing autosomal regions (e.g. Avila-Arcos *et al.* 2011; Burbano *et al.* 2010), complete mitochondrial genomes (e.g. Krause *et al.* 2010), including the oldest DNA from a hominin (Meyer *et al.* 2014) and recently, enrichment methods for whole-genome capture have also been proposed (Carpenter *et al.* 2013; Enk *et al.* 2014). Given the extreme DNA degradation of aDNA samples, target enrichment methods will probably pave the way to the analysis of degraded DNA samples in a forensic identification.

5.5 Future Prospects

It is clear that degradation of DNA is a complex process influenced by biological and environmental factors, which makes it hard to predict whether a biological sample is of sufficient quality to be analysed. While the prospect of analysing DNA from recent biological samples is much higher than with DNA from ancient or archaeological specimens, the methodology used will be decisive if DNA results are to be obtained. The rapid progress in HTS methodologies observed in aDNA research will lead to novel applications in forensic identification. In particular, the targeted enrichment of specific genomic or mitochondrial regions by in-solution capture methods is very promising, as it captures even short DNA fragments that cannot be amplified with revised PCR methods. Another development might be the selection of SNPs in regions of the human genome that could escape the process of DNA degradation (Thanakiatkrai and Welch 2011). The DNA sequence in the nucleus of the cell is wrapped twice around histones forming complexes called nucleosomes (Figure 5.2). The nucleosomes act as a barrier against DNA degradation from natural cell death in addition to bacterial and environmental degradation. Combining the efficiency of SNP typing with shorter sequences and the greater resistance to DNA degradation by using nucleosome-protected SNPs provides an assay that is more robust than traditional methods (Freire-Aradas *et al.* 2012). However, a recent study on Drosophila has shown that genetic variation within nucleosome protected DNA regions are not always neutral and could be under selective pressure, which makes these variations not applicable in forensic DNA analysis (Langley *et al.* 2014).

In vitro DNA repair has been considered as a potential solution to improve the analysis of aDNA (Mitchell *et al.* 2005). While the success of this strategy has been demonstrated in several aDNA studies (Di Bernardo *et al.* 2002; Pusch *et al.* 1998), widespread introduction into aDNA research has not been reached. The main reason for this lack of interest might be the extra steps involved in this procedure, which increases the chance for the introduction of contamination. *In vitro* DNA repair methods have recently attracted interest from the forensic field with the introduction of a commercial repair

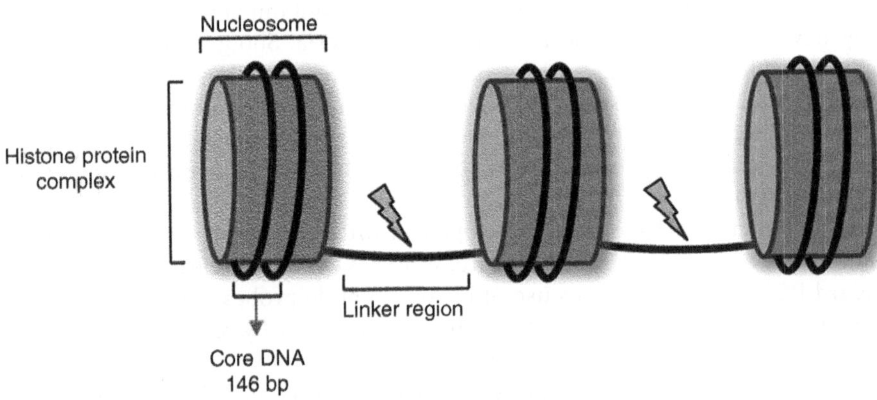

Figure 5.2 Nucleosomes and DNA degradation protection. Nucleosomes provide protection from DNA degradation when the DNA strand is wrapped around the histone protein complex. DNA strands in the linker region are unprotected and most vulnerable to DNA degradation by endonucleases (indicated by lightning flashes).

kit (PreCR™ Repair Mix). An initial study (Diegoli *et al.* 2012) showed an improvement in STR typing after using the repair procedure, but recent studies concluded that additional work is necessary in order to implement this kit in forensic case work as a general approach (Ambers *et al.* 2014; Robertson *et al.* 2014). In particular, the combination of certain repair enzymes might be crucial to ensure an efficient repair of the damaged DNA (Tie and Uchigasaki 2013). However, as these repair strategies are mainly focused on the repair of UV lesions and the removal of apurinic/apyrimidinic sites, fragmentation might not be overcome, which is still the main complication for analysing degraded DNA. Future methodologies for analysing degraded DNA samples will therefore still rely on advanced HTS methods, either with or without a DNA repair protocol prior to the analysis.

5.6 Conclusion

Though our understanding of the biochemical and physical processes of DNA degradation has improved over the past decade, predicting the survivability of DNA in biological remains is still in its infancy. Many environmental factors influence DNA degradation but it is difficult to reconstruct these factors when human remains are recovered. However, the rapid advancements in technology in the past few years have revolutionised genetic identification. Especially with regard to the analysis of difficult and highly degraded biological samples, HTS strategies have proven to overcome the limitations of degraded DNA and to be able to generate genetic data, even from minimum amounts of human DNA in a background of non-human DNA (e.g. microbial). Therefore, we expect that HTS methodologies will become the standard procedure for genetic identification of human remains if traditional procedures fail to produce results.

References

Alaeddini, R., Walsh, S.J. and Abbas, A. (2010) Forensic implications of genetic analyses from degraded DNA – a review. *Forensic Science International: Genetics*, **4**: 148–157.

Allentoft, M.E., Collins, M., Harker, D., Haile, J., Oskam, C.L. *et al.* (2012) The half-life of DNA in bone: measuring decay kinetics in 158 dated fossils. *Proceedings of the Royal Society B: Biological Sciences*, **279**: 4724–4733.

Allouche, M., Hamdoum, M., Mangin, P. and Castella, V. (2008) Genetic identification of decomposed cadavers using nails as DNA source. *Forensic Science International: Genetics*, **3**: 46–49.

Ambers, A., Turnbough, M., Benjamin, R., King, J. and Budowle, B. (2014) Assessment of the role of DNA repair in damaged forensic samples. *International Journal of Legal Medicine*, **128**: 913–921.

Avila-Arcos, M.C., Cappellini, E., Romero-Navarro, J.A., Wales, N., Moreno-Mayar, J.V. *et al.* (2011) Application and comparison of large-scale solution-based DNA capture-enrichment methods on ancient DNA. *Scientific Reports*, **1**: 74.

Bekaert, B., Massoli, C., Anandarajah, A., Van de Voorde, W. and Decorte, R. (2013) Multiplex DNA amplification and barcoding in a single reaction for 454 Roche sequencing: a comprehensive study on the control region of the mitochondrial genome. *Forensic Science International: Genetics Supplement Series*, **4**: e111–e112.

Bengtsson, C.F., Olsen, M.E., Brandt, L.O., Bertelsen, M.F., Willerslev, E. *et al.* (2012) DNA from keratinous tissue. Part I: Hair and nail. *Annals of Anatomy*, **194**: 17–25.

Bennett, E.A., Massilani, D., Lizzo, G., Daligault, J., Geigl, E.M. and Grange, T. (2014) Library construction for ancient genomics: single strand or double strand? *Biotechniques*, **56**: 289–290, 292–296, 298, passim.

Berger, C. and Parson, W. (2009) Mini-midi-mito: adapting the amplification and sequencing strategy of mtDNA to the degradation state of crime scene samples. *Forensic Science International: Genetics*, **3**: 149–153.

Briggs, A.W., Stenzel, U., Johnson, P.L., Green, R.E., Kelso, J. *et al.* (2007) Patterns of damage in genomic DNA sequences from a Neandertal. *Proceedings of the National Academy of Sciences of the United States of America*, **104**: 14616–14621.

Brown, T.A. and Brown, K. (2011) *Biomolecular Archaeology: An introduction.* Wiley-Blackwell: Chichester, UK.

Budowle, B. and van Daal, A. (2008) Forensically relevant SNP classes. *Biotechniques*, **44**: 603–608, 610.

Burbano, H.A., Hodges, E., Green, R.E., Briggs, A.W., Krause, J. *et al.* (2010) Targeted investigation of the Neandertal genome by array-based sequence capture. *Science*, **328**: 723–725.

Butler, J.M. (2009) *Fundamentals of Forensic DNA Typing*. Elsevier Academic Press: San Diego.

Butler, J.M., Shen, Y. and McCord, B.R. (2003) The development of reduced size STR amplicons as tools for analysis of degraded DNA. *Journal of Forensic Science*, **48**: 1054–1064.

Campos, P.F., Craig, O.E., Turner-Walker, G., Peacock, E., Willerslev, E. and Gilbert, M.T. (2012) DNA in ancient bone – where is it located and how should we extract it? *Annals of Anatomy*, **194**: 7–16.

Carpenter, M.L., Buenrostro, J.D., Valdiosera, C., Schroeder, H., Allentoft, M.E. *et al.* (2013) Pulling out the 1%: whole-genome capture for the targeted enrichment of ancient DNA sequencing libraries. *American Journal of Human Genetics*, **93**: 852–864.

Champlot, S., Berthelot, C., Pruvost, M., Bennett, E.A, Grange, T. and Geigl, E.-M. (2010) An efficient multistrategy DNA decontamination procedure of PCR teagents for hypersensitive PCR applications. *PLoS One*, **5**: e13042.

Collins, M.J., Penkman, K.E., Rohland, N., Shapiro, B., Dobberstein, R.C. *et al.* (2009) Is amino acid racemization a useful tool for screening for ancient DNA in bone? *Proceedings of the Royal Society B: Biological Sciences*, **276**: 2971–2977.

Colson, I.B., Bailey, J.B., Vercauteren, M., Sykes, B. and Hedges, R. (1997) The preservation of ancient DNA and bone diagenesis. *Ancient Biomolecules*, **1**: 109–117.

Cooper, A. and Poinar, H.N. (2000) Ancient DNA: do it right or not at all. *Science*, **289**: 1139.

Derheimer, F.A., O'Hagan, H.M., Krueger, H.M., Hanasoge, S., Paulsen, M.T. and Ljungman, M. (2007) RPA and ATR link transcriptional stress to p53. *Proceedings of the National Academy of Sciences of the United States of America*, **104**: 12778–12783.

Di Bernardo, G., Del Gaudio, S., Cammarota, M., Galderisi, U., Cascino, A. and Cipollaro, M. (2002) Enzymatic repair of selected cross-linked homoduplex molecules enhances nuclear gene rescue from Pompeii and Herculaneum remains. *Nucleic Acids Research*, **30**: e16.

Diegoli, T.M., Farr, M., Cromartie, C., Coble, M.D. and Bille, T.W. (2012) An optimized protocol for forensic application of the PreCR Repair Mix to multiplex STR amplification of UV-damaged DNA. *Forensic Science International: Genetics*, **6**: 498–503.

Enk, J.M., Devault, A.M., Kuch, M., Murgha, Y.E., Rouillard, J.M. and Poinar, H.N. (2014) Ancient whole genome enrichment using baits built from modern DNA. *Molecular Biology and Evolution*, **31**: 1292–1294.

Fregeau, C.J., Vanstone, H., Borys, S., McLean, D., Maroun, J.A. *et al.* (2001) AmpFlSTR Profiler Plus and AmpFlSTR COfiler analysis of tissues stored in GenoFix, a new tissue preservation solution for mass disaster DNA identification. *Journal of Forensic Science*, **46**: 1180–1190.

Freire-Aradas, A., Fondevila, M., Kriegel, A.K., Phillips, C., Gill, P. *et al.* (2012) A new SNP assay for identification of highly degraded human DNA. *Forensic Science International: Genetics*, **6**: 341–349.

Gansauge, M.T. and Meyer, M. (2014) Selective enrichment of damaged DNA molecules for ancient genome sequencing. *Genome Research*, **24**: 1543–1549.

Gansauge, M.T. and Meyer, M. (2013) Single-stranded DNA library preparation for the sequencing of ancient or damaged DNA. *Nature Protocols*, **8**: 737–748.

Gilbert, M., Rudbeck, L., Willerslev, E., Hansen, A., Smith, C. *et al.* (2005) Biochemical and physical correlates of DNA contamination in archaeological human bones and teeth excavated at Matera, Italy. *Journal of Archaeological Science*, **32**: 785–793.

Gilbert, M.T.P., Bandelt, H.-J., Hofreiter, M. and Barnes, I. (2005) Assessing ancient DNA studies. *Trends in Ecology & Evolution*, **20**: 541–544.

Gnirke, A., Melnikov, A., Maguire, J., Rogov, P., LeProust, E.M. *et al.* (2009) Solution hybrid selection with ultra-long oligonucleotides for massively parallel targeted sequencing. *Nature Biotechnology*, **27**: 182–189.

Goodwin, W., Linacre, A. and Haddi, S. (2010) *An Introduction to Forensic Genetics*, 2nd edition, John Wiley & Sons: Chichester, UK.

Götherström, A., Collins, M.J., Angerbjörn, A. and Lidén, K. (2002) Bone preservation and DNA amplification. *Archaeometry*, **44**: 395–404.

Green, R.E., Briggs, A.W., Krause, J., Prufer, K., Burbano, H.A. *et al.* (2009) The Neandertal genome and ancient DNA authenticity. *EMBO Journal*, **28**: 2494–2502.

Haile, J., Holdaway, R., Oliver, K., Bunce, M., Gilbert, M.T., Nielsen, R. *et al.* (2007) Ancient DNA chronology within sediment deposits: are paleobiological reconstructions possible and is DNA leaching a factor? *Molecular Biology and Evolution*, **24**: 982–989.

Hansen, A., Willerslev, E., Wiuf, C., Mourier, T. and Arctander, P. (2001) Statistical evidence for miscoding lesions in ancient DNA templates. *Molecular Biology and Evolution*, **18**: 262–265.

Hedges, R.E.M. (2002) Bone diagenesis: an overview of processes. *Archaeometry*, **44**: 319–328.

Heyn, P., Stenzel, U., Briggs, A.W., Kircher, M., Hofreiter, M. and Meyer, M. (2010) Road blocks on paleogenomes – polymerase extension profiling reveals the frequency of blocking lesions in ancient DNA. *Nucleic Acids Research*, **38**: e161.

Higuchi, R., Bowman, B., Freiberger, M., Ryder, O.A. and Wilson, A.C. (1984) DNA sequences from the quagga, an extinct member of the horse family. *Nature*, **312**: 282–284.

Jans, M.M.E., Nielsen-Marsh, C.M., Smith, C.I., Collins, M.J. and Kars, H. (2004) Characterisation of microbial attack on archaeological bone. *Journal of Archaeological Science*, **31**: 87–95.

Jehaes, E., Toprak, K., Vanderheyden, N., Pfeiffer, H., Cassiman, J.J. *et al.* (2001) Pitfalls in the analysis of mitochondrial DNA from ancient specimens and the consequences for forensic DNA analysis: the historical case of the putative heart of Louis XVII. *International Journal of Legal Medicine*, **115**: 135–141.

Jennings, R.B., Ganote, C.E. and Reimer, K.A. (1975) Ischemic tissue injury. *American Journal of Pathology*, **81**: 179–198.

Kilpatrick, C.W. (2002) Noncryogenic preservation of mammalian tissues for DNA extraction: an assessment of storage methods. *Biochemical Genetics*, **40**: 53–62.

Kim, N.Y., Lee, H.Y., Park, S.J., Yang, W.I. and Shin, K.J. (2013) Modified midi- and mini-multiplex PCR systems for mitochondrial DNA control region sequence analysis in degraded samples. *Journal of Forensic Science*, **58**: 738–743.

Koon, H.E.C., Nicholson, R.A. and Collins, M.J. (2003) A practical approach to the identification of low temperture heated bone using TEM. *Journal of Archaeological Science*, **30**: 1393–1399.

Krause, J., Briggs, A.W., Kircher, M., Maricic, T., Zwyns, N. *et al.* (2010) A complete mtDNA genome of an early modern human from Kostenki, Russia. *Current Biology*, **29**: 231–236.

Langley, S.A., Karpen, G.H. and Langley, C.H. (2014) Nucleosomes shape DNA polymorphism and divergence. *PLoS Genetics*, **10**: e1004457.

Lazaridis, I., Patterson, N., Mittnik, A., Renaud, G., Mallick, S. *et al.* (2014) Ancient human genomes suggest three ancestral populations for present-day Europeans. *Nature*, **513**: 409–413.

Leonard, J.A., Shanks, O., Hofreiter, M., Kreuz, E., Hodges, L. *et al.* (2007) Animal DNA in PCR reagents plagues ancient DNA research. *Journal of Archaeological Science*, **34**: 1361–1366.

Lindahl, T. (1993) Recovery of antediluvian DNA. *Nature*, **365**: 700.

Lindahl, T. and Karlstrom, O. (1973) Heat-induced depyrimidination of deoxyribonucleic acid in neutral solution. *Biochemistry*, **12**: 5151–5154.

Lindahl, T. and Nyberg, B. (1972) Rate of depurination of native deoxyribonucleic acid. *Biochemistry*, **11**: 3610–3618.

Margulies, M., Egholm, M., Altman, W.E., Attiya, S., Bader, J.S. *et al.* (2005) Genome sequencing in microfabricated high-density picolitre reactors. *Nature*, **437**: 376–380.

Mayhew, T.M., Myklebust, R., Whybrow, A. and Jenkins, R. (1999) Epithelial integrity, cell death and cell loss in mammalian small intestine. *Histology and Histopathology*, **14**: 257–267.

Meyer, M., Fu, Q., Aximu-Petri, A., Glocke, I., Nickel, B., Arsuaga, J.L. *et al.* (2014) A mitochondrial genome sequence of a hominin from Sima de los Huesos. *Nature*, **505**: 403–406.

Meyer, M., Kircher, M., Gansauge, M.-T., Li, H., Racimo, F. *et al.* (2012) A high-coverage genome sequence from an archaic Denisovan individual. *Science*, **338**: 222–226.

Mikkelsen, M., Frank-Hansen, R., Hansen, A.J. and Morling, N. (2014) Massively parallel pyrosequencing of the mitochondrial genome with the 454 methodology in forensic genetics. *Forensic Science International: Genetics*, **12**: 30–37.

Milos, A., Selmanovic, A., Smajlovic, L., Huel, R.L., Katzmarzyk, C. *et al.* (2007) Success rates of nuclear short tandem repeat typing from different skeletal elements. *Croatian Medical Journal*, **48**: 486–493.

Mitchell, D., Willerslev, E. and Hansen, A. (2005) Damage and repair of ancient DNA. *Mutation Research*, **571**: 265–276.

Nielsen-Marsh, C.M. and Hedges, R.E.M. (1999) Bone porosity and the use of mercury intrusion porosimetry in bone diagenesis studies. *Archaeometry*, **41**: 165–174.

Olsen, M.E., Bengtsson, C.F., Bertelsen, M.F., Willerslev, E. and Gilbert, M.T. (2012) DNA from keratinous tissue. Part II: Feather. *Annals of Anatomy*, **194**: 31–35.

Orlando, L., Ginolhac, A., Zhang, G., Froese, D., Albrechtsen, A. *et al.* (2013) Recalibrating Equus evolution using the genome sequence of an early Middle Pleistocene horse. *Nature*, **499**: 74–78.

Ottoni, C., Koon, H.E., Collins, M.J., Penkman, K.E., Rickards, O. and Craig, O.E. (2009) Preservation of ancient DNA in thermally damaged archaeological bone. *Naturwissenschaften*, **96**: 267–278.

Pääbo, S. (1985) Molecular cloning of Ancient Egyptian mummy DNA. *Nature*, **314**: 644–645.

Pääbo, S., Poinar, H., Serre, D., Jaenicke-Despres, V., Hebler, J. *et al.* (2004) Genetic analyses from ancient DNA. *Annual Review of Genetics*, **38**: 645–679.

Pääbo, S. and Wilson, A.C. (1991) Miocene DNA sequences – a dream come true? *Current Biology*, **1**: 45–46.

Parson, W., Strobl, C., Huber, G., Zimmermann, B., Gomes, S.M. *et al.* (2013) Evaluation of next generation mtGenome sequencing using the Ion Torrent Personal Genome Machine (PGM). *Forensic Science International: Genetics*, **7**: 543–549.

Pilli, E., Modi, A., Serpico, C., Achilli, A., Lancioni, H. *et al.* (2013) Monitoring DNA contamination in handled vs. directly excavated ancient human skeletal remains. *PLoS One*, **8**: e52524.

Poinar, H.N., Hofreiter, M., Spaulding, W.G., Martin, P.S., Stankiewicz, B.A. *et al.* (1998) Molecular coproscopy: dung and diet of the extinct ground sloth *Nothrotheriops shastensis*. *Science*, **281**: 402–406.

Poinar, H.N., Hoss, M., Bada, J.L. and Pääbo, S. (1996) Amino acid racemization and the preservation of ancient DNA. *Science*, **272**: 864–866.

Poinar, H.N. and Stankiewicz, A.B. (1999) Protein preservation and DNA retrieval from ancient tissues. *Proceedings of the National Academy of Sciences of the United States of America*, **96**: 8426–8431.

Prinz, M., Carracedo, A., Mayr, W.R., Morling, N., Parsons, T.J. *et al.* (2007) DNA Commission of the International Society for Forensic Genetics (ISFG): recommendations regarding the role of forensic genetics for disaster victim identification (DVI). *Forensic Science International: Genetics*, **1**: 3–12.

Proskuryakov, S.Y., Konoplyannikov, A.G. and Gabai, V.L. (2003) Necrosis: a specific form of programmed cell death? *Experimental Cell Research*, **283**: 1–16.

Prufer, K., Racimo, F., Patterson, N., Jay, F., Sankararaman, S. *et al.* (2014) The complete genome sequence of a Neanderthal from the Altai Mountains. *Nature*, **505**: 43–49.

Pruvost, M., Grange, T. and Geigl, E.-M. (2005) Minimizing DNA-contamination by using UNG-coupled quantitative real-time PCR (UQPCR) on degraded DNA samples: application to ancient DNA studies. *Biotechniques*, **38**: 569–575.

Pruvost, M., Schwarz, R., Correia, V.B., Champlot, S., Braguier, S. *et al.* (2007) Freshly excavated fossil bones are best for amplification of ancient DNA. *Proceedings of the National Academy of Sciences of the United States of America*, **104**: 739–744.

Pusch, C.M., Giddings, I. and Scholz, M. (1998) Repair of degraded duplex DNA from prehistoric samples using *Escherichia coli* DNA polymerase I and T4 DNA ligase. *Nucleic Acids Research*, **26**: 857–859.

Raghavan, M., Skoglund, P., Graf, K.E., Metspalu, M., Albrechtsen, A. et al (2014) Upper Palaeolithic Siberian genome reveals dual ancestry of Native Americans. *Nature*, **505**: 87–91.

Rasmussen, M., Li, Y., Lindgreen, S., Pedersen, J.S., Albrechtsen, A. *et al.* (2010) Ancient human genome sequence of an extinct Palaeo-Eskimo. *Nature*, **463**: 757–762.

Robertson, J.M., Dineen, S.M., Scott, K.A, Lucyshyn, J., Saeed, M. *et al.* (2014) Assessing PreCR repair enzymes for restoration of STR profiles from artificially degraded DNA for human identification. *Forensic Science International: Genetics*, **12**: 168–180.

Rockenbauer, E., Hansen, S., Mikkelsen, M., Borsting, C. and Morling, N. (2014) Characterization of mutations and sequence variants in the D21S11 locus by next generation sequencing. *Forensic Science International: Genetics*, **8**: 68–72.

Sanchez, J.J., Phillips, C., Borsting, C., Balogh, K., Bogus, M. *et al.* (2006) A multiplex assay with 52 single nucleotide polymorphisms for human identification. *Electrophoresis*, **27**: 1713–1724.

Sawyer, S., Krause, J., Guschanski, K., Savolainen, V. and Pääbo, S. (2012) Temporal patterns of nucleotide misincorporations and DNA fragmentation in ancient DNA. *PLoS One*, **7**: e34131.

Scorrano, G., Valentini, F., Martinez-Labarga, C., Rolfo, M.F., Fiammenghi, A. *et al.* (2015) Methodological strategies to assess the degree of bone preservation for ancient DNA studies. *Annals of Human Biology*, 1–10.

Seo, S.B., King, J.L., Warshauer, D.H., Davi, s C.P., Ge, J. and Budowle, B. (2014) Single nucleotide polymorphism typing with massively parallel sequencing for human identification. *International Journal of Legal Medicine*, **127**: 1079–1086.

Shapiro, B. and Hofreiter, M. (2014) A paleogenomic perspective on evolution and gene function: new insights from ancient DNA. *Science*, **343**: 1236573.

Shapiro, R. (1981) Damage to DNA caused by hydrolisis. In: Seeberg, E. and Kleppe, K. (eds), *Chromosome Damage and Repair*. Plenum Press: New York, pp. 3–18.

Smith, C.I., Chamberlain, A., Riley, M.S., Stringer, C. and Collins, M.J. (2003) The thermal history of human fossils and the likelihood of successful DNA amplification. *Journal of Human Evolution*, **45**: 203–217.

Thanakiatkrai, P. and Welch, L. (2011) Evaluation of nucleosome forming potentials (NFPs) of forensically important STRs. *Forensic Science International: Genetics*, **5**: 285–290.

Tie, J. and Uchigasaki, S. (2013) DNA repair and STR PCR amplification from damaged DNA of human bloodstains. *Molecular Biology Reports*, **40**: 1505–1510.

Tomita, Y., Nihira, M., Ohno, Y. and Sato, S. (2004) Ultrastructural changes during in situ early postmortem autolysis in kidney, pancreas, liver, heart and skeletal muscle of rats. *Legal Medicine (Tokyo)*, **6**: 25–31.

Tucker, T., Marra, M. and Friedman, J.M. (2009) Massively parallel sequencing: the next big thing in genetic medicine. *American Journal of Human Genetics*, **85**: 142–154.

Van Neste, C., Van Nieuwerburgh, F., Van Hoofstat, D. and Deforce, D. (2012) Forensic STR analysis using massive parallel sequencing. *Forensic Science International: Genetics*, **6**: 810–818.

Willerslev, E., Cappellini, E., Boomsma, W., Nielsen, R., Hebsgaard, M.B. *et al.* (2007) Ancient biomolecules from deep ice cores reveal a forested southern Greenland. *Science*, **317**: 111–114.

Wyllie, A.H., Morris, R.G. and Smith, A.L. (1984) Chromatin cleavage in apoptosis: associated with condensed chromatin morphology and dependence on macromolecular synthesis. *Journal of Pathology*, **142**: 67–77.

Zeng, X., King, J.L., Stoljarova, M., Warshauer, D.H., La Rue, B.L. *et al.* (2014) High sensitivity multiplex short tandem repeat loci analyses with massively parallel sequencing. *Forensic Science International: Genetics*, **16C**: 38–47.

6

Taphonomic Alterations to Hair and Nail

Andrew S. Wilson

6.1 Introduction

This chapter explores the nature of changes that hair and nail can undergo in different depositional environments, drawing upon archaeological, forensic and experimental observations. It is important to distinguish between circumstances where naturally shed, forcibly removed fibres or cut fingernails may be found isolated from a body, and those instances where a body is encountered, for which broader taphonomic variables affecting the differential decomposition of body tissues can help to explain changes (Janaway *et al.* 2009; Wilson 2008; Wilson *et al.* 2007b).

Both hair and nail grow incrementally, yet these cellular structures are in essence dead once they emerge from the skin as hardened 'keratinised' structures. The only living portion of hair – the follicle – is seen to undergo distinct changes of morphology. The pattern of development follows predictable phases of growth (anagen), transition (catagen) and resting (telogen) that give rise to the hair growth cycle (Paus 1998). This cyclic pattern of hair growth, together with the fact that we do not moult, instead having a mosaic pattern of growth, explains the fact that roughly a hundred hairs are naturally shed from the body each day (Courtois *et al.* 1996).

Normal development of the nail plate, which grows at different incremental rates between fingernails and toenails (Kapickis 2003; Yaemsiri *et al.* 2010), will continue unchecked unless traumatic injury affects the nail bed. In cases of crush or avulsion injury, the nail may be shed with regrowth, which can take between 6 and 9 months, depending on the integrity of the nail bed (Zook 1985). Growth of both hair and nail is usually kept in check through normal grooming practice, which means that shed hair and nail clippings are often recoverable from domestic dwellings and in association with personal effects, which may be particularly relevant as ante-mortem reference samples as part of a missing persons investigation, or Disaster Victim Identification (DVI).

Hair and nail are relatively robust tissues and so long as the depositional environment is relatively dry and stable, isolated fibres and nail clippings can survive indefinitely given the right conditions. Of course, a multitude of environmental conditions can be expected in different depositional environments, which justifies using archaeological experience to consider variables affecting hair and nail degradation over extended timescales. The fact that within the archaeological record, hair and nail will normally only survive under extreme environmental conditions, emphasises the dominant role that microbial biodeterioration plays in their destruction. Keratin is recognised as being recalcitrant to many common proteolytic enzymes, and as such, only keratinolytic microorganisms, which produce keratinase enzymes, have the capacity to exploit keratin as a sole nutrient source, unless these structures have already undergone some alteration (Gupta and Ramnani 2006). Furthermore, the age of the specimen is largely irrelevant in relation to taphonomic alteration, since it is the localised

Taphonomy of Human Remains: Forensic Analysis of the Dead and the Depositional Environment, First Edition.
Edited by Eline M.J. Schotsmans, Nicholas Márquez-Grant and Shari L. Forbes.

environment that will determine the extent of biological activity, based on the key variables of temperature, light, aeration, moisture, salinity and pH. This normally means that within the wider environment, these tissues survive long term where they are shielded from light and as a consequence of desiccation, waterlogging or extreme cold, which are all conditions under which microbial activity is retarded or ceases altogether.

Hair and nail are recognised as valuable repositories of information (Wilson 2005; Wilson and Gilbert 2007). Traditional methods of morphological characterisation of hair (Tridico *et al.* 2014) use comparison of external features, such as cuticle scale pattern and fibre diameter, and internal features, such as medulla, pigment density and cortical fusi, using light microscopy of fibre whole mounts, scale casts and fibre cross-sections. Whilst the follicle used to be the preferred source of DNA, the hair shaft and nail plate are now recognised as a source of biomolecular information using both DNA and proteomics (Bengtsson *et al.* 2012; Edson *et al.* 2013; Parker *et al.* 2016; Solazzo *et al.* 2013). Furthermore, hair and nail are important because of the incremental way in which these tissues develop. Of key importance is the fact that once formed, these tissues do not undergo biogenic alteration. In the case of terminal scalp hair, it grows at a fairly constant rate of roughly 1 cm per month (Wilson and Gilbert 2007), although this varies between population groups (Loussouarn 2001). The incremental nature of hair growth offers a timeline of recent lifeways information, such as sequential data on health, physiology nutrition and starvation, using stable light isotopes and on chronic drug use with mass spectrometry (Thompson *et al.* 2014; Wilson *et al.* 2013). Ultimately, the amount of potential information is dependent on the fibre or nail length and the sample requirements of different analytical methods. It is worthwhile also noting that by harnessing an understanding of the formation times of different body tissues – from hair/nail and muscle (recent), to bone (lifetime average) and teeth (childhood) – it may be possible to create a composite picture of lifeways information that can augment a biological profile for unidentified remains.

6.2 Structure of Hair and Nail

Although markedly different in appearance, hair and nail share a common chemistry and origin, which are detailed elsewhere (de Berker 2013; McCarthy 2004; Robbins 2002; Ryder 1973). Both tissues derive from the ectoderm during late embryonic development and have a heterogeneous structure based on the arrangement of keratinised cells.

The nail plate, which comprises multiple layers of flattened keratinised cells, varies markedly in thickness (Mogensen *et al.* 2007) and rate of growth, between fingernails and toenails. Both have a hard resistant structure, with some elasticity and translucency. The nail plate comprises three main layers – ranging from the hard, dense, smooth outer (dorsal) surface (~200 μm thick), only a few cells thick, to the thinnest lower (ventral) layer that connects the nail plate with the underlying nail bed. The main bulk of the nail plate comprises the intermediate layer, with a fibrous structure that is oriented perpendicular to the direction of nail growth.

Terminal human scalp hair shares features common with fibres from other mammalian species (Thomas *et al.* 2012) – comprising a protective outer cuticle, responsible also for the optical properties of the fibre; the cortex, the main bulk of the hair shaft, offering strength, resilience and flexibility to the fibre and the central medulla, which may be continuous, discontinuous or absent. Key distinctions between species include variations in fibre diameter; the thickness or number of cells comprising the cuticle and the diameter and form of the medulla. Outwardly, protection of the hair fibre is afforded by the lipid-protein complex of the exocuticle, which conveys hydrophobicity (Bringans *et al.* 2007).

The three-dimensional architecture of macrofibrils within individual cortical cells gives rise to the mechanical properties of human hair (Harland *et al.* 2014). The bilateral arrangement of cortical cells into orthocortex and paracortex, which is more distinct in wool, results from the concentration of cysteine and the higher proportion of ultra-high sulphur proteins in the tightly packed paracortex, compared with the less densely packed orthocortex (Plowman *et al.* 2007). In physical terms, these distinctions give rise to the amount of curl in a fibre, with the paracortex on the concave inside of the crimp wave and the orthocortex on the convex outside of the crimp wave. A third, intermediate type of cell has also been described as the mesocortex (Plowman *et al.* 2007). A further distinction is the amount of matrix material in each, with greater electron density of the matrix relative to the intermediate filaments, observed under transmission electron microscopy and attributed to more disulphide bonds within the matrix.

6.3 Changes to Hair and Nail

Nutritional deficiency, especially protein intake, can affect the growth of hair and nail (Cashman and Sloan 2010; Goldberg and Lenzy 2010). Diseases of the hair/scalp and nailbed can affect the strength of hair and nail, including dermatophytic infections, or relatively rare developmental conditions with associated hair fragility, such as monilithrix, which results in changes to hair proteins comparable to oxidative damage due to chemical insult from cosmetics (Sinclair *et al.* 2012). Both disease and aggressive grooming practice can affect the condition of hair in life and make these tissues more susceptible to changes that can occur within the depositional environment.

6.3.1 Physical Alteration

Hair can undergo physical change in living individuals – largely as a direct result of aggressive grooming practice. Frequent washing and brushing of hair can result in physical abrasion of the outer cuticle, initially causing damage to the margins of individual cuticle cells. Aggressive brushing and combing will lead ultimately to breakage and loss of the cuticle. Where the cuticle is lost in its entirety to expose the underlying cortex, there is little to safeguard against separation of cortical cells – essentially the changes responsible for split ends. Hair and nail have a significant water content, and the use of heat tongs at the wrong setting is known to cause swelling and thus physical damage to hair, due to the effect of excess heat on this moisture (Christian *et al.* 2011). Because of the incremental nature of hair, growth changes are more pronounced towards the distal end due to greater cumulative damage to these, the oldest parts of the hair shaft. Such progressive changes are termed 'weathering' (Bottoms *et al.* 1972; Dawber 2002) and can physically weaken the fibre, exposing it to a broader range of insults – including chemical and biological attack. Weathering has been demonstrated to have an effect on stable light isotope values in cattle tail hair (Auerswald *et al.* 2011). The progress of morphological change can be seen using various histological means of assessment, combining fibre cross-section techniques, such as high resolution light microscopy and transmission electron microscopy, and fibre whole mounts, using both light microscopy and fluorescence microscopy with different staining techniques and scanning electron microscopy (Wilson *et al.* 2010b).

6.3.2 Chemical Alteration

The over-use of hair care/cosmetic products, including bleach, chemical straighteners, perming, colourants or highlights, can have a deleterious effect on hair (Gavazzoni Dias 2015; Miranda-Vilela *et al.* 2013; Tate *et al.* 1993). Whilst many hair care product ingredients are intended to provide positive benefits, such as improved tensile strength and hydrophobicity (Oshimura *et al.* 2007), even seemingly innocuous styling sprays and mousses that are alcohol-based, can have a drying effect on hair in the long term.

Hair and nail can tolerate a wide range of pH conditions. Since the skin is mildly acidic, it is not surprising to note that alkalis have a more marked effect on keratin structures, although both strong acids and strong alkalis can denature hair and nail. Under controlled parameters, high pH conditions are used within cosmetic treatment, as with the use of sodium hydroxide to bring about chemical straightening of hair. Given that such chemicals can also be found in many cleaning products, including drain cleaners, the potential dramatic effect on hair and nail is noteworthy. The structural changes that can be brought about have been seen to affect hair differently, according to race (Kuzuhara 2005; Lee *et al.* 2014).

Given that hair and nail are normally found associated with bodies in the archaeological record where other biomaterials also survive (bone, teeth and potentially other soft tissues), there is often comparative data on how aggressive conditions have been within the depositional environment, by examining the extent of differential decomposition across these tissues.

There are exceptional circumstances where all that remain are keratotics, such as hair, nail and proteinaceous clothing items (woollen textiles and hides). These situations usually occur where low temperature and/or waterlogged acidic pH conditions persist, and include findings of cut hair in organic-rich deposits, such as at Deer Park Farms in Ireland (Wilson 2010a) and from permafrost in Greenland (Rasmussen *et al.* 2010). Specialised microenvironments may develop, such as within oak coffin burials where the acidic conditions, brought about by formation of tannic acids derived from the oak coffin, destroy mineralised structures such as bone and teeth. Examples include the remains of a woman found at Quernmore, Lancashire in the UK, where only hair, fingernails and a woollen cloak survived (Turner 1995) and with the Egtved woman from Denmark (Frei *et al.* 2015), where hair, textile and a hide cloak were all that remained.

These rare situations also emphasise the robust nature of hair in relation to putrefactive change and mild acidic conditions that are otherwise destructive to other tissues. However, these observations do not mean that hair and nail is immune from degradative change. These structures are subject to hydrolytic and oxidative change and this is evidenced by work on wool fibres from wet depositional environments (von Holstein *et al.* 2014). It is evident that variations in localised depositional conditions are responsible for different degrees of chemical breakdown, such as deamidation of the alpha keratin structure (Solazzo *et al.* 2014).

Gerontobiology shows us that in addition to fundamental changes to the hair growth cycle (Messenger 2011; Van Neste and Tobin 2004), the underlying substructure of the fibre is affected by ageing – with hair follicles reprogramming matrix keratinocytes to 'increase production of medullary, rather than cortical keratinocytes', as evidenced by increased growth and medullation to fibres alongside decreased pigmentation (Trueb 2009). These physical rearrangements to the hair shaft can offer a greater surface area to chemical and biological attack, as well as reducing the quantity of pigment, which is also more resistant to microbial attack.

All hair contains a mixture of eumelanin and phaeomelanin, which are responsible for the black-brown and red-yellow colouration of hair respectively, alongside factors such as pigment density. Whilst there is a sound basis to explain potential changes to hair colouration, based on chemical alteration to hair pigmentation under both oxidising and reducing conditions – this generally requires either extreme desiccating conditions or extreme waterlogging, which even under archaeological conditions accounts for a small proportion of the surviving examples. In each case, the less stable eumelanin, either decolourises (oxidising conditions) or turns red (reducing conditions), resulting in an overall enhancement of the red-yellow phaeomelanin (Wilson *et al.* 2001). Of course, other parameters need to be taken into account, such as changes to the optical properties of the fibre, based on cuticle condition and the infiltration of material from the depositional environment, for example humic material from waterlogged conditions. Many examples of dark pigmented hair have been recovered from the archaeological record (Wilson and Tobin 2010).

6.3.3 Biological Alteration

Although only keratinolytic species can exploit hair and nail in its native state as a sole nutrient source, these organisms have fairly widespread geographic distribution, having been linked to contact with animals and other humans (Chermette *et al.* 2008; Nweze 2011; Okafor and Ada 2000; Spiewak and Szostak 2000; Weitzman and Summerbell 1995) and a wide range of different soil environments (Abdel-Fattah *et al.* 1982; Deshmukh and Verekar 2014; Filipello Marchisio *et al.* 1991; Kaul and Sumbali 1997). Infections caused by Dermatophytes (typically members of the *Microsporum, Trichophyton* and *Epidermophyton* genera) and non-dermatophytic infections affecting hair and nail, have been extensively reported within the clinical literature (Nenoff *et al.* 2014a; Segal and Frenkel 2015; Shemer *et al.* 2015) for which targeted therapies are recommended (Nenoff *et al.* 2014b, 2015). Some bacteria and actinobacteria can also exploit keratin as a sole nutrient source, of importance in managing keratinous waste – such as rendering waste poultry feather (Brandelli *et al.* 2010; Kornillowicz-Kowalska and Bohacz 2010, 2011).

One distinctive feature of keratinolytic fungi is that they produce boring hyphae. These penetrating organs, often with an 'anvil-shaped' form, produce keratinase enzymes that attack the disulphide bonds of the keratin substrate (Deshmukh and Agrawal 1982, 1985; English 1963; Kunert and Krajci 1981). The term keratinolytic fungi emphasises their lytic activity that results in characteristic focal destruction (Figure 6.1). These ovoid lesions have erosive margins and the openings of so-called 'fungal tunnels' (DeGaetano *et al.* 1992) that initially run perpendicular to the main fibre axis, before allowing the hyphae to exploit inherent weaknesses as they branch out laterally within the cortex and medulla (Figure 6.2). Microbial alteration to hair will change the appearance of the fibre in several ways – by either destroying tissue or physically disrupting the layered structure of the fibre, particularly the outer cuticle, which is largely responsible for the optical properties of the fibre. The structures have varied resistance to enzymatic attack, with melanin pigment granules being most resistant (Figure 6.3) (Wilson *et al.* 2007a). Once either biological or chemical change has been initiated, this physically opens these tissues up to exploitation by a wider range of bacteria and fungi, which can then gain access past the protective outer cuticle, and can make use of the chemically less-resistant structures and breakdown products (Wilson 2010b; Wilson *et al.* 2007a).

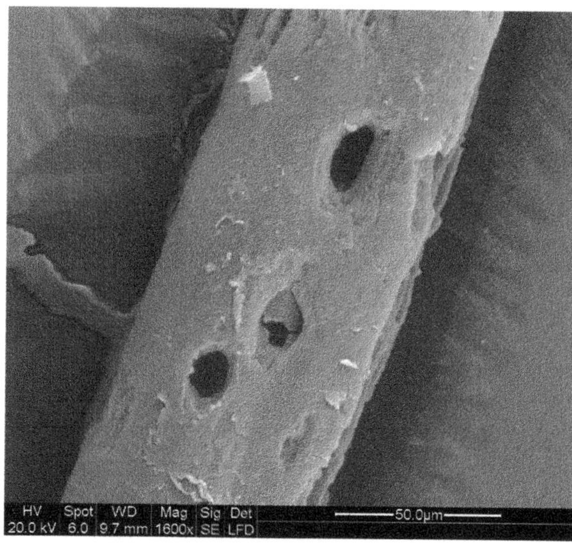

Figure 6.1 Scanning electron micrograph of scalp hair affected by keratinolytic fungi, evident from characteristic ovoid lesions created by fungal tunnelling. Bar = 50 μm

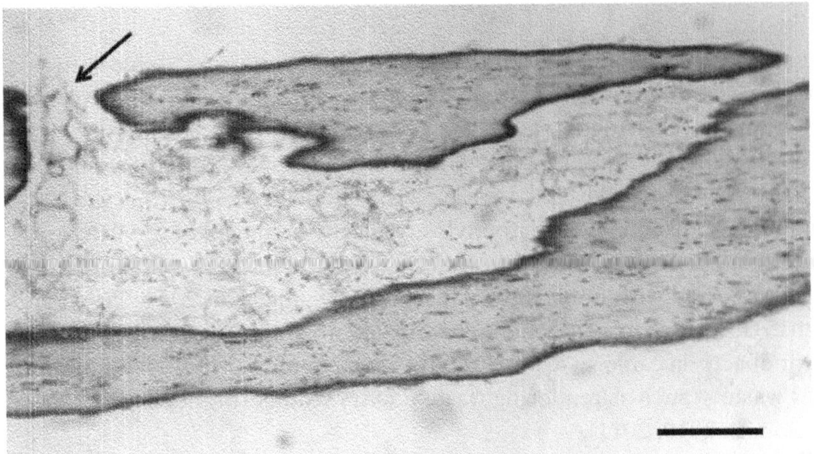

Figure 6.2 Transverse semi-thin section of scalp hair stained with toluidine blue in borax showing fungal tunnelling in progress (arrow), with fungal hyphae extending within the hair shaft. Bar = 15 μm

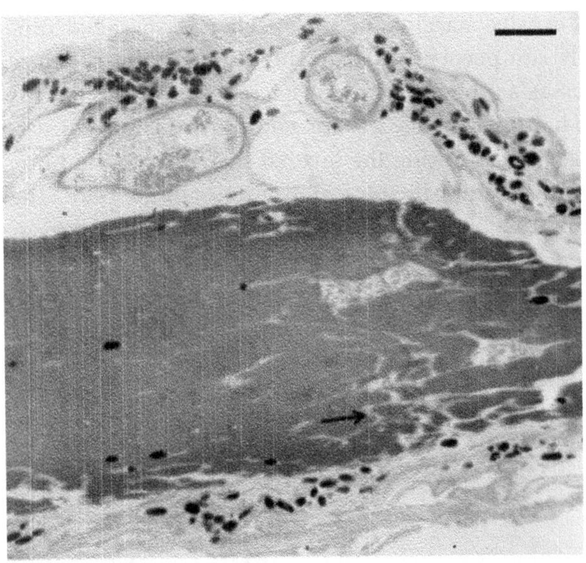

Figure 6.3 Transverse ultra-thin transmission electron micrograph, showing enzymatic attack resulting in separation of macrofibrils (arrow). The circular black structures aggregated within the fungal hyphae are melanin pigment granules which are chemically distinct from keratin and more resistant to enzymatic attack. Bar = 5 μm

6.3.4 Changes Associated with Body Decomposition

During active putrefactive change, the integument undergoes a process commonly termed skin slippage (Dix and Graham 2000; Janaway *et al.* 2009). During this wet phase of decomposition, the hair and nail can be lost as the skin is weakened and sloughs off the body.

Hair recovered from decomposed or partially decomposed human remains has been shown to undergo alteration, with characteristic changes evident to the proximal end of fibres that were in anagen and catagen (Koch *et al.* 2013). Post-mortem root banding is a feature that is associated with putrefactive changes and is visible in the 'soft' unkeratinised region of the hair shaft (Koch *et al.* 2013). The onset of post-mortem root banding, which is hastened by conditions conducive to putrefaction such as warm temperatures, has also been observed to have been delayed where putrefaction is similarly retarded in aqueous environments and conditions which influence desiccation, such as air-conditioning and cold weather (Koch *et al.* 2013).

The phenomenon of post-mortem banding is influenced by staining from putrefactive changes to the skin, and the infiltration of degradative products to the porous structure of the developing proximal fibre. It is a function of the structural differentiation during hair shaft formation, where initially intermediate filaments are aggregated into fibrils. These regions of the developing fibre have a more open structure, prior to the synthesis and insertion of matrix proteins that have been shown to aggregate as 'blocks', which subsequently disperse between the intermediate filaments as differentiation advances within the zone of keratinisation (Rogers 2004).

In archaeological cases where hair is encountered with human remains, it is often devoid of scalp tissue (particularly in temperate 18/19th century contexts). Commonly, short embrittled fibre lengths may be encountered without discernible root, their embrittled nature characteristic of breakage caused by fungal tunnelling action by keratinolytic fungi, which produce ovoid lytic lesions disrupting the hair shaft. In the best surviving examples involving exceptionally preserved bodies in archaeology, principles of conservation often override the potential for using invasive methods, such as plucking hair or excising tissue that will potentially damage the remains, and are in favour instead of cutting hair close to the scalp. With both situations, it is unlikely that the most proximal portion of the fibre will be available and so post-mortem root banding will not be evident on examination.

In terms of entomology, late stage arrivals to a corpse include insects from the family Dermistidae (e.g. *Anthrenus spp.* – carpet beetles; *Dermestes maculatus* – the hide beetle) and the family Tineidae (the clothes' moths). The common names for these insects emphasise the special adaptations that their larvae have in order to be able to exploit keratin – including use of chewing mouthparts and keratinolytic enzymes in order to digest keratin (Cohen 2015). It is possible to clearly distinguish between breakage of fibres due to forcible trauma and entomological activity using SEM (Mazzarelli *et al.* 2015).

6.4 Processing and Storage of Hair

Despite the range of possible insults to hair and nail, dry samples can generally be stored under stable conditions at room temperature. Acid-free paper bags are preferable to plastic, since biomolecular evidence is an important consideration, with long-term contact with plasticisers a potential issue for analysis by chromatography.

Hair and nails can retain valuable microscopic evidence, including particulates, such as gunshot and explosives residues or testate amoebae, pollen and soil that serve as valuable ecological indicators. Recommendations exist for processing hair for this type of evidence at autopsy (Wiltshire 2006).

When hair and nail is recovered from a body in casework, it is possible for hair to be saturated in blood, putrefactive by-products or other moisture/nutrient-laden sources, depending on the circumstances of the case. If it is recovered damp, it is important that this hair is either processed immediately or frozen on recovery. Since this text is intended both for forensic practitioners and those in other related disciplines such as archaeology, it is important to highlight that poor practice in terms of packaging and curation has seen fungal activity re-established on samples stored damp from excavation, where soft tissue or putrefactive fluids were present with the hair (Wilson and Tobin 2010).

6.5 Conclusion

The evidential or research value of hair and nail continues to expand with new biomolecular approaches, many of which exploit the incremental nature of hair and nail growth. Hair and nail are robust biomaterials that will persist over considerable time depths unless exposed to various different taphonomic variables. Only a discrete range of 'keratinolytic' organisms can exploit hair and nail as a sole nutrient source. Characteristic biological and chemically induced changes to hair are usually readily identifiable as the cause, and can be distinguished from weathering in life. These alterations can provide access to a wide range of insults when the protective structures such as the cuticle are breached, hastening further alteration.

Acknowledgements

The author wishes to thank Professor Des Tobin and the support of colleagues in the Centre for Skin Sciences at the University of Bradford, as well as Rob Janaway, Professor Mark Pollard, Dr Hilary Dodson and colleagues in the School of Archaeological Sciences.

References

Abdel-Fattah, H.M., Moubasher, A.H. and Maghazy, S.M. (1982) Keratinolytic fungi in Egyptian soils. *Mycopathologia*, **79**: 49–53.

Auerswald, K., Rossmann, A., Schaufele, R., Schwertl, M., Monahan, F.J. and Schnyder, H. (2011) Does natural weathering change the stable isotope composition ((2)H, (1)(3)C, (1)(5)N, (1)(8)O and (3)(4)S) of cattle hair? *Rapid Communications in Mass Spectrometry*, **25**: 3741–3748.

Bengtsson, C.F., Olsen, M.E., Brandt, L.O., Bertelsen, M.F., Willerslev, E. *et al.* (2012) DNA from keratinous tissue. Part I: Hair and nail. *Annals of Anatomy*, **194**: 17–25.

Bottoms, E., Wyatt, E. and Comaish, S. (1972) Progressive changes in cuticular pattern along the shafts of human hair as seen by scanning electron microscopy. *British Journal of Dermatology*, **86**: 379–384.

Brandelli, A., Daroit, D.J. and Riffel, A. (2010) Biochemical features of microbial keratinases and their production and applications. *Applied Microbiology and Biotechnology*, **85**: 1735–1750.

Bringans, S.D., Plowman, J.E., Dyer, J.M., Clerens, S., Vernon, J.A. and Bryson, W.G. (2007) Characterization of the exocuticle a-layer proteins of wool. *Experimental Dermatology*, **16**: 951–960.

Cashman, M.W. and, Sloan, S.B. (2010) Nutrition and nail disease. *Clinical Dermatology*, **28**: 420–425.

Chermette, R., Ferreiro, L. and Guillot, J. (2008) Dermatophytoses in animals. *Mycopathologia*, **166**: 385–405.

Christian, P., Winsey, N., Whatmough, M. and Cornwell, P.A. (2011) The effects of water on heat-styling damage. *Journal of Cosmetic Science*, **62**: 15–27.

Cohen, A.C. (2015) *Insect Diets: Science and Technology*. Boca Raton: CRC Press.

Courtois, M., Loussouarn, G., Hourseau, S. and Grollier, J.F. (1996) Periodicity in the growth and shedding of hair. *British Journal of Dermatology*, **134**: 47–54.

Dawber, R. (2002) Cosmetic and medical causes of hair weathering. *Journal of Cosmetic Dermatology*, **1**: 196–201.

de Berker, D. (2013) Nail anatomy. *Clinical Dermatology*, **31**: 509–515.

DeGaetano, D.H., Kempton, J.B. and Rowe, W.F. (1992) Fungal tunneling of hair from a buried body. *Journal of Forensic Science*, **37**: 1048–1054.

Deshmukh, S.K. and Agrawal, S.C. (1982) *In vitro* degradation of human hair by some keratinophilic fungi. *Mykosen*, **25**: 454–458.

Deshmukh, S.K. and Agrawal, S.C. (1985) Degradation of human hair by some dermatophytes and other keratinophilic fungi. *Mykosen*, **28**: 463–466.

Deshmukh, S.K. and Verekar, S.A. (2014) Isolation of keratinophilic fungi from selected soils of Sanjay Gandhi National Park, Mumbai (India). *Journal de Mycologie Medicale*, **24**: 319–327.

Dix, J. and Graham, M. (2000) *Time of Death, Decomposition and Identification: An atlas*. CRC Press: Boca Raton.

Edson, J., Brooks, E.M., McLaren, C., Robertson, J., McNevin, D. et al (2013) A quantitative assessment of a reliable screening technique for the STR analysis of telogen hair roots. *Forensic Science International Genetics*, **7**: 180–188.

English, M.P. (1963) The saprophytic growth of keratinophilic fungi on keratin. *Sabouraudia*, **2**: 115–130.

Filipello Marchisio, V., Curetti, D., Cassinelli, C. and Bordese, C. (1991) Keratinolytic and keratinophilic fungi in the soils of Papua New Guinea. *Mycopathologia*, **115**: 113–119.

Frei, K.M., Mannering, U., Kristiansen, K., Allentoft, M.E., Wilson, A.S. *et al*. (2015) Tracing the dynamic life story of a Bronze Age Female. *Scientific Reports*, **5**: 10431.

Gavazzoni Dias, M.F. (2015) Hair cosmetics: an overview. *International Journal of Trichology*, **7**: 2–15.

Goldberg, L.J. and Lenzy, Y. (2010) Nutrition and hair. *Clinical Dermatology*, **28**: 412–419.

Gupta, R. and Ramnani, P. (2006) Microbial keratinases and their prospective applications: an overview. *Applied Microbiology and Biotechnology*, **70**: 21–33.

Harland, D.P., Walls, R.J., Vernon, J.A., Dyer, J.M., Woods, J.L. and Bell, F. (2014) Three-dimensional architecture of macrofibrils in the human scalp hair cortex. *Journal of Structural Biology*, **185**: 397–404.

Janaway, R.C., Percival, S.L. and Wilson, A.S. (2009) Decomposition of human remains. In: Percival, S.L. (ed.), *Microbiology and Aging*. Springer: New York; pp. 313–334.

Kapickis, M. (2003) Rate of fingernail growth. *Plastic Reconstruction Surgery*, **112**: 1501.

Kaul, S. and Sumbali, G. (1997) Keratinolysis by poultry farm soil fungi. *Mycopathologia*, **139**: 137–140.

Koch, S.L., Michaud, A.L. and Mikell, C.E. (2013) Taphonomy of hair – a study of postmortem root banding. *Journal of Forensic Science*, **58**: S52–S59.

Kornillowicz-Kowalska, T. and Bohacz, J. (2010) Dynamics of growth and succession of bacterial and fungal communities during composting of feather waste. *Bioresource Technology*, **101**: 1268–1276.

Kornillowicz-Kowalska, T. and Bohacz, J. (2011) Biodegradation of keratin waste: theory and practical aspects. *Waste Management*, **31**: 1689–1701.

Kunert, J. and Krajci, D. (1981) An electron microscopy study of keratin degradation by the fungus *Microsporum gypseum in vitro*. *Mykosen*, **24**: 485–496.

Kuzuhara, A. (2005) Analysis of structural change in keratin fibers resulting from chemical treatments using Raman spectroscopy. *Biopolymers*, **77**: 335–344.

Lee,Y., Kim, Y.D., Pi, L.Q., Lee, S.Y., Hong, H. and Lee, W.S. (2014) Comparison of hair shaft damage after chemical treatment in Asian, White European and African hair. *International Journal of Dermatology*, **53**: 1103–1110.

Loussouarn, G. (2001) African hair growth parameters. *British Journal of Dermatology*, **145**: 294–297.

Mazzarelli, D., Vanin, S., Gibelli, D., Maistrello, L., Porta, D. *et al*. (2015) Splitting hairs: differentiating between entomological activity, taphonomy and sharp force trauma on hair. *Forensic science, Medicine, and Pathology*, **11**: 104–110.

McCarthy, D.J. (2004) Anatomic considerations of the human nail. *Clinics in Podiatric Medicine and Surgery*, **21**: 477–491.

Messenger, A.G. (2011) Hair through the female life cycle. *British Journal of Dermatology*, **165** Suppl **3**: 2–6.

Miranda-Vilela, A.L., Botelho, A.J. and Muehlmann, L.A. (2013) An overview of chemical straightening of human hair: technical aspects, potential risks to hair fibre and health and legal issues. *International Journal of Cosmetic Science*, **36**: 2–11.

Mogensen, M., Thomsen, J.B., Skovgaard, L.T. and Jemec, G.B. (2007) Nail thickness measurements using optical coherence tomography and 20-MHz ultrasonography. *British Journal of Dermatology*, **157**: 894–900.

Nenoff, P., Kruger, C., Ginter-Hanselmayer, G. and Tietz, H.J. (2014a) Mycology – an update. Part 1: Dermatomycoses: causative agents, epidemiology and pathogenesis. *Journal der Deutschen Dermatologischen Gesellschaft*, **12**: 188–209.

Nenoff, P., Kruger, C., Schaller, J., Ginter-Hanselmayer, G., Schulte-Beerbuhl, R. and Tietz, H.J. (2014b) Mycology – an update. Part 2: Dermatomycoses: clinical picture and diagnostics. *Journal der Deutschen Dermatologischen Gesellschaft*, **12**: 749–777.

Nenoff, P., Kruger, C., Paasch, U. and Ginter-Hanselmayer, G. (2015) Mycology – an update. Part 3: Dermatomycoses: topical and systemic therapy. *Journal der Deutschen Dermatologischen Gesellschaft*, **13**: 387–410.

Nweze, E.I. (2011) Dermatophytoses in domesticated animals. *Revista do Instituto de Medicina Tropical de Sao Paulo*, **53**: 94–99.

Okafor, J.I. and Ada, N. (2000) Keratinolytic activity of five human isolates of the dermatophytes. *Journal of Communicable Diseases*, **32**: 300–305.

Oshimura, E., Abe, H. and Oota, R. (2007) Hair and amino acids: the interactions and the effects. *Journal of Cosmetic Science*, **58**: 347–357.

Paus, R. (1998) Principles of hair cycle control. *Journal of Dermatology*, **25**: 793–802.

Parker, G.J., Leppert, T., Anex, D.S., Hilmer, J.K. and Matsunami, N. *et al.* (2016) Demonstration of protein-based human identification using the hair shaft proteome. *PLoS ONE*, **11**: e0160653.

Plowman, J.E., Paton, L.N. and Bryson, W.G. (2007) The differential expression of proteins in the cortical cells of wool and hair fibres. *Experimental Dermatology*, **16**: 707–714.

Rasmussen, M., Li, Y., Lindgreen, S., Pedersen, J.S., Albrechtsen, A. *et al.* (2010) Ancient human genome sequence of an extinct Palaeo-Eskimo. *Nature*, **463**: 757–762.

Robbins, C.T. (2002) *Chemical and Physical Behavior of Human Hair*. Springer-Verlag: New York.

Rogers, G.E. (2004) Hair follicle differentiation and regulation. *The International Journal of Developmental Biology*, **48**: 163–170.

Ryder, M.L. (1973) *Hair*. The Institute of Biology: London.

Segal, E. and Frenkel, M. (2015) Dermatophyte infections in environmental contexts. *Research in Microbiology*, **166**: 564–569.

Shemer, A., Gupta, A.K., Farhi, R., Daigle, D. and Amichai, B. (2015) When is onychomycosis onychomycosis? A cross-sectional study of fungi in normal-appearing nails. *British Journal of Dermatology*, **172**: 380–383.

Sinclair, R., Flagler, M.J., Jones, L., Rufaut, Nm and Davism M,G, (2012) The proteomic profile of hair damage. *British Journal of Dermatologym* **166 Suppl 2**: 27–32.

Solazzo, C., Wadsley, M., Dyer, J.M., Clerens, S., Collins, M.J. and Plowman, J. (2013) Characterisation of novel alpha-keratin peptide markers for species identification in keratinous tissues using mass spectrometry. *Rapid Communications in Mass Spectrometry*, **27**: 2685–2698.

Solazzo, C., Wilson, J., Dyer, J.M., Clerens, S., Plowman, J.E. *et al.* (2014) Modeling deamidation in sheep alpha-keratin peptides and application to archeological wool textiles. *Analytical Chemistry*, **86**: 567–575.

Spiewak, R. and Szostak, W. (2000) Zoophilic and geophilic dermatophytoses among farmers and non-farmers in Eastern Poland. *Annals of Agricultural and Environmental Medicine*, **7**: 125–129.

Tate, M.L., Kamath, Y.K. and Ruetsch, S.B. (1993) Quantification and prevention of hair damage. *Journal of the Society of Cosmetic Chemists*, **44**: 347–371.

Thomas, A., Harland, D.P., Clerens, S., Deb-Choudhury, S., Vernon, J.A. *et al.* (2012) Interspecies comparison of morphology, ultrastructure, and proteome of mammalian keratin fibers of similar diameter. *Journal of Agricultural Food Chemistry*, **60**: 2434–2446.

Thompson, A.H., Wilson, A.S. and Ehleringer, J.R. (2014) Hair as a geochemical recorder: ancient to modern. In: Cerling, T.E. (ed.), *Treatise on Geochemistry: Archaeology and Anthropology*. Elsevier: Cambridge, pp. 371–393.

Tridico, S.R, Houck, M.M., Kirkbride, K.P., Smith, M.E. and Yates, B.C. (2014) Morphological identification of animal hairs: myths and misconceptions, possibilities and pitfalls. *Forensic Science International*, **238**: 101–107.

Trueb, R.M. (2009) Oxidative stress in ageing of hair. *International Journal of Trichology*, **1**: 6–14.

Turner, R.C. (1995) Gazetteer of bog bodies in the British Isles. In: Turner, R.C. and Scaife, R.G. (eds), *Bog Bodies, New Discoveries and New Perspectives*. British Museum Press: London, pp. 205–234.

Van Neste, D. and Tobin, D.J. (2004) Hair cycle and hair pigmentation: dynamic interactions and changes associated with aging. *Micron*, **35**: 193–200.

von Holstein, I.C., Penkman, K.E., Peacock, E.E. and Collins, M.J. (2014) Wet degradation of keratin proteins: linking amino acid, elemental and isotopic composition. *Rapid Communications in Mass Spectrometry*, **28**: 2121–2133.

Weitzman, I. and Summerbell, R.C. (1995) The dermatophytes. *Clinical Microbiology Reviews*, **8**: 240–259.

Wilson, A.S. (2005) Hair as a Bioresource in Archaeological Study. In: Tobin, D.J. (ed.), *Hair in Toxicology: an Important Biomonitor*. Royal Society of Chemistry: Cambridge, pp. 321–345.

Wilson, A.S. (2008) The decomposition of hair in the buried body environment. In: Tibbett, M. and Carter, D.O. (eds), *Soil Analysis in Forensic Taphonomy: Chemical and biological effects of buried human remains*. CRC Press: Boca Raton, pp. 123–151.

Wilson, A.S. (2010a) The condition of the Deer Park Farms hair and its potential for stable isotope investigation. In: McDowell, J. (ed.), *Deer Park Farms*. Department of the Environment, Northern Ireland, pp. 490–496.

Wilson, A.S. and Gilbert, M.T.P. (2007) Hair and nail. In: Thompson, T. and Black, S. (eds), *Forensic Human Identification: An introduction*. CRC Press: Boca Raton, pp. 147–174.

Wilson, A.S. and Tobin, D.J. (2010) Hair after death. In: Trueb, R.M. and Tobin, D.J. (eds), *Aging Hair*. Springer: New York, pp. 249–261.

Wilson, A.S., Dixon, R.A., Dodson, H.I., Janaway, R.C., Pollard, A.M. *et al*. (2001) Yesterday's hair-human hair in archaeology. *Biologist (London)*, **48**: 213–217.

Wilson, A.S., Dodson, H.I., Janaway, R.C., Pollard, A.M. and Tobin, D.J. (2007a) Selective biodegradation in hair shafts derived from archaeological, forensic and experimental contexts. *British Journal of Dermatology*, **157**: 450–457.

Wilson, A.S., Janaway, R.C., Holland, A.D., Dodson, H.I., Baran, E. *et al*. (2007b). Modelling the buried human body environment in upland climes using three contrasting field sites. *Forensic Science International*, **169**: 6–18.

Wilson, A.S., Dodson, H.I., Janaway, R.C., Pollard, A.M. and Tobin, D.J. (2010b) Evaluating histological methods for assessing hair fibre degradation. *Archaeometry*, **52**: 467–481.

Wilson, A.S., Brown, E..L, Villa, C., Lynnerup, N., Healey, A. et al, (2013) Archaeological, radiological and biological evidence offer insight into Inca child sacrifice. *Proceedings of the National Academy of Sciences*, **110**: 13322–13327.

Wiltshire, P.E.J. (2006) Hair as a source of forensic evidence in murder investigations. *Forensic Science International*, **163**: 241–248.

Yaemsiri, S., Hou, N., Slining, M.M. and He, K. (2010) Growth rate of human fingernails and toenails in healthy American young adults. *Journal of the Eurean Academy of Dermatology and Venereology*, **24**: 420–423.

Zook, E.G. (1985) Nail bed injuries. *Hand Clinics*, **1**: 701–716.

7

Taphonomy of Teeth

Christopher W. Schmidt, Robin Quataert, Fatma Zalzala and Ruggero D'Anastasio

7.1 Introduction

7.1.1 Dental Tissues in Forensic and Archaeological Contexts

It is generally the case that teeth preserve well in forensic and archaeological contexts, because of their high mineral content (e.g. Bowers 2004; Schmidt *et al.* 2015a). In forensic contexts, teeth are used primarily for positive identification and are particularly strong indicators of age (Adams *et al.* 2014; Bowers 2004; Christensen *et al.* 2014; Senn and Weems 2013). Archaeologically, dental studies that incorporate teeth include, for example, dietary reconstruction, biological distance, stable isotope analysis and pathology (e.g. Hillson 1996; Kelley and Larsen 1991; Scott and Irish 2013). They are also sound reservoirs for (ancient) DNA (Benazzi *et al.* 2015). There are instances, however, when taphonomic events/factors are significant enough to damage teeth to an extent that certain analyses are hampered or even obviated.

This chapter provides examples where extreme post-mortem mechanical and thermal events affected the conditions of teeth in terms of presence and appearance. Mechanical processes need not be severe to fracture teeth; traumata, such as those seen in forensic settings where high-speed projectiles or blunt objects impact the face, can lead to dental fractures (e.g. Veevers *et al.* 2009). However, even when major events such as mass disasters occur, it is possible that teeth will be available for study. Therefore, it is important to understand dental anatomy and the physical properties of teeth in order to properly recover and study them.

7.1.2 Dental Anatomy

Teeth are comprised primarily of three dental tissues: enamel, dentin and cement. Enamel is that part exposed in the mouth upon eruption. It is around 99% mineral and acellular. Dentin makes up the bulk of the tooth; it underlies the enamel and forms the root. At its centre, the pulp chamber that houses nerves and blood vessels is found. Dentin is around 75% mineral and, although it does not have cell bodies distributed throughout, it does have a layer of living cells lining the pulp cavity making it a living tissue. Cementum is around 65% mineral; its primary function in humans is to surround the root and to help maintain teeth firmly in their sockets (Ten Cate 1994).

Both enamel and dentin are harder and more mineralised than bone, which is around 65% mineral. Their hardness means they are strong and resistant to many of the forces they encounter in life. Consider the constant mechanical forces they encounter via mastication. Human bite forces are comparable to other similarly sized hominoids (Wroe *et al.* 2005), and as such, generate substantial

Taphonomy of Human Remains: Forensic Analysis of the Dead and the Depositional Environment, First Edition.
Edited by Eline M.J. Schotsmans, Nicholas Márquez-Grant and Shari L. Forbes.

mechanical loads on the teeth. Some human populations routinely chip their teeth because of the excessive demands they put on them, for example the Inuit, who use their teeth as tools (Hylander 1977; Scott and Winn 2010), but for the most part, human teeth are sturdy enough to deal with both masticatory and extramasticatory demands. Their sturdiness, however, also means they are brittle, particularly the enamel. Teeth fail when their elastic abilities (i.e. their ability to bend and return to their original shapes) are exceeded by the forces put upon them (Natali 2003). Collagen, which is the non-mineral component of dentin, is highly elastic and allows for some deformation. Enamel, in contrast, is almost entirely mineral and has little ability to bend. In fact, enamel depends on the underlying dentin to provide a somewhat elastic foundation so that it does not fracture when the teeth are in use (Ten Cate 1994).

7.2 Mechanical Damage: Forensic Case Study

Mechanical damage to teeth can be expressed in a variety of ways. It may result in the breakage of individual teeth or it may refer to fragmentation of the dental arches so that teeth, normally in contact with each other, become dispersed. An example of both of these conditions comes from a tragic airplane crash. On 31 October 1994, American Eagle flight 4184 was preparing for its scheduled landing at O'Hare International Airport in Chicago, Illinois. The craft was instructed to descend to 4,000 feet by air traffic controllers. In the course of this manoeuvre, the plane rolled twice and lost lift, possibly the result of icing on the wings. It crashed into an agricultural field near the town of Roselawn in northern Indiana, striking the ground, nose first, in an inverted position, at approximately 804.7 kph (500 mph). There were no survivors among the 68 passengers and crew aboard, and the fragmentation of the human remains was extraordinary. Recovery personnel found few elements from the upper aspects of the bodies, and the relatively few teeth they recovered were usually molars because, for the most part, only the posterior aspects of the jaws were encountered. In fact, only 9% of the teeth were ever found. Two teeth, determined to be from the same individual, were found 76.2 m (250 feet) apart (McGue 2006). It is likely that a certain percentage of the teeth were unaccounted for because they were driven deep into the ground; however, it is also clear that a sizable percentage of the teeth were simply damaged to such an extent that they were either missed by the forensic recovery teams or unidentifiable in the field. This sort of destruction is not common and underscores the enormity of the forces generated by the speed and angle of impact.

Recovery efforts took several days and over that time a dispersal pattern was recognised. Remains from the front end passengers clustered just north of the impact crater, remains from those passengers in the middle third of the plane were found in the crater, and those sitting in the rear third were found in a line east of the crater (McGue 2006). This sort of patterning has been documented in other plane crash sites (e.g. Dirkmaat 2012) and its understanding has helped to improve remains recovery and analysis.

Despite the extraordinary tooth and jaw fragmentation resulting from this tragedy, of the 198 teeth recovered, 163 were identified by tooth type and those were used to positively ID 34 people (McGue 2006). Thus, half of the passengers were identified dentally, even though fewer than 10% of the teeth were available for study. The teeth used for identification came from those found in isolation as well as those from jaw fragments that included multiple teeth; identifications were made via dental morphology as well as dental restorations. While this is an atypical case of taphonomic damage, it underscores the usefulness of teeth and the value of their recovery, even when circumstances significantly affect their availability.

7.3 Effects of Thermal Damage

Thermal damage to bones and teeth is usually documented in two ways: colour changes and fracturing. The colour changes are related to moisture and collagen loss and start out as a mottled tan. Bones with this colour probably did not reach temperatures above 100° to 200°C. The next colour is brown followed by black. Blackened elements are charred and indicate temperatures around 300°C. Bones and teeth then turn dark blue, blue grey and grey as temperatures near 600°C. Around 700°C bone starts to calcine, or turn white, as nearly all of the collagen has burned away (Symes *et al.* 2015) (Chapter 21). Teeth may calcine somewhat faster than bone because they have less water and collagen to lose. But, in general, dentin discolours in ways similar to bone in that it first darkens then becomes grey and white (see Sandholzer 2015). Enamel will darken, but usually colour changes are greater in developing crowns, because they have a greater non-mineralised content (Schmidt 2015).

Although temperature tends to be the more important causative factor when interpreting colour changes, duration does play an important role, because it takes time for skeletal elements to reach any particular temperature. Circumstances, ranging from tissue shielding to whether or not an element is facing toward or away from a heat source, determine the time it takes for heat to affect a particular element. Therefore, even though analysts have developed temperature-based standards like those described here for interpreting colour changes, studies like that of Sandholzer (2015) have found that thermally-induced colour changes can be accelerated or inhibited by the duration of thermal exposure at a particular temperature.

Thermal fractures result from micro-temperature differences along a bone or tooth (Symes *et al.* 2015) (Chapter 21). For example, a living tooth exposed to a high temperature has much of its corpus (mainly the roots) protected by its bony crypt. The exposed crown and its underlying dentin get hotter faster. As the tissues heat up, water and collagen are driven out, shrinking them noticeably. Burned teeth (primarily the dentin) can shrink as much as 30% if heated to around 700°C (e.g. Sandholzer 2015; Shipman *et al.* 1984). As the hot crown shrinks, the cooler root end keeps its original size longer. A crack forms where these areas of different temperature meet. Additional cracks form as the heated area expands into cooler areas, and the cracks deepen as the heat penetrates the tooth. Eventually the entire tooth reaches a high temperature and fragments as a result of its ongoing fracturing (e.g. Mahoney and Miszkiewicz 2015; Sandholzer 2015). Root fractures are commonly circumferential and look like dentin rings when found in isolation, the hollow middle being the pulp chamber. Crowns tend to fracture along cusp grooves, but not always; fractures can form anywhere, and localised shrinking or a temperature gradient creates a point of weakness. In incisors, these are often manifested as vertical fractures, while on molars they may be vertical or horizontal.

Ultimately, thermal changes are both chemical and mechanical. In experimental burning events, thermal fractures can be observed and often happen suddenly. Teeth, however, do not explode. Because dentin shrinks more than enamel, it may appear that a crown has exploded off from its dentin foundation, but this is not the case (Schmidt 2015).

Thermal changes in teeth are also evident in their microstructures when viewed histologically (e.g. Mahoney and Miszkiewicz 2015; Thompson 2015). Mahoney and Miszkiewicz found teeth experimentally exposed to temperatures at or above 250°C had carbon deposits and microfracturing that obscured neonatal lines, Striae of Retzius and cross-striations. However, the authors were still able to determine formation timing of these features until the enamel reached temperatures above 472°C. Around 500°C, they found that enamel detached from the dentin and fractured macroscopically. Taken together, their findings indicate that ageing burned enamel fragments histologically is possible, up to the point where enamel begins to transition to a calcined state and/or visibly breaks down.

7.4 Thermal Damage: Archaeological Case Study

7.4.1 Introduction

In AD 79, Mount Vesuvius destroyed the town of Herculaneum. The eruption, which also buried Pompeii, created a number of pyroclastic events, one of which overcame Herculaneum as the people huddled in boathouses and on the shore, while waiting to be rescued. The fatal surge hit at a speed nearing 160 kph (100 mph) and contained hot gases and debris, perhaps as high as 600°C (Schmidt *et al.* 2015b). It is suspected that the heat killed people instantly because it was 6 times greater than the boiling point of water. The victims were gradually buried by 20 m (65.6 feet) of material.

Evidence from the skeletons indicates that although the initial temperatures of the surge were approaching 600°C, the maximum temperature reached by most bones did not exceed 300°C. This disparity comes from several factors including soft tissue shielding, people shielding each other as they huddled together, and a rapid drop off of gas temperatures after the initial blast passed through the population. Both the people on the beach and in the boathouses have evidence of being burned, indicating the latter offered little protection.

For most people, thermally damaged bones were those covered by the least soft tissue. Of the bones of the cranium, the frontal and parietals were often the most burned. The maxilla and mandible were also frequently burned. In contrast, the more protected areas of the orbits and the cranial base were infrequently burned (Oakley 2015). The teeth, being protected only by the soft tissues of the mouth, should have been directly impacted fairly quickly. However, for most individuals, thermal damage to the teeth was limited to darkening of the roots (to either brown or black), adherence of charred soft tissues on the enamel and orange staining of the enamel. A preliminary inspection, focused on gross enamel appearance, found that only about 18% of the adults had distinctive thermal fracturing of their teeth. Nearly all of these instances accompanied blackened alveoli and blackened roots (Figure 7.1).

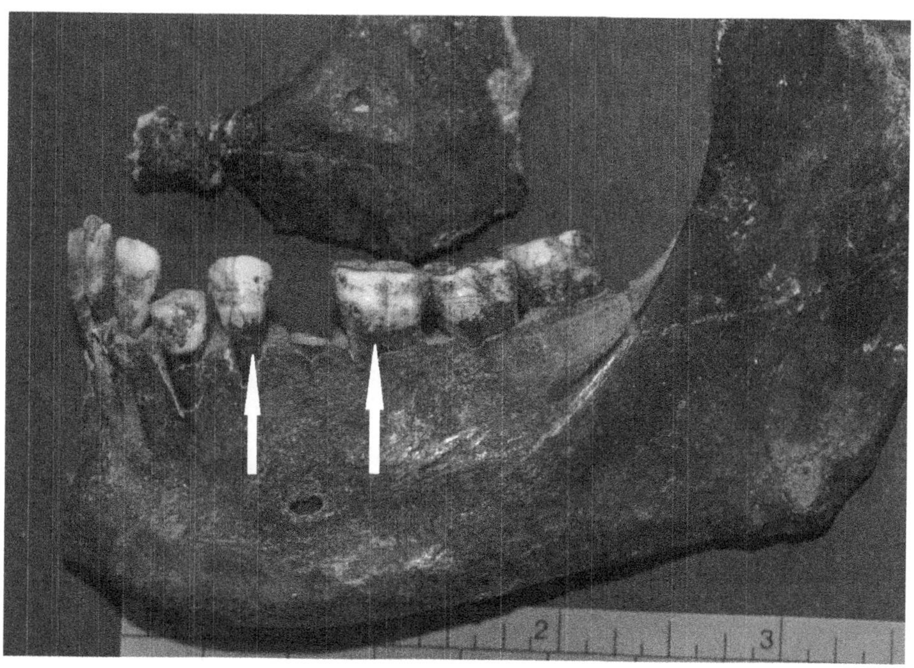

Figure 7.1 Teeth from Herculaneum individual E 41 having blackened roots (arrows).

In all cases at Herculaneum, the dentin initiated thermal change before the enamel. Recall that blackened bone indicates it reached a minimum temperature of around 300°C. Therefore, dentin that has blackened probably reached a comparable temperature, although not necessarily the same as bone (e.g. Sandholzer 2015). Thermally damaged teeth lacking enamel fractures typically had brown to dark brown roots, which is what one would expect for teeth that have not yet blackened.

While the dentin of the people of Herculaneum had changed considerably in those cases where the bones reached 300°C, their enamel had changed little. Small fractures appeared on the labial surfaces, which were largely linear and running vertically, although some fractures coursed horizontally (Figure 7.2). The fractures got deeper presumably as the heat continued; for some that meant the labial enamel flaked away once the cracks reached the dentin. For others, the cracks proceeded through the dentin and led to the flaking of enamel and dentin crown segments. A number of individuals had their crowns sheared at the cervix, presumably because of the temperature gradient between the exposed crowns and the protected roots. In other instances, however, it is possible the loss of the crown was due to peri-mortem or post-mortem trauma that severed the thermally-weakened cervix.

The enamel did not blacken or calcine in any of the adults. This is in contrast to findings by Schmidt *et al.* (2015a), who found brown, grey and calcined enamel among early to middle Holocene cremains from Indiana. In that study, the thermally discoloured enamel came from developing teeth, both permanent and deciduous. The Herculaneum population did have children with developing teeth, but colour changes were uncommon. This circumstance may be due to at least two related factors; the first being that the developing teeth were protected by their surrounding maxillary and mandibular bones; the second being the short-lived nature of the highest temperatures of the surge, which subsided soon after the surge passed through.

7.4.2 Changes in Colour

A condition of the bones of Herculaneum that was unlike what is typically seen in intentionally burned bones was the adherence of thin veneers of charred soft tissue. At times this tissue was also located on the teeth. It is thought the tissue was gingiva or those surrounding the oral cavity. No effort was made here to identify cell type in order to determine tissue types. An additional discolouration, which occurred more frequently on people who exhibited some charring, was a stark orange colour. This staining occurred on the bones and was particularly common inside cranial vaults. The origin of the stain is under investigation, but recent Scanning Electron Microscope-based elemental analysis

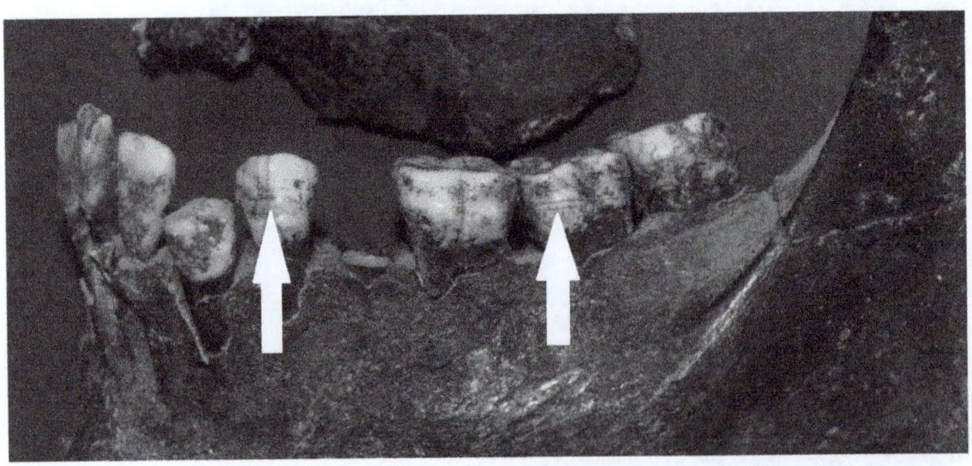

Figure 7.2 Detail of teeth from Figure 7.1. Notice vertical (left arrow) and horizontal (right arrow) fracturing.

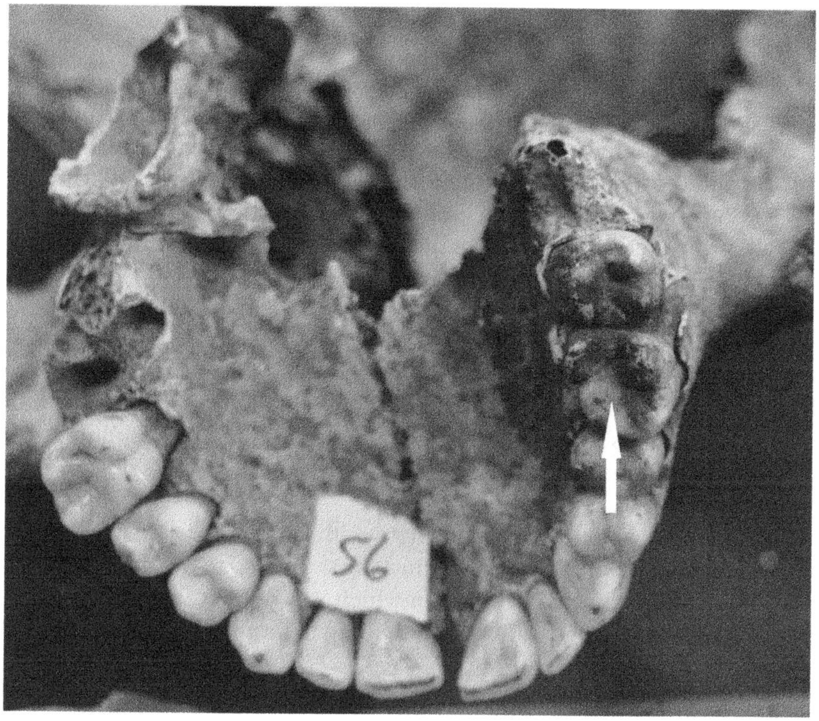

Figure 7.3 Orange staining (arrow) on teeth of Herculaneum individual E56 adjacent to areas with charred soft tissue. The staining is due to oxidation of soil near to a charred area.

found the stains contain silicon, sodium, sulphur, aluminium and iron, which are known to exist in appreciable levels in the Vesuvian volcanic ash (Horwell *et al.* 2010). Iron artefacts have been found on and near a number of the victims, but the orange staining on the teeth is not of this origin. The iron staining from the artefacts was darker and often had small bits of the artefacts still present (e.g. the skeletal individuals E52 and E30 present, respectively, iron deposits on the mandible and an iron hair clip fastened to the skull) (Capasso 2001). Moreover, the orange staining does not appear to be of a biological origin. Its endocranial co-occurrence with charred soft tissues hinted that it came from the body, but the elemental study indicates that the staining appeared as the ash around the remains oxidised. On the teeth, it is a superficial discolouration found commonly, but not always, adjacent to areas of charred soft tissue (Figure 7.3).

Observations of the charred tissues on the teeth indicate that their presence is directly related to the temperature of the surge and the gradual means by which the heat subsided. It is plausible that the initial heat of the surge burned superficial soft tissues and that the burning progressed steadily to deeper tissues over a period of time. However, in some individuals, the bones reached a temperature of around 300°C, which charred them and desiccated the soft tissues. For some people, the desiccation was enough to help preserve the soft tissues. For most people, however, their bones were not charred and their soft tissues eventually decayed.

7.5 Caveats

While this chapter has argued that teeth generally survive even significant taphonomic processes, there are cases where teeth are damaged to a point where they are no longer suitable for study. For example, soil chemistry can play a major role in preservation; sediments with a pH below 5.3 can demineralise hard tissues to the point where almost nothing remains (Gordon and Buikstra 1981). Bethell (1989) carried out chemical analysis of so-called 'shadow burials' where only imprints of the bodies remained, apart from tooth enamel in some cases. Another unpublished example of such an instance comes from the excavation of an adult female grave from a mid-19th century cemetery, located in southern Indiana (USA), and carried out by archaeologists from the University of Indianapolis. Although agricultural activity had removed much of the soil above the burial, it was clear the soil's acidity had destroyed all of the teeth and bones. In fact, all that remained at the bottom of the burial shaft was a necklace and an organic stain marking the outline of the body.

Another extremely damaging taphonomic event is commercial cremation; it involves both mechanical and thermal changes that drastically alter dental remains. Bodies are exposed to temperatures approaching 900°C for several hours. After burning, the remains are calcined and brittle but not thoroughly fragmented and some elements are still several centimetres in length. The remains are then passed through a pulveriser that reduces them to fragments of no more than a few millimetres in length (Schultz *et al.* 2015). Modern cremations are capable of damaging teeth so severely that their study is very limited.

These examples serve as reminders that while teeth are likely to withstand any particular taphonomic insult, they are not indestructible. Recognising the circumstances that led to the deposition of a body, either ancient or modern, as well as the environment in which it is recovered, allows one to better understand the likelihood of recovering teeth and understanding their condition once found.

7.6 Conclusion

The extraordinary cases described here make it clear that even severe taphonomic events often leave teeth in a condition sound enough for study. Changes may be in the quality or quantity of teeth, which may be radically fragmented, commingled and dispersed, as was the case in the plane crash example; they may be discoloured by thermal changes and/or ground staining, as was the case for the teeth from Herculaneum. It is therefore recommended for those recovering human remains that they have a strategy for collecting teeth, because they are likely to be present and available for constructing biological profiles and performing bioarchaeological analyses. Finally, the overview provided here should not imply that all is understood regarding tooth taphonomy. Despite advances in recent years of our understanding of thermal changes in dentin and enamel (particularly concerning changes in microanatomy led by researchers like P. Mahoney, M. Sandholzer and T. Thompson), much remains to be learned. One such area with notable deficiencies concerns changes related to very long exposures to high temperatures, such as that which occurred to the people of Herculaneum, who may have experienced temperatures hot enough to affect bone for days. It is hoped the research presented here and the new questions these studies raise will stimulate further research in dental taphonomy.

References

Adams, C., Carabott, R. and Evans, S. (2014) *Forensic Odontology: An essential guide*. Wiley Blackwell: Oxford.

Benazzi, S., Slon, V., Talamo, S., Negrino, F., Peresani, M. *et al.* (2015) The makers of Protoaurignacian and implications for Neanderthal extinction. *Science*, **348**: 793–796.

Bethell, P.H. (1989) Chemical analysis of shadow burials. In: Roberts, C.A., Lee, F. and Bintliff, J.J. (eds), *Burial Archaeology: Current research, methods and developments*. BAR British Archaeological Reports Series 211: Oxford, pp. 205–214.

Bowers, C.M. (2004) *Forensic Dental Evidence*. Elsevier: Amsterdam.

Capasso, L. (2001) *I Fuggiaschi di Ercolano. Paleobiologia delle vittime dell'eruzione vesuviana del 79 d.C.* L'Erma di Bretchneider: Rome.

Christensen, A.M., Passalacqua, N.V. and Bartelink, E.J. (2014) *Forensic Anthropology*. Academic Press: Amsterdam.

Dirkmaat, D.C. (2012) Forensic anthropology at the mass fatality incident (commercial airliner) crash scene. In: Dirkmaat, D.C. (ed.), *A Companion to Forensic Anthropology*. Wiley-Blackwell: Hoboken, pp. 136–156.

Gordon, C.C. and Buikstra, J.E. (1981) Soil pH, bone preservation, and sampling bias at mortuary sites. *American Antiquity*, **46**: 566–571.

Hillson, S.W. (1996) *Dental Anthropology*. Cambridge University Press: Cambridge.

Horwell, C.J., Stannett, G.W., Andronico, D., Bertagnini, A., Fenoglio, I. and Fubini, B. (2010) A physico-chemical assessment of the health hazard of Mt Vesuvius volcanic ash. *Journal of Volcanology and Geothermal Research*, **191**: 222–232.

Hylander, W.L. (1977) The adaptive significance of Eskimo craniofacial morphology. In: Dahlberg, A.A. and Graber. T.M. (eds), *Orofacial Growth and Development*. Mouton: Paris, pp. 129–170.

Kelley, M.A. and Larsen, C.S. (1991) *Advances in Dental Anthropology*. Wiley-Liss: New York.

Mahoney, P. and Miszkiewicz, J. (2015) Formation times in thermally altered enamel. In: Schmidt, C.W. and Symes, S.A. (eds), *The Analysis of Burned Human Remains*. Elsevier: New York, pp. 355–364.

McGue, B.C. (2006) Dental identification of American Eagle Flight 4184. *Journal of the Indiana Dental Association*, **85**: 6–12.

Natali, A.N. (2003) *Dental Biomechanics*. CRC Press: New York.

Oakley. E.R. (2015) Analysis of thermal changes among the people of Herculaneum. Unpublished MS Thesis, University of Indianapolis.

Sandholzer, M. (2015) Influence of heating regimes on dimensional and colorimetric changes of teeth. In: Schmidt, C.W. and Symes, S.A. (eds), *The Analysis of Burned Human Remains*. Elsevier: New York, pp. 365–380.

Schmidt, C.W. (2015) Burned human teeth. In: Schmidt, C.W. and Symes, S.A. (eds), *The Analysis of Burned Human Remains*. Elsevier: New York, pp. 61–82.

Schmidt, C.W., Tomak, C.H., Lockhart, R.A., Greene, T.R. and Reinhardt, G.A. (2015a) Early archaic cremations from Southern Indiana. In: Schmidt, C.W. and Symes, S.A. (eds), *The Analysis of Burned Human Remains*. Elsevier: New York, pp. 247–258.

Schmidt, C.W., Oakley, E., D'Anastasio, R., Brower, R., Remy, A.J. and Viciano, J. (2015b) Herculaneum. In: Schmidt, C.W. and Symes, S.A. (eds), *The Analysis of Burned Human Remains*. Elsevier: New York, pp. 149–162.

Schultz, J.J., Warren, M.W. and Krigbaum, J.S. (2015) Analysis of human cremains. In: Schmidt, C.W. and Symes, S.A. (eds), *The Analysis of Burned Human Remains*. Elsevier: New York, pp. 83–104.

Scott, G.R. and Winn, J.R. (2011) Dental chipping: contrasting patterns of microtrauma in Inuit and European populations. *International Journal of Osteoarchaeology*, **21**: 723–731.

Scott, G.R. and Irish, J.D. (2013) *Anthropological Perspectives on Tooth Morphology*. Cambridge University Press: Cambridge.

Senn, D.R. and Weems, R.A. (2013) *Manual of Forensic Odontology*, 5th edition. CRC Press: Boca Raton.

Shipman, P., Foster, G. and Schoeninger, M. (1984) Burnt bones and teeth: an experimental study of color, morphology, crystal structure and shrinkage. *Journal of Archaeological Science*, **11**: 307–325.

Symes, S.A., Rainwater, C.W., Chapman, E.N., Gipson, D.R. and Piper, A.L. (2015) Patterned thermal destruction in a forensic setting. In: Schmidt, C.W. and Symes, S.A. (eds), *The Analysis of Burned Human Remains*. Elsevier: New York, pp. 17–59.

Ten Cate, A.R. (1994) *Oral Histology*. Mosby: St Louis.

Thompson, T.J. (2015) The analysis of heat-induced crystallinity change in bone. In: Schmidt, C.W. and Symes, S.A. (eds), *The Analysis of Burned Human Remains*. Elsevier: New York, pp. 323–338.

Veevers, A.E., Lawler, W. and Rutty, G.N. (2009) Walk and die: an unusual presentation of head injury. *Journal of Forensic Sciences*, **54**: 1466–1469.

Wroe, S., McHenry, C. and Thomason, J. (2005) Bite club: comparative bite force in big biting mammals and the prediction of predatory behaviour in fossil taxa. *Proceedings of Royal Society B*, **272**: 619–625.

8

The Taphonomy of Natural Mummies

Dario Piombino-Mascali, Heather Gill-Frerking and Ronald G. Beckett

8.1 Introduction

The shorter the timescale between interment and recovery, the more likely soft tissue will be preserved, but the presence of extensive soft tissue does not always indicate a recent death. Decomposition processes are largely dependent on the individual circumstances of the burial. The unique combination of several different factors will determine whether a body decomposes or remains preserved. These factors help establish the meaning of 'taphonomy'. Although meanings vary between authors, depending on the intention of the publication, taphonomy is generally defined as '…the study of the processes that operate on organic remains after death…' (Micozzi 1991). For the purposes of this chapter, taphonomy refers to both natural and anthropogenic processes that affect human remains after death. In particular, this chapter will focus on taphonomic processes that lead to, and affect, mummified human remains.

Human mummies are remains with preservation of soft tissue, such as muscle, skin, fat or connective tissue. The word mummy is derived from the Persian word *múmiyá* (*mûm* in Arabic) meaning bitumen (Ikram 2010). It could be argued that the term should be reserved for cases of anthropogenic preservation of soft tissue, also called artificial mummification, although it is widely applied to all preserved bodies, including those found in natural environments. Today, mummification can be interpreted by its strict definition of natural or spontaneous mummification, arrested decay by moisture loss and tissue desiccation, or by the broader common usage of the word; survival of soft tissue by any mechanism including artificial processes (Aufderheide 2003). Furthermore, within the various definitions for the term 'mummy', there is no clear distinction between a skeleton with some preserved elements, such as ligaments, skin and a well-preserved body (Lynnerup 2007). In general, the term is typically employed to define corpses with an overall preservation of soft tissues, which may include skin, fasciae, ligaments or even muscles and internal organs. The mummification process can lead to different states of preservation. Internal organs, especially those of the digestive tract, may be completely decomposed, while others undergo changes that make them morphologically indistinguishable and dislocated (Lynnerup 2007).

Mummification is a widespread phenomenon in both bioarchaeological and forensic contexts. Discoveries of spontaneously preserved remains are well known to forensic pathologists and may shed light on present-day social isolation, especially amongst the elderly. Cases have been reported of subjects being found days, weeks or even years after death (Campobasso *et al.* 2009; Introna *et al.* 2011; Jit *et al.* 2001; Ventura *et al.* 2013). Notwithstanding the occurrence of such findings, the factors that

Taphonomy of Human Remains: Forensic Analysis of the Dead and the Depositional Environment, First Edition.
Edited by Eline M.J. Schotsmans, Nicholas Márquez-Grant and Shari L. Forbes.

lead to the processes of natural mummification are only partly known. Furthermore, few experimental studies in natural mummification have been carried out (Garcia *et al.* 2014; Gill-Robinson 2001; Gill-Frerking and Healey 2011), as opposed to the various projects that have examined the processes of artificial mummification (e.g. Brier and Wade 2001; Panzer *et al.* 2013; Zimmerman 1979). This chapter will provide an overview of natural mummification processes and the taphonomy of such bodies, applicable to both the archaeological and forensic settings.

8.2 Post-Mortem Decay

Mummies are unusual in that they do not generally experience typical post-mortem processes of decomposition. Both putrefaction, caused by anaerobic degradation, and decay, caused by aerobic degradation (Micozzi 1991) usually occur immediately after death, breaking down soft tissues such as internal organs and muscles first and eventually hard tissues such as bone. Natural mummies are preserved because putrefaction or decay, or both, is impeded by the surrounding environmental conditions.

Human tissues are basically formed by three components: lipids, carbohydrates and proteins. Each is responsible for specific chemical purposes (Aufderheide 2011). Autolysis is an enzymatic process that commences immediately after death (Chapters 1 and 2). Chemical reactions within a body are enhanced by enzymes, which possess a very specific mechanism only used to impact their targets. Some of them are even designed to break molecules into smaller fragments. After death, cadavers undergo three waves of enzymatic action derived from intracellular enzymes, bacteria or animal activity. The final result consists of small molecules that react with the environment, or are ingested by other living organisms that will use enzymes to transform them into new compounds. The first chemical change occurs within the cell cytoplasm as many of the cells contain hydrolases, that is, enzymes aimed at destroying large molecules through a process called hydrolysis. These enzymes are contained in organelles known as lysosomes within the cytoplasm of living cells. In the living, the enzymes of the lysosome help digest or break down worn out or excess organelles, food particles and invading materials, such as bacteria. At death, due to hypoxic conditions and altered intracellular pH, the membranes surrounding the lysosomes lose their integrity, releasing their digestive enzymes into the cell, which generates self-digestion, a process known as autolysis, ultimately leading to liquefaction. The following phase of the decay process is represented by the spread of bacteria, both aerobic and anaerobic, which expand from the gut to other tissues, secreting further destructive enzymes. The process is also gravity-regulated; the most dependent areas will be heavily colonised by anaerobic bacteria. At this stage, bloating of the abdomen can occur due to gas formation, which may result in purging of the fluids or rectal/uterine prolapse. An additional phase of the decomposition process is represented by the colonisation of insects and other arthropods, which may appear shortly after death and feed on the cadaver, consuming the majority of soft tissue (Aufderheide 2003). Mummification, both natural and artificial, represents an interruption of the decomposition process, producing a state of arrested decay.

8.3 Natural or Spontaneous Mummification

Most enzymes operate within an aqueous environment (Aufderheide 2011). Therefore, natural removal of water slows down the decomposition process, eventually resulting in its cessation. In spontaneous mummification, the process of natural body water loss occurs more rapidly than does the advance of enzymatic activity. Body water loss can be expedited when the body experiences environments that will enhance desiccation, as seen in body fluids passing through the skin by means of heat, osmosis, evaporation and exposure to a given external environment. Removing the internal tissue water through the cutis will ensure dehydration at its maximal rate. In this respect, permeable clothing lying on the skin surface may contribute to the process through a wicking action (Aturaliya and Lukasewycz 1999). Ventilation and fine, humidity-absorbing soil may also impact the rate of tissue dehydration. This mechanism of water removal can determine changes to the corpse itself, such as the lack of epidermis in the torso region due to enzyme-rich residual water from the abdomen, or the lack of substance in gravity-dependent areas. Internal organs are also affected; some, such as the heart, are slower to desiccate, while others decompose more rapidly due to their structural characteristics (Aufderheide 2011). It should also be noted that enzymatic action may be influenced by a number of additional environmental factors, including acidity, temperature and various inhibiting substances. Alterations from the optimum pH level or temperature, both of which vary according to the environment, can slow down this destructive enzymatic activity, while the presence of, for example, heavy metal ions in the soil, may retard the enzymatic action as well.

8.4 Soft Tissue Changes

While most of the forensic literature has generally focused on the processes of skeletonisation in different environments, much of what is known about changes in ancient human mummies is due to the scholarly work of Arthur Carl Aufderheide (2003), whose pioneering research on modern mummy studies provided a considerable body of information on taphonomic processes affecting soft tissue. There is a high degree of variability in the state of soft tissue preservation, due primarily to the environmental conditions associated with the remains. Often, miniscule differences in localised microclimates lead to significant variation in preservation, even within the same body. For example, the famous Iron Age bog body from Denmark, Tollund Man, has exceptionally well-preserved head and feet, but the hands and arms are skeletonised. A spontaneously mummified corpse appears shrunken and is lighter in weight, often flat at the areas in contact with a level surface. Impressions of fibres and textiles can occasionally be observed in the preserved tissue. Eyes may be present, collapsed into the orbit, while lips may be retracted, displaying anterior teeth. Gravity-dependent areas, such as the back, or if the position of the body is vertical, the inner thighs, may show substantial lack of tissue. External genitalia are usually recognizable, more often in men than in women. Preserved penises are a common find as are the scrota. Erect penises and anal and vaginal prolapse can sometimes be observed, due to gas formation. In women, breasts are generally collapsed due to chemical changes of the fat contained in them. However, areolae and nipples are often visible. Hair and nails are commonly present due to their high keratin and low water content. Areas of the body in close contact, such as an arm resting on a thigh or the genital region of a mummy in a foetal position, may have decayed tissue, due to the impedance of enzyme-rich water removal. As far as internal organs are concerned, the gastrointestinal tract may be present in a collapsed form, and the stomach may appear distended. If the heart is preserved, its basic structures with fibrous/elastic components may be identifiable; in some cases, it is possible to identify the auricles and ventricles. Lungs may appear contracted and collapsed and fibrous membranes may be observed, reflecting visceral pleurae and those that subdivide the lobe into smaller units. The liver may be present, although reduced in size, while the spleen and kidneys generally decompose rapidly. Similarly, the pancreas and adrenals undergo rapid autolysis. Organs inside the pelvic cavity such as the urinary bladder, the pelvic colon and the rectum, may be affected by visceral decay (Aufderheide 2003). The preservation of the brain varies among natural mummies. One may find a completely desiccated brain reduced in size, a few structures remaining, such as the *dura mater*, or nothing at all (Chapter 30).

A method was devised in order to roughly quantify the presence of soft tissue, hair and internal organs in mummified remains (Aufdherheide 2003; Wittmers *et al.* 2008). Assessment of the percentage of bones, hair and bodily parts is measured by assigning a numeric value between 1 and 5 to five anatomical districts including head, thorax, abdomen, upper limbs and lower limbs. The total provides a soft tissue index. In contrast, the visceral index can be obtained by an assessment of 10 internal organs, valued 10 points if present. The total equates to the percentage of organ preservation. While it can be argued that this method focuses on the quantity of residual tissue, rather than on the quality, this calculation provides a more objective estimate for comparative purposes. The preservation indices are seldom applied in publications discussing mummies and mummification. If further indices could be developed to account for qualitative assessment of preserved tissue, these indices could greatly enhance quantitative research in mummy studies, possibly allowing for inter- and intrasite comparison of mummies.

8.5 Environment, Culture or Both?

Understanding the impact of both the environment and cultural practices is critical when assessing naturally mummified remains. Considering the tendency for normal decomposition, the disruption of typical taphonomic changes to human remains due to varied, and often co-contributory, environmental forces, can result in wide variation in the state of mummification. It is important to keep these forces in mind when studying spontaneous natural mummies. The importance of knowing the environment from which the mummified remains were recovered, and the climatic conditions from the time period that the individual was alive, are key factors in understanding the study of such mummies. During the study of mummified remains, it is also essential to consider additional bioarchaeological information about culture, including funerary and mortuary practices that may impede the natural decomposition process. For example, traditional placement of a body in a well-ventilated dry cave may have a profound impact on the condition of the remains. When the cave environment is combined with the presence of textiles that may wick fluids from the body, the rate of desiccation will be markedly different from a similarly wrapped body that was interred in a subterranean tomb (Guillen 2004). The process of determining the efficacy of the mummification environment is challenging. When assessing the state of preservation of natural mummies, the potential impact of the conditions and environment surrounding the burial or deposition of the deceased and post-depositional changes, must also be considered. Furthermore, since it is not always possible to examine mummies while they are *in situ*, many specimens that are examined have been held in museum collections for a century or more. It is not uncommon for these mummies to have experienced post-acquisition modification in the form of conservation with resins, paints or other substances; reinforcement with rods or other support structures, or treatments with pesticides and other chemical substances that have damaged the soft tissue (Gill-Frerking 2014).

8.6 Dry Environments

Desiccation can occur rapidly if an environment conducive to this process is present. Burials in North Africa, Peru and Chile, for instance, are suited to this type of mummification. Areas with little fluid, such as fingers, toes and scrotum, dehydrate quicker. Forensic evidence suggests that a body can mummify in as little as two weeks when left exposed in hot, arid environments, and about one to three months when in an enclosed area, such as a structure (Galloway *et al.* 1989). In contrast, temperate environments generally require at least three months. Examples of dry mummies include those found

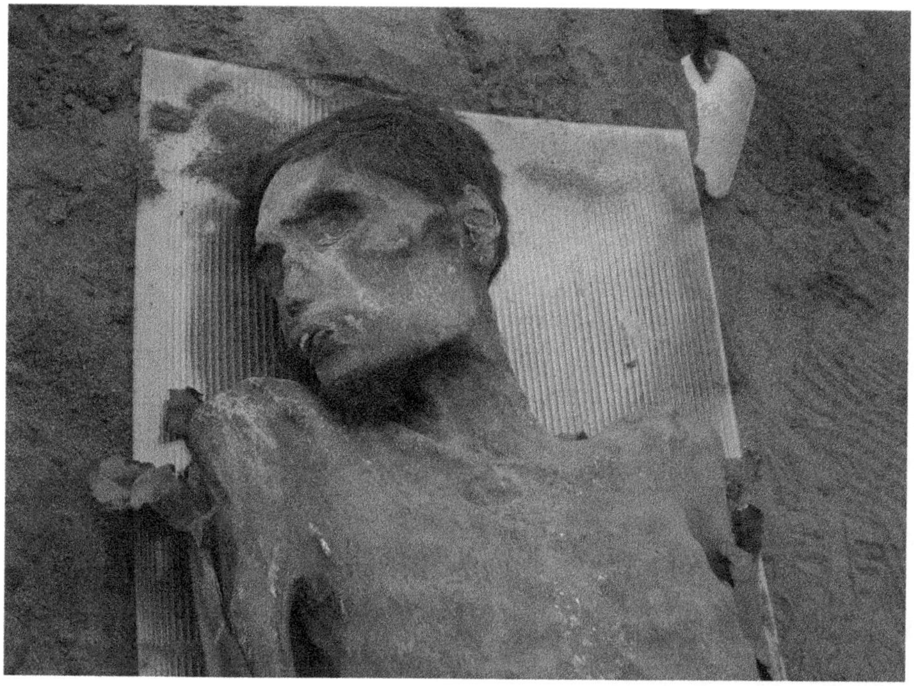

Figure 8.1 Isla San Lorenzo, Peru. This naturally mummified individual was buried in a wooden coffin in the sands of the desert island, Isla San Lorenzo, off of the coast of Callao, Peru. Although the island is typically surrounded with fog, the high degree of preservation is a testament to the environmental conditions of the burial.

in Egypt, dating to the pre-Dynastic period, when bodies were interred in sandy pits with a few grave goods (Ikram and Dodson 1998). The arid conditions of the sand desiccated a number of these corpses naturally, a factor which may have influenced subsequent anthropogenic treatments. Furthermore, dry prehistoric mummies such as the Chiribaya and Tiwanaku, are found in great numbers in Peru. While not all of them have been scientifically investigated, information seems to confirm that most of those bodies mummified spontaneously, due to burial in arid, sandy soil and envelopment in textiles (Figure 8.1) (Guillen 2004). There are also many spontaneous mummies of the Chinchorro culture who were buried in the Atacama Desert of northern Chile, where the mechanisms of mummification include the area's aridity, little groundwater and sandy soil. Moreover, the soil contains nitrates and arsenic, which may have contributed to the mummification process through osmosis and chemical variations that impede decomposition (Aufderheide 2003; Garcia *et al.* 2014). The process of osmosis is also known to have occurred in the cases of the salt men, several human corpses found in the Chehrabad salt mine of the Zanjan province, in Iran, which consists of an outcrop made of nearly pure sodium chloride (Niknami *et al.* 2014). This highly hydrophilic substance interacted with the bodies reducing water volume, preventing chemical reactions and bacterial growth.

Those who died 'in odour of sanctity' and were located in burials such as crypts provide another example of natural mummification (Figure 8.2). In these locations, the human remains were often protected from humidity and rainwater, and found to be in pristine condition (Figures 8.3 to 8.5) (Cardin 2014). One example of natural crypt mummies comes from Guanajuato, Mexico. The mummies, displayed at the Museo de las Momias, resulted from the regional dry mountain air, which enhanced desiccation, and interment in limestone-rich, above ground burial vaults was also a co-contributing factor (Figures 8.6 and 8.7) (Beckett and Conlogue 2010; Cardin 2014). Finally, another group of thousands of spontaneous mummies is located in Sicily, Italy. This group of mummies was created by

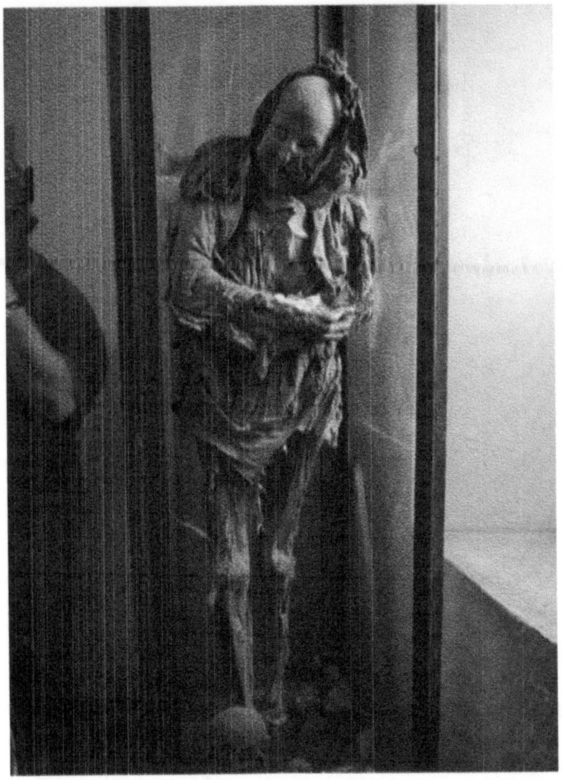

Figure 8.2 Fray Lazaro de Santofimia. The naturally mummified remains of Fray Lazaro de Santofimia were discovered after an earthquake exposed his coffin, which was encased in a stone windowsill of the Church of la Asuncion in Guano, Ecuador. Fray Lazaro was a Spanish missionary who undertook religious conversion work in the region during the 16th century.

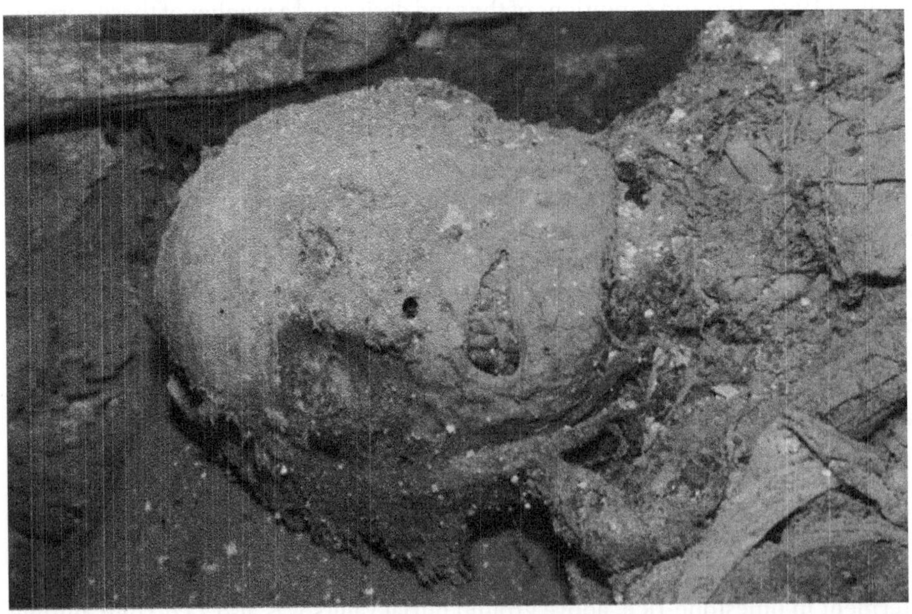

Figure 8.3 Popoli, Italy. This mummy was discovered in a crypt under a side room off the main altar area of the Church of the Holy Trinity in the village of Popoli, in the Abruzzo region of Italy. The dry, sealed crypt held multiple burials.

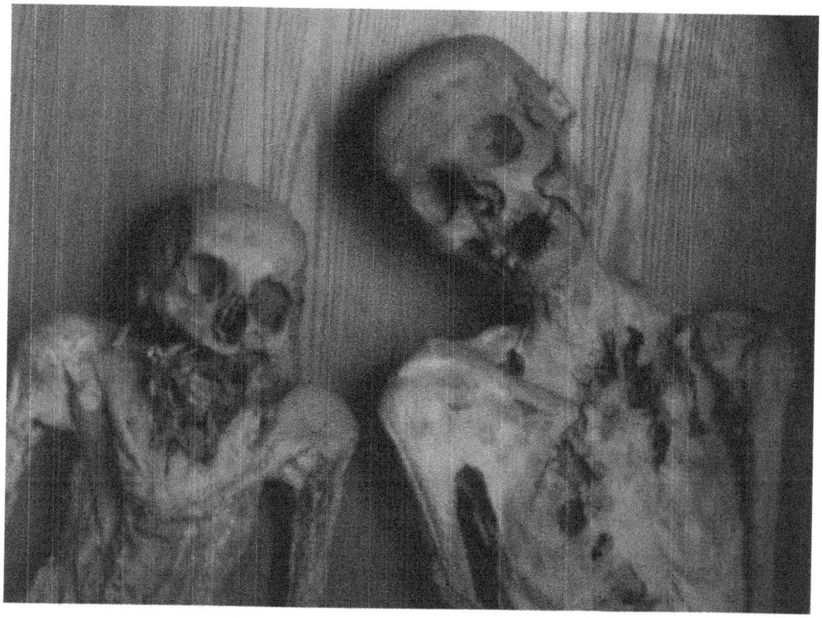

Figure 8.4 Urbania, Italy. Church of the Good Death. These bodies were discovered when a cemetery was relocated in Urbania, Italy. The individuals were thought to be beneficiaries of the burial provided to the poor by the Brotherhood of the Good Death. It is possible that some of the bodies were buried wrapped in a linen shroud, which would serve to wick fluids away from the body. The fluids were probably absorbed by the burial matrix, resulting in natural mummification.

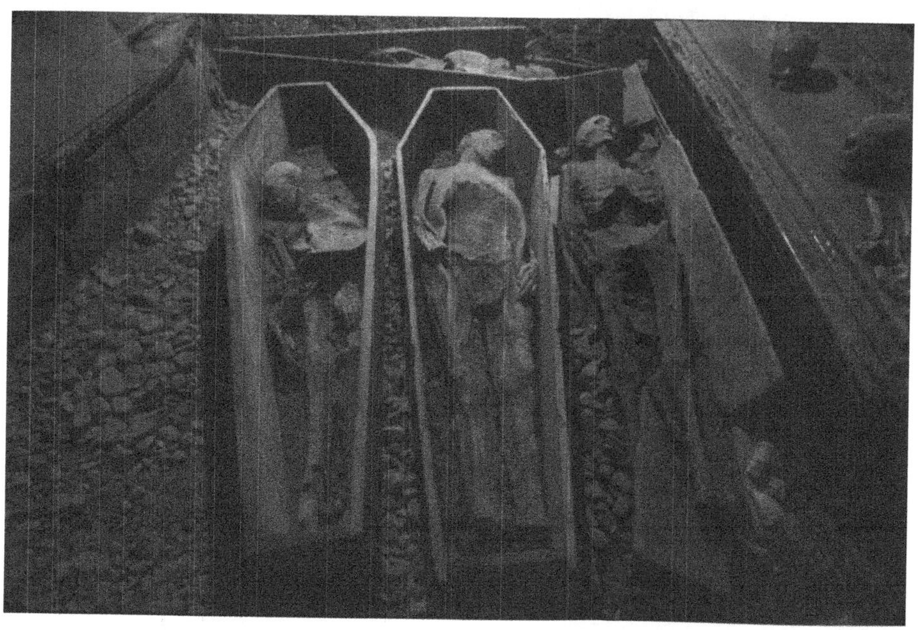

Figure 8.5 The Big Four, St Michan's Church, Ireland. These four individuals were discovered in the catacombs beneath St Michan's Church in Dublin, Ireland. They provide excellent examples of natural mummification in crypt environments.

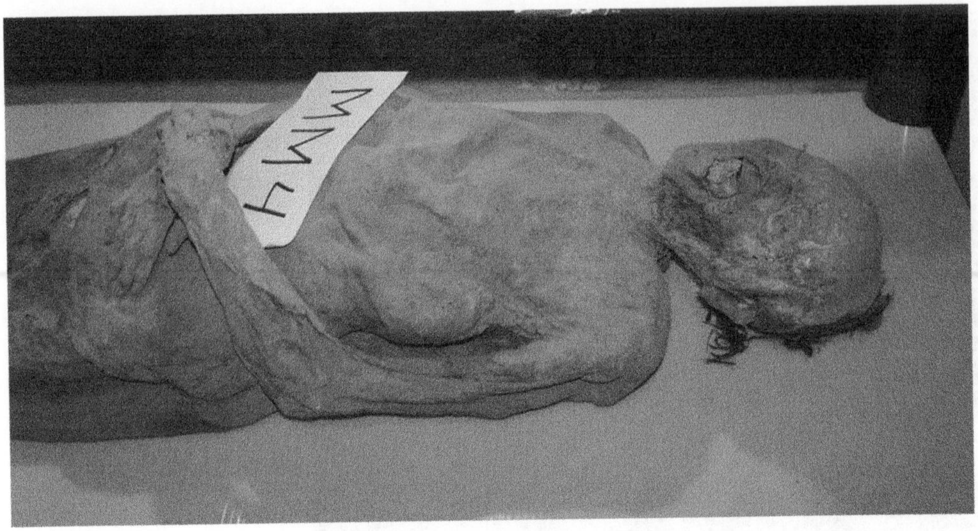

Figure 8.6 Guanajuato, Mexico. This is an example of natural mummification occurring in an above-ground mausoleum crypt in the sierra region of Guanajuato, Mexico. The natural mummification was likely the result of burial in the dry season, reduction of the surrounding humidity by the limestone structure, and interment in a location where water was less likely to bleed into the vault (Museo de las Momias).

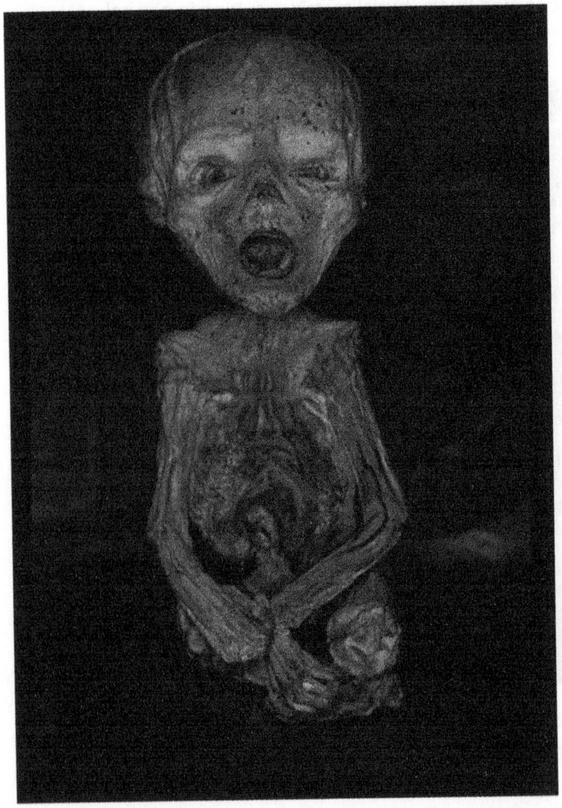

Figure 8.7 Guanajuato foetus. Another example of natural mummification is that of a foetus, which is said to have been buried with the mother, who apparently perished from an attempted Caesarean section. The natural mummification was likely the result of burial in the dry season, reduction of the surrounding humidity by the limestone structure, and interment in a location where water was less likely to bleed into the vault (Museo de las Momias).

enhancing the dehydration process via special architectural structures aimed at gathering the bodily fluids, promoting desiccation of the tissues, together with the dry and aerated chambers that facilitated a long-term preservation of the bodies (Panzer *et al.* 2010).

8.7 Bog Environments

The natural mummification category also includes mummies from wet environments. Historical bodies from bogs provide excellent examples of this category of spontaneous preservation. The bog bodies are preserved human corpses found in wetland pit deposits, specifically acidic peat bogs (Figure 8.8). There are two types of peat environments; although human remains have been recovered from both types of peat, the type and extent of preservation is very different. Ombrotrophic sites, also referred to as 'peat bog', are acidic (pH 3.2–5) wetlands, the water for which is derived only from precipitation. Bodies preserved in ombrotrophic peat frequently have well-preserved soft tissue, but bones are severely demineralised or sometimes even absent. These bodies often appear flattened, as a result of the weight of the overlying peat putting pressure on the starkly demineralised skeletal material (Crowther 2002). Minerotrophic wetlands, also referred to as 'fens', are generally alkaline environments (pH 5.5–7.8). Bodies preserved in fens are typically completely skeletonised, with no remaining soft tissue (Healy and Housley 1992). These peats are commonly found in various geographic areas, but remains have been located primarily in Northern Europe (Britain, Ireland, Denmark, Germany, The Netherlands), although excavation of the 8,000-year-old Windover site near Titusville, Florida, revealed 168 skeletons, 91 of which had well-preserved brain tissue in the skulls (O'Connor *et al.* 2011).

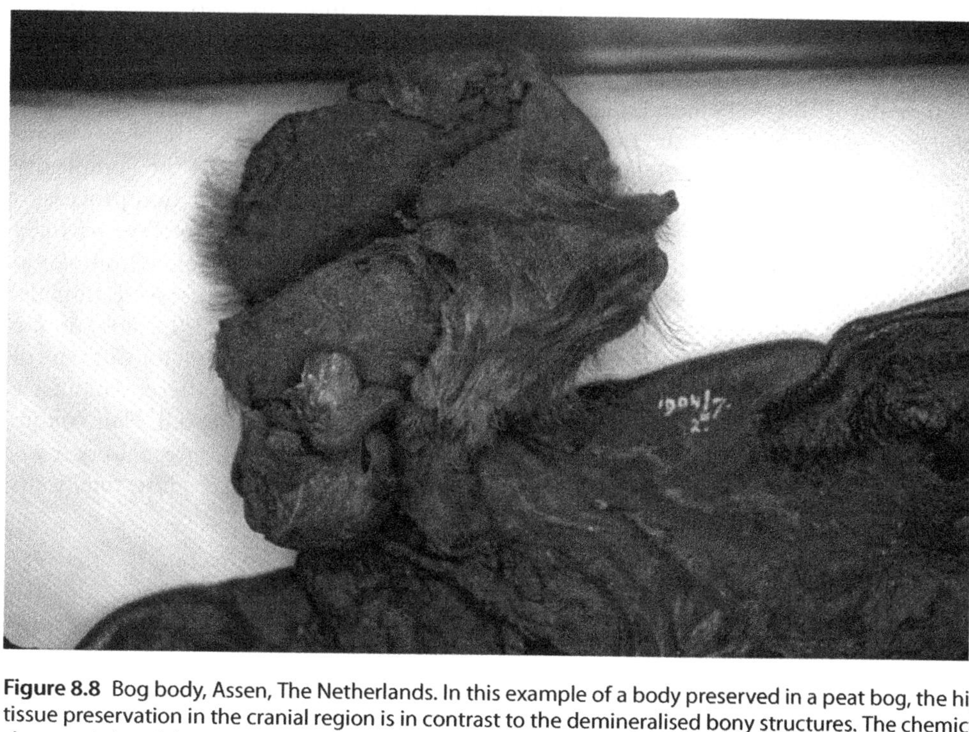

Figure 8.8 Bog body, Assen, The Netherlands. In this example of a body preserved in a peat bog, the high level of soft tissue preservation in the cranial region is in contrast to the demineralised bony structures. The chemical characteristics of the peat bog leach calcium, magnesium and other minerals from the bone over time, leading to compression of the entire body from the weight of the overlying peat. The soft tissues retain a high degree of preservation.

Most of the European bog bodies were discovered accidentally, often during the extraction of peat for fuel and later, on an industrial scale, for horticulture. There are several factors specific to bog environments that contribute to the creation of mummified remains (Brothwell and Gill-Robinson 2002). Peat bogs are generally cold, acidic and anaerobic. One key factor is the vegetation that is specific to the peat bogs. The sites are characterised by the presence of *Sphagnum* moss, which grows on the surface (Painter 1991); the lower layers of the bog consist of decomposed *Sphagnum*. When the plant dies, it releases a polysaccharide called 'sphagnan', which possesses chelating properties, allowing the removal of metal ions from a solution. As a result of this process, some metal ions such as iron, copper or zinc, are no longer available to bacteria, depriving them of an important source of nourishment. This lack of nourishment slows down microbial activity. Furthermore, calcium chelation results in calcium being leached out of the bones, which dissolve or become pliable, often leaving only collagen. This is not necessarily a uniform phenomenon, but based on experimental archaeology research, it is clear that the demineralisation process occurs very rapidly. The bones of piglets buried in peat were completely demineralised in less than six months. The bones were rubbery and could be compressed completely flat with ease (Gill-Robinson 2001).

A 'Maillard reaction' between sphagnan, ammonia, amino acids and polypeptide amino-groups, also occurs in bogs. The humic acids resulting from this biodegradation, which are among the major organic substances of the bog pit, are extremely resistant to microbial attack due to the lack of nitrogen, which becomes unavailable to microorganisms (Painter 1991). Significantly, the above-mentioned reaction also creates cross-linking of the collagen fibres, which expels water from the interstices and confers resistance to bacterial attack. Sphagnan and its holocellulose (the polysaccharide component of the fibrous peat, consisting of both the cellulose and any associated hemicelluloses) also inhibit the activity of the enzymes secreted by bacteria, further contributing to the preservation of the human remains (Aufderheide 2011). Tannins are also present in the bog, and it is plausible to believe that they also play a role in the mummification process (Painter 1991). Tannins and the substances involved in the Maillard reaction also cause the bodies to turn a dark brown, often almost black, colour. Experimental research also identified the importance of the water level for the preservation of the body. Where water levels were higher, there was more soft tissue preservation (Gill-Robinson 2001). This same research also highlighted the complexity of interpreting microenvironmental variation in preservation in natural mummification processes. Within a small area (~1 m^2), two piglet specimens were nearly decomposed, two were partially skeletonised and two retained substantial well-preserved soft tissue. Although the environmental conditions were nearly identical, the water levels were higher near the well-preserved animals, suggesting the importance of the water to the retention of soft tissue. Observations of taphonomic changes reveal that preservation of the connective tissue such as skin is most common for this type of mummy. Other features typical of bog bodies are a lack of epidermis, and little or differential muscle preservation. The skin collagen and keratin of hair and nails are usually well preserved. Hair colour, however, is modified, as melanin oxidises to a reddish tone. Preservation of the internal organs is most common in those with a mainly collagenous content, such as the lungs and the intestinal walls (Brothwell and Gill-Robinson 2002).

8.8 Cold Environments

Another special environment that can produce spontaneous natural mummification is the extreme cold found at very high altitudes, or where a body can be locked in a glacial flow, such as with the 5,300-year-old Iceman (Dickson 2011). It is important to note that there are two different forms of mummies produced by extreme cold conditions, frozen and freeze-dried. Freeze-drying occurs when

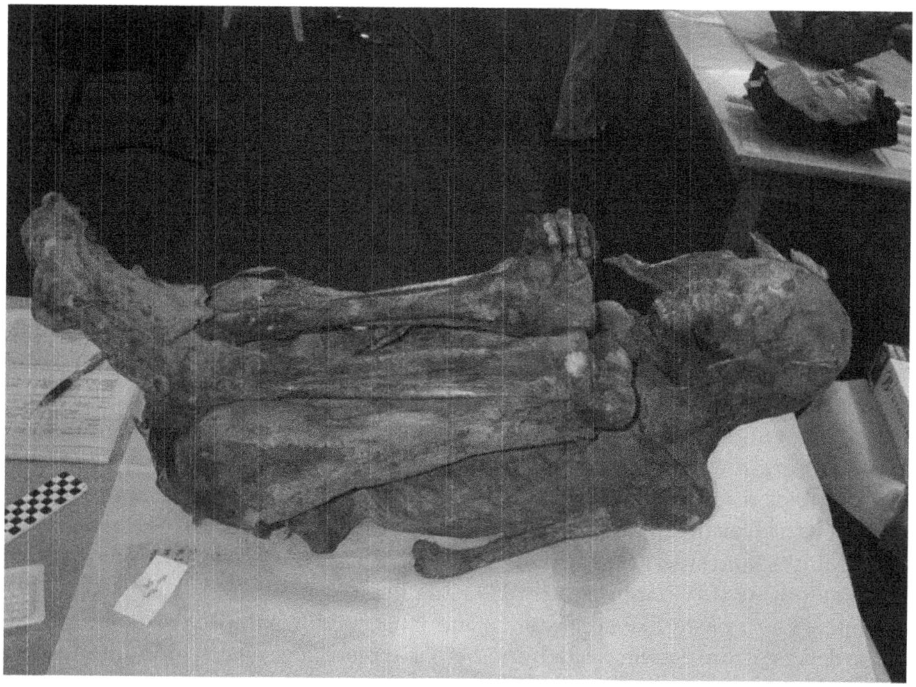

Figure 8.9 Inca mummy, Cusco, Peru. A combination of dry air, high altitude and burial in caves or niches, enabled some Inca mummies to spontaneously desiccate through evaporation and convection, without external treatment.

the body is first frozen in a high altitude environment where the atmospheric pressure is very low (Figure 8.9). The low pressure allows the frozen water in the subject to sublimate, or pass directly from the solid state of matter to a gaseous state. The ice leaves the body prior to liquefying, thus reducing the possibility of microbial action, even if the body is returned to a reasonable temperature. The freeze-dried body is essentially desiccated. In contrast, a frozen body still has its water content and when returned to temperatures above the freezing point has a greater potential of continuing along the process of decay. Clearly, in either category, mummies found in these environments must be very carefully conserved or the body could rapidly be lost to decomposition.

Well-known ice mummies include the Inca child mummies of the Andes discovered in 1999, and the Iceman found in the Alps between Austria and Italy in 1991, known as 'Ötzi'. The Llullaillaco mummies are three frozen sub-adults individually entombed near the summit of the homologous volcano (6,739 m), Argentina, in the context of Inca human sacrifice (Wilson *et al.* 2013). Their exceptional preservation can be attributed to the freezing temperature, although other factors must have contributed. These bodies were buried 50 cm underground, and the tomb's space became filled with protective volcanic ash, which created a barrier to external moisture while maintaining the internal, still-frozen water associated with the bodies. This specific environment transformed the bodily fats into adipocere (see below) as a layer of snow minimised environmental oxygen (Corthals *et al.* 2012). Ötzi, the Iceman, is particularly unusual because he dates back to the end of the Neolithic era. When discovered, he was associated with a number of artefacts including clothes, tools and weapons, which have opened a new window into prehistoric life (Dickson 2011). A recent atomic force microscopic study has shed new light on the mummification process, indicating evidence that preservation occurred by freeze-drying and inclusion in a glacier. Reportedly, the Iceman's skin had played a protective role, and prevented decomposition of the connective tissue (Janko *et al.* 2010). This suggested that the body was covered in snow almost immediately after death, and as a consequence of thawing and freezing, underwent physical damage, possible adipocere formation (see below), loss of the epidermis and desiccation.

8.9 Anaerobic Environments

As Aufderheide (2003) noted, anaerobiasis has often been used as an explanation for the natural mummification phenomenon; however, no study has been carried out to support this interpretation. It has been reported that enclosure of bodies in metal caskets has occasionally resulted in the preservation of the remains (Owsley and Compton 1997), possible as a result of a generally anoxic environment. As the human colon normally hosts some anaerobes, it may be expected that they can proliferate and destroy tissue, even in an anoxic environment. While air-deprived contexts should be experimentally investigated for understanding their impact on soft tissue preservation, the formation of adipocere (also known as 'grave wax' or 'fatty wax') appears to be related. Adipocere is a product of body fat decomposition that results from the processes of hydrolysis and hydrogenation of adipose tissue. The defining characteristic of adipocere formation is the transformation of unsaturated fatty acids. The levels of palmitic and stearic acids increase, and hydroxystearic acid forms during the conversion of the fats to adipocere (O'Connor *et al.* 2011) (Chapter 2).

Adipocere initially appears as a paste-like consistency and later solidifies until it resembles hard wax. It is generally regarded as a consequence of a humid environment, but is also found in diverse contexts including dry and watery environments. Its formation is most common in individuals with high body fat content and is commonly promoted by various types of soils and clothes with absorbent properties. Major factors contributing to the development of adipocere include an alkaline pH, warm temperature, anoxic conditions and adequate humidity, and the post-mortem presence of bacteria of the *Clostridria* group that facilitate its production. Adipocere has been reported to form within hours after death, but in reality takes several weeks or months to form (Forbes *et al.*, 2005a; 2005b; 2005c; O'Connor *et al.* 2011; Ubelaker and Zarenko 2011). If the environmental conditions do not change, the composition of the adipocere can remain intact for centuries, although the presence of anaerobic bacteria and oxygen will lead to rapid decay (O'Connor *et al.* 2011). Adipocere formation has a similar impact to mummification, in that the process may preserve the external morphology of the subjects affected, leading to their positive identification in a forensic context. Furthermore, adipocere may serve as a protective coating, preserving underlying tissues.

The 'Soap Lady', the 'Soap Man', the body from Lake Brienz and the Meenybraddan bog body are a few examples of mummies that have significant evidence of adipocere formation. In 1875, during road construction, Joseph Leidy, a prominent Pennsylvania physician in Philadelphia (USA), exhumed two bodies, later nicknamed the 'Soap Lady' and the 'Soap Man' (Figure 8.10). The Soap Lady eventually became curated by the Mütter Museum in Philadelphia, while the Soap Man was displayed in the National Museum of Natural History in Washington. The identities of the bodies were questioned, and subsequent radiological investigations refuted the information collected in the museum records (Conlogue *et al.* 1997). These unusual mummies, and their supposed identities, demonstrate the importance of considering the post-depositional context when examining any human remains, whether in a bioarchaeological or forensic context. Another example of a soap mummy was recovered from Lake Brienz, Switzerland in 1996 (Thali *et al.* 2011) (Chapter 17, Figure 17.1). The remains, in variable condition, with the presence of adipocere, consisted of a headless human torso with three partial extremities, mostly skeletonised. Some external parts were encrusted with vivianite, a mineral associated with a context of organic archaeological and geological materials and a rare occurrence in modern bodies. Investigations revealed that the remains belonged to a 25- to 30-year-old male,

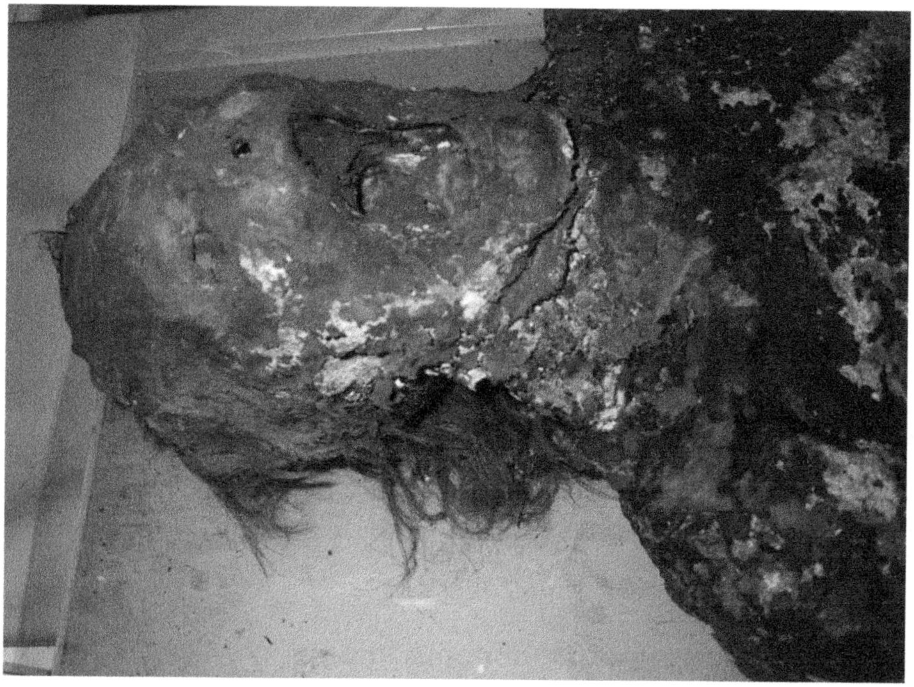

Figure 8.10 Soap Lady. An example of extensive adipocere formation is seen here in the mummy known as the 'Soap Lady', curated at the Mütter Museum in Philadelphia, Pennsylvania. This special type of natural mummification occurs when the body fats convert to a waxy soap-like substance due to contact with alkaline environments

most probably from the 18th century, who drowned in the area and was incorporated into the sediment under anoxic conditions. Ancient mummies may also have substantial adipocere. The bog body known as the 'Meenybraddan Woman', radiocarbon dated to around 1200 AD, had substantial adipocere formation, which protected underlying soft tissue structures (Delaney and O'Floinn 1995).

Finally, it is worth noting that adipocere is commonly found in association with preserved brain due to their high fat content, even when the rest of the body has decomposed. A recent example of preserved brain was identified in a 13th century burial from Quimper in Bretagne, France, where the presence of a salty and fresh water environment combined with acidic clay soil played a role in the preservation process, and adipocere was identified (Papageorgopoulou *et al.* 2010).

8.10 Differential Decomposition

Natural mummification due to dehydration of the cadaver and adipocere formation is often described as a dichotomous phenomenon. However, slight adipocere formation can occur in combination with desiccation, if the bodily water is sufficient to hydrolyse the fat but insufficient to allow for decomposition. Recently, the remains of a small, thin, 65-year-old male were found in coniferous woodland in Belgium; the corpse displayed both adipocere and dry tissue (Schotmans *et al.* 2011). The deceased, who had gone missing some seven months earlier, had been a victim of a homicide and was buried in a shallow pit. The tissue was well preserved, with minor deterioration at the level of the temporal bone, which appeared skeletonised. The phalanges of the left hand were missing, probably due to the activity of scavengers. The head, neck, right shoulder, upper torso and left leg were covered in adipocere, while the right leg appeared mummified. The rest of the torso and the arms appeared still fresh, as if the subject had died recently. Delayed putrefaction had left the body in the bloating state of decomposition. Except for some organs, most of the internal tissues were still preserved, as were the muscles. Hair was also present. According to the investigation results, the victim had been undressed, covered with plastic bags, rolled in a mattress and kept for about two days in a windowless room, after which time he was transported to the wood, uncovered and buried. While the pre-burial conditions were too vague to allow for a proper assessment of the post-depositional changes, the environment in which the body was interred provided clues. First of all, the cadaver was probably buried in a rather dry period, within an area protected by the coniferous woodland that impeded temperature fluctuations and sun exposure. Additionally, relatively cold weather and low precipitation may have played a role in tissue preservation. The sandy soil and the shallowness of the grave must have provided excellent drainage and a low pH must have limited bacterial decay, while favouring adipocere formation. Finally, the right leg protruding from the soil became desiccated due to exposure to airflow, as opposed to the rest of the body, which was shielded by burial. Of course, some physical characteristics of the subject must also have played a role in this case, including his thin build and the small body size. This case demonstrates how different factors can be responsible for differential preservation on the same cadaver (Schotsmans *et al.* 2011).

8.11 Post-Depositional Factors and Taphonomic Impact

Various environments and conditions have the potential to disrupt the natural stages of decomposition, resulting in different states of preserved remains. Once mummification has occurred, the taphonomic impact is still apparent, regardless of the extent or degree of mummification. While it is often assumed that mummies are stable at a specific stage of preservation, they continue to decompose, usually at a much reduced and varied rate. When considering the condition and characteristics of mummified remains, whether in a bioarchaeological or forensic setting, what happens to these remains following natural mummification is critical. Two broad categories of taphonomic impact need to be considered: the environment and regional fauna. The environment in which the remains are interred or discovered influences the post-depositional characteristics of these remains. Precipitation; climate (temperature, humidity, exposure to wind) over time; gravity; running water; repeated freeze-thaw cycles; sun exposure; soil conditions and regional topography all influence continued taphonomic change (Behrensmeyer 1978; Ubelaker 1997). Local fauna also affect mummified remains, or bodies with the potential to mummify. Modification of remains by animal activity is always a possibility (Moraitis and Spiliopoulou 2010). The type and extent of faunal modification is dependent upon the surroundings in which the body is placed. Although scavenging is the most common form of animal activity considered in taphonomic analyses, additional impact by animals, including insects, needs to be considered. Trampling, gnawing, pecking and consumption of the remains greatly alter the condition of the remains and may create routes of access to the body cavities initially protected by the mummified integument (Klippel and Synstelien 2007; Marean 1991). These disruptions in the mummified body increase the rate of taphonomic change by increasing the environmental exposure described above.

There are many examples of exposed remains that exhibit signs of gnawing, and indeed infestation of internal body cavities by vermin or insects (Figure 8.11) (Beckett *et al.* 2011). Dermestids are typically scavengers that feed on dry flesh (Huchet *et al.* 2013). Given the right conditions for development, the dermestid can create significant and numerous openings in mummified flesh, exposing the internal body cavities to the external environment and enhancing the potential for decay. Therefore,

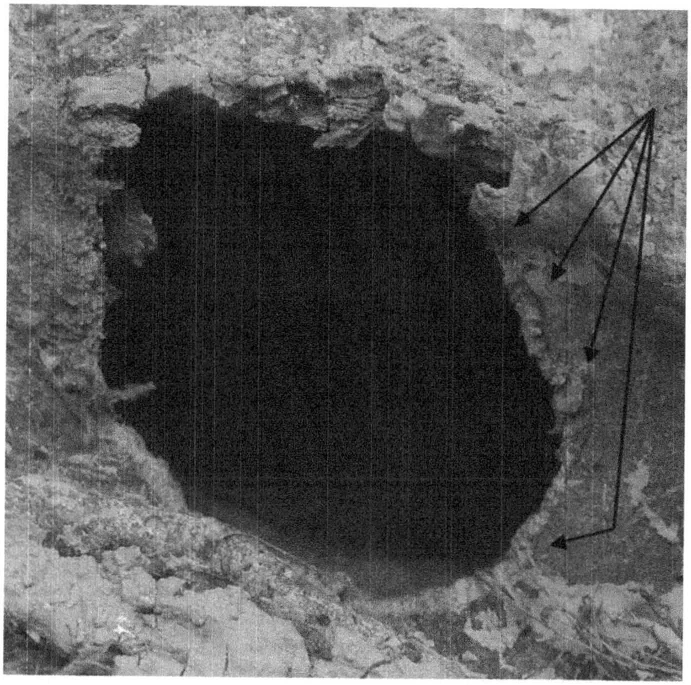

Figure 8.11 Post-depositional change at the lateral side of the torso of an individual. Evidence of vermin activity along the right lateral abdominal surface of the individual at the mid-axillary line resulted in post-depositional changes. Note the chew marks indicated by the arrows.

it is critical to gain an understanding of the context associated with the remains, in other words, the conditions when they mummified. It is also important to consider the regional environment at the time of mummification and develop a reconstructed environmental time-map ranging from the time of death to the present, identifying possible changes in environmental conditions. Furthermore, any peri- and post-mortem events that would result in the exposure of the internal body cavities to external forces of the environment or regional fauna must be taken into account during analysis to ensure the accuracy of the interpretation (Haglund 1997). It is often very difficult to determine human- versus nature-induced changes to the body, and ante-mortem, peri-mortem and post-mortem trauma is easily misinterpreted.

Since as much bioarchaeological information as possible needs to be obtained to develop the most probable explanation for the condition of the remains (e.g. Arriaza 1995), the archaeological, cultural and environmental context of the site provides a reasonable starting point in the assessment of post-depositional changes to accurately interpret the current condition of the naturally mummified remains. Burial typologies also influence the creation of natural mummies, such as surface versus interment in a burial pit, cave, tomb, coffin or crypt (Fornaciari *et al.* 2015; Piombino-Mascali *et al.* 2014). Each of these factors impacts the processes of natural mummification. Funerary traditions and burial artefacts, such as textiles, shrouds, clothing, objects and coffin materials, as well as the physical and chemical composition of the environment all make significant contributions to the preservation, or decomposition, of a body. Bioanthropological information, such as the age at death and the presence of palaeopathology, is also important when considering the taphonomic change over time (Chen *et al.* 2013; Ortner 2003).

Bone composition, and the taphonomic changes seen, involves collagen proteins and calcium compounds, which can be reduced as a part of the normal ageing process (Lau and Adachi 2011). After death, calcium may further be reduced by an acidic pH and water percolation, where soaking tends to decrease the calcium in bones (Dent *et al.* 2004). Higher temperatures also serve to dehydrate the bony structures, rendering them brittle. The decreased bone density may influence the interpretation of skeletonised material.

Of critical note is the potential for the development of less than accurate bioarchaeological assumptions when taphonomic changes, both intrinsic and extrinsic, are not considered. The diagenesis of prehistoric bone is often used to approximate dietary reconstructions. If taphonomy is not considered in these investigations, false assumptions may arise (Price *et al.* 1992; Wittmers *et al.* 2008). The conditions that produced the natural mummy, the extended period of environmental variation, sometimes millennia, and the impact of these variables must always be considered during the process of interpretation. Most mummies, no matter how effective the natural forces were in producing that mummy, are still on their taphonomic journey back to the elements (e.g. Piñar *et al.* 2013).

8.12 Conclusion

Natural, or spontaneous, preservation is of tremendous scientific importance. When making interpretations, it is important to consider both the original context and the environmental change over time as the extended context associated with the remains. Although largely neglected in many research reports, soft tissue taphonomy is of vital importance for interpretation of findings. Changes in gross anatomical and chemical features should always be kept in mind in both historical and forensic contexts. Finally, the state of arrested decay can change if the depositional environment changes, or if the mummy is removed from the original preservation environment.

References

Arriaza, B.T. (1995) Chinchorro bioarchaeology: chronology and mummy seriation. *Latin American Antiquity*, **6**: 35–55.

Aturaliya, S. and Lukasewycz, A. (1999) Experimental forensic and bioanthropological aspects of soft tissue taphonomy. Part 1: Factors influencing postmortem tissue desiccation rate. *Journal of Forensic Sciences*, **44**: 893–896.

Aufderheide, A.C. (2003) *The Scientific Study of Mummies*. Cambridge University Press: Cambridge.

Aufderheide, A.C. (2011) Soft tissue taphonomy: a paleopathology perspective. *International Journal of Paleopathology*, **1**: 75–80.

Beckett, R.G. and Conlogue, G.J, (2010) *Paleoimaging: Field applications for cultural remains and artifacts*. Boca Raton: CRC Press.

Beckett, R.G., Lohmann, U. and Bernstein, J. (2011) A unique field mummy conservation project in Papua New Guinea. *Yearbook of Mummy Studies*, **1**: 19–27.

Behrensmeyer, A.K. (1978) Taphonomic and ecologic information from bone weathering. *Paleobiology*, **4**:150–162.

Brier, B. and Wade, R.S. (2001) Surgical procedures during ancient Egyptian mummification. *Chungará*, **33**: 117–123.

Brothwell, D. and Gill-Robinson, H. (2002) Taphonomic and forensic aspects of bog bodies. In: Haglund, W.D. and Sorg, M.H. (eds), *Advances in Forensic Taphonomy*. CRC Press: Boca Raton, pp. 119–132.

Campobasso, C.P., Falamingo, R., Grattagliano, I. and Vinci, F. (2009) The mummified corpse in a forensic setting. *American Journal of Forensic Medicine and Pathology.* **30**: 307–310.

Cardin, M. (2014) *Mummies around the world: An encyclopedia of mummies in history, religion, and popular culture.* ABC Clio: Santa Barbara.

Chen, H., Zhou, X., Fujita, H., Onozuka, M. and Kubo, K. (2013) Age-related changes in trabecular and cortical bone micro-structure. *International Journal of Endocrinology,* Article ID 213234

Conlogue, G., Forcier, D., Airo, M., Kilosky, J., Gambardella, S. *et al.* (1997) Radiographic evaluation of the Soap man mummy. *Radiologic Technology,* **68**: 391–398.

Corthals, A., Koller, A., Martin, D.W., Rieger, R., Chen, E.I. *et al.* (2012) Detecting the immune system response of a 500-year-old Inca mummy. *PLoS ONE,* **7**: e41244.

Crowther, J. (2002) The experimental earthwork at Wareham, Dorset after 33 years: retention and leaching of phosphate released in the decomposition of buried bone. *Journal of Archaeological Science,* **29**: 411–505.

Delaney, M. and O'Floinn, R. (1995) A bog body from Meenybraddan Bog, County Donegal, Ireland. In: Turner, R.C. and Scaife, R.G. (eds), *Bog Bodies: New discoveries and new perspectives.* British Museum Press: London, pp. 123–132.

Dent, B.B., Forbes, S.L. and Stuart, B.H, (2004) Review of human decomposition processes in soil. *Environmental Geology,* **45**: 576–585.

Dickson, J.H. (2011) *Ancient Ice Mummies.* The History Press: Stroud, UK.

Forbes, S.L., Stuart, B.H. and Dent, B.B. (2005a) The effect of the burial environment on adipocere formation. *Forensic Science International,* **154**: 24–34.

Forbes, S.L., Dent, B.B. and Stuart, B.H. (2005b) The effect of soil type on adipocere formation. *Forensic Science International,* **154**: 35–43.

Forbes, S.L., Stuart, B.H. and Dent, B.B. (2005c) The effect of the method of burial on adipocere formation. *Forensic Science International,* **154**: 44–52.

Fornaciari, G., Giuffra, V., Bortolotti, F., Gottardo, R., Marvelli, S. et al (2015) A medieval case of digitalis poisoning: the sudden death of Cangrande della Scala, Lord of Verona (1291–1329). *Journal of Archaeological Science,* **54**: 162–167.

Galloway, A., Birkby, W.H., Jones, A., Henry, T. and Parks, B. (1989) Decay rates of human remains in an arid environment. *Journal of Forensic Sciences,* **34**: 607–616.

Garcia, A.M.B, Beckett, R.G. and Watson, J.T. (2014) Internal environmental characteristics of a Chiribaya style tomb holding swine remains and their taphonomic impact on decomposition delay, a requisit for mummification. *Papers on Anthropology,* **23**: 45–62.

Gill-Frerking, H.C. (2014) The impact of historical post-excavation modifications on the re-examination of human mummies. *Papers on Anthropology,* **23**: 63–75.

Gill-Frerking, H.C. and Healey, C. (2011) Experimental archaeology for the interpretation of taphonomy related to bog bodies: lessons learned from two projects undertaken a decade apart. *Yearbook of Mummy Studies,* **1**: 69–74.

Gill-Robinson, H.C. (2001) People and piglets: peat and preservation. In: Millard, A. (ed.), *Archaeological Sciences '97: Proceedings of the Conference held at the University of Durham, 2–4 September 1997.* British Archaeological Reports International Series 939 (BAR S939). Archaeopress: Oxford, pp. 160–163.

Guillen, S. (2004) Artificial mummies from the Andes. *Collegium Antropologicum,* **28**, **Supplement 2**: 141–157.

Haglund, W.D. (1997) Dogs and coyotes: postmortem involvement with human remains. In: Haglund, W.D. and Sorg, M.H. (eds), *Forensic Taphonomy: The postmortem fate of human remains.* CRC Press: Boca Raton, pp. 367–381.

Healy, F. and Housley, R.A. (1992) Nancy was not alone: human skeletons of the Early Bronze Age from the Norfolk peat fen. *Antiquity*, **66**: 948–955.

Huchet, J.B., Le Mort, F., Rabinovich, R., Blau, S., Coqueugniot, H. and Arensburg, B. (2013) Identification of dermestid pupal chambers on Southern Levant human bones: inference for reconstruction of Middle Bronze Age mortuary practices. *Journal of Archaeological Science*, **40**: 3793–3803.

Ikram, S. (2010) Mummification. In: Dieleman, J. and Wendrich, W. (eds), *UCLA Encyclopedia of Egyptology*. UEE: Los Angeles.

Ikram, S. and Dodson, A. (1998) *The Mummy in Ancient Egypt: Equipping the Dead for Eternity*. American University in Cairo Press: Cairo.

Introna, F., De Donno, A., Santoro, V., Corrado, S. *et al.* (2011) The bodies of two missing children in an enclosed underground environment. *Forensic Science International*, **207**: e40–e47.

Janko, M., Zink, A., Gigler, A.M., Heckl, W.M. and Stark, R.W. (2010) Nanostructure and mechanics of mummified type I collagen from the 5,300-year-old Tyrolean Iceman. *Proceedings of the Royal Society B*, **227**: 2301–2309.

Jit, I., Sehgal, S. and Sahni, D. (2001) An Indian mummy: a case report. *Forensic Science International*, **117**: 57–63.

Klippel, W.E. and Synstelien, J.A. (2007) Rodents as taphonomic agents: bone gnawing by brown rats and grey squirrels. *Journal of Forensic Science*, **52**: 765–773.

Lau, A.N. and Adachi, J.D. (2011) Bone aging. In: Nakasato, Y. and Young, R.L. (eds), *Geriatric Rheumatology: A comprehensive approach*. Springer: New York, pp. 11–16.

Lynnerup, N. (2007) Mummies. *Yearbook of Physical Anthropology*, **50**: 162–190.

Marean, C.W. (1991) Measuring the post-depositional destruction of bone in archaeological assemblages. *Journal of Archaeological Science*. **18**: 677–694.

Micozzi, M. (1991) *Postmortem Change in Human and Animal Remains*. Charles C. Thomas: Springfield, IL.

Moraitis, K. and Spiliopoulou, C. (2010) Forensic implications of carnivore scavenging on human remains recovered from outdoor locations in Greece. *Journal of Forensic and Legal Medicine*, **17**: 298–303.

Niknami, K.A., Masoumian, M. and Nekouei, P. (2014) Saltification process of human body in the Chehrabad salt mine using XRF and Psychrometric test. *International Journal of Archaeology*, **2**: 45–50.

O'Connor, S., Ali, E., Al-Sabah, S., Anwar, D., Bergström, E. *et al.* (2011) Exceptional preservation of a prehistoric human brain from Heslington, Yorkshire, UK. *Journal of Archaeological Science*, **38**: 1641–1654.

Ortner, D.J. (2003) *Identification of Pathological Conditions in Human Skeletal Remains*. Academic Press: San Diego.

Owsley, D.W. and Compton, B.E. (1997) Preservation in late 19th century iron coffin burials. In: Haglund, W.D. and Sorg, M.H. (eds), *Forensic Taphonomy: The postmortem fate of human remains*. CRC Press: Boca Raton, pp. 511–526.

Painter, T.J. (1991) Lindow Man, Tollund Man and other peat-bog bodies: the preservative and antimicrobial action of Sphagnan, a reactive glycuronoglycan with tanning and sequestering properties. *Carbohydrate Polymers*, **15**: 123–142.

Panzer, S., Zink, A. and Piombino-Mascali, D. (2010) Radiologic evidence of anthropogenic mummification in the Capuchin Catacombs of Palermo, Sicily. *RadioGraphics*, **30**: 1123–1132.

Panzer, S., Borumandi, F., Wanek, J., Papageorgopoulou, C., Shved, N. *et al.* (2013) Modeling ancient Egyptian embalming: radiological assessment of experimentally mummified human tissue by CT and MRI. *Skeletal Radiology*, **42**: 1527–1535.

Papageorgopoulou, C., Rentsch, K., Raghavan, M., Hofmann, M.I., Colacicco, G. *et al.* (2010) Preservation of cell structures in a medieval infant brain: a paleohistological, paleogenetic, radiological and physico-chemical study. *NeuroImage*, **50**: 893–901.

Piñar, G., Piombino-Mascali, D., Maixner, F., Zink, A. and Sterflinger, K. (2013) Microbial survey of the mummies from the Capuchin Catacombs of Palermo, Italy: biodeterioration risk and contamination of the indoor air. *FEMS Microbiology Ecology*, **86**: 341–356.

Piombino-Mascali, D., Jankauskas, R., Tamošiūnas, A., Valančius, R., Thompson, R.C. and Panzer, S. (2014) Atherosclerosis in mummified human remains from Vilnius, Lithuania (18th–19th centuries AD): a computed tomographic investigation. *American Journal of Human Biology*, **26**: 676–681.

Price, T.D., Blitz, J., Burton, J. and Ezzo, J.A. (1992) Diagenesis in prehistoric bone: problems and solutions. *Journal of Archaeological Science*, **19**: 513–529.

Schotsmans, E.M.J, Van de Voorde, W., De Winne, J. and Wilson, A.S. (2011) The impact of shallow burial on differential decomposition to the body: a temperate case study. *Forensic Science International*, **206**: e43–e48.

Thali, M.J., Lux, B., Lösch, S., Rösing, F.W., Hürlimann, J. *et al.* (2011) Brienzi – the blue Vivianite man of Switzerland: time since death estimation of an adipocere body. *Forensic Science International*, **211**: 34–40.

Ubelaker, D.H. (1997) Taphonomic applications in forensic anthropology. In: Haglund, W.D. and Sorg, M.H. (eds), *Forensic Taphonomy: The postmortem fate of human remains*. CRC Press: Boca Raton, pp, 77–90.

Ubelaker, D.H. and Zarenko, K.M. (2011) Adipocere: what is known after over two centuries of research. *Forensic Science International*, **208**: 167–172.

Ventura, F., Portunato, F., Pizzorno, E., Mazzone, S., Verde, A. and Rocca, G. (2013) The need for an interdisciplinary approach in forensic sciences: perspectives from a peculiar case of mummification. *Journal of Forensic Sciences*, **58**: 831–836.

Wilson, A.S., Brown, E.L., Villa, C., Lynnerup, N., Healey, A. *et al.* (2013) Archaeological, radiological and biological evidence offer insight into Inca child sacrifice. *Proceedings of the National Academy of Sciences*, **110**: 13322–13327.

Wittmers, L.E. Jr., Aufderheide, A.C., Pounds, J.G., Jones, K.W. and Angel, J.L. (2008) Problems in determination of skeletal lead burden in archaeological samples: an example from the First African Baptist Church population. *American Journal of Physical Anthropology*, **136**: 379–386.

Wittmers, L.E. Jr., Aufderheide, A.C. and Buikstra, J.E. (2011) Soft tissue preservation system: applications. *International Journal of Paleopathology*, **1**: 150–154.

Zimmerman, M.R. (1979) Paleopathologic diagnosis based on experimental mummification. *American Journal of Physical Anthropology*, **51**: 235–254.

9

Degradation of Clothing in Depositional Environments

Barbara H. Stuart and Maiken Ueland

9.1 Introduction

Clothing has long been present as part of everyday life and, as a consequence, provides a valuable source of information in forensic and archaeological contexts (Bier and Dusenbury 2008; Goffer 2007; Robertson and Grieve 1999; Taupin and Cwiklik 2011). In forensic scenarios, textiles are a common source of evidence and can provide valuable insight into a crime. In the field of forensic taphonomy, the nature and condition of textiles collected from a crime scene can assist investigators in determining the nature of the death (e.g. examination of stab wounds) and in the identification of the victim. The presence of clothing and other body coverings at the deposition site can have a significant effect on the estimation of the post-mortem interval. In an archaeological context, clothing provides insight into past costumes, socio-economic status and technologies. Therefore, the state of preservation is important in the retention of this particular source of cultural heritage.

The fibres used to produce clothing are varied in composition. Traditionally, natural plant- and animal-based fibres such as wool and cotton have been used, but the development of synthetic polymer fibres during the 20th century saw the diversification of fibre types in use. The variety of available structures also means a variety of responses to degradation agents, as the mechanism will depend on the chemical structure of the fibres. This chapter provides an overview of commonly encountered material types and their associated degradation mechanisms.

Clothing damage has been the subject of a number of forensic and archaeological investigations. Some studies have focused on particular cases or finds, while others have been carried out on model systems to gain a greater understanding of the parameters that control clothing degradation in burial environments (e.g. Janaway 2008). Representative examples of forensic and archaeological clothing studies are provided in this chapter. The collection of damaged or preserved clothing from burial environments requires special care, therefore forensic and archaeological protocols have been established to avoid further damage. An overview of the protocols for forensic and archaeological clothing collection is also provided in this chapter.

9.2 The Structures and Properties of Clothing Materials

Fibres are used in many artefacts, especially textiles (woven fabric), and are made of both natural and synthetic materials (Hearle and Schwaller 2011; Mather and Wardman 2011). Fibres of natural origin have been used for thousands of years for the production of textiles. Natural fibres are derived from

Taphonomy of Human Remains: Forensic Analysis of the Dead and the Depositional Environment, First Edition.
Edited by Eline M.J. Schotsmans, Nicholas Márquez-Grant and Shari L. Forbes.

plant and animal sources and are generally converted into yarns by a spinning process. Once fibres are produced, they are woven into textiles, with the specific technology employed depending on the end use. Leather objects have also long been used for clothing, shoes and coverings.

A range of man-made polymer fibres are used for textile production (Hearle and Mather and Wardman 2011; Schwaller 2011). Synthetic textile production emerged during the mid-20th century and the use of synthetic and natural-synthetic fibre blends expanded in textile manufacture. Synthetic fibres grew in popularity because of a variety of attractive properties, which included crease and chemical resistance, colour fastness, resistance to microorganisms and good mechanical properties. A range of organic synthetic reactions is standardly employed to produce the polymers that are utilised in synthetic fibre manufacture. The choice of reaction (e.g. chain or step polymerisation, copolymerisation) will depend on the class of fibre. Once the polymer has been synthesised, the molten polymer is usually extruded using a device called a spinneret containing small holes, which produce filaments that are solidified.

During or after processing, textile fibres commonly undergo a range of treatments, depending on the end use of the material (Clark 2011; Wayland 2012). Fibres are principally coloured by dyes, colouring agents that are soluble in the solvent employed in an application. There is an extensive range of commercial synthetic dyes, which can be classified by their structure type or the method of application. Some common structural types used as dyes include azos, phthalocyanines and anthraquinones. A wide range of finishing agents is used after dying and may involve physical, chemical or biological processes. Physical processes, such as brushing, mechanically alter the textile surface. Chemical processes are utilised to add agents (e.g. silicones are used for waterproofing) or remove agents (e.g. bleaching removes the existing colour of natural fibres). Biological processes involve the use of enzymes, which react with the fibre surface, modifying the physical appearance.

9.2.1 Natural Fibres

Cellulosic fibres, such as cotton and linen, are derived from plants. Cotton is the most widely used natural textile and has been in use for cloth since antiquity. It is used in its pure form as well as in synthetic blends (Goffer 2007; Janaway 2002). Cotton fibre is obtained from the seed hair of the cotton seed and is predominantly comprised of cellulose (90–99%), a polysaccharide made up of glucose residues (the structure is illustrated in Figure 9.1). Cotton undergoes several finishing procedures prior to use in textiles. Desizing is usually carried out using enzymes. Scouring is a process that involves boiling in an alkali to remove wax and other impurities. Cotton is usually bleached prior to use and oxidising agents such as hydrogen peroxide or sodium hypochlorite can be used for this purpose. Linen is produced from flax plant stems – generally accepted as the first fibres to be used by humans (Janaway 2002; Goffer 2007). Linen fibres are extracted by a bacterial process known as retting, in which fungi degrade the woody tissue and the remaining linen fibres are removed and dried. In addition to containing a substantial amount of cellulose (of the order of 70%), flax also contains hemicellulose, lignin and pectin, which produce a matrix that imparts more strength and rigidity when compared to cotton.

Protein-based fibres from animal sources include wool and silk. Wool is the fibre obtained from the fleece of the sheep and has been utilised in textiles for thousands of years, being the dominant fibre used for clothing until the emergence of the cotton industry in the 19th century (Goffer 2007; Janaway 2002; Zahn *et al.* 2003). Although the relatively high cost of wool production has reduced its application, wool is still in wide use for knitwear. It is predominantly composed of the protein keratin. Keratin is a fibrous protein with a high degree of sulphur–sulphur cross-linking between the cysteine amino acid residues in its structure. The extensive hydrogen bonding and α-helical structures formed result in stable protein chains of keratin, which group together to form fibrils. Wool also

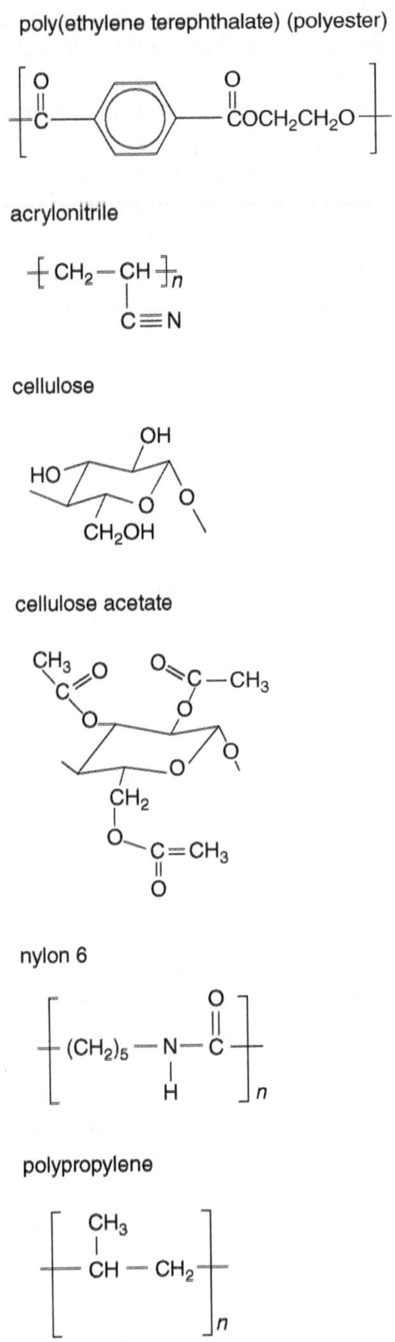

Figure 9.1 Chemical structures of some common textile fibre components.

contains small quantities of lipids, with the fibres protected by a layer of lanolin, which is usually removed prior to use as it attracts dirt. Silk is secreted by the larvae of a particular species of moth and its use as a highly prized textile fibre dates back several thousand years in China (Goffer 2007; Janaway 2002, 2008). It is primarily composed of the fibrous protein fibroin, resulting in a strong fibre.

9.2.2 Synthetic Fibres

Four types of synthetic fibres dominate in textile production – polyester, nylon, acrylic and polyolefin (Fenichell 1997; Mather and Wardman 2011). The chemical structures of some of the most common synthetic fibre materials are shown in Figure 9.1. Polyester accounts for about 60% of synthetic fibre production and Terylene and Dacron are common trade names. Poly(ethylene terephthalate) (PET) is the major form and finds use in clothing and furnishings. Polyester is used on its own or in cotton mixtures for textile manufacture and has advantageous mechanical properties, minimal shrinkage and good colour retention. The development of nylon was the result of a deliberate process to produce a material which could replace silk. The first applications of nylon were as fibres in fabric for parachutes and stockings and the polymer is now in widespread use for ropes, tents and carpets, as well as clothing. Nylon is a polyamide and a variety of nylons are produced based on the length and sequence of the repeat unit. Some examples of nylons that are popular for use in textile manufacture include nylon 6, nylon 11 and nylon 6,6. Acrylic fibres are copolymers comprised of at least 85% acrylonitrile. Acrylonitrile is copolymerised with other monomers such as vinyl acetate or methyl acetate to produce acrylic fibres. The light and soft properties of acrylic fibres make them a suitable substitute for wool and they are used for applications such as jumpers, hats and socks, as well as in home furnishings. Olefin fibres include polyethylene and polypropylene. Polyethylene is used mainly for ropes and twines, while polypropylene is used for carpets, sportswear and thermal clothing.

Some examples of other types of synthetic polymers that find use in textiles include regenerated cellulose, acetates and urethanes. Regenerated cellulose is cellulose precipitated from acidic solution and when prepared as a fibre; it is known as viscose, rayon or viscose rayon. The development of cellulose acetate was a result of the esterification of cellulose. When complete acetylation is carried out, cellulose triacetate is formed, but the acetylation reaction may also be reversed to a point where cellulose diacetate is formed, which is more suitable for use as a fibre. Urethane fibres (elastane) are highly elastic and therefore are popular for the production of flexible textiles used for stockings and swimwear.

Metallic fibres are comprised of pure metals or of a polymer fibre coated in metal. Gold and silver have been used since antiquity as decorative high status yarns. Aluminium has replaced gold and silver in more recent time and is layered in a polyester or acetate film.

9.2.3 Leather

Animal skin has traditionally been used to produce leather and is composed of the proteins collagen and keratin that require a preservation process (Cronyn 1990; Goffer 2007; Kite and Thomson 2006). Tanning is a chemical procedure for preserving skin that alters the protein structure and makes the skin pliable and impermeable to water. Prior to tanning, flesh, fat and hair are removed using agents such as lime. A traditional approach is vegetable tanning, which utilises tannins, polyphenol compounds that occur naturally in a variety of plants. Tannins bind to proteins and create a structure that is less water-soluble. Lubricating oils or fats are applied to make the material pliable. A common mineral tanning technique is chrome tanning, which utilises chromium (III) sulphate as a tanning agent. Prior to chromium treatment, the skin is treated with sulphuric acid to lower the pH, which modifies the protein structure and ensures that the chromium complex is introduced. Once the chrome has been incorporated, the pH is raised by treatment with sodium bicarbonate. Another form of mineral tanning involves the use of aluminium and potassium sulphates (alums) and is known as tawing.

9.3 Decomposition Mechanisms of Clothing Materials in Depositional Environments

9.3.1 Decomposition Agents

In addition to the activity of insects and scavenging animals, there is a number of environmental factors that are critical to the degradation or preservation of clothing in burial sites. These include the presence of microorganisms, body decomposition fluids, moisture content, temperature, pH, electrochemistry and surface treatments (Cronyn 1997; Janaway 1996, 2002, 2008). How these factors affect clothing is dependent on the structural nature of the fibres that make up materials, because the biodegradation or chemical degradation mechanism will depend on the fundamental chemistry.

Biodegradation is a major source of deterioration of textiles in soil environments. Microorganisms, including bacteria and fungi, produce enzymes that are capable of attacking the molecular structures of the polymers, both natural and synthetic, that form the principal components of textile fibres. The availability of oxygen in the burial environment determines the nature of the biological agents that are present and, therefore, determines the type of biodegradation. Certain biodegradation mechanisms require aerobic conditions, while other microorganisms thrive in anaerobic conditions. For instance, oxygen is required for fungal metabolism, thus it will be anaerobic bacteria that attack textile materials in anaerobic environments.

During the natural decomposition process, lipids, proteins and carbohydrates are broken down into smaller molecules. These decomposition by-products are the major components in decomposition fluid. The presence of decomposing remains may inhibit or delay textile degradation in a burial environment, but there has been very little research on the specific mechanisms that prevent or delay textile degradation when in contact with decomposing remains. The difference in degradation rate, or lack thereof, is likely due to the leaching of the decomposition fluid, which then becomes embedded within the textiles.

The amount of water in the burial environment is also a determining factor in the biodegradation of textiles. Bacteria require moisture to flourish. However, waterlogged soils are not conducive to most bacteria, due to the reduction in available oxygen. Likewise, very dry environments reduce the microbial population and so inhibit biodegradation.

Microorganisms are also sensitive to temperature. Bacteria usually exist in the range 10–40°C (and proliferate at 25–35°C). Extreme temperatures will affect the biodegradation agents, with very cold conditions inhibiting bacterial activity. Where soil conditions are below freezing, biodeterioration can be prevented for a long period of time. Likewise, under very hot conditions, the biological agents are unable to thrive.

Bacterial populations are also affected by pH and most soil bacteria exist in the range pH 4–10, so particular biodegradation processes will be inhibited or prevented in highly acidic or basic environments. Highly acidic low pH burial environments can include peat marshes. High pH alkaline soil environments are usually due to high concentrations of carbonates. Where chemical degradation mechanisms are feasible, extreme pH can result in destructive reactions, such as hydrolysis.

The presence of particular metals in contact with textiles can interfere with degradation processes and, in fact, preserve organic materials (Chen 1998; Janaway 1987, 1996, 2002, 2008). Copper alloys may undergo an electrochemical process to produce copper ions, depending on the environmental pH. Copper ions can be transported into a textile and in a high enough concentration, act as a biocide that inhibits microbial decay. Ferrous metals also affect the degradation process of certain textile materials, but do so by forming corrosion products such as iron oxides, hydroxides and soil minerals that encapsulate the textile. The textile degradation process is not inhibited, but instead a hollow cast of the material remains, provided that the iron corrosion product is deposited prior to significant textile degradation.

Various types of fibre treatments used in textile production also influence the degradation process. For instance, the class of dye used may prevent decay by microorganisms – for example, mordant dyes that utilise metal ions (such as iron or copper) to enable fibre adhesion can be toxic for microorganisms (Janaway 2002). The application of antimicrobial finishes will also play an important role in the rate of decay (Heywood 2003). Antimicrobial agents are applied via chemical finishing and are designed to inhibit the microorganisms that are responsible for decay.

The type of production method used to produce a textile also has a potential effect on the ability of the material to degrade in a burial environment. Different weaving methods will result in a textile allowing more or less access to degradation agents. For example, a carpet is made by interlacing fibres through a woven cloth, thus creating a substantially more protected material than a simple woven fabric produced from the sample fibre type, for say, clothing production.

9.3.2 Degradation of Natural Fibres

Cotton is particularly susceptible to decomposition due to its high cellulose content (Cardamone *et al.* 1991; Janaway 2002; Raschle 1989). Examples of the visual changes that can occur are illustrated in Figure 9.2, which shows an example of a cotton textile that has been exhumed from an acidic and sandy soil surface environment after a period of one year. Cotton is very absorbent and swells in a wet or moist environment. Microbial agents readily break down the cellulose component, and the

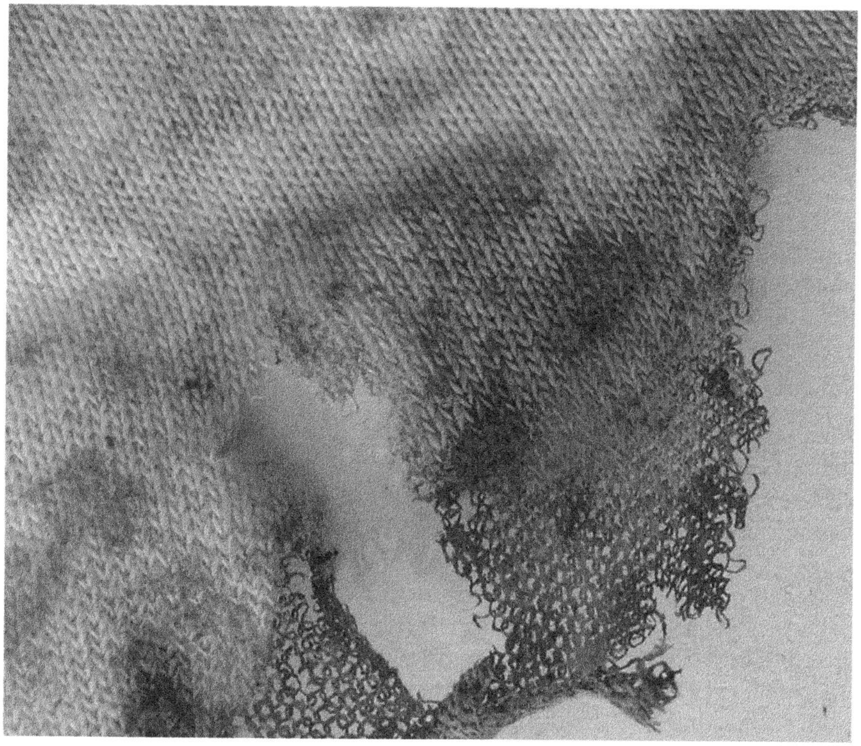

Figure 9.2 Visual damage to cotton after one year of burial in an acidic sandy soil.

presence of water is important for these processes. Enzymatic processes are catalysed by cellulase enzymes, and result in the destruction of the linkages between the glucose components. Cotton is highly vulnerable to hydrolysis in acidic environments. The glycosidic link in cellulose can hydrolyse, and oxidation of hydroxyl groups may occur to form oxycellulose. Both mechanisms result in a reduction of mechanical properties. It is possible for cotton to survive in high pH alkaline, very dry or frozen burial environments, as these conditions inhibit the processes responsible for the breakdown of the cellulose structure. As cotton can readily absorb water and dissolved cations, this fibre may be preserved when in association with copper.

Like cotton, linen is susceptible to degradation in many burial environments, but may survive in frozen or desiccated environments (Cronyn 1990; Janaway 2002). Linen also readily absorbs water and is easily broken down by microorganisms. However, it is somewhat more resistant to degradation in acidic environments and less resistant to alkaline environments compared to cotton.

Wool shows more resistance to chemical degradation than cotton due to the more stable proteins making up the principal component of keratin (Janaway 2002, 2008; Solazzo 2013). However, wool is susceptible to strongly alkaline environments. In such environments, the hydrogen bonding within protein molecules is disrupted leading to denaturation. Disulphide bridges in keratin react with alkalis to form a weaker lanthionine link with a single sulphur atom. Under more severe conditions, the lanthionine also breaks down and peptide bonds may also be broken, resulting in a weakening of the fibres. Wool is more resistant to acidic environments, with the disulphide links in protein resistant to acids above pH 2. However, when exposed to very strong acids, hydrogen bonding will be disrupted and hydrolysis of the peptide bonds can occur. Degradation of wool may also occur as a result of the attack of particular microorganisms. The protein is degraded by keratinolytic microorganisms in soil, which produce enzymes that specifically attack keratin. When the hydrogen bonding and disulphide bonds in keratin are disrupted, proteolytic enzymes are able to gain access and attack the protein. Such biodegradation is inhibited in environments that are not conducive to bacteria or fungi, such as cold wet burials and peat bogs, salty or very dry environments (Peacock 1996). The physical changes, observed as a result of degradation of wool, are discolouration, surface pitting and/or defibrillation. Generally, metal preserved wool textiles are more likely when in contact with ferrous metals (Janaway 2002).

Silk behaves in a similar way to wool in burial environments, but is less resistant to decay (Janaway 2002, 2008). Silk is very hygroscopic, therefore like wool, does not decay rapidly. It has been observed to survive for long periods in anaerobic soils and in water logged anoxic conditions (Janaway 2002; Sibley and Jakes 1984). Silk will, however, discolour and disintegrate in aerobic soils.

9.3.3 Degradation of Synthetic Fibres

Synthetic fibres are regarded as considerably more resistant to deterioration when compared to their natural counterparts (Janaway 2008; Quye 2014; Szostak-Kotowa 2004). However, some classes of synthetic fibres are subject to degradation, due to the presence of functional groups that are vulnerable to oxidation and enzymatic attack.

Polyester fibres show a very good resistance to biological and chemical factors, but if certain finishes (such as starch) are used in production, fungal growth may occur on the surface and result in discolouration.

Nylons used in fibres are quite resistant to biodegradation. However, nylons tend to be susceptible to light degradation and thermo-oxidation, which results in discolouration and embrittlement. Thus, changes may be observed in surface burials. The resulting photo-oxidation reactions include chain scission, cross-linking and secondary oxidative reactions. The degradation rate will be affected by the presence of dyes or pigments or the addition of ultraviolet absorbers or anti-oxidants added during manufacture. Thermo-oxidation mechanisms involve the production of peroxy radicals that react with the methylene group adjacent to the amide linkage in nylon.

Acrylic fibres are very resistant to biodegradation and ultraviolet radiation. The dominant acrylonitrile group within the structure of this class of fibre is particularly stable.

Polyolefin fibres, such as polypropylene and polyethylene, are very resistant to biodegradation. They do, however, degrade when exposed to ultraviolet radiation.

Regenerated cellulose fibres tend to absorb moisture in wet conditions and swell due to the presence of hydroxyl groups. Consequently, fibres such as viscose rayon are susceptible to fungal growth and hydrolytic degradation. Cellulose acetate fibres are less water absorbent than regenerated cellulose fibres due to the substitution of hydroxyl groups with acetate groups during production. This makes acetate fibres more resistant to biodegradation mechanisms.

Urethane fibres may undergo degradation hydrolysis. Polyurethanes containing ester groups are susceptible to both chemical and microbiological degradation. Ether-based polyurethanes are more resistant to biodegradation.

9.3.4 Leather

Modern leathers tend to be more resistant than archaeological leathers due to the chrome tanning process employed. Leather will appear more brittle and darkened as it deteriorates (Cronyn 1990; Kite and Thomson 2006; Strzelczyk 1997). Surface fats or oils can oxidise and cause the leather to stiffen. The preservation of leather is dependent on the moisture content of the environment. In dry environments, moisture is lost from the leather and shrinkage and cracking will occur. Where the moisture content is high, leather may hydrolyse into a black resinous material. Leather buried in a wet site can be well preserved, but the nature of the wet environment will influence the preservation. For instance, environments high in organic matter are known to preserve, because they can undergo anaerobic microbial decomposition to produce compounds that inhibit the microorganisms that could degrade leather. Leaching of oils or tannins and reaction with organic compounds or salts in the soil will influence this degradation process. Darkening of leather indicates an increase in pH.

9.4 The Influence of Clothing on the Decomposition Processes

The presence of clothing will have a significant influence on the decomposition of a cadaver (Anderson 2010; Forbes *et al.* 2005; Kelly *et al.* 2009; Mann *et al.* 1990; Voss *et al.* 2011). Clothing or body wrappings have been observed to have different effects on the decomposition rate – the process may be accelerated or delayed. Clothing may slow down the rate of cooling of the body and provide an environment that is warmer and more humid and thus is favourable to insects. Clothing may also protect insects from predators and environmental factors such as sunlight and rain. However, sometimes clothing acts as a barrier for colonising insects and so inhibits decomposition. Adipocere formation may also be enhanced by the presence of clothing, depending on the material's ability to retain moisture. The formation of adipocere has been observed to be more likely in dressed bodies (Forbes *et al.* 2005; Mant 1987).

The nature of the material used for body coverings plays an important role in the decomposition process. As synthetic fibres are significantly more resistant to degradation in a burial environment, they provide protection of the body for a longer period of time and therefore change the rate of body decomposition. Adipocere formation has been shown to be dependent on the type of material present. For example, the presence of polyester clothing is observed to enhance the formation of adipocere, most likely due to the ability to retain moisture as well as its resistance to biodeterioration (Forbes *et al.* 2005).

9.5 Forensic and Archaeological Studies of Clothing Degradation

Studies of the degradation of clothing in forensic and archaeological contexts have been widely reported. Both case reports and model experimental studies have been described in the literature. Examples of reported studies, which demonstrate the influence of the nature of the fibre and the burial environment on the deterioration of natural and synthetic fibres and leather objects, are provided in this section.

9.5.1 Natural Fibre Studies

Valuable information about the behaviour of common natural textile materials has been provided by the Experimental Earthworks Project in the UK (Bell *et al.* 1996; Janaway 2002, 2008). A component of the project, which began in 1960, involved the burial of a range of textiles of archaeological and forensic interest for long periods at two contrasting sites. The study demonstrated the importance of considering the nature of the burial environment when assessing the degradation of textiles. For example, natural textiles buried in sites conducive to biological activity (in a pH range 4.8–5.3) were vulnerable to decomposition when compared to an environment of high pH 7.5. Of the natural textiles studied, undyed cotton was the most vulnerable to decomposition in biologically active soil, with dyed cotton such as denim still vulnerable, but less so than the undyed material. Wool and silk were shown to be more resistant to decay in such an environment over a period of 36 months.

Metal preservation of natural textiles has been widely reported for archaeological materials (Janaway 2002). The phenomenon was even reported for Roman artefacts during the 19th century by Michael Faraday (Faraday 1836). In a wide range of archaeological sites, textiles associated with metals such as copper or iron have been preserved, and have enabled the nature of the textile to be characterised, otherwise the material would have been lost (Janaway 1983, 1987, 2002). An important observation from relevant studies has been that the metal preservation of organic materials is favoured in burial environments conducive to corrosion of the associated metal, with a resulting transport of corrosion products onto the textile.

A model pig burial study carried out in Bradford in the UK has provided insight into the effect of decomposition fluids on textile preservation (Janaway 2008; Wilson *et al.* 2007). It was observed that while natural fibres including cotton, denim and wool were susceptible to decay in the well-drained and biologically active soil utilised when positioned above the pigs, some preservation was afforded to the same textiles when placed below the pigs in the same environment. A more recent study utilising gas chromatography-mass spectrometry (GC-MS) and infrared spectroscopy techniques supported these observations, demonstrating a greater stability for cotton when in contact with a decomposing pig carcass (Lowe *et al.* 2013; Ueland *et al.* 2015).

Freezing conditions have also been responsible for the preservation of archaeologically significant textiles. Numerous sites have been excavated in the Arctic region, with one of the best-preserved sites being that of the Sir John Franklin's 1845 expedition to Canada's Northwest Passage (Kerr and Schweger 1989). A gravesite of one of the first sailors to die on this expedition, John Torrington, provides an example of well-preserved textiles in freezing conditions. Torrington was buried in a wooden coffin, below the permafrost, with water within the coffin remaining frozen until specimens were collected in the 1980s. Wool, cotton and linen fibres within the coffin were very well preserved (along with Torrington's body itself), while textiles located outside the coffin and in contact with soil were considerably degraded.

9.5.2 Synthetic Fibre Studies

A number of studies on the degradation of the behaviour of synthetic textile materials in a forensic burial context have been reported. The focus has been on the examination of the degradation of the most common synthetic textiles materials in model burial soil environments (Lowe *et al.* 2013; Mitchell *et al.* 2012; Morse 1983; Morse and Dailey 1985; Rowe 1997).

Studies of the effect of the burial on a series of clothing materials in model trenches in Florida have been reported (Morse 1983; Morse and Dailey 1985). The synthetic fibres examined in these studies included rayon, cellulose triacetate, nylon, acrylic and a polyester/cotton blend. The cloth specimens were examined periodically for a period of 60 months and monitored using microscopy and tensile strength tests. Rayon was the textile that was the most readily deteriorated in these studies, even more so when compared to the natural textiles examined – cotton, silk and wool. The polyester/cotton blend and cellulose triacetate showed moderate stability. Nylon and acrylic textiles were shown to be resistant to burial damage.

The deterioration of synthetic clothing textiles in model burial environments was subsequently studied utilising chromatographic and spectroscopic techniques (Northrop and Rowe 1987; Rowe 1997; Singer and Rowe 1989). The use of these techniques enables biodeterioration processes to be monitored. In these studies, the regenerated cellulose fibres underwent biodeterioration rapidly, while the purely synthetic fibres, such as nylon, polyester and acrylic, were very resistant to biodeterioration. Table 9.1 gives the relative resistance of various synthetic fibres in a soil burial environment (Northrop and Rowe 1987; Rowe 1997; Singer and Rowe 1989).

The influence of body decomposition on polyester textiles has been investigated in several studies (Lowe *et al.* 2013; Spennemann and Franke 1995). Polyester and polyester/cotton items were collected from human burials during an exhumation in the Marshall Islands (Spennemann and Franke 1995). The materials that had been used for clothing and coffin linings showed very good preservation in the tropical conditions. A model study utilising the controlled burial of pigs clothed with polyester/cotton showed evidence of degradation at 14 months of burial, either when in contact with the body or when in direct contact with the soil (Lowe *et al.* 2013).

Table 9.1 The deterioration of man-made fibres buried in well-watered soil (Northrop and Rowe 1987; Rowe 1997; Singer and Rowe 1989).

	Time / Months								
Fibre type	1	2	3	4	5	6	7	8	9
Rayon	N	SL	SL	DF	DF	DF	DF	SD	SD
Cellulose acetate	N	SL	SD	SD	SD	SD	SD	NR	NR
Cellulose triacetate	N	N	N	N	N	N	N	N	N
Nylon	N	N	N	N	N	N	N	N	N
Polyester	N	N	N	N	N	N	N	N	N
Acrylic	N	N	N	N	N	N	N	N	N

N: no deterioration
SL: slight deterioration (some pitting or fibre splitting)
DF: definite deterioration (extensive pitting and fibre splitting)
SD: severe deterioration (extensive fibre fragmentation and disintegration)
NR: not recoverable (textile completely decomposed)

9.5.3 Leather Studies

There are many examples of preserved archaeological leather goods surviving under optimum conditions, with goods dating back to the Neolithic period, the Bronze Age, the Roman period and the Middle Ages, making up collections worldwide (Kite and Thomson 2006). Leather survives best in what may be regarded as extreme environments – very wet or very dry. More commonly, leather finds are located in waterlogged environments and covered with organic plant matter. Multiple examples of preserved leather artefacts, such as boots and belts, have been collected from World War I sites in Europe (Robertshaw and Kenyon 2008). However, an example of well-preserved leather is a shoe excavated from a cave in Armenia (Pinhasi *et al.* 2010). The shoe is regarded as the world's oldest shoe, dating to around 3500 BC. The cave's very stable protected cool and dry conditions were conducive to preservation in this case.

Modern leather is well known to be a surviving grave good in forensic investigations – items such as shoes and belts can remain in the environment where other clothing has disintegrated. As part of the Experimental Earthwork's Project, modern tanned leather has been demonstrated to be more resistant to degradation than vegetable tanned leather, in a range of soil burial conditions (Bell *et al.* 1996; Janaway 2002).

9.6 Protocols for Forensic and Archaeological Clothing Collection and Analysis

For both forensic and archaeological clothing specimens, there is a similar strategy for collection and analysis. An appropriate strategy to protect the items will involve retrieval, cleaning, examination and stabilisation steps (Adovasio 2008; Cronyn 1990; Kite and Thomson 2006). The approach taken will also depend on the nature of the burial environment – different approaches are required for wet and dry burial sites.

The retrieval of clothing artefacts from burial sites requires care due to the fragile nature of such materials. For dry sites, it is recommended that specimens are removed with surrounding soil to prevent damage and the samples should be well supported. For wet sites, more specialist extraction techniques involving hydraulics may be required, and specimens should be maintained in a wet state until transported to the laboratory. Generally, specimens are stored in plastic or paper bags or rigid plastic containers.

Once transported to the laboratory, specimens should be cleaned and examined. Water is the best option as a cleaning agent. Wet materials should be air-dried and specimens should preferably be stored in a refrigerator or freezer. An initial visual examination of artefacts, using microscopy, can provide valuable information about the state of degradation as well the construction of the item, such as the type of weave. Further information may be obtained via examination using infrared and ultraviolet light. The application of chemical tests, such as pH measurements and the application of analytical techniques, such as infrared spectroscopy, may assist in the identification of the fibre type and the degree of deterioration.

Although the priority with archaeological specimens should be to do as little as possible, stabilisation agents can be applied if it is apparent that further deterioration is likely to occur. A variety of commercial preparations are available that are suitable for clothing specimens and include Parylene (based on poly(p-xylylene polymers). Leather specimens are commonly conserved using a freeze-drying procedure after treatment with polyethylene glycol or glycerol. Following treatment, specimens should be maintained at a stable temperature, with relative humidity and light exposure minimised. Microscopic techniques are used to inspect the condition of archaeological specimens.

In addition, other analytical techniques, such as chromatography to investigate dyes, may be applied if required prior to any conservation treatments.

9.7 Conclusion and Future Research

In forensic science, textiles are a common source of evidence and can provide valuable insight into a crime. The broad range of depositional conditions that exist worldwide provide a challenge when attempting to understand the taphonomy of clothing in forensic or archaeological cases. Future studies of the influence of such environments on the degradation of the ever-increasing variety of clothing types will provide a valuable source of information for forensic practitioners, as the material composition plays a significant role in degradation behaviour. The broad range of surface treatments that are employed during manufacture also adds complexity to the understanding of degradation mechanisms and further studies are required. A greater understanding of textile degradation and the deterioration mechanisms in burial environments will also be enhanced by the expanding application of modern analytical techniques, such as chromatography and spectroscopy.

References

Adovasio, J.M. (2008) Fibre artefacts. In: Pearsall, D.M. (ed.), *Encyclopaedia of Archaeology*. Elsevier: Amsterdam, pp. 1375–1386.

Anderson, G.S. (2010) Factors that influence insect succession on carrion. In: Byrd, J.H. and Castner, J.I. (eds), *Forensic Entomology: The utility of arthropods in legal medicine*. CRC Press: Boca Raton, pp. 201–250.

Bell, M., Fowler, P.W. and Hillson, S.W. (1996) *The Experimental Earthwork Projects, 1960–1992*. Council for British Archaeology: York.

Bier, C. and Dusenbury, M.M. (2008) Textiles. In: Pearsall, D.M. (ed.), *Encyclopaedia of Archaeology*. Elsevier: Amsterdam, pp. 2119–2125.

Cardamone, J.M., Keister, K.M. and Osareh, A.H. (1991) Degradation and conservation of cellulosics and esters. In: Allen, N.S., Edge, M. and Horis, C.V. (eds), *Polymers in Conservation*. Royal Society of Chemistry: London, pp. 108–124.

Chen, H.L., Jakes, K.A. and Foreman, D.W. (1998) Preservation of archaeological textiles through fibre mineralisation. *Journal of Archaeological Science*, **25**: 1015–1021.

Clark, M. (2011) *Handbook of Textile and Industrial Dyeing, vol. 1: Principles, processes and types of dyes*. Woodhead Publishing: Oxford.

Cronyn, J.M. (1990) *The Elements of Archaeological Conservation*. Routledge: Abingdon.

Faraday, M. (1836) Letter on 'Recent discovery of Roman sepulchral relics in one of the greater barrows at Batlow, in Ashdon, Essex'. *Archaeologia*, **16**: 30–31.

Fenichell, S. (1996) *Plastic: The making of a synthetic century*. Harper: New York.

Forbes, S.L., Stuart, B.H. and Dent, B.B. (2005) The effect of method of burial on adipocere formation. *Forensic Science International*, **154**: 44–52.

Goffer, Z. (2007) *Archaeological Chemistry*. Wiley-Interscience: Hoboken.

Hearle, J.W.S. and Schwaller, D. (2011) Fibres. Part 2: Structure. In: Elvers, B. (ed.), *Ullmann's Encyclopaedia of Industrial Chemistry*. Wiley-VCH: Weinheim.

Heywood, D. (2003) *Textile Finishing*. Society of Dyers and Colourists: Bradford.

Janaway, R.C. (1983) Textile fibre characteristics preserved by metal corrosion: the potential of SEM studies. *The Conservator*, **7**: 48–52.

Janaway, R.C. (1987) The preservation of organic materials in association with metal artefacts deposited in inhumation graves. In: Boddington, A., Garland, A.N. and Janaway, R.C. (eds), *Death, Decay and Reconstruction*. Manchester University Press: Manchester, pp. 127–148.

Janaway, R.C. (1996) The decay of buried human remains and their associated materials. In: Hunter, J., Roberts, C.A. and Martin, A. (eds), *Studies in Crime: An introduction to forensic archaeology*. BT Batsford: London, pp. 58–85.

Janaway, R.C. (2002) Degradation of clothing and other dress materials associated with buried bodies in both archaeological and forensic interest. In: Haglund, W.D. and Sorg, M.H. (eds), *Advances in Forensic Taphonomy. Method, theory and archaeological perspectives*. CRC Press: Boca Raton, pp. 379–402.

Janaway, R.C. (2008) The decomposition of materials associated with buried cadavers. In: Tibbett, M. and Carter, D.O. (eds), *Soil Analysis in Forensic Taphonomy: Chemical and biological effects of buried human remains*. CRC Press: Boca Raton, pp. 153–202.

Kelly, J.A., van der Linde, T.C. and Anderson, G.S. (2009) The influence of clothing and wrapping on carcass decomposition and arthropod succession during the warmer seasons in Central South Africa. *Journal of Forensic Sciences*, **54**: 1105–1112.

Kerr, N. and Schweger, B. (1989) Survival of archaeological textiles in an arctic environment. In: O'Rear, C.E. and Llewellyn, G.C. (eds), *Biodeterioration Research 2*. Plenum Press: New York, pp. 19–38.

Kite, M. and Thomson, R. (2006) *Conservation of Leather and Related Materials*. Butterworth-Heinemann: London.

Lowe, A.C., Beresford, D.V., Carter, D.O., Gaspari, F., O'Brien, R.C. *et al.* (2013) The effect of soil texture on the degradation of textiles associated with buried bodies. *Forensic Science International*, **231**: 331–339.

Mann, R.W., Bass, W.M. and Meadows, L. (1990) Time since death and decomposition of the human body: variables and observations in case and experimental field studies. *Journal of Forensic Sciences*, **35**: 103–111.

Mant, A.K. (1987) Knowledge acquired from post-war exhumation. In: Garland, A.N. and Janaway, R.C. (eds), *Death, Decay and Reconstruction: Approaches to archaeology and forensic science*. Manchester University Press: Manchester, pp. 65–78.

Mather, R.R. and Wardman, R.H. (2011) *The Chemistry of Textile Fibres*. Royal Society of Chemistry: Cambridge.

Mitchell, J.L., Carr, D.J., Niven, B.E., Harrison, K. and Girvan, E. (2012) Physical and mechanical degradation of shirting fabrics in burial conditions. *Forensic Science International*, **222**: 94–101.

Morse, D. (1983) The degree of deterioration of associated death scene material. In: Mores, D., Duncan, J. and Stoutamire, J. (eds), *Handbook of Forensic Archaeology and Anthropology*. Florida State University Press: Tallahassee, pp. A1–A15.

Morse, D. and Dailey, R.C. (1985) The degree of deterioration of associated death scene material. *Journal of Forensic Sciences*, **30**: 119–127.

Northrop, D.M. and Rowe, W.F. (1987) Effect of the soil environment on the biodeterioration of man-made textiles. In: Llewellyn, G.C. and O'Rear, C.E. (eds), *Biodeterioration 1*. Plenum Press: New York, pp. 7–16.

Peacock, E.E. (1996) Characterisation and simulation of water-degraded archaeological textiles: a review. *International Biodeterioration and Biodegradation*, **38**: 35–47.

Pinhasi, R., Gasparian, B., Areshian, G., Zardaryan, D., Smith, A. *et al.* (2010) First direct evidence of Chalcolithic footwear from the Near Eastern Highlands. *PLoS ONE*, **5**: e10984.

Quye, A. (2014) Factors influencing the stability of man-made fibres: a retrospective view for historical textiles. *Polymer Degradation and Stability*, **107**: 210–218.

Raschle, P. (1989) Microbial influence on cellulosic textiles and microbiological testing. *International Biodeterioration*, **25**: 237–244.

Robertshaw, A. and Kenyon, D. (2008) *Digging the Trenches: The archaeology of the Western Front*. Pen and Sword: Barnsley.

Robertson, J. and Grieve, M. (1999) *Forensic Examination of Fibres*. Taylor & Francis: London.

Rowe, W.F. (1997) Biodeterioration of hairs and fibres. In: Haglund, W.D. and Sorg, M.H. (eds), *Forensic Taphonomy: The postmortem fate of human remains*. CRC Press: Boca Raton, pp. 337–352.

Sibley, L.R. and Jakes, K.A. (1984) Survival of protein fibres in archaeological contexts. *Science and Archaeology*, **26**: 17–27.

Singer, S.M. and Rowe, W.F. (1989) Biodeterioration of man-made textiles in various soil environments. In: Llewellyn, G.C. and O'Rear, C.E. (eds), *Biodeterioration Research 2*. Plenum Press: New York, pp. 81–89.

Solazzo, C., Dyer, J.M., Clerens, S., Plowman, J., Peacock, E.E. and Collins, M.J. (2013) Proteomic evaluation of the biodegradation of wool fabrics in experimental burials. *International Biodeterioration and Biodegradation*, **80**: 48–59.

Spenneman, D.H.R. and Franke, B. (1995) Decomposition of buried human bodies and associated death scene materials on coral atolls in the tropical Pacific. *Journal of Forensic Sciences*, **40**: 356–367.

Strzelczyk, A.B., Bannach, L. and Kurowska, A. (1997) Biodeterioration of archaeological leather. *International Biodeterioration and Biodegradation*, **39**: 301–309.

Szostak-Kotowa, J. (2004) Biodeterioration of textiles. *International Biodeterioration and Biodegradation*, **53**: 165–170.

Taupin, J.M. and Cwiklik, C. (2011) *Scientific Protocols for Forensic Examination of Clothing*. Taylor and Francis; Boca Raton.

Ueland, M., Nizio, K., Forbes, S.L. and Stuart, B.H. (2015) The interactive effect of the degradation of cotton clothing and decomposition fluid production associated with decaying remains. *Forensic Science International*, **255**: 56–63.

Voss, S.C., Cook, D.F. and Dadour, I.R. (2011) Decomposition and insect succession of clothed and unclothed carcasses in Western Australia. *Forensic Science International*, **211**: 67–75.

Wayland, R.L. (2012) Textile auxiliaries, 7. Finishing agents. In: Elvers, B. (ed.), *Ullmann's Encyclopaedia of Industrial Chemistry*. Wiley-VCH: Weinheim.

Wilson, A.S., Janaway, R.C., Holland, A.D., Dodson, H.I., Buran, E. et al, (2007) Modelling the buried human body environment in upland climes using three contrasting field sites. *Forensic Science International*, **169**: 6–18.

Zahn, H., Wortmann, F.J., Wortmann, G., Schaefer, G., Hoffmann, R. and Finch, R. (2003) Wool. In: Elvers, B. (ed.), *Ullmann's Encyclopaedia of Industrial Chemistry*. Wiley-VCH: Weinheim.

10

Post-Mortem Interval Estimation: an Overview of Techniques

Tal Simmons

10.1 Introduction

When human remains are discovered, one of the key questions investigators ask of forensic anthropologists is, 'how long ago did he/she die?' or 'how long has the body/skeleton been here?' Of all the areas in which forensic anthropologists can contribute concerning the identification and analysis of human remains, the estimation of time since death is, arguably, the most difficult. Whilst forensic pathologists are generally comfortable with estimating the early post-mortem interval (PMI) from particular signs, e.g. *rigor mortis* onset and decline, appearance of *tâche noire*, greenish discoloration of the abdomen, abdominal bloating, etc., once a body begins to show more advanced signs of decomposition or is approaching skeletonisation, estimates are given with more caution or not ventured. In the past, PMI estimation after this initial period has been the sole purview of the forensic entomologist, who used either oviposition, eclosion and larval development in the early stages or insect succession patterns in the later stages to arrive at a PMI range. Traditionally, the ability of the forensic anthropologist to estimate PMI was based on his/her familiarity with decomposition patterns in the region in which the anthropologist worked and, from seeing a number of cases over the years, a rough estimate of days, months or years could be hazarded. Only within the last ten years, however, have forensic anthropologists had a specific, novel method from which to estimate the PMI when confronted with decomposed remains.

10.2 Why Estimating the PMI is Important

Estimations of the PMI may be used in investigations in three important ways. First, it is most commonly used in the process of identification of the decomposed body. By estimating the time since death, it is possible to narrow down the window in which the individual was killed and deposited where the corpse was found. A list of persons reported missing during that interval might narrow the potential leads to identification and result in a positive identification of the corpse. Second, once this is known, it may lead investigators to include or exclude persons of interest in their investigation by virtue of verified alibis for the period in question. Third, although much less commonly employed, PMI estimation is useful in projecting what a body might be expected to look like when searchers are engaged to find a missing person, who is presumed dead. In the reverse of predicting when the individual died and was deposited, one can calculate the accumulated degree-days (ADD) from the time the individual went missing (and/or was presumed dead) to the date of the search, in order to

Taphonomy of Human Remains: Forensic Analysis of the Dead and the Depositional Environment, First Edition.
Edited by Eline M.J. Schotsmans, Nicholas Márquez-Grant and Shari L. Forbes.

predict the total body score, which provides a descriptive range for the appearance of the body. This may be quite helpful, as searchers generally assume that they will recognise 'a body', but may not be prepared to recognise it in whatever state of decomposition the body might be in at the time of the search. This is particularly true if temperatures have been hot enough or scavengers active enough to effect considerable change.

10.3 Scientific Method versus Anecdote in PMI Estimation

Based on their observations of cadavers at the University of Tennessee's Anthropological Research Facility, Mann *et al.* (1990) subjectively rated the factors influencing the rate of decay (either increasing or decreasing). The authors rated three variables as most influential: temperature, access by insects and burial depth. The last of the three is, of course, actually an interaction of the first two, temperature and insect access, for example the deeper the burial the cooler the temperatures and the less insect access. They rated carnivores/rodents, trauma (penetrating/crushing) and humidity/aridity as the next most important; rainfall, body size/weight and embalming were somewhat less important, with clothing even less so, while the surface on which the remains were placed was rated as the least influential and the pH of the soil as having an unknown degree of influence. As noted by the authors themselves, these were indeed subjective ratings with no data presented to corroborate their logical, albeit anecdotal findings. Mann *et al.* (1990) also discussed the difference between patterns (the manifestation of decomposition in the body) and rate (– the length of time it takes for the body to decompose), an issue that became muddled in much subsequent literature.

10.3.1 Mythology and Fallacy in PMI Estimation

Caution is warranted when reading the taphonomic literature, as many statements concerning decay rates are rather sweeping generalisations, which have been perpetuated in the literature; when the citations listed in support of these statements are scrutinised, it is interesting to note that the original data corroborating these are scant, if extant at all. As one example, numerous authors have stated that it takes a buried body, on average, eight times longer to decompose than one on the ground surface; whilst intuitively this makes sense, what is invariably cited for example in Rodriguez (1997) and/or Turner and Wiltshire (1999), presents no data actually comparing surface and burial cohorts of experimental subjects and the sample size in the Turner and Wiltshire study consisted of three pigs. Similarly, whilst Mann *et al.* (1990) suggested that penetrating trauma influences decomposition rates, this was a visual observation, which indicated that a wound to the thorax seemed to attract insects preferentially, as the chest showed tissue destruction caused by maggot activity. Mann *et al.* (1990) state that this corpse decomposed more rapidly; however, this is unsubstantiated by quantitative data and the basis for the conclusion was a single case with a gunshot to the chest compared to a single case with no gunshot wounds. Mann *et al.* (1990) state that trauma might explain the increased rate of decay observed, but no further work with quantitative data to confirm this one-off observation was conducted. In contrast, 20 years later, Cross and Simmons (2010) showed in a controlled experiment with a larger sample size ($n = 34$) that decomposition rates in individuals with penetrating trauma did not differ from those without penetrating trauma. Thus, as should always be the case, works by authors stating far reaching conclusions need to be read carefully and a thorough review of the references cited by them conducted as well.

10.3.2 Ideal versus Real – Limitations of PMI Studies

Ideally, studies concerning the estimation of PMI in humans would be conducted on human cadavers. What one sees is what one gets; results would be transferable to casework, particularly in the realm of patterns of decomposition. The process of decomposition has been presented by many authors (e.g. Galloway *et al.* 1989), and while the overall progression of decay is equivalent, the stages named and the divisions of various stages have been represented differently by many (Adlam and Simmons 2007).

Unfortunately, as far as the conduct of controlled experimental research is concerned, the ability to use human cadavers is subject to the ebb and flow of body donations, shipping delays of donated cadavers in which decomposition is not halted and the accrued temperature is unknown, and problems with the storage of cadavers at temperatures which arrest decomposition but do not alter the subsequent decomposition process (Roberts and Dabbs 2015). Thus, although numerous facilities exist in the USA (and one in Australia) for the study of decomposition in human remains, the research conducted at these is fraught with difficulties in conducting truly controlled research. Very few studies, apart from individual case examples, concern decomposition in actual humans and these are predominantly anecdotal in nature, since there are no significant sample sizes, treatment and control groups, statistical analyses or data presented. They are interesting in their own right, providing general principles of decay rate and pattern, but ultimately do little to provide investigators or the legal system with scientifically valid results.

Research conducted using animal models provides the antithesis; reasonably tightly controlled experiments using large sample sizes, cohorts and repeats, where a single variable can be tested whilst keeping all others the same – yet, while these results provide excellent information concerning what does and does not affect the rate of decay, they may be difficult to 'translate' to human terms due to innate differences in weight, limb proportions, etc. and a formula derived from an animal model cannot unequivocally be applied to humans.

10.3.3 Experimental Studies

In ensuing years, many of the factors purported to influence decomposition highlighted by Mann *et al.* (1990) – as well as others – have been experimentally tested and differences (and the relationship) between rate and pattern explored more fully: repeated disturbance of remains (Adlam and Simmons 2007); decomposition rates in burial (Bachmann and Simmons, 2010); the influence of insects in buried and surface remains (Simmons *et al.* 2010); penetrating trauma (Cross and Simmons 2010); pre-decomposition charring (Gruenthal *et al.* 2012); presence/absence of clothing (Card *et al.* 2015); decomposition in hanging remains (Lynch-Aird *et al.* 2015); the influence of maggot-generated heat on decomposition (Heaton *et al.* 2014); differential decomposition with mass graves (Troutman *et al.* 2014); etc. The majority of these have shown little, if any, significant difference in rate of decomposition, although some have shown a slight difference in the pattern, and some effects of different treatments have caused a delay to the start of the decomposition process, whilst the rate remained the same (Moffatt and Simmons 2015). All of these studies have similarities in the experimental design utilised, for which the underlying considerations will be outlined here.

A solid experimental study needs to have, first of all, a reasonable sample size. This ensures that any effect(s) seen are real, as opposed to one-time events related to unknown factors. Many of the early experiments in decomposition used only one or two, or at most six, animals and frequently used different treatments on each one. In studies such as this it is impossible to reach any scientifically valid conclusions (i.e. defensible in court), since it is impossible to assess the statistical significance of the results, as samples sizes of one or two are too small to test robustly and determine accuracy of prediction.

Second, an experiment should be designed to test the effect of a single variable (e.g. clothing – as opposed to no clothing) on decomposition. It is not helpful to try to test decomposition with four animals (wearing clothing, wrapped in a blanket, wrapped in plastic and unclothed), while at the same time each animal is placed in either sun, shade, buried or in a rubbish bin. Is the effect witnessed because of sun – or because the body was wrapped in carpet? Does this effect really compare in any meaningful way to that seen in the plastic wrapped and buried animal? This may seem absurd, but many manuscripts have been submitted to journals for review where experiments were not designed much better than this, unfortunately.

Third, the experiment must have controls. In other words, if one is testing the effect of clothing (to continue the analogy), one must have an equal number of animals which remain unclothed whilst all other variables are kept the same (e.g. all placed in woodland, positioned with heads facing North).

Fourth, one must decide upon protocols for data collection – these have consequences with regard to sample size. For example, if one is studying decomposition in clothed versus unclothed pigs, what data are to be collected? If one is simply observing the carcasses and using a system which scores the visual decomposition, then one can use fewer animals (although an equal number of treatment versus control animals), as they will not be disturbed in the process of the experiment. If, on the other hand, one wishes to take soil samples from under the carcass or weigh the carcass on a regular basis as it decomposes, one needs to design the experiment with enough animals to allow removal of at least three (to obtain an average) at any data collection point from the experiment – never to be used again – because disturbing carcasses alters their rate of decomposition since it disturbs the insect masses (Adlam and Simmons 2007; Cross and Simmons 2010). Thus, an experiment on clothed and unclothed pigs taking weight data, may require 30 pigs in each group (treatment or control) if 10 data collection points are planned. It must also be noted that if carcasses are going to be scored (or other data collected from them) repeatedly, one needs to plan for a statistical model that accounts for repeated measures (e.g. a mixed effects model where 'pig' is the random variable), rather than a simple regression of scores on time, temperature, etc.

Fifth, data collection intervals need to be determined ahead of time; this allows both the calculation of the duration of the experiment itself and determines the number of animals required. By using known equations (Megyesi *et al.* 2005; Vass *et al.* 1992), or data from other published experiments, how long the experiment should run and how many animals needed can usually be estimated with good accuracy, if not precision (Ousley 1995). Thus, if it is known that the average daily temperature where the experiment will be done is roughly 20 °C for the duration of the experiment and one wishes to collect data, for example every 100 ADD (5 days × 20 °C), and one wants to run the experiment until the ADD is, for example 1000, then one would need to have 10 data collection points (every 5 days for a total of 50 days, or 2⅔ months) and 3 animals per data collection point in each group (e.g. 6 total each time) if they will be discarded after each data collection point. Thus, 60 animals would be needed in total for this experiment.

Ideally, the experiment should also be repeated under equivalent conditions several times. Repetition ensures that the results obtained were genuine and also allows comparison of even larger groups of treatment and control animals. Unfortunately, it has proved very rare indeed for data concerning repetition to have been published or presented, and only a single abstract concerning this type of study exists (Simmons and Moffatt 2013).

10.4 Methods for Estimating PMI

The method for estimating the PMI in cases where the body is no longer fresh – and hence techniques used in the early PMI by pathologists are no longer useful – was developed by Megyesi *et al.* (2005) based in part on concepts published earlier by Vass *et al.* (1992). The Vass *et al.* (1992) publication, using the concentration of volatile fatty acids in the soil underneath cadavers to estimate time since death, introduced the concept of ADD as a means to combine the variables of time and temperature. By using accumulated temperature over time to describe the progression of decomposition, this concept allows the comparison of multiple geographic regions, seasons, etc. where using chronology alone (e.g. 'days') does not. Until ca. 2010, it was common for papers to report that it took 'XX days' for the corpse to reach the bloat stage, the wet decomposition stage, and on to reaching skeletonisation. The drawback, of course, was that 5 days in the northwest of England in the summer, where the average daily temperature is 15 °C, is rather different to 5 days in east Tennessee, where the average daily temperature might be 30 °C on those same days. The former 5 days would be 75 ADD, and the latter double the ADD at 150. Two corpses deposited the same day in each location would look radically different after five days. On the other hand, a corpse deposited in the same location in England might be expected to look very similar indeed to the one in Tennessee after ca. 10 days at a 15 °C daily average (also 150 ADD).

10.4.1 Retrospective Studies

Much useful information has also come from retrospective studies of human cadavers, where multiple cases with known date of disappearance/death and date of body recovery have been paired with historical temperature data to create equations for the estimation of PMI. Megyesi *et al.* (2005) examined surface deposition cases derived from medical examiner office files in (primarily) the Midwestern United States. This was a ground-breaking study for two reasons: first, it used known PMI to calculate the ADD, and second, it quantified decomposition by assigning a progressive numerical value to descriptive decomposition stages (total body score, or TBS). The authors presented a formula for estimating ADD from TBS which, in practice, allowed for the continuous subtraction of known average daily temperatures from the estimated ADD, until one arrived at zero, which corresponded with the date of death (within a range of error). Although, subsequently, the entomological estimates of time since death and the formula itself have been shown to be flawed (Moffatt *et al.* 2016), the Megyesi *et al.* (2005) article provided a methodology with the use of ADD and TBS, thus opening the door for substantive experimental research allowing the comparison of decomposition rates in different geographical and climatological regions.

Dabbs (2010) has added a caveat concerning the use of data from national weather service stations; care should be taken when choosing a weather station near to the site of body discovery, as it may not necessarily reflect the temperatures at the site correctly. Practitioners are urged to examine the temperature fluctuations at the crime scene over a period of several days and only then choose which of the local weather stations parallels its temperatures most closely. No correction of weather station data should be attempted using regression to compensate for differences, as these methods were shown to create more significant differences than using data from the weather station with the closest approximation to the site data within 15.3 km of the crime scene (Dabbs 2015).

Heaton *et al.* (2010) used the ideas presented in Megyesi *et al.* (2005) and applied the concept of decomposition as quantifiably temperature dependent to water deposition cases in UK waterways. This study compared decomposition in the River Clyde (Scotland) with the River Mersey and the Mersey canals (Northwest England) using the same variables – witnessed dates of entry into the water (resulting in death) and known dates of body recovery from the waterway, coupled with known historical water temperature data. Using an inverse prediction model, the authors also presented a formula for predicting the ADD from the Total Aquatic Decomposition Score (TADS), a decomposition scale for bodies in water based on the idea of Megyesi *et al.*'s (2005) TBS. There were no statistically significant differences among the three waterways studied, and the formula shows a slower rate of decomposition in water than for bodies deposited on the ground surface.

It is important to note that both these retrospective studies, and the TBS and TADS scales provided, function much in the same way as skeletal (and some dental) forensic morphological age estimation systems. Age estimation essentially provides estimates based on 'age at phase'. Each of these models (e.g. Brooks and Suchey 1990; Iscan and Loth 1994; Lovejoy *et al.* 1985; etc.) assigns morphological status to implicitly progressive phases, the underlying assumption for which is that every individual must have passed through all the previous phases, in order to be classified as displaying the current phase at death. Each of these models acknowledges that not every bone will display all the characteristics of each phase, but that assignment to phase is on a 'best fit' basis. The TBS and TADS systems operate under the same principals for assessing stage of decomposition at ADD interval; each stage (PBS for each region, and hence the summary TBS) represents an accumulation of bacterially- and insect-mediated changes correlated to having reached an accumulation of the catalyst, heat, which drives the reaction. The nature of the changes is mosaic, with not every cadaver reaching the full set of descriptive components in each phase, but where the majority of characteristics dictate which phase is assigned.

More recently in 2011, Vass published a paper entitled 'The elusive universal post-mortem interval formula' in the journal *Forensic Science International*, in which several formulae are presented for PMI estimation in buried and surface-deposited remains, based on 20 years of (unpublished) data from the University of Tennessee's Anthropological Research Facility (Vass 2011). The method presented by Vass requires an estimation of the percentage of the body showing decomposition, although guidelines for approximating an accurate percentage are not provided and there appears to be a range of flexibility in this process. Other than a few abstracts presented at the American Academy of Forensic Science meetings (e.g. Inoue and Carter 2015), no other researchers have tested Vass's formulae for either aerobic or anaerobic decomposition. The Inoue and Carter (2015) abstract indicates that the formula for surface deposition provided accurate results for only 50% of cases, valid for cadavers exhibiting little decomposition, but increasingly inaccurate when subjective estimates of tissue loss must be estimated.

10.5 Case Example

The following case is derived from a published source and provides an example of how to apply the Megyesi *et al.* (2005) technique, based on the revised scale and formula presented in Moffatt *et al.* (2016). The question posed by human rights workers was, 'could the body in the photograph be this decomposed if the individual had been killed 21–25 days prior?' In order to answer this question, two things are required:

1) an evaluation of the photograph using the TBS system to score decomposition stage of the head/neck, torso and limb regions; and
2) a record of the average daily temperatures for the location where the body was found.

In this particular case, the photographs (Free Burma Rangers 2006) of the bodies were provided by a non-government organization (NGO) and had been taken by a Free Burma Rangers relief team on 19 April 2006. The individuals were purportedly killed by the Burmese Army on 27 March 2006 and in 'early April' 2006. Photographs of the body were not of the best quality and the limbs in particular were difficult to assess. Therefore, only the photograph depicting the most complete individual was evaluated. For all descriptions below, see Megyesi *et al.* (2005) and for all point values assigned to these stages, see Moffatt *et al.* (2016). For the head/neck region, the best match for the decomposition scale was a PBSH score of Category D Stage 3, or 'bones largely dry, but retaining some grease', which is equal to 11 points; this judgement was reached based on the photograph showing a skeletonised cranium where light is clearly shining off a greasy area in a way it would not do if the bone was dry. For the torso region, the PBST was Category C, Stage 3, or 'mummification with bone exposure of less than one half that of the area being scored', which is equal to 7 points; this judgement was reached based on the photographic depiction of dried skin partially covering the torso, but with the lower ribs exposed. For the limbs, as always, a combination of lower and upper limb appearance was evaluated. The PBSL was Category D, Stage 1, or 'bone exposed over one half the area being scored, some decomposed tissue and body fluids remaining', equal to 7 points; this judgement was reached based on the combination of desiccation and bone exposure in the upper limbs and greater bone exposure in both lower limbs. The sum of the regions yielded a TBS of 25 points. The new formula provides a point estimate of 1182 ADD and a 95% Prediction Interval range of 534–2963 ADD or, a 75% Prediction Interval range of 752–1930 ADD. Since the PMI equals the ADD divided by the average daily temperatures, this information was needed for the location in which the body was found.

The report provided a description of the topography of the area as well as the GPS coordinates for the location of the remains, and reference to a topographic map of the area confirmed that this was a hilly region on the border of the valley. Since access to weather station data originating in Burma was impossible to obtain at the time, the NGO requested assistance with this case, as the only climatic information that was available were monthly climate guides reporting high and low average temperatures for lowland and highland Burma. Since the region was borderline, the calculations were performed for both lowland and highland regions.

For the months of March and April, in low altitude areas, the daytime high was 35.6°C and the night-time low was 23.9°C, yielding an average daily temperature of 29.8°C. For high altitude areas in the same months, the daytime high was 31.7°C and the night-time low was 16.7°C, or an average daily temperature of 24.2°C. In order to calculate the 95% Prediction Interval for low altitude areas, the minimum ADD of 534 is divided by the average daily temperature of 29.8°C, giving 18.3 days (the minimum time it would take a body to reach a TBS of 25 at that temperature). The maximum amount of time is the maximum ADD of 2963 divided by 29.8°C, or 99 days. Thus, if the environment could be classified as lowland, a PMI estimate of 18.3–99 days agrees with the time in question, that is 21–25 days from death to discovery. If on the other hand, the environment could be classified as highland, the 95% Prediction Interval is calculated from the minimum 534/24.2°C (the average daily temperature) and the maximum 1963/24.2 °C. This provides a PMI interval of 22–122 days, which is also concordat with the 21–25 days from death to discovery.

Of course, even though the time intervals from purported killing to photographic documentation claimed by the witnesses are consistent with and do not contradict those provided by the 95% Prediction Interval based on the average daily temperatures, this merely corroborates that death *could have occurred* at the time the witnesses claim it did. It does not speak to broader issues of who (or what entity) killed the individuals, and such evidence would have to derive from witness testimony, documentary evidence detailing troop movements, etc. The estimate of PMI merely shows the possibility that death occurred during the time frame in question; it does not prove that individual perpetrators committed the murder.

10.6 Conclusion and Future Research

For the future, the most important research for the estimation of PMI should focus on the following areas, about which little of a quantifiable nature is known – to name only a few:

1) if the rate at which temperature is accrued affects decomposition rate more than simply the sum of temperatures
2) how the role of fluctuating temperatures affects ADD and insect development

3) how the role of scavenging affects the estimation of PMI
4) how differences in insect communities may (or may not) account for varied decomposition rates
5) how the heat generated by maggot masses of varying sizes (and composed of varying taxa) affects ADD and the rate of decomposition

In reality, the estimation of PMI by visual observation correlated to temperature is only the first – and probably rather crude – step in attaining better accuracy for assessing the time since death. Work in complimentary disciplines, for example DNA degradation, DNA markers of age, DNA of the necromicrobiome, characterisation of the volatile sulphur compounds given off by the corpse relative to ADD, etc. may supplant current techniques.

The hope remains that future studies will move beyond a solely observational approach and explore the control and quantification of a greater number of well-defined and objectively measureable variables – and this holds true for both retrospective and experimental studies, for both human and non-human models – in the quest to derive a more accurate PMI formula.

References

Adlam, R. and Simmons, T. (2007) The effect of repeated physical disturbance on soft tissue decomposition – are taphonomic studies an accurate reflection of decomposition? *Journal of Forensic Sciences*, **52**: 1007–1010.

Bachmann, J. and Simmons, T. (2010) The influence of pre-burial insect access on the decomposition rate. *Journal of Forensic Sciences*, **55**: 893–900.

Brooks, S. and Suchey, J. (1990) Skeletal age determination based on the os pubis: a comparison of the Acsadi-Nemeskeri and Suchey-Brooks methods. *Human Evolution*, **5**: 227–238.

Card, A., Cross, P., Moffatt, C. and Simmons, T. (2015) The effect of clothing on the rate of decomposition and *Diptera* colonization on *Sus scrofa* carcasses. *Journal of Forensic Sciences*, **60**: 979–982.

Cross, P. and Simmons, T. (2010) The influence of penetrative trauma on the rate of decomposition. *Journal of Forensic Sciences*, **55**: 295–301.

Dabbs, G. (2010) Caution! All data are not created equal: the hazards of using National Weather Service data for calculating accumulated degree days. *Forensic Science International*, **202**: e49–e52.

Dabbs, G. (2015) How should forensic anthropologists correct National Weather Service temperature data for use in estimating the postmortem interval? *Journal of Forensic Sciences*, **60**: 581–587.

Free Burma Rangers (2006) www.freeburmarangers.org/2006/04/19/fbr-report-relief-team-finds-bodies-of-murdered-idps/#2 (Accessed 30 July 2015).

Galloway, A., Birkby, W., Jones, A., Henry, T. and Parks, B. (1989) Decay rates of human remains in an arid environment. *Journal of Forensic Sciences*, **34**: 607–616.

Gruenthal, A., Moffatt, C. and Simmons, T. (2012) Differential decomposition patterns in charred versus uncharred remains. *Journal of Forensic Sciences*, **57**: 12–18.

Heaton, V., Lagden, A., Moffatt, C. and Simmons, T. (2010) Predicting the post-mortem submersion interval for human remains recovered from UK waterways. *Journal of Forensic Sciences*, **55**: 302–307.

Heaton, V., Moffatt, C. and Simmons, T. (2014) Quantifying the temperature of maggot masses and its relationship to decomposition. *Journal of Forensic Sciences*, **59**: 676–682.

Inoue, C. and Carter, D. (2015) Validating an equation to estimate postmortem interval on Oahu, Hawaii. *Proceedings of the American Academy of Forensic Sciences*, **21**: 925.

Iscan, M., Loth, S. and Wright, R. (1994) Age estimation from the rib by phase analysis: white males. *Journal of Forensic Sciences*, **29**: 1094–1104.

Lovejoy, C., Meindl, R., Pryzbeck, T. and Mensforth, R. (1985) Chronological metamorphosis of the auricular surface of the ilium: a new method for the determination of adult skeletal age at death. *American Journal of Physical Anthropology*, **68**: 15–28.

Lynch-Aird, J., Moffatt, C. and Simmons, T. (2015) Decomposition rate and pattern in hanging pigs. *Journal of Forensic Sciences*, **60**: 1155–1163.

Mann, R., Bass, W. and Meadows, L. (1990) Time Since Death and decomposition of the human body: variables and observations in case and experimental field studies. *Journal of Forensic Sciences*, **35**: 103–111.

Megyesi, M., Nawroki, S. and Haskell, N. (2005) Using accumulated degree days to estimate the postmortem interval from decomposed human remains. *Journal of Forensic Sciences*, **50**: 618–626.

Moffatt, C. and Simmons, T. (2015) Forensic entomology research at the University of Central Lancashire's TRACES decomposition facility. *Antenna (Journal of the Royal Entomological Society)* Special Edition: 114–115.

Moffatt, C., Simmons, T. and Lynch-Aird, J. (2016) An improved equation for TBS and ADD: establishing a reliable postmortem interval Framework for Casework and Experimental Studies. *Journal of Forensic Sciences*, **61**: S201–S207.

Ousley, S. (1995) Should we estimate biological or forensic stature? *Journal of Forensic Sciences*, **40**: 768–773.

Roberts, L.G. and Dabbs, G. (2015) A taphonomic study exploring the differences in decomposition rate and manner between frozen and never frozen domestic pigs (*Sus scrofa*). *Journal of Forensic Sciences*, **60**: 588–594.

Rodriquez, W. (1997) Decomposition of buried and submerged bodies. In: Haglund, W.D. and Sorg, M.H. (eds), *Forensic Taphonomy: The postmortem fate of human remains*. CRC Press: Boca Raton, pp. 459–467.

Rodriguez, W.C. and Bass, W.M. (1985) Decomposition of buried bodies and methods that may aid in their location. *Journal of Forensic Sciences*, **30**: 836–852.

Simmons, T. and Moffatt, C. (2013) The consistency of ADD, TBS and decomposition rate: a validation study spanning five years. *Proceedings of the American Academy of Forensic Sciences*, **19**: 457–458.

Simmons, T., Adlam, R. and Moffatt, C. (2010) Debugging decomposition data – comparative taphonomic studies and the influence of insects and carcass size on decomposition rate. *Journal of Forensic Sciences*, **55**: 8–13.

Simmons, T., Cross, P. and Moffatt, C. (2010) The influence of insects on decomposition rate in buried and surface remains. *Journal of Forensic Sciences*, **55**: 889–892.

Troutman, L., Moffatt, C. and Simmons, T. (2014) A preliminary examination of differential decomposition patterns in mass graves. *Journal of Forensic Sciences*, **59**: 621–626.

Turner, B. and Wiltshire, P. (1999) Experimental validation of forensic evidence: a study of the decomposition of buried pigs in a heavy clay soil. *Forensic Science International*, **101**: 113–122.

Vass, A., Bass, W., Wolt, J., Foss, J. and Ammons, J. (1992) Time since death determinations of human cadavers using soil solution. *Journal of Forensic Sciences*, **37**: 1236–1253.

Vass, A. (2011) The elusive universal post-mortem interval formula. *Forensic Science International*, **204**: 34–40.

Part II

The Depositional Environment

11

Relationships between Human Remains, Graves and the Depositional Environment

Emily N. Junkins and David O. Carter

11.1 Introduction

The purpose of this chapter is to review our current understanding of the interactions between graves, human remains and decomposition, which are many and complex. The definitions of these three variables can be equally complex, but hereafter decomposition is defined as a chemical, biological and/or physical process that contributes to the cycling of energy and nutrients (Swift *et al.* 1979). Human remains are corpses, or components of corpses, which are discovered during decomposition at some time point after death. For the purpose of this chapter, a grave is defined as any location at which human remains are located; a grave can be above-ground, below-ground, indoors, outdoors, aquatic, or within any other possible natural or anthropogenic habitat. In a forensic context, many graves are anthropogenic and can be as varied as the boot of a car, a suitcase or a bathtub. It is also recognised that graves can vary significantly in their temporal persistence; the age of a grave can range from seconds to millennia.

This chapter focuses on the decomposition of human remains that have been buried in soil. The disposition of human remains can be the result of criminal activity or activities associated with non-criminal anthropology, including belief systems. Regardless of the means that brought remains to their final resting place, the decomposition patterns will remain relatively similar, excluding any significant disturbance with the remains (e.g. religious beliefs that introduce foreign material into a burial, or mutilation).

11.2 The Taphonomy of Buried Human Remains

The decomposition of all organic resources is ultimately mediated by three primary factors (Swift *et al.* 1979):

1) the decomposer community that has access to the remains
2) the physical and chemical environment of the grave
3) the biophysicochemical properties of the organic material itself

Human remains are highly nutritious resources that attract the attention of many organisms. These organisms include insects (particularly flies and beetles), mammals, birds, reptiles and microorganisms. The primary contribution that burial makes to the decomposer community is that it selects for a decomposer community that is predominantly microbial, because burial often inhibits

Taphonomy of Human Remains: Forensic Analysis of the Dead and the Depositional Environment, First Edition.
Edited by Eline M.J. Schotsmans, Nicholas Márquez-Grant and Shari L. Forbes.

the activity of insect and vertebrate scavengers, which tends to slow the rate of decomposition (Turner and Wiltshire 1999). Thus, the analysis of taphonomy in soil requires the understanding that decomposition is a function of burial depth and soil texture, because these variables influence the temperature, pH, moisture content and bioavailable oxygen within a grave. This means that, following burial in soil, the taphonomy of human remains is driven primarily by autolysis, putrefaction and aerobic catabolism; the rates of these processes are regulated by the environment, particularly burial depth and soil texture.

11.3 Factors that Influence Decomposition: Environmental and Intrinsic Variables

A buried body will still experience the stages of decomposition, as discussed in Chapters 1 and 2 of this book. However, the rate at which these stages progress will differ. It has been suggested that a buried body decomposes at a rate eight times slower than an exposed body (Casper 1861; Rodriguez 1997), but this is not necessarily the case (Carter *et al.* 2010). It is true that burial tends to slow decomposition, and the lesser rate of decomposition following burial is attributed to three primary factors:

1) a decrease in insect activity and scavengers
2) a decrease in temperature relative to the above-ground atmosphere
3) soil characteristics that influence pH and bioavailable moisture and oxygen

11.3.1 The Decomposer Community

Arguably, the most significant effect that burial has on taphonomy is that burial selects for a decomposer community that is dominated by microorganisms, with the exclusion of insects and vertebrate scavengers. Insects and scavengers can access buried remains (Pastula and Merritt 2013) but they do not always do so. Although microorganisms are the most abundant decomposer organisms, they are the least efficient decomposers relative to insects and scavengers. Insects, for example, play an important role in decomposition by using the remains as a nursery and food source for their developing young; fly larvae are particularly important in this process. A decomposer community that is primarily microbial will be associated with significantly slower decomposition, because insects and scavengers can consume 80–90% of a carcass much faster than bacteria, fungi and other microbial eukaryotes. With limited or no access to insects and scavengers, human remains will not undergo rapid decomposition.

11.3.2 Temperature

There are only two aspects to the decomposition of human remains, taxonomy and taphonomy. To understand the decomposition of human remains, it is necessary to understand the taxonomy (what organisms are there?) and taphonomy (what processes are occurring?). While burial generally selects the taxonomy of the decomposer community, temperature primarily regulates the taphonomy of human remains. It is possible that temperature will also select for certain microbial taxa (Carter *et al.* 2015; Iancu and Purcarea 2015). For example, Carter *et al.* (2015) observed a flush of bacterial genus *Psychrobacter* in soils associated with decomposing swine in the winter. This was an insightful finding, because *Psychrobacter* is a cold-tolerant microbe that was not observed during the summer (Carter *et al.* 2015), that is temperature can select for certain decomposer microbes. However, the primary role of temperature is probably to regulate decomposer activity.

An increase in temperature has been repeatedly demonstrated to drive biological and chemical reactions, which break down the body into the compounds that will eventually enter the surrounding soil (e.g. Carter and Tibbett 2008). Furthermore, it is commonly accepted that a temperature increase will facilitate faster decomposition (Carter *et al.* 2007; Mann *et al.* 1990; Vass *et al.* 1992). Conversely, cooler temperatures decrease the rate of decomposition by slowing the decomposition processes. This is primarily the result of slowing microbial metabolism associated with taphonomy: putrefaction (largely fermentation), anaerobic respiration and aerobic respiration. Research by Carter *et al.* (2008) showed that microbial activity increased significantly when temperature increased. A similar response was observed following the burial of much simpler remains: a 1.5 g cube of mammalian skeletal muscle tissue (Carter and Tibbett 2006). These observations have several implications for forensic taphonomy. First, they show that temperature plays a critical role in taphonomy due to its direct effect on autolysis and putrefaction. These observations also show us that the placement of human remains in soil, regardless of whether they are complete corpses or single pieces of soft tissue, stimulate significant microbial activity that is regulated by temperature. In other words, an increase in temperature results in an increase in decomposer microbial activity and the rate of decomposition.

11.3.3 Soil Texture, Moisture and Oxygen

Soil texture, moisture and oxygen also have a direct effect on taxonomy and taphonomy (e.g. Wilson *et al.* 2007). It is important to consider these three parameters together, as moisture and oxygen are a function of soil texture (the relative abundance of sand, silt and clay particles). To give two extreme examples, first consider a clayey soil that comprises at least 40% clay particles (<0.002 μm diameter) (Soil Science Society of America 1997). The small particle size of clay restricts gas diffusion, which eventually results in the depletion of oxygen and the proliferation of anaerobic microorganisms. Furthermore, the small size of clay particles allows clayey soils to hold more moisture than sandy soils, even though the moisture is bound by greater matric potential in clayey soils. In contrast, consider a sandy soil that comprises at least 85% sand particles. The large sand particles (0.05–2.0 mm diameter) (Soil Science Society of America 1997) will allow gas to diffuse at a greater rate and retain relatively little moisture (Janaway 1996).

Soil texture, moisture and oxygen modulate both biotic and abiotic decomposition processes. The high rate of gas diffusivity and lack of moisture observed in sandy soils promotes desiccation of soft tissue, which can restrict the decomposition process (Carter *et al.* 2010). The lack of gas diffusivity observed in clayey soils creates an anaerobic environment in which the aerobic microorganisms cannot effectively decompose the body. This then leaves the task of decomposition to the anaerobic community that is not as proficient a decomposer compared to aerobic microorganisms (Carter *et al.* 2010). Clayey soil can also promote the formation of adipocere, which slows decomposition as well (Forbes 2008).

11.3.4 Soil pH

The texture of soils is also related to the pH, a soil parameter that is much less studied from an experimental perspective. It is generally accepted that remains will shift from an alkaline state to a more acidic state during the early post-mortem period (Clark *et al.* 1997). This could be attributed to the breakdown of macromolecules to their molecular constituents. For example, proteins will break down into amino acids, lipids will break down into triglycerides and then further degrade to fatty acids, and carbohydrates will decompose into organic acids, all lowering the pH (Dent *et al.* 2004). However, the decomposition of remains tends to increase the pH of soil (Vass *et al.* 1992), unless the soil is already alkaline (Benninger *et al.* 2008; Van Belle *et al.* 2009). To highlight one common process, the conversion of ammonia (NH_3) to ammonium (NH_4^+) ions will decrease the concentration of free H^+, thereby increasing the pH (Carter *et al.* 2009; Haslam and Tibbett 2009; Meyer *et al.* 2013). Soil will eventually return to its basal pH, exhibiting the self-regulating characteristic of most soils (Carter *et al.* 2009; Jhonson 2009). Whatever the effect the body has on the soil, pH will directly affect the function of the decomposer community. It is typically observed that bacteria thrive in neutral soils, whereas fungi thrive in acidic and more alkaline soils (Carter *et al.* 2009; Haslam and Tibbett 2009; Jhonson 2009). Recent research by Haslam and Tibbett (2009) compared the decomposition of ovine muscular tissue buried in soils of varying pH. It was observed that decomposition rates were three times greater in acidic soil compared to alkaline soil (Haslam and Tibbett 2009).

Using an empirical approach, the effect of soil pH on human remains is relatively well established, particularly from an archaeological perspective. Bones tend to be less well preserved in acidic soils ($pH < 7$). This can even result in the formation of soil stains, or silhouettes, with no survival of bone (Bethell and Carver 1987; Mays 1998). Conversely, skeletal remains in alkaline soils ($pH < 7$) tend to be much better preserved than in acidic soils, attributed to the relative insolubility of hydroxyapatite at an alkaline pH (Mays 1998).

11.3.5 Intrinsic Properties

The intrinsic properties of the human remains can also affect decomposition and include drug use (Chapter 20), artificial mummification and mass burial (Chapter 18). Age at death, sex and mass can also have an effect on the decomposition of human remains in soil. This is because each of these properties has an effect on the nutritional quality of the remains (most decomposition is biologically mediated), the structure of the associated decomposer community and the physicochemical properties of the burial environment.

The influence of intrinsic properties on decomposition is difficult to study experimentally. This requires the acquisition of cadavers or carcasses that are of similar age, sex, mass or physical state at the time of burial. This can be very difficult because of the limited availability of materials, particularly human remains. However, a great deal has been learned from empirical studies and the archaeological record, and it is clear that the physical condition of the body at the time of burial has a significant effect on decomposition (Janaway 1996; Janaway *et al.* 2009; Mant 1950, 1987). This has allowed some generalisations to be made, but individual circumstances must be considered when interpreting taphonomy. For example, thin corpses tend to skeletonise more rapidly than more fleshy corpses (Mant 1953). A similar phenomenon has been observed with surface decomposition (Spicka *et al.* 2011), probably because a thinner corpse requires less mass to be decomposed.

The presence of physical trauma can also result in a greater rate of decomposition, probably because it enhances the colonisation of decomposer organisms (Janaway 1996). Similarly, more rapid decomposition is associated with bodies that have been left on the surface and colonised by decomposers prior to burial; the activity of many of these organisms will continue after burial (Bachmann and Simmons 2010; Janaway 1996). Somewhat related to the influence of perimortem wounding is the influence of internal pathologies that develop later in life, like osteoporosis. These changes in the density of bone can result in differential decomposition, because less dense bone may be more prone to decay (Janaway 1996).

Age can also influence the decomposition of human remains of those that died early in life. Infant and juvenile bones are smaller and less dense, which makes them more prone to decomposition. In fact, the size and shape of bones can also influence their decomposition. The skull is prone to crushing while long bones, such as the femur and humerus, can be more resistant to breakdown because of their shape (Janaway 1996). The smaller phalanges, carpals and tarsals appear to be particularly prone to breakdown (Waldron 1987). Overall, the influence of these intrinsic factors is not well established and forensic taphonomy would benefit greatly from more research in this area.

11.4 Decomposition Processes: Autolysis, Putrefaction and Decay

A buried body will exhibit the standard stages of decomposition, as described in Chapters 1 and 2. The chapter considers three broad processes of decomposition: autolysis, putrefaction and decay, and how they potentially differ when remains are buried.

11.4.1 Autolysis

Depending on the scene of death, the body could begin decomposing before it is buried; however, our perspective is focused on remains that are buried shortly after death so that decomposition largely occurs underground. Two phenomena, autolysis and the mortis triad characterise this initial stage. Autolysis, or cellular self-destruction by self-enzymes, is a series of biochemical reactions that break down the body. These microscopic changes manifest in macroscopic post-mortem changes observed in the mortis triad. *Algor mortis, livor mortis* and *rigor mortis* are changes in the body's temperature, vascular structure and muscular structure, respectively (Chapters 1 and 2). Ultimately, during the initial stage of decomposition, exposed bodies and buried bodies will undergo the same biological and chemical breakdown.

11.4.2 Putrefaction

Putrefaction describes the rise in mostly anaerobic microbial activity following death (Chapters 1 and 2). During this process, the body releases carbon dioxide, methane, nitrogen, ammonia, sulphuric acid and hydrogen sulphide (Chapters 1–3). For an exposed body, this diffuses into the atmosphere. A portion of these released compounds serves as a chemical signal to flies, attracting them to the source (Tomberlin *et al.* 2014). This process is not as prevalent with a buried body. The gases released diffuse into the soil, where many compounds are utilised by the soil microorganisms' metabolic pathways (Carter *et al.* 2009). Some compounds are released into the atmosphere, depending on grave depth and chemical structure (Vass *et al.* 2008), but the diffusion of gases from the body, into the soil and into the atmosphere, is regulated by soil texture, moisture and oxygen. Ultimately, during the putrefactive process, exposed bodies and buried bodies will undergo the same biological and chemical breakdown, resulting in the release of various compounds. The destinations of these compounds, however, potentially differ between the two circumstances.

11.4.3 Decay

Decay describes the decomposition processes that are not autolysis or putrefaction. Decay includes the activity of aerobic decomposer organisms and weathering processes, such as freezing and thawing due to changes in temperature or shrinking and swelling due to changes in moisture content. One of the major effects that burial has on decomposition is the prevention of vast insect colonisation and scavenger activity that aids in the decomposition. Second only to microbial mediated decomposition, insect colonisation is a major contributor to the recycling of the body through the environment, particularly by the fly species (Carter *et al.* 2007). Fly larvae, or maggots, are major contributors to the breakdown of the body and the process of decay. As previously mentioned, the release of certain compounds from the putrefactive process is believed to attract flies and other insects or scavengers (Tomberlin *et al.* 2014). With buried remains, many of the organisms that aid in decomposition of exposed remains are unable to reach them. This restricted access to the resource results in the decomposition of buried remains being largely achieved by microorganisms. This greatly decreases the rate of decomposition compared to exposed remains.

11.5 The Forensic Application of Taphonomy

Taphonomy is a remarkably valuable form of physical evidence for the justice system. Not only does taphonomic analysis facilitate the spatial reconstruction of a death scene, such as locating clandestine graves or remains resulting from a mass disaster, but taphonomy is also one of the few forms of physical evidence that facilitates the temporal reconstruction of a death scene. These data are typically presented as estimates of post-mortem interval, but taphonomy might also be applied to cases of abuse and neglect. An understanding of the processes associated with the decomposition and preservation of organic materials is of great importance to forensic science and archaeology, because they can be used to identify the deceased, establish cause and manner of death, locate human remains and estimate post-mortem interval.

11.5.1 Locating Human Remains

Forensic taphonomy plays an important role in the location of clandestine graves due to the effect that decomposition has on the burial site, and vice versa, it can be used to locate these sites. Human remains can serve as a significant source of nutrients for plants, but some time is required before this effect can be observed on the soil surface. Initially, a burial will result in the clearing of vegetation and produce a void area in the soil surface (Hunter and Martin 1996). These voids can be used to identify areas of interest before progressing with the use of geophysical techniques (Duncan 1983; Dupras *et al.* 2006; Hunter and Martin 1996; Killam 1990; Stoutamire 1983) or a full excavation. Eventually, the burial of remains will result in a flush of plant growth as plant communities establish themselves in the disturbed soil by taking advantage of the energy and nutrients released from the body. It is important to note that these gravesoil plant communities can differ from surrounding vegetation by containing a greater proportion of weedy pioneer species that can rapidly consume these newly available nutrients (Watson and Forbes 2008). Indications of clandestine graves can vary between climate, season and soil type. For instance, in temperate forests during cooler, wetter months, one might expect to observe the proliferation of post-putrefaction fungi growing above and around the gravesite, indicating the presence of active decomposition. These organisms can also form mushrooms in response to the presence of latrines and burrowing animals (Sagara *et al.* 2008). Forensic chemistry can also be employed to locate clandestine graves as they decompose and release their component parts into surrounding soils.

11.5.2 Identification of the Deceased

The relationship between decomposition, soils and human remains is complex and can have significant implications on the ability to identify the deceased. Remains that are placed in well-drained, aerated soils could increase the likelihood of desiccation and preservation of soft tissues. This process can be enhanced if it coincides with a high or low temperature. However, these types of soils are also typically associated with the poor preservation of bones, which are greatly affected by soil pH (e.g. Bethell 1989; Grupe 1995). In contrast, poorly drained, poorly aerated, clayey soils can result in the formation of adipocere and extended anaerobic metabolism, like that observed with putrefaction. This can make identification more difficult, because these processes do not tend to result in the preservation of identifiable characteristics. Partly because of this, one of the most valuable means of identification is through the use of dental records. Furthermore, using the decomposition process to reconstruct a scene could also aid in the identification of the deceased, using context clues and/or secondary effects of decomposition.

11.5.3 Establishing Cause and Manner of Death

Primarily done at the Coroner or Medical Examiner's office, establishing a cause and manner of death of a partially decomposed body becomes much easier when the cause of death resulted in the formation of a wound that has been preserved due to burial. In cases such as this, decomposition patterns could be altered, focusing on the wounds as new points of origin for decomposition. Not only does this aid in establishing the cause of death, but also the reconstruction of the events leading to death.

11.5.4 Estimating Post-Mortem Interval

Many recent taphonomy-based estimates of PMI are achieved by measuring Total Body Score (Megyesi *et al.* 2005) (Chapter 10). Additionally, forensic entomology is used to study a secondary mediator of decomposition, insects. Entomology is widely recognised as a method to estimate PMI. However, limitations of this method are inhibitive to a quick death investigation, the most obvious being the time factor. Identifying the larval stages and correlating those with time varies among species of fly. Upon collecting samples at a death scene, an entomologist must determine species, scene temperature and the age ranges of larvae found in the body. This takes time and is not always conducive for a death investigation, which has the primary goal of determining PMI quickly. Another problem is the death scene environment. Cold temperatures and burial will limit, if not inhibit, insect activity. Furthermore, recent attempts to correlate temporal changes to chemical and biological taphonomy are being studied. As a corpse decomposes, it will undergo biochemical breakdown yielding pH shifts observed in the soil (Rodriguez and Bass 1985; Carter *et al.* 2010). This phenomenon can be further applied to an additional decomposition environment. Chun *et al.* (2015) demonstrated that the maggot mass in particular exhibits unique chemical shifts in terms of pH and oxidation-reduction potential. These data suggest that maggot masses, a common occurrence at death scenes, provide much greater information to a forensic investigation than PMI estimations via entomology. This illustrates that taphonomy is an integral discipline in forensic science. Humans are comprised of common compounds that will degrade and decompose in similar patterns. Once the factors altering the patterns are understood, decomposition and taphonomy will play a much larger role in accurate and fast PMI estimations across the field of forensic science.

11.6 Conclusion

In conclusion, the relationships between human remains, soils and the burial environment are numerous and complex. Remains will progress through autolysis, putrefaction and decay, but these processes are influenced greatly by the burial environment and the intrinsic properties of the remains at the time of burial. Temperature, moisture, soil texture and pH are all environmental factors that greatly influence the breakdown of human remains. In addition, age at death, trauma/pathology and bone size can influence the decomposition of human remains. Although forensic taphonomy has made great strides in the last few decades, this field will benefit from much more empirical and experimental research that draws from the perspectives of archaeology, anthropology, ecology and medicolegal death investigation.

References

Bachmann, J. and Simmons, T. (2010) The influence of preburial insect access on the decomposition rate. *Journal of Forensic Sciences*, **55**: 893–900.

Benninger, L.A., Carter, D.O. and Forbes, S.L. (2008) The biochemical alteration of soil beneath a decomposing carcass. *Forensic Science International*, **180**: 70–75.

Bethell, P.H. (1989) Chemical analysis of shadow burials. In: Roberts, C., Lee, F. and Bintliff, J. (eds), *Burial Archaeology: Current research, methods and developments*. BAR: Oxford, pp. 205–214.

Bethell, P.H. and Carver, M.O.H. (1987) Detection and enhancement of decayed inhumations at Sutton Hoo. In: Boddington, A., Garland, A.N. and Janaway, R.C. (eds), *Death, Decay and Reconstruction: Approaches to archaeology and forensic science*. Manchester University Press: Manchester, pp.10–21.

Carter, D.O., Forbes, S.L. and Tibbett, M. (2009) Soil microbial ecology as forensic taphonomy. In: Wecht, C.W. (ed.), *Forensic Sciences*, vol, **1**. LexisNexis Matthew Bender: Albany, pp. 23B1–23B47.

Carter, D.O., Metcalf, J.L., Bibat, A. and Knight, R. (2015) Seasonal variation of postmortem microbial communities. *Forensic Science, Medicine, and Pathology*, **11**: 202–207.

Carter, D.O. and Tibbett, M. (2006) Microbial decomposition of skeletal muscle tissue (*Ovis aries*) in a sandy loam soil at different temperatures. *Soil Biology and Biochemistry*, **38**: 1139–1145.

Carter, D.O. and Tibbett, M. (2008) Cadaver decomposition and soil: processes. In: Tibbett, M. and Carter, D.O. (eds), *Soil Analysis in Forensic Taphonomy: Chemical and biological effects of buried human remains*. CRC Press: Boca Raton, pp. 29–51.

Carter, D.O., Yellowlees D. and Tibbett M. (2007) Cadaver decomposition in terrestrial ecosystems. *Naturwissenschaften*, **94**: 12–24.

Carter, D.O., Yellowlees, D. and Tibbett, M. (2010) Moisture can be the dominant environmental parameter governing cadaver decomposition in soil. *Forensic Science International*, **200**: 60–66.

Casper, J.L. (1861) *A Handbook of the Practice Of Forensic Medince: Based upon personal experience*. The New Sydenham Society: London.

Chun, L.P., Miguel, M.J., Junkins, E.N., Forbes, S.L. and Carter, D.O. (2015) An initial investigation into the ecology of culturable aerobic postmortem bacteria. *Science & Justice*, **55**: 394–401.

Clark, M.A., Worrell, M.B. and Pless, J.E. (1997) Postmortem changes in soft tissue. In: Haglund, W.D. and Sorg, M.H. (eds), *Forensic Taphonomy: The postmortem fate of human remains*. CRC Press: Boca Raton, pp. 151–164.

Dent, B.B., Forbes, S.L. and Stuart, B.H. (2004) Review of human decomposition processes in soil. *Environmental Geology*, **45**: 576–585.

Duncan, J. (1983) Search Techniques. In: Morse, D., Duncan, J. and Stoutamire, J. (eds), *Handbook of Forensic Archaeology and Anthropology*. Rose Printing: Tallahassee, pp. 4–19.

Dupras, T.L., Schultz, J.J., Wheeler, S.M. and Williams, L.J. (2006) *Forensic Recovery of Human Remains: Archaeological approaches*. CRC Press: Boca Raton.

Forbes, S.L. (2008) Decomposition chemistry in a burial environment. In: Tibbett, M. and Carter, D.O. (eds), *Soil Analysis in Forensic Taphonomy: Chemical and biological effects of buried human remains*. CRC Press: Boca Raton, pp. 203–223.

Grupe, G. (2005) Preservation of collagen in bone from dry, sandy soil. *Journal of Archaeological Science*, **22**: 193–199.

Haslam, T.C. and Tibbett, M. (2009) Soils of contrasting pH affect the decomposition of buried mammalian (*Ovis aries*) skeletal muscle tissue. *Jounal of Forensic Sciences*, **54**: 900–904.

Hunter, J.R. and Martin, A.L. (1996) Locating buried remains. In: Hunter, J., Roberts, C. and Martin, A. (eds), *Studies in Crime: An introduction to forensic archaeology*. Routledge: London, pp. 86–100.

Iancu, L., Carter, D.O., Junkins, E.N. and Purcarea, C. (2015) Using bacterial and necrophagous insect dynamics for post-mortem interval estimation during cold season: Novel case study in Romania. *Forensic Science International*, **254**: 106–117.

Janaway, R.C. (1996) The decay of buried remains and their associated material. In: Hunter, J., Roberts, C. and Martin, A. (eds), *Studies in Crime: An introduction to forensic archaeology*. Routledge: London, pp. 58–85.

Janaway, R.C., Percival, S.L. and Wilson, A.S. (2009) Decomposition of human remains. In: Percival, S.L. (ed.), *Microbiology and Aging*. Springer: Berlin, pp. 313–334.

Jhonson, C. (2009) *Biology of Soil Science*. Oxford Book Company: Jaipur.

Killam, E.W. (1990) *The Detection of Human Remains*. Charles C. Thomas: Springfield.

Mann, R.W., Bass, M.A. and Meadows, L. (1990) Time since death and decomposition of the human body: variables and observations in case and experimental field studies. *Journal of Forensic Sciences*, **35**: 103–111.

Mant, A.K. (1950) A study in exhumation data. Unpublished MD thesis, University of London.

Mant, A.K. (1953) Adipocere: a review. *Journal of Forensic Medicine*, **4**: 18–35.

Mant, A.K. (1987) Knowledge acquired from post-war exhumations. In: Boddington, A., Garland, A.N., and Janaway, R.C. (eds), *Death, Decay and Reconstruction: Approaches to archaeology and forensic science*. Manchester University Press: Manchester, pp. 65–78.

Mays, S. (1998) *The Archaeology of Human Bones*. Routledge: London.

Megyesi, M.S., Nawrocki, S.P. and Haskell, N.H. (2005) Using accumulated degree-days to estimate the postmortem interval from decomposed human remains. *Journal of Forensic Sciences*, **50**: 618–626.

Meyer, J.D., Anderson, B.F. and Carter, D.O. (2013) Seasonal variation of carcass decomposition and gravesoil chemistry in a cold (Dfa) climate. *Journal of Forensic Sciences*, **58**: 1175–1182.

Pastula, E.C. and Merritt, R.W. (2013) Insect arrival pattern and succession on buried carrion in Michgan. *Journal of Medical Entomology*, **50**: 432–439.

Rodriguez, W.C. (1997) Decomposition of buried and submerged bodies. In: Haglund, W.D. and Sorg, M.H. (eds), *Forensic Taphonomy: The postmortem fate of human remains*. CRC Press: Boca Raton.

Rodriguez, W.C. and Bass, W.M. (1985) Decomposition of buried bodies and methods that may aid in their location. *Journal of Forensic Sciences*, **30**: 836–852.

Sagara, N., Yamanaka, T. and Tibbett, M. (2008) Soil fungi associated with graves and latrines: toward a forensic mycology. In: Tibbett, M. and Carter, D.O. (eds), *Soil Analysis in Forensic Taphonomy*. CRC Press: Boca Raton.

Soil Science Society of America (1997) *Glossary of Soil Science Terms*. Soil Science Society of America: Madison.

Spicka, A., Johnson, R., Bushing, J., Higley, L.G. and Carter, D.O. (2011) Carcass mass can influence rate of decomposition and release of ninhydrin-reactive nitrogen into gravesoil. *Forensic Science International*, **209**: 80–85.

Stoutamire, J. (1983) Excavation and recovery. In: Morse, D., Duncan, J. and Stoutamire, J. (eds), *Handbook of Forensic Archaeology and Anthropology*. Rose Printing: Tallahassee, pp. 20–47.

Swift, M.J., Heal, O.W. and Anderson, J.M, (1979) *Decomposition in Terrestrial Ecosystem*. Blackwell Scientific: Oxford.

Tomberlin, J.K., Crippen, T.L., Benbow, M.E. and Tarone, A.M. (2014) *Development and Validation of Standard Operating Procedures for Measuring Microbial Populations for Estimating a Postmortem Interval*. Report 2010-DN-BX-K23, US Department of Justice: Washington.

Turner, B.D. and Wiltshire, P.E.J. (1999) Experimental validation of forensic evidence: a study of the decomposition of buried pigs in a heavy clay soil. *Forensic Science International*, **101**: 113–122.

Van Belle, L.E., Carter, D.O. and Forbes, S.L. (2009) Measurement of ninhydrin reactive nitrogen influx into gravesoil during above-ground and below-ground carcass (*Sus scrofa domesticus*) decomposition. *Forensic Science International*, **193**: 37–41.

Vass, A.A. (2011) The elusive universal post-mortem interval formula. *Forensic Science International*, **204**: 34–40.

Vass, A.A., Bass, W.M., Wolt, J.D., Foss, J.E. and Ammons, J.T. (1992) Time since death determination in human cadavers using soil solution. *Journal of Forensic Sciences*, **37**: 1236–1253.

Vass, A.A., Smith, R.R., Thompson, C.V., Burnett, M.N., Dulgerian, N. and Eckenrode, B.A. (2008) Odor analysis of decomposing buried remains. *Journal Forensic Sciences*, **53**: 384–391.

Waldron, T. (1987) The relative survival of the human skeleton: implications for palaeopathology. In: Boddington, A., Garland, A.N. and Janaway, R.C. (eds), *Death, Decay and Reconstruction: Approaches to archaeology and forensic science*. Manchester University Press: Manchester, pp. 55–64.

Watson, C.J. and Forbes, S.L. (2008) An investigation of the vegetation associated with grave sites in southern Ontario. *Canadian Society of Forensic Science Journal*, **41**: 199–207.

Wilson, A.S., Janaway, R.C., Holland, A.D., Dodson, H.I., Baran, E. *et al.* (2007) Modelling the buried human body environment in upland climes using three contrasting field sites. *Forensic Science International*, **169**: 6–18.

12

Bacterial Symbionts and Taphonomic Agents of Humans

Franklin E. Damann

12.1 Introduction

Microbially mediated decomposition is an important process in ecology and it is second only to photosynthesis for the production of energy in a given ecosystem (McGuire and Treseder 2010). Cadaver decomposition creates a resource patch utilised by a myriad of decomposer organisms that facilitate nutrient and energy transformations, which are fundamental concepts in ecosystem ecology (Carter *et al.* 2007). Applying high-throughput sequencing to identify patterns of microbial communities associated with cadaver decomposition is a significant advancement for understanding ecological processes of decomposition. Studies that investigate the communities of bacteria associated with decomposing cadavers have implications in taphonomy, as bacterial community succession is a promising indicator of the post-mortem interval.

High-throughput sequencing and open access to microbial ecology data are transforming the way we understand our relationship to the microbial worlds that live in and around us. Greater insight is being achieved through majorly funded microbial ecology projects such as the Human Microbiome Project (http://www.hmpdacc.org/), Earth Microbiome Project (http://www.earthmicrobiome.org/) and the Microbiome of the Built Environment (http://microbe.net/). Protocols and standards for sample extraction and analyses can be found on each of these websites.

Each of these research consortia and associated projects are producing data on a scale not previously possible. Studies in microbial ecology are not only revealing relationships among human microbes, health and disease, but they are also providing new data on the diversity and abundance of microbes associated with decomposing mammals. Moreover, producing and sharing large data sets is becoming standard practice in microbial ecology, which necessitates standardisation of methods. Detailed descriptions of molecular methods and data analyses can be found on the websites of the major projects listed above.

This chapter applies a bacteriocentric perspective on the decomposition of human remains. First, basic concepts of bacterial growth and metabolism, and factors that govern growth are presented. The factors that govern the growth and metabolism of bacteria will be familiar to the reader, who understands the limiting factors of macroscopic decomposition (i.e. temperature, moisture, etc.). Second, a brief discussion on the microbiome of living humans is presented, because any discussion on bacterially mediated decomposition should include reference to the symbiotic organisms of the human body. Finally, recent projects that have explored bacterial communities associated with the decomposition of humans and model organisms will be discussed.

Taphonomy of Human Remains: Forensic Analysis of the Dead and the Depositional Environment, First Edition.
Edited by Eline M.J. Schotsmans, Nicholas Márquez-Grant and Shari L. Forbes.

12.2 Bacterial Growth and Metabolism

Bacteria are ubiquitous. They are present around the globe and in our bodies. A single gram of soil contains 10^9 bacterial cells (Paul 2007), while an adult human is composed of roughly 10^{14} prokaryotic cells (Wilson 2008). Taken by mass, bacteria account for approximately 2% of an individual's body weight, which is roughly equivalent to the mass of a human liver. Broadly speaking, an individual's microbiome can be considered a separate functioning organ system. Sequencing and subsequent analyses of the human genome have identified approximately 20,000 protein-coding genes, while the functional genes of the human microbiome contribute orders of magnitude greater than our own eukaryotic genome (Turnbaugh *et al.* 2007). Perhaps our 20,000 functional genes are a mere suite of house-keeping genes that support microorganisms and their specialised functions, permitting humans to thrive and adapt to various environmental contexts.

Under ideal physical and nutrient conditions, the vegetative state of bacterial species follows an exponential population growth curve that includes an initial lag phase, which encompasses a period of time sufficient for bacteria to adjust to a new environment. The length of the lag phase is extended or shortened based on the organism itself, nutrient availability and the physicochemical environment (e.g. temperature, moisture, pH, oxygen). The lag phase is followed by an exponential growth phase where the bacteria reproduce by binary fission. Continuous growth does not go unchecked, however. In a closed system such as a culture tube, or a cecum of a dead human, available nutrients may become scarce, waste products accumulate, pH levels drop and O_2 availability decreases, eliciting a stationary phase of growth for a specific bacterial species where death and reproduction rates equalise. The final stage of bacterial growth is not growth at all, but exponential decline (Pommerville 2004). As bacteria grow, they continuously reduce the available nutrient content of a substrate and their metabolic products change the conditions of the environment. In polybacterial environments, like a living human or a decomposing corpse, these changes promote succession to taxonomically and physiologically different bacteria.

The diversity and specificity of bacteria to various human habitats (i.e. guts, mouth, skin, etc.) are attributable to the various chemical pathways by which they acquire energy and carbon so that they may grow, maintain cellular stability and replicate (Jurtshuk 1996). Chemotrophs are organisms that oxidise organic compounds in order to acquire energy, and thus depend on oxidation-reduction reactions. Fundamentally, energy acquisition is about the movement of electrons in a system. If a substance is losing or gaining electrons it is being oxidised or reduced, respectively. Carbon and other nutrients are acquired through dissimilatory reactions, where autotrophs acquire carbon primarily from CO_2 and heterotrophs utilise organic compounds, such as carbohydrates, proteins, lipids and nucleic acids as a carbon source.

12.3 Limiting Factors of Bacterial Growth and Function

The physicochemical parameters that govern the rate of macroscopic change of a decomposing corpse (Damann and Carter 2014) are similar to cofactors that either limit or facilitate bacterial growth. Primary factors include temperature, water activity, substrate pH, oxygen availability, nutrient content and the physical structure of the substrate. Across various anatomical structures, these factors combine to create multiple environments conducive to different bacterial types. For example, pH in the human gastrointestinal tract varies from ≤ 2 in the stomach to ≥ 7.3 in the ileum, and to approximately 5.7 in the cecum (Wilson 2008). Similarly, oxygen availability fluctuates across the length of the gastrointestinal tract, where the stomach, small intestines, cecum and colon contain 29, 22, 19 and 23% of the oxygen content of air, respectively (Wilson 2008). These differences are the result of both normal human anatomical structure and the metabolic products of the resident bacterial communities. Understanding how these factors govern community membership and how particular communities may alter the microstructure of human remains may provide insight into the burial context in which the human remains were initially deposited.

12.3.1 Temperature

Bacteria have a minimum, maximum and optimal temperature range that allows for growth by directly affecting an organism's generation time and lag period. Temperatures on the low end of an organism's spectrum will reduce enzyme activity and transport across cell walls, while high temperatures will cause internal cellular components to denature (Tortora *et al.* 1995). Bacteria can be classified by their temperature tolerance. From cold to warm they are described as psychrophiles, psychrotrophs, mesophiles, thermophiles and extreme thermophiles (Tortora *et al.* 1995). Most heterotrophic bacteria function over the mesophilic range (25–40°C), which is why a refrigerator works well to preserve a corpse prior to autopsy.

12.3.2 Moisture

Moisture is essential for bacterial growth and activity as it facilitates microbial motility, diffusion of nutrients and waste, and enzyme function. Carter *et al.* (2010) present data indicating that moisture is one of the most prominent environmental parameters governing decomposition of a corpse in soil. Reducing moisture precludes microbial movement and activity, while water saturated soils reduce gas diffusion and promote less efficient anaerobic metabolism (Carter *et al.* 2010).

12.3.3 Substrate pH

Just as bacteria have optimal temperature and moisture ranges that support growth and function, the same is true for pH. Substrate pH is a measure of the hydrogen ion concentration in a solution and is measured on a logarithmic scale. Along the pH scale, bacteria are named appropriately as acidophiles, neutrophiles and alkaliphiles. For each of these three types of bacteria, they have a minimum and maximum pH at which point they do not grow and an optimal pH where they grow best. For example, acidomicrobia were well represented in soils at the University of Tennessee Anthropology Research Facility, but their presence was reduced in soil samples that had increased pH as a result of active human decomposition (Damann 2010).

12.3.4 Redox Potential

Reduction and oxidation (redox) potential is a ratio of oxidising to reducing power of a substance and is a measure of electron availability (Jay 2000). Common electron donors are organic and reduced inorganic compounds (e.g. NH_4^+, Fe^{2+}, Mn^{2+}, S^{2-}, CH_4 and H_2), while common electron acceptors are O_2, NO_3^-, MnO_2, SO_4^{2-} and HCO_3^- (DeLaune and Reddy 2005). In environments where oxygen is plentiful, aerobic bacteria use oxygen as a terminal electron acceptor. Typically, an anaerobic environment is limited by electron acceptors; however, electron donors are plentiful (DeLaune and Reddy 2005). Facultative anaerobes may use oxygen when available, but can use non-oxygen compounds, whereas oxygen is poisonous to obligate anaerobes. Redox potentials are measured in millivolts (mV). Aerobic metabolism occurs under oxidised more positive (more than +350 mV) redox conditions, anaerobic metabolism occurs in highly reduced more negative (less than −200 mV) redox conditions, and facultative anaerobic metabolism typically occurs under moderately reduced redox conditions, between −100 and +300 mV (DeLaune and Reddy 2005).

12.3.5 Nutrient Requirements

There are a dozen essential nutrients that bacteria require from the environment in order to build necessary cellular structures. The major requirements for biosynthesis include carbon, oxygen, hydrogen, nitrogen, sulphur and phosphorus. Potassium, calcium, magnesium, iron, copper and zinc constitute the micronutrients, which are also required but in lesser amounts than the macronutrients. Carbohydrates, proteins, nucleic acids and enzymes are synthesised from these elements. Organisms that grow in environments with limited nutrients are oligotrophs. Copiotrophs are present in ecological niches where nutrient availability is abundant (Koch 2001) and follow a feast or famine pattern of growth.

12.4 Bacteria as Symbiotic Organisms

Human-associated bacteria have been the subject of much study and relatively recent advances in high-throughput sequencing technology have provided greater insight into the unique community fingerprints of our personalised microbiomes across multiple body habitats (Costello *et al.* 2009). These fingerprints have indicated how bacterial communities contribute to human health and disease, such as obesity (Turnbaugh *et al.* 2009; Ley 2010; Greenblum *et al.* 2012), inflammatory bowel disease (Joossens *et al.* 2011), the formation of kidney stones (Kaufman *et al.* 2008), acute wheezing in children (Hyde *et al.* 2014) and how endogenous bacterial communities protect hosts against invading pathogens (Ravel *et al.* 2011; Stumpf *et al.* 2013).

Among the various body sites explored, the alimentary system and the gastrointestinal tract (GIT) in particular have received significant attention (Eckburg *et al.* 2005; Gill *et al.* 2006; Ley *et al.* 2006; Li *et al.* 2008; Nicholson *et al.* 2005). Resident microorganisms of the human gut help digest food and maintain our immune systems, while also providing vitamins K, B and folate via specific metabolic pathways (Morgan *et al.* 2013).

The GIT is a specialised environment rich in nutrients, but membership to the resident community is selective. Along the nearly 5 m of the human GIT, oxygen availability and pH govern the resident bacterial population in living persons. The oesophagus and stomach are aerobic environments, and while the pH of the stomach is low, ranging between pH 1 and 5, the negative effects on local bacteria can be buffered by ingested food. Introduced foods and liquids, along with host secreted mucins, salivary proteins and dead microbes serve as a nutrient source for the resident microbiota (Wilson 2008). The pH of the small intestines increases with the addition of alkaline fluids from bile and pancreatic juices, while the availability of oxygen is further reduced by bacterial catabolism of chyme, creating a redox potential as low as −150 mV in the ileum (Wilson 2008). The lumen of the large intestine has a redox potential in the range of −200 to −300 mV (Wilson 2008), which facilitates communities of facultative and obligate anaerobes.

While there are hundreds of unique prokaryotic taxa that reside in the human GIT, only seven bacterial divisions at the phylum level have been identified (Eckburg *et al.* 2005). Ley *et al.* (2006) contrast this relatively low number of phyla against 20 different bacterial phyla found in soil that basically perform the same catalysis of organic compounds. The dominant bacteria represented in the human cecum, colon, rectum and faeces belong to the Firmicutes, Bacteroidetes, Proteobacteria, Verrucomicrobia, Fusobacteria, Actinobacteria and Cynobacteria. Firmicutes and Bacteroidetes are the dominant divisions and account for ≥95% of all taxonomically identified taxonomic units (Costello *et al.* 2009; Eckburg *et al.* 2005; Li *et al.* 2008). Within these two phyla, the most frequently observed genera included anaerobic Firmicutes of *Clostridia* and *Mollicutes*, with the majority of Bacteroidetes represented by *B. vulgatus* and *Prevotellaceae* (Eckburg *et al.* 2005). Despite the trillions of bacterial inhabitants of the human gut, their potentially deleterious effects are kept at bay, because normal GIT anatomy provides sufficient antimicrobial defences in life. Approximately 200 billion epithelial cells are shed into the lumen each day and coupled with the intestinal mucous layer, the low pH of the stomach, the presence of bile and proteolytic enzymes that are active against gram-positive organisms, microbial invasion of the gut wall is typically precluded in the healthy gut of living humans (Wilson 2008). However, the same cannot be stated for the gut of dead humans, as the resident bacteria represent one of the first taphonomic agents of human decomposition.

12.5 Bacteria as Taphonomic Agents

Death results in the cessation of respiratory and circulatory systems causing oxygen depletion in tissue (Perper 1993). Without oxygen, mitochondria swell and internal cellular organelles rupture (Evans 1963); consequently, membrane pumps fail and cell membranes are destroyed. Without protection of normal homeostatic mechanisms, the intestinal mucosal layer degrades, permitting initial bacterial transmigration from the GIT across the internal mucosa, allowing microbes to move along vascular and lymphatic systems (Kellerman *et al.* 1976; Melvin *et al.* 1984) and then along tissue planes to whole organ systems (Evans 1963). The rich nutritive substratum of the human body is then used for the growth of enteric microorganisms. Bacteria have been detected in the liver of a cadaver 20 hours after death and blood, heart, brain and spleen all contained bacteria 58 hours after death (Can *et al.* 2014).

Similar to macroscopic observations of decomposition, bacterial growth in the early post-mortem period is limited only by environmental factors such as temperature and moisture (Garcia-Lopez *et al.* 1998). Inside the body, bacteria invade new environments and logarithmic growth occurs once they have adjusted their metabolism and have adapted to their new environment (Marshall and Bal'a 2001). The depletion of oxygen in tissues with high metabolic demand (i.e. heart, kidneys, brain, liver and skeletal muscle) forces the use of different electron acceptors. This change causes a shift in bacterial metabolism from aerobic to predominantly anaerobic. Evans (1963) described this transition as one that is exemplified by a change from coliform, staphylococcal and *Proteus* bacteria to *Clostridia*.

Dominant organisms occur in a particular decomposing substrate because of higher growth rates, and the increased growth is due to metabolic advantages or greater tolerance to limiting factors (Garcia-Lopez *et al.* 1998). Bacteria first grow on the surfaces of internal tissues at the expense of water-soluble low molecular weight compounds, such as glucose and glycolysis intermediates (Gill 1983). Simple sugars are preferentially consumed, producing lactic acid and lowering substrate pH, which in turn supports the growth of *Lactobacillus* and other organisms unaffected by low pH (Gill 1983). This pattern continues until substrate-carrying capacity is reached, which is typically cited as 10^8 cells g^{-1} of muscle tissue (Gill 1983; Ingram and Dainty 1971; Marshall and Bal'a 2001; Standbridge and Davies 1998). After glucose is depleted, bacteria catabolise high molecular weight compounds such as proteins, as a source of carbon and energy.

12.6 Putrefaction

The microbially mediated process of putrefaction leads to bloating and active decomposition (Damann and Carter 2014). Onset of putrefaction is variable, as the catabolic processes specific to putrefaction are regulated by an array of limiting factors that affect bacterial growth and metabolism.

As water-soluble sugars are consumed at the surface of tissue planes, bacteria move into deeper tissue spaces to catabolise amino acids. Bacterially-induced dissimilatory reactions of protein and amino acids mark the onset of putrefaction (Marshall and Bal'a 2001). This is accomplished by obligate and facultative anaerobic microorganisms, represented by the *Clostridium, Bacteroides* and *Lactobacilli, Staphylococcus* genera, plus the Enterobacteriaceae family (Carter *et al.* 2007; Gill-King 1997; Melvin *et al.* 1984). Utilisation of the amino acids ornithine and arginine produce putrescine, and cadaverine is released by the catalysis of lysine (Gill-King 1997; Nychas *et al.* 1998). The sulphur-containing amino acids cysteine, cystine and methionine, may be reduced in the presence of water by bacterial cysteine desulfhydrase, producing hydrogen sulphide, ammonia and pyruvic acid (Marshall and Bal'a 2001). In addition to being a source of sulphur for bacteria, hydrogen sulphide creates the rotten-egg odour of decomposition. Hydrogen sulphide reacts with iron ions forming ferrous sulphide, a black precipitate found in the capillaries near the skin surface of a decomposing corpse (Gill-King 1997; Love and Marks 2003). Biliary acids form sulpha-haemoglobin complexes, which appear as a green discoloration of the skin near the left anterior abdominal wall (Clark *et al.* 1997; Gill-King 1997). In the presence of myoglobin, hydrogen sulphide forms sulph-myoglobin, which produces the green discoloration of muscle tissue (Standbridge and Davies 1998). These chemical changes initiated by bacterial metabolism produce the macroscopic appearance often referred to as marbling. Cadaverine, putrescine, ammonia, hydrogen sulphide, pyruvic acid, methane, carbon dioxide and other volatile organic compounds (Chapter 3) not only cause the body to blister and swell, but are also partly responsible for the odoriferous milieu associated with human decomposition (Evans 1963; Marshall and Bal'a 2001; Vass *et al.* 1992).

Blistered epidermis, bloat and subsequent rupture and collapse of the abdominal region are macroscopic changes often observed during decomposition. Gas from anaerobic metabolism and the liquefaction of internal tissues produces frothy exudate of the eyes, nose, mouth and anus. The build-up of gas causes the body to blister and bloat. When the internal pressure exceeds the structural integrity of remaining tissues, rupture occurs. Rupture causes a purge of nutrient-rich body fluids to surrounding grave soils (Carter *et al.* 2010) and promotes additional aerobic decay (Gill-King 1997; Micozzi 1991). It is a long-held hypothesis that rupture forces the transition from anaerobically dominated bloat to the aerobic decay stage of decomposition (Payne 1965; Reed 1958), which coincides with a shift in the metabolic and taxonomic structure of enteric and edaphic bacterial communities (Lauber *et al.* 2014; Metcalf *et al.* 2013). Through culture-independent sequencing methods, Metcalf *et al.* (2013) confirm this notion by evaluating microbial community membership and structure of 40 decomposing mice and their associated grave soils. Pre-rupture enteric communities were dominated by Firmicutes and Bacteroidetes, which included the families of Lactobacillaceae and Bacteroidaceae, respectively (Metcalf *et al.* 2013). After rupture, the abundance of these taxa decreased, and were replaced by aerobic bacteria from the families Phyllobacteriaceae, Hyphomicrobiaceae and Brucellaceae (Alphaproteobacteria), and facultative anaerobes of the family Enterobacteriaceae (Gammproteobacteria), including *Serratia, Escherichia, Klebsiella* and *Proteus* (Metcalf *et al.* 2013). Similarly, bacterial taxa of associated grave soils changed between pre- and post-rupture. The release of nutrients into soil is associated with a rise in soil pH (Vass *et al.* 1992; Haslam and Tibbett 2009) that creates a succession from the Acidobacteria of normal pre-rupture soils to a community where members of Alphaproteobacteria increased, as they outcompeted slower-growing Acidobacteria for corpse-derived nutrients (Metcalf *et al.* 2013). Decline in Acidobacteria abundance in response to increased soil pH was observed by Lauber *et al.* (2009) and was similarly observed in areas of concentrated human decomposition at the University of Tennessee outdoor decomposition facility (Damann 2010).

Hyde *et al.* (2013) sampled the GIT from two decomposing humans and analysed the bacterial communities present at the end of the bloat stage via culture-independent methods. When compared to their early pre-bloat oral swab samples, the end-bloat period was dominated by *Clostridia* and *Bacteroides*, which transitioned from the aerobic *Staphylococcus* and Enterobacteriacae. Despite slight variation in the relative abundance among sample locations within the GIT, as a whole, members of Firmicutes, Bacteroidetes and Proteobacteria dominated the end-of-bloat samples; a finding consistent with studies using pigs (Pechal *et al.* 2014) and mice (Metcalf *et al.* 2013) as model organisms.

After bloat and purge, the efflux of nutrients to the surrounding grave soils may become immobilised in the surrounding community of living organisms, mineralised, leached into the burial substrate, and/or evolved as volatile compounds (Swift *et al.* 1979), while the mostly recalcitrant tissues of poly-phenolic humus, bone, ligaments and hair remain. Relative to the copiotrophic environment of the GIT and early phases of soft tissue decomposition, bone tissue itself presents a different decomposing resource, where its intrinsic quality hosts a limited nutrient pool of primarily calcium and phosphorus that is physically protected within the bone microstructure. That said, microbially mediated effects on bone tissue have been observed in forensic, archaeological and laboratory contexts (Turner-Walker 2008). Bacteria and microeukaryotes with collagenases use collagen as a source of C and N to meet metabolic demands. Through culture enrichment and biochemical staining techniques, 17% of the total microbial isolates of archaeological bone and soil contained an identifiable collagenase, but attempts to demonstrate specific isolates as the taphonomic agents of bone bioerosion failed to produce reliable results (Child 1995).

Recent application of culture-independent sequencing of bacteria from decaying human bone recovered from bodies decomposing on the surface at the University of Tennessee Anthropology Research Facility, identified Proteobacteria, Firmicutes, Bacteroidetes, Actinobacteria and Acidobacteria as the dominate communities (Damann *et al.* 2015). With advancing time, Firmicutes and Bacteroidetes decreased in bone samples, while Alpha-, Gamma-proteobacteria and Actinobacteria increased over the four-year decay period. Acidobacteria from the families Solibacteraceae and Koribacteraceae appeared in bone samples exposed on the ground surface for more than two years and were also observed in a similar soil not exposed to cadaver decomposition.

The most abundant bacterial taxa present in bone were members of Pseudomonadaceae, Clostridiaceae and Tissierellaceae (Table 12.1). While the presence of specific bacterial taxa in decaying bone has been documented (Damann *et al.* 2015), no simple relationship exists among taxa identified during decomposition of a corpse to the source (e.g. human or soil-derived organisms) of bacteria present in late-stage decomposition (Lauber *et al.* 2014); nor have the functional attributes of those taxa in decaying bone been concluded; a finding in part due to the complex polymicrobial edaphic and enteric environments of human decomposition.

12.7 Microbiology in Forensic Medicine

Estimating the post-mortem interval accurately is difficult and only becomes more so with advancing time and decay. Early post-mortem chemical changes in vitreous potassium levels and the evaluation of the mortis triad (e.g. *algor*, *livor* and *rigor mortis*) are unreliable indicators of PMI due to extreme individual variation. Forensic entomology provides significant improvement to PMI estimates, but necessitates the presence of insects. Bacteria on the other hand are always present.

Recent projects are demonstrating the possibility of a universal model with limited error for estimating PMI based on the presence and succession of microbial communities (Metcalf *et al.* 2013; Pechal *et al.* 2013). The samples in these studies were collected from decomposing animal models and associated soils. In each event, the preferred collection technique used a sterile cotton swab. Duplicate samples were taken from the exposed skin surface and the location of the sample site was recorded. In addition to the body samples, swabs of associated decomposition soils and a control soil swab were also collected. Data from bone samples were obtained by destructive sampling of field-collected tissue (Damann *et al.* 2015). Once collected, swabs and bones were refrigerated (4°C)

Table 12.1 Rank-order abundance of the top 12 most abundant bacterial families identified in bone and non-corpse soils (Damann *et al.* 2015). Types are listed in order from most abundant to least abundant.

Bone	Non-corpse soil
Pseudomonadaceae (Gammaproteobacteria)	Hyphomicrobiaceae (Alphaproteobacteria)
Clostridiaceae (Firmicutes)	Koribacteraceae (Acidobacteria)
Tissierellaceae (Firmicutes)	Solibacteraceae (Acidobacteria)
Caulobacteraceae (Alphaproteobacteria)	Flavobacteriaceae (Bacteroidetes)
Sphingobacteriaceae (Bacteroidetes)	Rhodospirillaceae (Alphaproteobacteria)
Flavobacteriaceae (Bacteroidetes)	Sphingobacteriaceae (Bacteroidetes)
Streptomycetaceae (Actinobacteria)	A4b (Chloroflexi, uncultured bacterium)
Xanthomonadaceae (Gammaproteobacteria)	Caulobacteraceae (Alphaproteobacteria)
Alcanivoracaceae (Gammaproteobacteria)	RB40 (Acidobacteria, uncultured bacterium)
Bacillaceae (Firmicutes)	Gaiellaceae (Actinobacteria)
Sphingomonadaceae (Alphaproteobacteria)	Hyphomonadaceae (Alphaproteobacteria)
Hyphomicrobiaceae (Alphaproteobacteria)	Nocardioidaceae (Actinobacteria)

(Source: Damann 2015. Reproduced with permission of John Wiley & Sons).

or frozen (−20°C), depending on when the samples were processed. Standard laboratory methods and analyses of microbial DNA can be found online (http://www.earthmicrobiome.org/) and in the respective publications.

Microbial community analyses of decaying animal models in the early post-mortem period (Carter *et al.* 2015; Metcalf *et al.* 2013; Pechal *et al.* 2013) and decaying human skeletal remains (Damann *et al.* 2015) are producing promising results for improving PMI estimations. This approach seems to be working, because the bacterial communities of a decedent are the sum of an individual's health, disease, diet and the environment in which they live and die. As the body changes as a result of decomposition, so will the underlying microbiome. By identifying predictable patterns of change in bacterial community membership and structure in response to environmental stimuli, the microbiomes of decomposition may be used to estimate the post-mortem interval.

As a body decomposes it undergoes multiple changes in its biochemical and anatomical components. Normal cellular functions terminate with death. Enteric bacterial populations undergo exponential growth; move over tissue surfaces and catabolise glucose, lactate and amino acids. Those organisms that do well in an oxygen-deprived environment with an abundance of nutrients thrive, until the local environment changes. These localised environmental changes coincide with shifting patterns in the members of the underlying microbial community (Figure 12.1). From death to advanced decay of swine (Pechal *et al.* 2014) and mice (Metcalf *et al.* 2013), the diversity of bacterial taxa decreased. In a complimentary project, bacterial taxon richness increased in decaying skeletal remains with advancing time (Damann *et al.* 2015).

Taken together, these studies suggest that taxon richness of sampled host tissues is reduced to the initial period of skeletal exposure, when the trajectory of taxon richness is reversed. Decreases in labile carbon sources with advancing time promotes oligotrophy, in which a different community of organisms are active due to their ability to gain carbon and nutrients from recalcitrant substrates

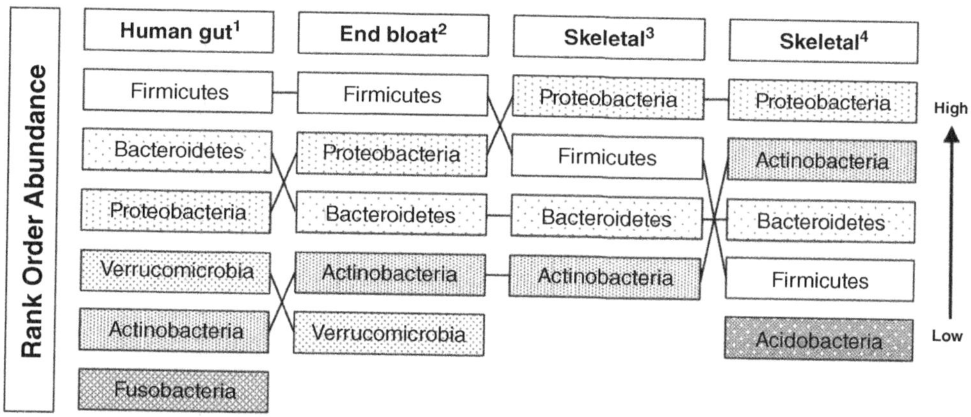

Figure 12.1 Average of the rank order abundances of dominate phyla in the human gut from 19 individuals presented in 3 separate studies (Costello *et al.* 2009; Eckburg *et al.* 2005; Li *et al.* 2008)[1]. Average of the rank order abundances of dominate phyla from the GIT of two individuals at the end of the bloat stage (Hyde *et al.* 2013)[2]. Dominate phyla recovered from lower ribs of eight individuals that decomposed for less than one year (Damann *et al.* 2015)[3]. Dominate phyla recovered from lower ribs of four individuals that decomposed for more than one year and less than four years (Damann *et al.* 2015)[4].

(Frey *et al.* 2013; Lauber *et al.* 2009, 2014). How this affects taxon richness in decomposing human tissue over longer time periods is not readily apparent in existing data.

When the availability of nutrients and energy are plentiful, survival of a few taxa may be the result of their ability to adapt quickly to the new environment and then out-compete all others. On the other hand, the massive efflux of liquefied tissues during purge and subsequent drying of the decomposition site creates a deleterious environment, forcing limitations on growth and migration of bacterial decomposers. Perhaps only those organisms with higher tolerances may survive. Over time, the decomposition site will be recolonised. As decaying bone weathers and delaminates, pore spaces enlarge and new avenues for bacterial infiltration are created. Primary colonisers may be replaced or augmented by additional organisms capable of acquiring nutrients and energy from bone, ligament and hair, thus increasing metabolic and taxonomic diversity.

These assumptions are based on a cursory review of recent projects that have evaluated the taxonomic diversity of microbial communities associated with mammalian decomposition. Functional analyses of microbiomes associated with human decomposition have yet to be performed and may provide insight into the interactions among myriad taxa and the usable substrate. The application of microbiome research to taphonomic studies of human remains are initiating many new questions and driving many new hypotheses about microbial involvement in energy and nutrient cycling. In doing so, these new data are applicable not only to microbial ecology, but also to taphonomy and medicolegal death investigations.

12.8 Conclusion

Microorganisms are primary constitutes that drive catabolic processes of decomposition. The metabolic specificity, functional diversity and ubiquitous distribution of bacteria make them a potentially significant contributor to forensic medicine. In life and death, bacteria are always present. By using molecular methods to investigate bacterial community succession over the course of decomposition, a novel approach for estimating post-mortem intervals is emerging.

DISCLAIMER: The views expressed are those of the author and should not be construed to represent the US government.

References

Can, I., Javan, G.T., Pozhitkov, A.E. and Noble, P.A. (2014) Distinctive thantomicrobiome signatures in the blood and internal organs of humans. *Journal of Microbiolology Methods*, **106**: 1–7.

Carter, D.O., Yellowlees, D. and Tibbett, M. (2007) Cadaver decomposition in terrestrial ecosystems. *Naturwissenschaften*, **94**: 12–24.

Carter, D.O., Yellowlees, D. and Tibbett, M. (2010) Moisture can be the dominant environmental parameter governing cadaver decomposition in soil. *Forensic Science International*, **200**: 60–66.

Carter, D.O., Metcalf, J.L., Bibat, A. and Knight, R. (2015) Seasonal variation of postmortem microbial communities. *Forensic Science, Medicine & Pathology*, **11**: 202–207.

Child, A.M. (1995) Towards an understanding of the microbial decomposition of archaeological bone in the burial environment. *Journal of Archaeological Science*, **22**: 165–174.

Clark, M.A., Worrell, M.B. and Pless, J.E. (1997) Postmortem changes in soft tissues. In: Haglund. W.D. and Sorg, M.H. (eds), *Forensic Taphonomy: The postmortem fate of human remains*. CRC Press: Boca Raton, pp. 151–164.

Costello, E.K, Lauber, C.L., Hamady, M., Fierer, N., Gordon, J.I. and Knight, R. (2009) Bacterial community variation in human body habitats across space and time. *Science*, **326**: 1694–1697.

Damann, F.E. (2010) Human decomposition ecology at the University of Tennessee Anthropology Research Facility. Unpublished PhD thesis, University of Tennessee, Knoxville.

Damann, F.E. and Carter, D.O. (2014) Human decomposition ecology and postmortem microbiology. In: Pokines, J. and Symes, S. (eds), *A Manual of Forensic Taphonomy*. CRC Press: Boca Raton, pp. 37–49.

Damann, F.E., Williams, D. and Layton, A. (2015) Potential use of bacterial community succession in decaying human bone for estimating postmortem intervals. *Journal of Forensic Science*. **60**: 844–850.

DeLaune, R.D. and Reddy, K.R. (2005) Redox potential. In: Hillel, D. (ed.), *Encyclopedia of Soils in the Environment*. Academic Press: Amsterdam. 366–371.

Earth Microbiome Project, http://www.earthmicrobiome.org/ (Accessed 15 December 2014).

Eckburg, P.B., Bik, E.M., Bernstein, C.N., Purdom, E., Dethlefsen, L. *et al*. (2005) Diversity of the human intestinal microbial flora. *Science*. **308**: 1635–1638.

Evans, W.E.D, (1963) *The Chemistry of Death*. Charles C. Thomas: Springfield.

Frey, S.D., Lee, J., Melillo, J.M. and Six, J. (2013) The temperature response of soil microbial efficiency and its feedback to climate. *Nature Climate Change*, **3**: 395–398.

Garcia-Lopez, M.L., Prieto, M. and Otero, A. (1998) The physiological attributes of gram-negative bacteria associated with spoilage of meat and meat products. In: Davies, A.R. and Board, R.G. (eds), *The Microbiology of Meat and Poultry*. Blackie Academic and Professional: London, pp. 1–34.

Gill, C.O. (1983) Meat spoilage and the evaluation of the potential storage life of fresh meat. *Journal of Food Protection*. **26**: 444–452.

Gill, S.R., Pop, M., Deboy, R.T., Eckburg, P.B., Turnbaugh, P.J. *et al*. (2006) Metagenomic analysis of the human distal gut microbiome. *Science*, **312**: 1355–1359.

Gill-King, H. (1997) Chemical and ultrastructural aspects of decomposition. In: Haglund, W.D. and Sorg, M.H. (eds), *Forensic Taphonomy: The postmortem fate of human remains*. CRC Press: Boca Raton, pp. 93–108.

Greenblum, S., Turnbaugh, P.J. and Borenstein, E. (2012) Metagenomic systems biology of the human gut microbiome reveals topological shifts associated with obesity and inflammatory bowel disease. *Proceeding of the National Academy of Sciences USA*, **109**: 594–599.

Haslam, T.C. and Tibbett, M. (2009) Soils of contrasting pH affect the decomposition of buried mammalian (*Ovis aries*) skeletal muscle tissue. *Journal of Forensic Science*, **54**: 900–904.

Human Microbiome Project, http://www.hmpdacc.org/ (Accessed 15 December 2014).

Hyde, E.R., Haarmann, D.P., Lynne, A.M., Bucheli, S.R. and Petrosino, J.F. (2013) The living dead: bacterial community structure of a cadaver at the onset and end of the bloat stage of decomposition. *PLoS One*, **8**: e77733.

Hyde, E.R., Petrosino, J.F., Piedra, P.A., Camargo, C.A. Jr.,, Espinola, J.A. and Mansbach, J.M. (2014) Nasopharyngeal Proteobacteria are associated with viral etiology and acute wheezing in children with severe bronchiolitis. *Journal of Allergy Clinical Immunology*, **133**: 1220–1222.

Ingram, M. and Dainty, R.H. (1971) Symposium on microbial changes in foods changes caused by microbes in spoilage of meats. *Journal of Applied Bacteriology*, **34**: 21–39.

Jay, J.M. (2000) *Modern Food Microbiology*. Aspen: Gaithersburg.

Joossens, M., Huys, G., Cnockaert, M., De Preter, V., Verbeke, K. *et al.* (2011) Dysbiosis of the faecal microbiota in patients with Crohn's disease and their unaffected relatives. *Gut*, **60**: 631–637.

Jurtshuk, P. Jr., (1996) Bacterial metabolism. In: Baron, S. (ed.), *Medical Microbiology*, 4th edition, University of Texas Medical Branch at Galveston: Galveston. Available from: http://www.ncbi.nlm.nih.gov/books/NBK7919/ (Accessed 30 October 2014).

Kaufman, D.W., Kelly, J.P., Curhan, G.C., Anderson, T.E, Dretler, S.P. *et al.* (2008) Oxalobacter formigenes may reduce the risk of calcium oxalate kidney stones. *Journal of the American Society of Nephrology*, **19**: 1197–1203.

Kellerman, G.D., Waterman, N.G. and Scharefenberger, L.F. (1976) Demonstration in vitro of postmortem bacterial transmigration. *American Journal of Clinical Pathology*, **66**: 911–915.

Koch, A.L. (2001) Oligotrophs versus copiotrophs. *Bioessays*, **23**: 657–661.

Lauber, C.L., Hamady, M., Knight, R. and Fierer, N. (2009) Pyrosequencing-based assessment of soil pH as a predictor of soil bacterial community structure at the continental scale. *Applied Environmental Microbiology*, **75**: 5111–5120.

Lauber, C.L., Metcalf, J.L., Keepers, K., Ackermann, G., Carter, D.O. and Knight, R. (2014) Vertebrate decomposition is accelerated by soil microbes. *Applied Environmental Microbiology*, **80**: 4920–4929.

Ley, R.E. (2010) Obesity and the human microbiome. *Current Opinions in Gastroenterology*, **26**: 5–11.

Ley, R.E., Peterson, D.A. and Gordon, J.I. (2006) Ecological and evolutionary forces shaping microbial diversity in the human intestine. *Cell*, **124**: 837–848.

Li, M., Wang, B., Zhang, M., Rantalainen, M., Wang, S. et al, (2008) Symbiotic gut microbes modulate human metabolic phenotypes. *Proceedings of the National Academy of Sciences USA*, **105**: 2117–2122.

Love, J.C. and Marks, M. (2003) Taphonomy and time: estimating the postmortem interval. In: Steadman, D.W. (ed.), *Hard Evidence: Case studies in forensic anthropology*. Prentice Hall: Upper Saddle River, pp. 160–175.

Marshall, D.L. and Bal'a, M.F.A. (2001) Microbiology of meats. In: Hui, Y.H. (ed.), *Meat Science and Applications*. Marcel Dekker: New York, pp. 149–169.

McGuire, K.L. and Treseder, K.K. (2010) Microbial communities and their relevance for ecosystem models: decomposition as a case study. *Soil Biology & Biochemistry*, **42**: 529–535.

Melvin, J.R. Jr, Cronholm, L.S., Simson, L.R. Jr., and Isaacs, A.M. (1984) Bacterial transmigration as an indicator of time of death. *Journal of Forensic Science*, **29**: 412–417.

Metcalf, J.L., Wegener Parfrey, L., Gonzalez, A., Lauber, C.L., Knights, D. *et al.* (2013) A microbial clock provides an accurate estimate of the postmortem interval in a mouse model system. *Elife*, **2**: e01104.

Micozzi, M. (1991) *Postmortem Change in Human and Animal Remains*. Charles C. Thomas: Springfield.

Microbiome of the Built Environment, http://microbe.net/ (Accessed 14 December 2014).

Morgan, X.C., Segata, N. and Huttenhower, C. (2013) Biodiversity and functional genomics in the human microbiome. *Trends in Genetics*, **29**: 51–58.

Nicholson, J.K., Holmes, E. and Wilson, I.D. (2005) Gut microorganisms, mammalian metabolism and personalized health care. *Nature Reviews Microbiology*, **3**: 431–438.

Nychas, G.-J.E., Drosinos, E.H. and Board, R.G. (1998) Chemical changes in stored meat. In: Davies, A.R. and Board, R.G. (eds), *The Microbiology of Meat and Poultry*. Blackie Academic and Professional: London, pp. 288–326.

Paul, E.A. (2007) *Soil Microbiology, Ecology and Biochemistry*, 3rd edition, Academic Press: Amsterdam.

Payne, J.A. (1965) A summer carrion study of the baby pig *Sus scrofa* Linnaeus. *Ecology*, **46**: 592–602.

Pechal, J.L., Crippen, T.L., Benbow, M.E., Tarone, A.M., Dowd, S. and Tomberlin, J.K. (2014) The potential use of bacterial community succession in forensics as described by high throughput metagenomic sequencing. *International Journal of Legal Medicine*, **128**: 193–205.

Perper, J. (1993) Time of death and changes after death. In: Spitz, W. (ed.), *Medicolegal Investigation of Death: Guidelines for the application of pathology to crime investigation*. Charles C. Thomas: Springfield, pp. 14–49.

Pommerville, J.C. (2004) *Alcomo's Fundamentals of Microbiology*, 7th edition. Jones & Bartlett: Sudbury.

Ravel, J., Gajer, P., Abdo, Z., Schneider, G.M., Koenig, S.S. *et al.* (2011) Vaginal microbiome of reproductive-age women. *Proceedings of the National Academy of Sciences USA*, **108 Suppl 1**: 4680–4687.

Reed, H.B. (1958) A study of dog carcass communities in Tennessee, with special reference to the insects. *American Midland Naturalist*, **59**: 213–245.

Standbridge, L.H. and Davies, A.R. (1998) The microbiology of chill-stored meat. In: Davies, A.R. and Board, R.G. (eds), *The Microbiology of Meat and Poultry*. Blackie Academic and Professional: London, pp. 174–219.

Stumpf, R.M., Wilson, B.A., Rivera, A., Yildirim, S., Yeoman, C.J. *et al.* (2013) The primate vaginal microbiome: comparative context and implications for human health and disease. *American Journal of Physical Anthropology*, **157**: 119–134.

Swift, M.J., Heal, O.W. and Anderson, J.M. (1979) *Decomposition in Terrestrial Ecosystems*. Blackwell Scientific: Oxford.

Tortora, G.J., Funke, B.R. and Case, C.L. (1995) *Microbiology: An introduction*. Benjamin Cummings Publishing: Redwood City.

Turnbaugh, P.J., Ley, R.E., Hamady, M., Fraser-Liggett, C.M., Knight, R. and Gordon, J.I. (2007) The human microbiome project. *Nature*. **449**: 804–810.

Turnbaugh, P.J., Hamady, M., Yatsunenko, T., Cantarel, B.L., Duncan, A. *et al.* (2009) A core gut microbiome in obese and lean twins. *Nature*. **457**: 480–484.

Turner-Walker, G. (2008) The chemical and microbial degradation of bones and teeth. In: Pinhasi, R. and Mays, S. (eds), *Advances in Human Paleopathology*. John Wiley & Sons: West Sussex, pp. 3–29.

Vass, A.A., Bass, W.M., Wolt, J.D., Foss, J.E. and Ammons, J.T. (1992) Time since death determinations of human cadavers using soil solution. *Journal of Forensic Sciences*, **37**: 1236–1253.

Wilson, M. 2008. *Bacteriology of Humans: An ecological perspective*. Blackwell: Malden.

13

Forensic Entomology and Funerary Archaeoentomology

Stefano Vanin and Jean-Bernard Huchet

13.1 Introduction

The association between decomposing bodies and insects has been a well-known topic since antiquity. This theme has been reported in numerous holy and literary books, as well as in paintings and sculptures (Benecke 2001).

The presence of insects on dead bodies has created many legends and beliefs; however, the development and modernisation of the scientific method, the confutation of the spontaneous generation theory by Francesco Redi in the 16th century and Louis Pasteur in the 19th century, plus the development of technology such as the invention of the microscope at the end of the 16th century, gave birth to a new forensic science: forensic entomology. This discipline applies the knowledge of insects to legal cases, in both civil and criminal law (Amendt *et al.* 2007). In addition, at the end of the 20th century, a new discipline emerged based on the same knowledge and related to the studies of archaeological human remains: funerary archaeoentomology (Huchet 1996).

During the decomposition process, insects are responsible for the removal of important parts of the soft tissue of the body and the alteration of other tissues such as bones and hair. The feeding activity of insects has two consequences:

1) insects can be used to obtain useful information about the circumstances surrounding death
2) they can produce alterations and modifications of the body that can be misinterpreted as a result of a violent act before death.

Both elements can be referred to as 'two sides of the same entomological coin' and they have an important value for present-day forensic entomology and funerary archaeoentomology.

Forensic entomology can be divided into three main fields: urban entomology, stored product entomology and forensic entomology *sensu stricto*, also called medico-legal entomology or medico-criminal entomology. The latter deals with the reconstruction of peri- and post-mortem events and with funerary archaeoentomology, all covered in this chapter. The main question, although not the only one, in which forensic entomology can make a contribution, concerns the estimation of time since death, the so-called post-mortem interval (PMI).

The analysis of insects from the body or crime scene can also provide useful information regarding body transfer or previous concealment. Furthermore, insects collected at the crime scene can be used to confirm 'cadaver presence' in cases where the body has been removed before the arrival of the investigators (Marchetti *et al.* 2013), or for the detection of drugs or poisons, also called entomotoxicology (Introna *et al.* 2001).

Taphonomy of Human Remains: Forensic Analysis of the Dead and the Depositional Environment, First Edition.
Edited by Eline M.J. Schotsmans, Nicholas Márquez-Grant and Shari L. Forbes.

The PMI of human cadavers can be estimated by forensic pathologists by looking at *algor, livor* and *rigor mortis*, vitreous potassium concentrations, electrical excitability of skeletal muscles and gastric content (Henssge *et al.* 2002). However, these methods can only be used accurately in the two to three days following death (Amendt *et al.* 2004), but are not useful in decomposed, burned and dismembered bodies (Vanin *et al.* 2013).

In these cases, the evaluation of the insect colonisation time plays an important role and is often the only method appropriate for the estimation of the minimum post-mortem interval (mPMI) or for the season of death where very old human remains are concerned (Vanin *et al.* 2009).

In order to better understand and apply the entomological approach correctly, in both forensic and archaeological contexts, considerations about insect biology, distribution and behaviour are necessary. These data are significant, not only in the analysis phase when the criminal events are reconstructed, but also operationally in the collection phase, both at a crime scene and during archaeological excavation.

13.2 Insects: Useful Information for Forensic Scientists and Archaeologists

Insects (Insecta) belong to the phylum Arthropoda, animals with jointed legs, which represent nearly 75% of the described living animals on Earth, and have colonised all the ecosystems including extreme environments. Even fly larvae, such as the carnivorous petroleum fly (*Helaemyia petrolei*), have the ability to develop in pools of crude petroleum (Thorpe 1931).

Insects are characterised by the presence of a chitinous exoskeleton, three pairs of legs and two pairs of wings (Figure 13.1). Wings can be absent in some species or transformed into rigid or semi-rigid structures (elytra and hemelytra), whereas legs can be absent in some larvae (Figure 13.2).

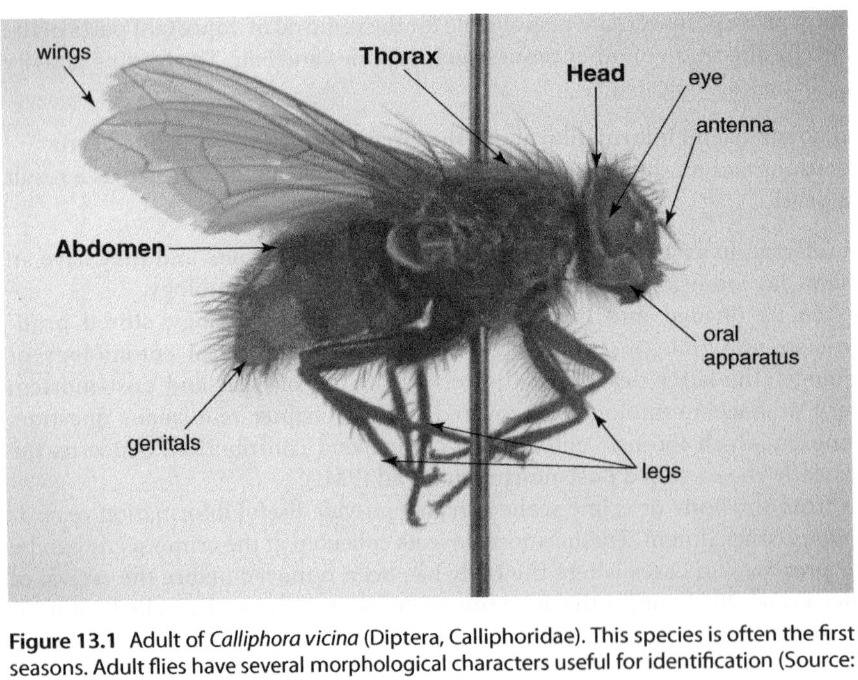

Figure 13.1 Adult of *Calliphora vicina* (Diptera, Calliphoridae). This species is often the first coloniser of a body in cold seasons. Adult flies have several morphological characters useful for identification (Source: S. Vanin).

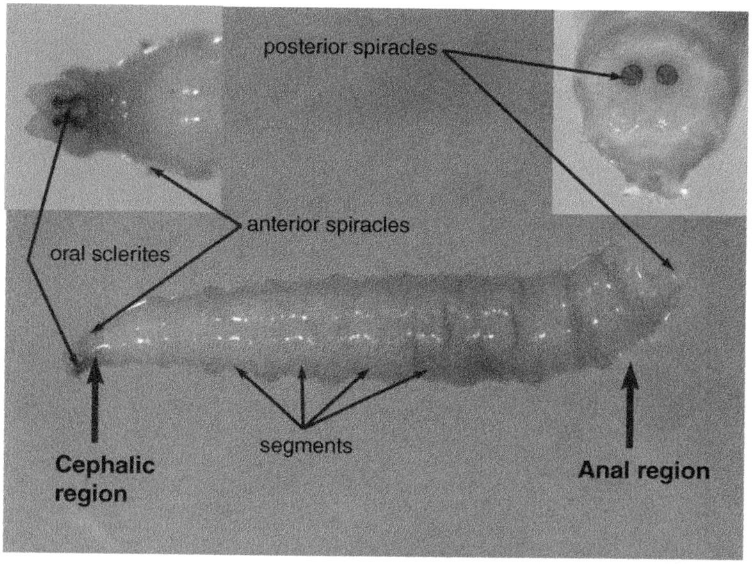

Figure 13.2 Larva of Calliphoridae. Only few characters are available for species identification if compared with the adults (Source: S. Vanin).

Chitin, an amino-polysaccharide, $(C_8H_{13}O_5N)_n$, is the main component of the insect cuticle. It is chemically stable and particularly resistant to decay. This robustness directly correlates to the preservability of insect remains in forensic and archaeological contexts (Speight 1974). Different modes of preservation occur and invertebrate exoskeletons may be preserved by anoxic waterlogging, dry environments, carbonisation or mineral replacement (mineralisation) (Huchet 2014a, 2014c).

The insects related to cadavers and carrion colonisation mainly belong to the Diptera (flies) and Coleoptera (beetles) orders. Species belonging to these taxa have a life cycle with complete metamorphosis called holometabolism, which includes four life stages: egg (embryo), larva, pupa – these three stages are called pre-imaginal or immature stages – and the final stage adult (imago) (Figure 13.3).

On a dead body or at a crime scene, all the developmental stages of the insect can be found (Figures 13.4 and 13.5), together with pupal cases. In fact, after metamorphosis of the Diptera species, the emerged adult will leave behind its pupal case, the last cuticles of its immature development, which is very resistant to decay, and therefore detectable many years later (Figure 13.6). As such, pupal cases are often found in archaeological burials (Huchet and Greenberger 2010) and have

Figure 13.3 Life cycle of Holometabolous insects.

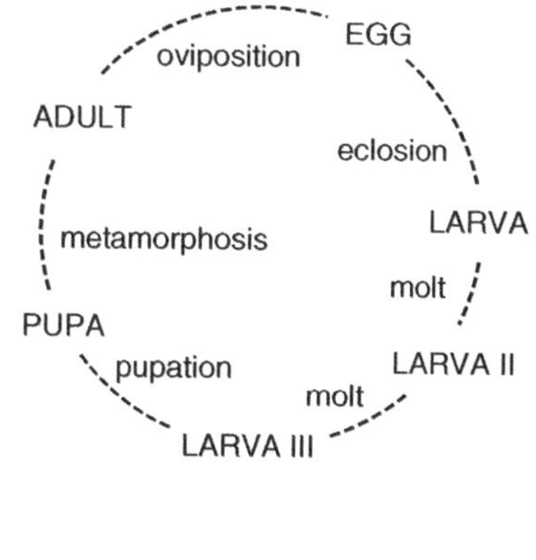

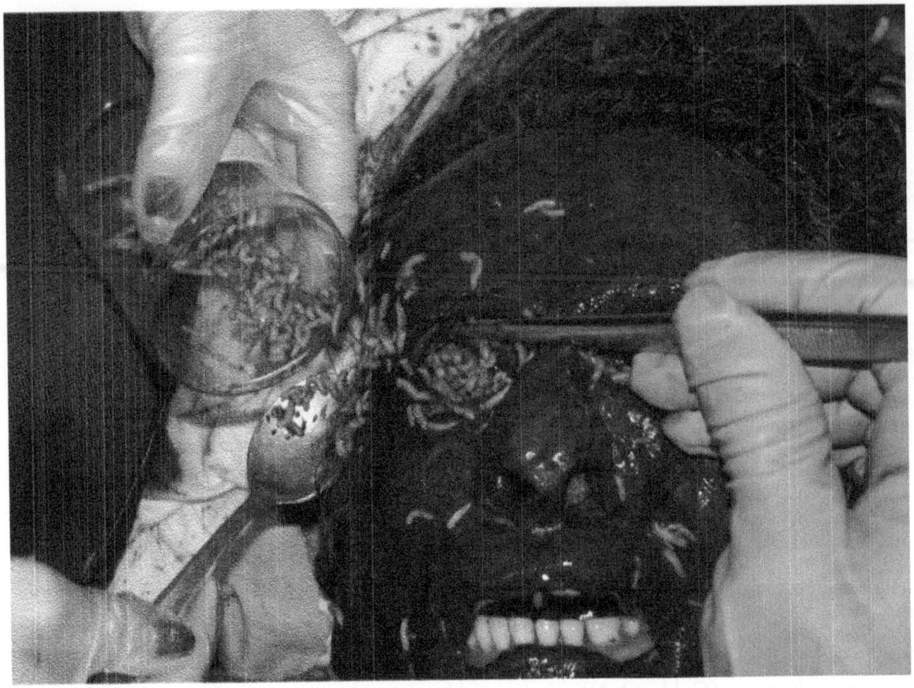

Figure 13.4 Diptera larvae collected from the ocular cavity of a cadaver in active decay (Source: Bassi 2014. Reproduced with permission of John Wiley & Sons).

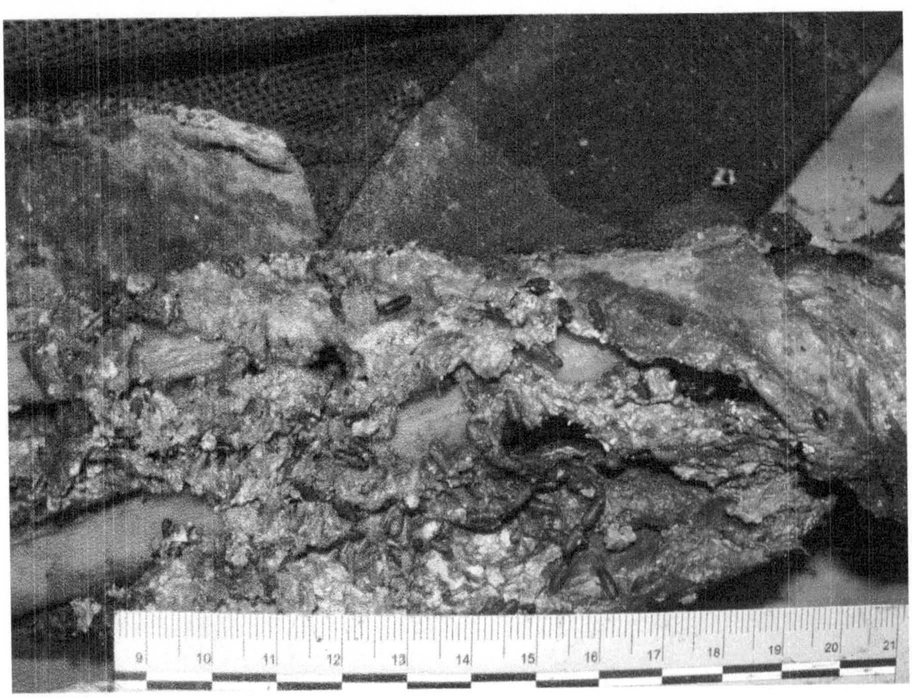

Figure 13.5 Pupae of Diptera species on a cadaver in advance decay (Source: S. Vanin/K. Bisogni).

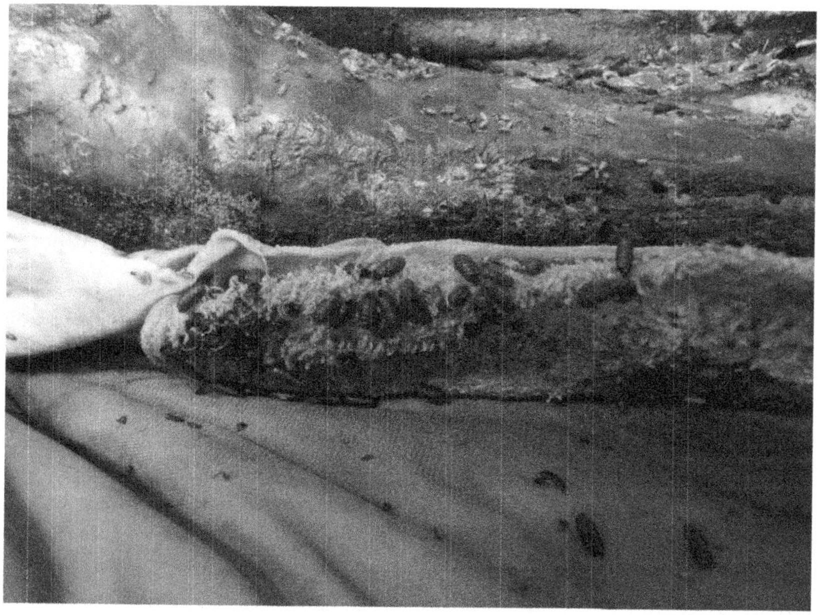

Figure 13.6 Empty puparia of Calliphoridae (dark-coloured in the foreground and mid-ground of the image) and pupae of Phoridae (white/yellow, mostly in the background) on a partially mummified body (Source: S. Vanin/K. Bisogni).

also been reported inside the skull of a Late Eemian bison (130,000–107,000 years ago) (Gautier and Schumann 1973), demonstrating the elevated preservability of their chemical composition.

As a generalised rule, taphocenoses[1] always imperfectly reflect past biocenoses[2] since, from the degree of sclerotisation of their exoskeletons, not all insect orders display the same aptitude for preservation. In most instances, adult beetles (Coleoptera), owing to the very resistant nature of their exoskeleton, can be remarkably preserved in archaeological sediments. Conversely, adult flies (Diptera), which are very helpful in current forensic entomological investigations, are fragile and usually do not stand the test of time. In archaeological contexts, the only exploitable fly remains consist of puparia, sclerotised barrel-shaped cases, inside which the fly has performed its metamorphosis. In most instances, archaeoentomologists refer to these tenuous remains in the taphonomical reconstitution of past events (Faulkner 1986; Dirrigl and Greenberg 1995; Gilbert 1966; Gilbert and Bass 1967; Huchet and Greenberg 2010; Nystrom *et al.* 2005; Vanin *et al.* 2009). Studies conducted on fragmented insect remains cannot match the precision and the predictability of forensic expertise on modern cadavers.

Whereas the adult insect body is composed of different structures with distinctive and diagnostic characters, the majority of the larvae, especially in Diptera of forensic interest, are, from a morphological point of view, very simple organisms. The general body of an adult insect is composed of a head with sensorial and feeding organs, a thorax with its locomotor appendixes and the abdomen containing digestive apparatus and reproductive organs.

Immature stages (larvae) are always wingless and often legless. In most larvae of forensic interest, the cephalic region is not sclerotised. Due to their simple structure, immature stages are difficult to

1 A group of fossil organisms brought together by sedimentary or other taphonomical processes after death (= death assemblage).

2 Association of different organisms forming a closely integrated community.

morphologically identify at the species level. In these cases, molecular identification plays a fundamental and crucial role. Several genes (*cytb, COI, COII, EF-1α, period, tRNA, 12S, 18S, 28S*) have been used for this purpose. Among them, *COI* is the most commonly analysed (Wells and Stevens 2008). The molecular approach has been used with success, including archaeological samples, despite the DNA extraction technique requiring some adjustments (Raoult *et al.* 2008).

Identifying the species both in a forensic and archaeological context is fundamental, because development, phenology, distribution and ecology are specific to single species or groups of species. The first step in any forensic or archaeological reconstruction, the so-called '6Ws' (Who, When, Where, What, How, Why), is based on correct species identification.

Insect development is species specific – sometimes population specific (Richards *et al.* 2008) – and temperature dependent. Insects are poikilothermic organisms, which means that their body temperature depends mainly on the environmental temperature. Temperature and the photoperiod[3] affect insect development as well as their activity such as flight, locomotion, food search and reproduction. Moreover, other parameters can affect the general biology and behaviour of the species, such as social interaction and food availability.

In general, insect development has a temperature range, called *optimum*, following a linear trend with a positive correlation between temperature and developmental rate. Above and below this range, temperature can cause death of the organism or the enhancement of diapause or aestivation, mechanisms evolved by the insect in order to guarantee survival during cold winters or hot summers.

In regions with clear and well-defined differences of temperature and photoperiod between seasons, insects show a very strong seasonality (phenology), with species only active in a specific season or only for short periods (weeks). Some species can be active in different periods of the year. Depending on the number of times they are active during the year, they are described as univoltine, bivoltine or multivoltine. A typical example of seasonality in first body colonisers is evident in Southern Europe, where the species of the genus *Lucilia* are active during the warmer season (summer) and those of the genus *Calliphora* are active during the colder seasons (spring and autumn) (Bugelli *et al.* 2015; Vanin *et al.* 2008).

Insects do not only have a temporal preference (*preferendum*) but also an environmental preference. The latter can be very different among species, with some taxa only present in very specific environments, such as *Lucilia ampullacea*, typical of forest environments, and others that are ubiquitous, such as *Lucilia sericata*, usually present in both urban and rural environments (Vanin *et al.* 2008). The same concept can be applied to their geographical distribution. Some species are endemic, widely distributed or cosmopolite. It is worth mentioning that over the last few years, both global warming and globalisation are contributing to an increased variation of the areal distribution of species. This also has an effect on species related to cadavers and carrions. Turchetto and Vanin (2010) reported that their shift from the southern to the northern regions is closely related to both the increase in temperature and their adventitious transportation performed during commercial trades (e.g. inside refrigerated containers) (Benelli *et al.* 2014).

A specific kind of environmental preference is the relationship of the insect species with humans, described as synantropic or asynantropic, depending on being typically associated with humans or occurring in non-urban environments.

Insects are not exclusive to sub-aerial environments. Some species are active in fresh water and others in caves. It is worth mentioning that aquatic insect species do not show specific

3 The daily duration of light and dark to which an organism is exposed with regard to its effect on development and behaviour.

saprophagous[4] habits, but are more generalist in food selection (Fenoglio *et al.* 2014). For this reason, it is not possible to define waves of colonisation in cadavers in water compared to terrestrial habitats. Moreover, aquatic species can show very well defined habitat preferences, with some characteristic of cold and oxygenated waters and others living in polluted waters. The parameters that affect the insect distribution in different aquatic environments are mainly temperature, oxygen availability, water turbulence, speed and the amount of organic matter.

Insects show not only specificity in their activity period and in the environment, but also in food preference, which includes species with a very specific diet (monophagous) and others more generalist (polyphagous). The nature of the water and the decomposition stage of a corpse are factors that mainly drive the arthropod carrion fauna to colonise exposed bodies. Fly larvae are typical of the first phases of decomposition of a body, when water is still abundant among the tissues, whereas some beetles (Coleoptera), moths (Lepidoptera) and mites (Ocarina) colonise a body during the last decay phases, when the tissues are drying and different kinds of fermentations (e.g. alcoholic, butyric, caseic, ammoniac) have happened (Figure 13.7). Some beetles and moths are also able to feed on bones and hair (Huchet *et al.* 2013a; Mazzarelli *et al.* 2015). Piophilid flies, for example, are typical of butyric and caseic fermentation of a body that happens during the active stage of decay.

Other factors can affect colonisation and the composition of colonising fauna (Table 13.1). These factors are related to the environment, the season of death, as well as the intrinsic condition of a body (i.e. size, cause of death, presence of wounds). Additionally, the accessibility of a body produces the first selection on the colonising species. Exposed bodies are commonly colonised by Calliphoridae, whereas flies of this family rarely colonise buried bodies. An indoor environment can also select the

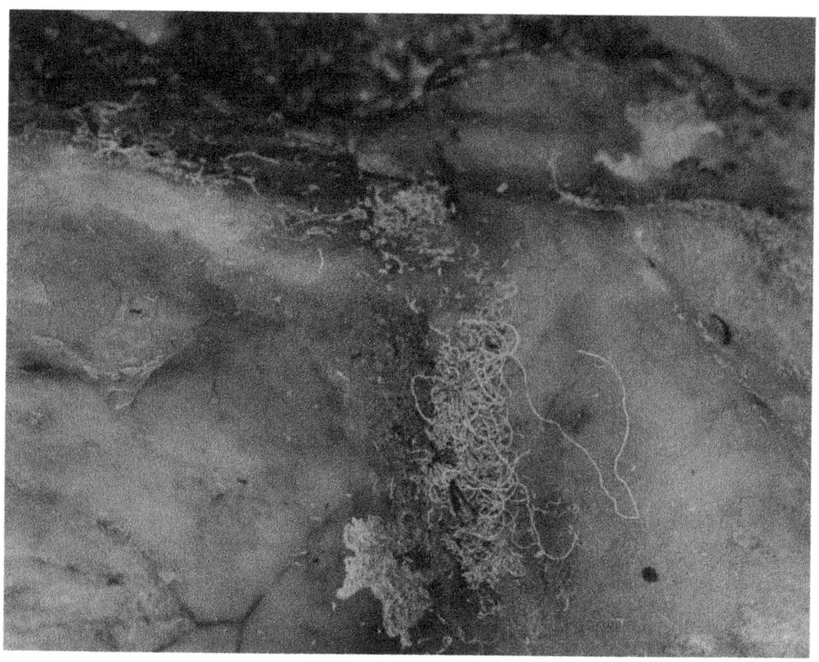

Figure 13.7 Excrements (frass) of dermestid beetles on mummified human skin (Source: K. Bisogni).

4 Saprophagous organisms feed on dead or decaying organic matter, whereas sarcophagous organisms feed on flesh of other animals. Sarco-saprophagous organisms feed both on fresh and decomposed flesh of other animals.

Table 13.1 Factors affecting the decomposition speed and the composition of the cadaver feeding fauna.

Factor	Effect on the speed of colonisation	Effect on the composition of the insect community
Temperature	In the optimum interval, the higher the temperature, the faster the colonisation. Too low and too high temperature stops or delays the colonisation	Depending on the temperature, frigophilous or xerophilous species will colonise the body
Rain	Precipitations delay the insect arrival and can have a 'flush out' effect on eggs and larvae on the body surface	Only a few species have been reported as able to fly under the rain (e.g. *Sarcophaga* species). This observation needs further investigation to be confirmed
Season	In summer the colonisation is faster compared to colder seasons	Different species are active in different seasons
Environment	Bodies in open spaces are colonised faster compared to body in confined environments (e.g. caves, indoor) Altitude as well can delay the insect's arrival on a body	Because of environmental specificity, the composition of the fauna differs in different environments (e.g. *Lucilia ampullacea* in forest environments, *Lucilia sericata* mainly in urban environments, *Lucilia illustris* and *Lucilia caesar* mainly along rivers and rural environments)
Indoors/outdoors	Indoor environments delay the colonisation	Domestic species (e.g. *Musca domestica*) and small species (e.g. *Megaselia scalaris*) are the first colonisers
Body concealment	Body burial and covering delay the colonisation. Burying of the body does not affect the speed of colonisation after the body reaches a thermal equilibrium with the environment	Only a few and specific species colonise buried remains Burying can create conditions for colonisation of several communities (waves) at the same time, depending of the water content of different body tissues
Clothes	Clothes and other fabrics in which the body can be wrapped delay the colonisation	No noticeable affect on community composition
Injuries	The presence of blood can accelerate the speed of colonisation	No noticeable affect on community composition
Cause of death	Presence of injuries can accelerate the speed of colonisation Hanging delays the colonisation Suicide with gas (e.g. car) delays the colonisation	Hanged bodies are not colonised by terrestrial fauna

first colonisers. When access to the indoor environment is limited, the scuttle fly *Megaselia scalaris* (Phoridae) is able to anticipate the larger Calliphorids (Reibe and Madea, 2010a; 2010b).

The insects present on a decomposing or decomposed body are not the only saprophagous species feeding on the remains, as predators and parasites can also be present, as well as opportunistic species.[5] In archaeological contexts, two other categories of insects can provide useful information: human ectoparasites (e.g. lice, fleas and ticks) and insects related with funerary offerings such as *Gnathocerus cornutus* (Coleoptera, Tenebrionidae), a pest of cereal grains recently recovered from South American mummies (McCaulay *et al.* 2014).

5 Organisms from the environment where the body is located but not interacting with the body as a source of food.

13.3 Forensic Entomology and the Application of Insect Knowledge in Forensic Contexts

Estimation of the mPMI is based on the two points previously discussed: the development duration (species specific and temperature dependent), and the waves of colonisation related to the food/water content preference. mPMI can be estimated depending on these two approaches: the first is applicable mainly for death occurring at maximum, in a temperate climate, days/weeks before the discovery of the body, and takes into account the development rate of the first coloniser species. Whereas the second method, used for longer times, considers the composition of the fauna collected from the body.

The first approach focuses on the developmental stage of fly species belonging mainly to the families Calliphoridae, Sarcophagidae and Muscidae. The determination of the developmental stage, correlated with the temperature at which the body has been exposed before its discovery, allows the estimation of the time since the deposition of the eggs. The correlation, developmental stage – temperature – time, can be obtained from tables of development, isomegalen and isomorphen diagrams[6] , or the ADD (Accumulated Degrees Days) method. An important parameter to consider in the latter method is the minimum temperature of development that is species specific. The correct reconstruction of the temperature history, as well as the correct species identification, is the basis for the correct estimation of the time of colonisation (= mPMI). Thermal reconstruction can be carried out using both temperature records from the closest meteorological station or temperature adjusted after recording meteorological data, using a data logger from the crime scene.

The estimation of the mPMI of cadavers found a long time after death is based on the study of the composition of the entomological community found on the body. A decomposing body is comparable to a changing environment, both from a physical and chemical point of view, where each decay stage is attractive to different communities of arthropods (insects, mites, etc.) representing the waves of colonisation. Because these communities colonise the body following a predictable order, despite differences related to the season and the geographical position, they can be used for mPMI estimation. Tables indicating the waves of colonisation have been published by several authors (e.g. Smith 1986; Wyss and Cherix 2006) and have to be considered at a regional scale after a meticulous analysis of the conditions in which the body was found. This approach provides only an approximation of the time since death.

Because of their strict phenology, some species can be used as an indicator of the season of death, or more precisely, of the season when the colonisation started. This application is particularly important in cases of cadavers found several months after death, as well as in archeological contexts. In all cases, the informative insects' remains are mainly the puparia belonging to the Diptera species of the first colonisation wave, which is better described in the following paragraphs.

The environmental specificity of the insects can reveal body displacement occurring after the beginning of colonisation. These kinds of conclusions can be supported by botanic and geo-pedological analyses that can provide more details on the area of origin of the body. This approach has been used in forensic contexts in order to detect the primary crime scene of a homicide or to discover the country of origin of illegally transported drugs (Smith 1986).

The species able to colonise an exposed in comparison to a buried body are completely different. This means that detailed analysis of the insects from the body can be used to detect if a body has been exposed before burying or contrarily first interred and later exposed. This approach was used in North Eastern Italy to detect a fraud dealing with false wild animal predation on sheep. The animals, dead of natural causes, were buried and later exhumed and bitten by the dogs of the sheep owner,

---

6 Isomegalen and isomorphen diagrams illustrate morphological (length or stage) changes during development of the fly depending on the time and temperature.

in order to simulate a wolf attack and obtain a regional compensation. The lack of vital infiltrations on the injuries, the presence of beetles belonging to Cholevidae and Scarabeidae and the lack of any larva of flies at the time of survey allowed reconstruction of the fraud, confirmed later by a confession (Vanin, unpublished).

Springtails (Collembola) are often collected from graves and buried bodies; these arthropods are an important component of the soil fauna (with nematodes and other invertebrates), and their presence in graves can be related to the presence of a high amount of decaying organic matter.

The presence of maggots on living persons (myasis) can be used in forensic entomology to identify cases of abandoned or neglected people (Benecke and Lessig 2001; Benecke *et al.* 2004).

With their capacity to store toxic molecules and products of their metabolism in their cuticle, insects can be used to detect the presence of drugs and poisons, even when soft tissues are not preserved (i.e. complete skeletonised or mummified bodies) (De Carvaho *et al.* 2010; Miller *et al.* 1994). An overview of information derived from the entomological community can be found in Table 13.2.

Standards and guidelines for the correct collection, preparation, storage and interpretation of the entomological evidence have been published by the European Association for Forensic Entomology (EAFE) (Amendt *et al.* 2007) and by other Forensic Associations for their members. In general, a correct sampling requires the collection of all the developmental stages present, not only on the body but also at the crime scene. Collection from the body can be performed during the body recovery and during the autopsy. A meticulous observation of the clothes can provide a more complete sample. Insect specimens can be fixed in hot water (>80°C for 30 sec) or immersed in different preservative solutions (e.g. KAA, XAA and Carnoy's solution[7], Ethanol, etc.). Species identification, as previously underlined, requires a specialist. It is worth mentioning that only a team where different specialists work together (i.e. forensic pathologist, forensic entomologist, forensic botanist, forensic anthropologist) can provide the best reconstruction of the event occurring in the peri-mortem period.

13.4 Insects Recovered from Graves or Associated with Human Remains in Archaeological Contexts

In archaeological contexts, the presence (or absence) of insect remains in the grave results from environmental, ecological, taphonomical and sometimes cultural events linked with specific past burial

Table 13.2 Information derived from the study of the entomological community.

Insect characteristic	Forensic cases	Archaeological cases
Development temperature dependent	mPMI (based on the developmental rate)	
Diet specificity	mPMI (based on the entomological community composition)	
Seasonality	Season of death	Season of death
Environmental specificity	Previous concealment or exposure	Immediate burial or corpse's exposure
Specific distribution	Post-mortem body displacement	Post-mortem body displacement
Storage of toxic molecule in the cuticle	Drugs and poison extraction	Drugs and poison extraction

7 KAA solution: 77% ethanol, 8% kerosene and 15% glacial acetic acid; XAA solution: 40% ethanol, 27% xylene and 33% glacial acetic acid; Carnoy's solution: 60% ethanol, 30% chloroform and 10% glacial acetic acid.

practices. Their recovery requires specific protocols typically implemented in the field of other bioarchaeological disciplines (i.e. palynology, carpology, palaeoparasitology), paleontological disciplines (ichnology) and forensic entomology. Based on their state of preservation, and on the possibility of identifying them subsequently, it might be possible to infer relevant information regarding the taphonomic 'history' of the human remains and the burial site.

It should, however, be borne in mind, that studies conducted on fragmented insect remains cannot match the precision and the predictability of forensic analysis. Furthermore, the intended objectives of archaeoentomological surveys are nevertheless distinct from those of the present-day forensic entomology discipline. Hence, no references will be made to the estimation of PMI. This section will describe how the subfossil entomofauna may provide information about the taphonomical processes in archeological contexts.

It is important to point out that the presence of insect necrofauna results from two distinct modes of colonisation. The 'pre-depositional' (or 'pre-burial') phase involves specific epigean necrophagous[8] insects invading human cadavers and animal carcasses shortly after death. Although mature larvae of some fly species have the ability to burrow at the post-feeding stage, they rarely exceed the soil surface layers (Gunn and Bird 2011). The second wave of invaders, namely the 'post-depositional' phase, occurs underground and involves both subterranean species and specialised ground-surface taxa morphologically adapted for colonising buried remains, sometimes at depths reaching 2 m (Bourel *et al.* 2004). Usually, these species, mainly belonging to the families Muscidae and Phoridae, intervene at a later stage of the decomposition process. The characterisation of these two ecological groups is of utmost importance in the reconstitution of the taphocenosis. Other relevant observations conducted in the field and subsequently in the laboratory must be taken into consideration to properly carry out the taphonomic analysis. These parameters include the numerical representation of preserved specimens, their location in the core of the burial site, their taxonomic diversity, and finally the fact that environmental factors have allowed or inhibited the completion of their life cycle (evidenced by the presence of empty or unhatched fly pupae).

Archaeoentomological surveys imply specific attention in the field. Particular caution should be paid to identify the exact location of the insect remains. To this end, the implementation of an internal grid (squares of 10 cm wide) is of great value in providing the exact location of each sample. Once the sampling has been done, it is first necessary to distinguish between the preserved insect remains resulting from initial infestation, and those from a potential subsequent underground colonisation. Such distinction, for a well-experienced forensic entomologist, is usually relatively easy to resolve from the ecological groups recovered within the burial place (Figures 13.8a, b and c).

Although it is not possible to generalise the following observations as an immutable rule, it appears that the size of the cadaver feeding species decreases as the body decay progresses. The usually large pioneer flies lay their eggs (or their larvae) directly upon fresh cadavers, especially around the natural openings or wounds. From the imperceptible size of their eggs or neonate larvae, they are frequently buried simultaneously with the cadaver. According to the mode of burial, they will have, or not, the opportunity to complete their life cycle underground. The presence of these typical 'open-air' taxa (mainly Calliphoridae and Sarcophagidae) is a good indicator of cadaver accessibility in the pre-sepulchral phase or after burial. Depending on the quantity of puparia remains and their specific diversity, it may sometimes be possible to advance hypotheses concerning the burial period (seasonality) (Gilbert and Bass 1967; Vanin *et al.* 2009) or the possibility of pre-depositional exposure (Huchet and Greenberg 2010; Teskey and Turnbull 1979). Inversely, the absence of any insect remains in a burial environment where organic material had propensity to be preserved should

8 Insects, which live on the surface (ground-surface insects) and feed on dead organisms.

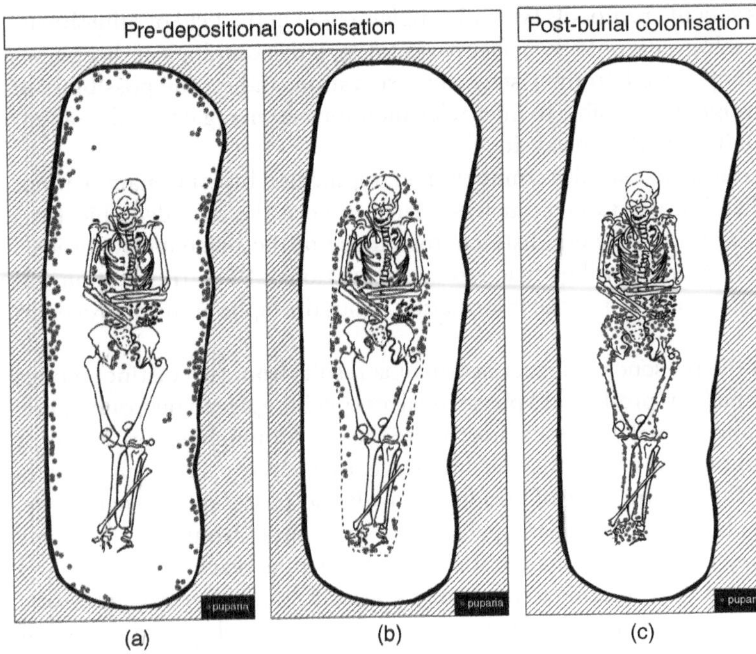

Figure 13.8 Modelled patterns of taphonomic reconstruction of a burial from the location of the insect remains. (a) Monospecific colonisation in a large pit in an empty space, allowing the third instar larvae to migrate from the body to pupate. (b) Entomological evidence of a decomposition of the body in a perishable structure, which has deteriorated by the time of excavation. (c) Patterns of colonisation by post-depositional flies (i.e. *Conicera*, *Ophyra* species), which pupate within the cadaver (initial drawing: P. Courtaud (PACEA, Bordeaux), modified by J.-B. Huchet).

raise questions: extreme climatic conditions (cold) at the time of death, taphonomic incidences, fast filling in of the burial, etc.

When decomposition occurs in an empty space, a large majority of pioneer fly larvae leave the cadaver to pupate in the perimeter delimited by the pit, grave or container (sarcophagus, coffin). Based on their location, relevant information can be learned from the initial structure of the burial, which usually has deteriorated by the time of excavation (Figure 13.8b). In the same way, the precise location of the fly puparia (in close contact with or at a distance from the skeleton), can thus provide pertinent data on inhumation modes (narrow pit, presence of clothing, etc.).

It should be stressed that the higher the species richness is, the more accurate information will be gleaned to provide a comprehensive reconstitution of taphonomic events. In this regard, the simultaneous presence of non-burrowing necrophagous, necrophile or parasitoid species would strongly support the possibility of a pre-depositional exposure and to advance hypotheses regarding its duration (Huchet and Greenberg 2010). Finally, other significant information could be inferred from the fly pupae, depending on whether the latter are empty (hatched) or complete (unhatched). The presence of empty puparia associated with human remains suggests that the complete cycle took place before burial, sometimes allowing for an estimation of the minimum duration of the pre-sepulchral phase. However, as the third instar larvae usually migrate from the nutritional source to pupate, only a non-representative sample of the original colonisation is generally available. Dead pupae are most often of less value as they only indicate that the environmental conditions or burial mode (mainly in open ground) inhibited the completion of their life cycle.

Different kinds of insects, with a significantly predominance of Diptera (Muscidae, Phoridae, Sphaeroceridae, Fanniidae, etc.), have propensity to colonise buried cadavers. Such species are

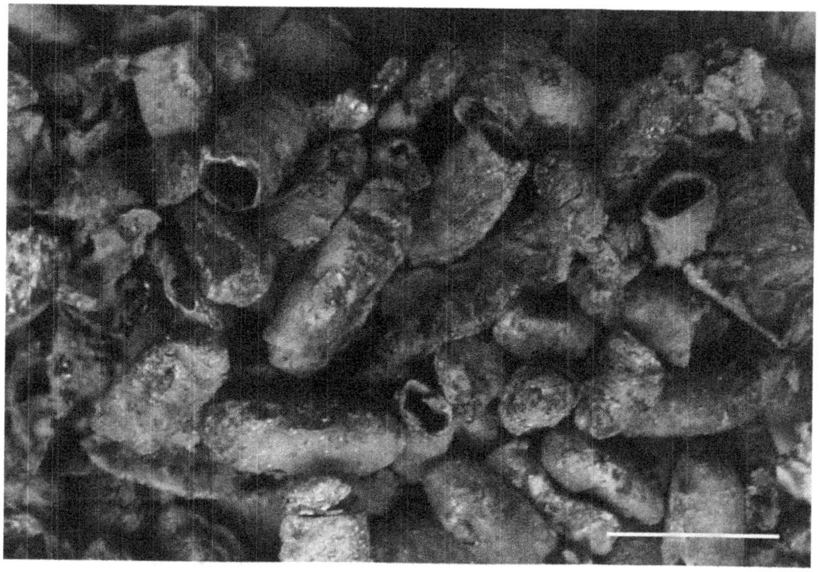

Figure 13.9 Puparia of the common post-burial fly *Ophyra capensis* (Wied.) (Diptera, Muscidae) associated with German soldier corpses of the First World War at the 'Kilianstollen' of Carspach (Haut-Rhin, France) (Huchet 2013). (Excavation: M Landolt; Photo: J.-B. Huchet) Scale = 5 mm. Note: the presence of this species with buried cadavers indicates that empty spaces (air pockets) persisted after the underground trench collapsed on the soldiers.

always found in very large numbers and several generations usually succeed underground (Bourel *et al.* 2004; Campobasso *et al.* 2004; Gaudry 2010). Their representation in myriads lead Mégnin (1887) to mention: '*...(les cadavres) en étaient couverts, comme des jambonneaux de chapelure*' ('... (the cadavers) were like a ham covered by breadcrumbs'). These species act as relevant indicators of burials in empty spaces or point towards the presence of non-filled burials in zones in contact with the cadavers at the time of colonisation (Figure 13.8c). Among the more representative taxa in our latitudes, *Ophyra capensis* (Muscidae) (Figure 13.9) and *Conicera tibialis*, the so-called 'coffin fly' (Phoridae) (Figures 13.10 and 13.11) are the most frequent post-depositional species in archaeological contexts (Couri *et al.* 2008, 2009; Masetti *et al.* 2008; Scharrer-Liska and Grassberger 2005; Turner-Walker and Scull 1997).

13.5 Body Alteration at the Crime Scene as a Result of Insect Activity

The whole process of decomposition of a body is an alteration of its original condition and insects play an important role in the removal of soft tissues. However, attention has to be paid to alterations of the body caused by insects, which can be misinterpreted as the result of violent acts that occurred before or around death. Certain post-mortem lesions may appear inflicted or non-inflicted ante- or peri-mortem injuries, with consequent potential problems in the interpretation during investigation. These kinds of alterations can be found both in terrestrial and aquatic environments (Campobasso *et al.* 2009; Vanin and Zancaner 2011). In bodies found in terrestrial environments, ants can produce different kinds of lesions: the classic irregular, serpiginous, scalloped areas and small white papulae (Bugelli *et al.* 2015; Campobasso *et al.* 2009).

Maggots moving from the body during the post-feeding stage can produce tracks on the ground that could be confused as tracks of dragging, whereas fly faecal and regurgitation artefacts can

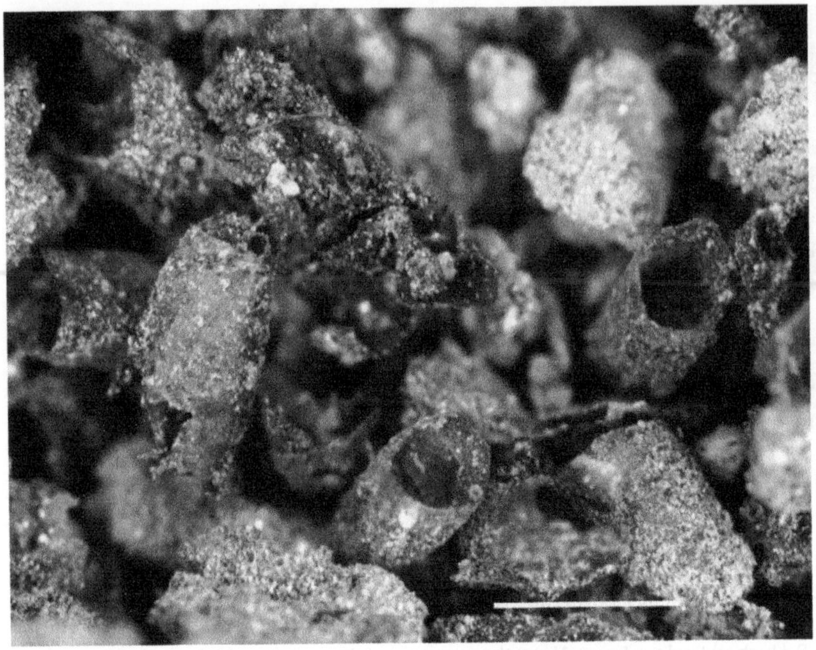

Figure 13.10 Puparia of typical 'coffin flies' (post-burial) (Phoridae) recovered from a mummified corpse buried in a wooden coffin (Church of Saint-Pierre d'Épernon, Eure-et-Loir, France) (Excavation: P Blanchard, INRAP, France; Photo: J.-B. Huchet) Scale = 1 mm.

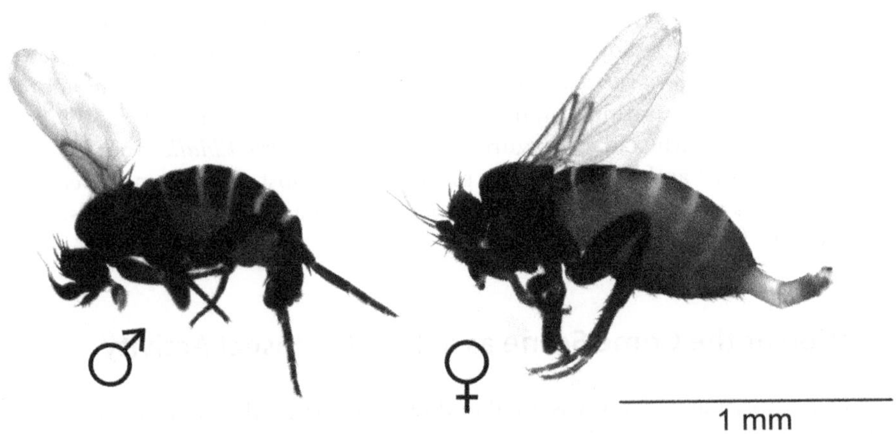

Figure 13.11 The 'Coffin Fly' *Conicera tibialis* Schmitz (Diptera: Phoridae). These specimens were recovered from the coffin of a buried individual exhumed 18 years after death in central Spain (image courtesy: D. Martín-Vega (NHM, London)).

interfere with the blood pattern analyses carried out on the crime scene (Durdle *et al.* 2013). Moreover, scavenger dung beetles feeding on a body can change its position as observed by Ururahy-Rodrigues *et al.* (2008) during an experiment with pig carcasses in Brazil.

In aquatic environments, the most important alterations of a body that can be misinterpreted, are related to the feeding activity of caddis flies (Trichoptera) (Holzer 1939) and aquatic amphipod species (Crustacea, Amphipoda) (Vanin and Zancaner 2011). More recently, damage to the skin and other tissues on experimental pig carcasses and on human bodies have been reported to be caused by the alloctonous species *Procambarus clarkii* (Decapoda, Cambaridae) in water ecosystems in Northern Italy (Manelli *et al.* 2014; Fais, P. personal communication).

13.6 Bone Modifications due to Insect Activity

The implication of different kinds of insects in the taphonomic processes of osteolytic degradation of human or faunal bones remains poorly documented. However, different orders of arthropods have the ability to impact bones and are responsible for significant bioerosion. In the current state of knowledge, four distinct orders of insects that can alter bone have been identified: Isoptera (subterranean termites), Coleoptera (beetles), Hymenoptera (wasps and burrowing bees) and Diptera (certain sarco-saprophagous fly larvae) (Huchet *et al.* 2011, 2013; Huchet 2014a, 2014b, 2014c). Among these taxa, subterranean termites are indisputably the most destructive agent worldwide. Typically known as wood-feeders, Thorne and Kimsey (1983) suggested that the occasional exploitation of bone remains by these insects might be a means to compensate for nitrogen deficiencies. Termites exploit indifferently buried or exposed bones and carcasses. The recognition of their traces on bones is of utmost importance, as their damage may sometimes mimic certain degenerative or infectious bone pathologies (pseudopathologies), traumatic damage, or even imitate certain peri- or post-mortem anthropic interventions (Huchet 2011, 2014a,b,c).

The larvae of different kinds of beetles (Dermestidae and Tenebrionidae) may also produce notable damage on bones. Recent studies conducted on Middle Bronze Age human bones from the Levant (c. 2100–1550 BC) (Huchet *et al.* 2013a) demonstrated that the multiple regular perforations (~3 mm wide) present on many long bones and skull fragments were linked with *Dermestes* activity at the time of pupation (Figure 13.12). The study of these traces allowed for detailed taphonomical hypotheses regarding the reconstruction of funerary practices of Middle Bronze Age collective burials.

Furthermore, Pittoni (2009) evidenced that different kinds of solitary wasps and wild bees caused significant damage on human bones in a Roman Necropolis (4th–5th century AD) in Sardinia. The author showed that the bone modification resulted from the post-burial nesting activity of Sphecidae and Halictidae (Hymenoptera), which continued until the time of excavation.

Finally, Gładykowska-Rzeczycka and Parafiniuk (2001) attributed enigmatic superficial lesions present on the internal surface of the cranial vault and the cervical vertebrae of an immature individual (Poland, 8th century) to the corrosive action of fly larvae gastric regurgitations.

Beyond the osteolytic lesions previously described, different kinds of insects (termites, ants, burrowing beetles, etc.) have propensity to produce notable soil bioturbations affecting the original position of the artefacts, but also causing destruction and/or distortion of archaeological data (Balek 2002; Fowler *et al.* 2004; McBrearty 1990; Ururahy-Rodrigues *et al.* 2008; Wood and Johnson 1978).

13.7 Conclusion

Insects or their remains can be found both at crime scenes and in archaeological contexts. If properly collected and analysed, insects act as a relevant tool in the reconstruction of past events, whether they are forensic or archaeological. The most important information that insects can provide about the circumstances surrounding death is the PMI and the season of death. Moreover, insects can provide information about body displacement, presence of drugs, pre-burial exposure and body concealment.

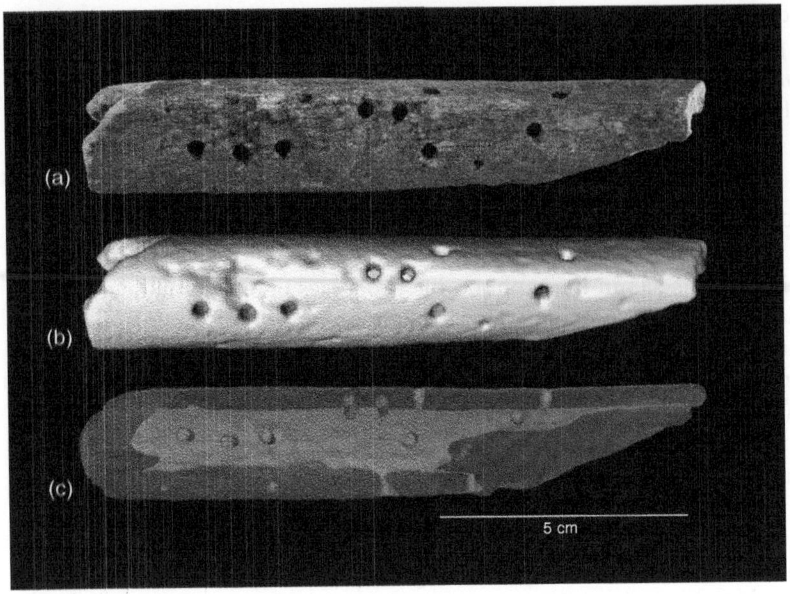

Figure 13.12 (a) Fragmented human bone from Middle Bronze Age (Munhata, Israel) bearing extensive perforations corresponding to dermestid pupal chambers. (b) Computed tomographic 3D reconstruction. (c) idem, with pupal chambers modelled (Source: Huchet *et al.* 2013).

A close interaction between all the specialists working at the crime scene or involved in archaeological research, is the '*conditio sine qua non*' for a better understanding and reconstruction of past events.

Acknowledgements

We are indebted to Daniel Martín-Vega (The Natural History Museum, London), who kindly allowed us to reproduce his illustrations of the coffin fly *Conicera tibialis* in this chapter.

References

Amendt, J., Campobasso, C.P., Gaudry, E., Reiter, C., Leblanc, H.N. and Hall, M.J.R. (2007) Best practice in forensic entomology-standards and guidelines. *International Journal of Legal Medicine*, **121**: 90–104.

Amendt, J., Krettek, R. and Zehner, R. (2004) Forensic entomology. *Naturwissenschaften*, **91**: 51–65.

Backwell, L.R., Parkinson, A., Roberts, E., d'Errico, F. and Huchet, J.B. (2012) Criteria for identifying bone modification by termites in the fossil record. *Palaeogeography, Palaeoclimatology, Palaeoecology*, **337–338**: 72–87.

Balek, C.L. (2002) Buried artifacts in stable upland sites and the role of bioturbation: A review. *Geoarchaeology*, **17**: 41–51.

Benecke, M. (2001) A brief history of forensic entomology. *Forensic Science International*, **120**: 2–14.

Benecke, M. and Lessig, R. (2001) Child neglect and forensic entomology. *Forensic Science International*, **120**: 155–159.

Benecke, M., Josephi, E. and Zweihoff, R. (2004) Neglect of the elderly: forensic entomology cases and considerations. *Forensic Science International*, **146**: S195–S199.

Bourel, B., Tournel, G., Hedouin, V. and Gosset, D. (2004) Entomofauna of buried bodies in northern France. *International Journal of Legal Medicine*, **118**: 215–220.

Bugelli, V., Forni, D., Bassi, L.A., Di Paolo, M., Marra, D. *et al.* (2014) Forensic entomology and the estimation of the minimum time since death in indoor cases. *Journal of Forensic Sciences*, **60**: 525–531.

Campobasso, C.P., Marchetti, D., Introna, F. and Colonna, M.F. (2009) Postmortem artifacts made by ants and the effect of ant activity on decompositional rates. *American Journal of Forensic Medicine and Pathology*, **30**: 84–87.

Campobasso, C.P., Di Vella, G. and Introna, F. (2001) Factors affecting decomposition and Diptera colonization. *Forensic Science International*, **120**: 18–27.

Campobasso, C.P., Disney, R.H.L. and Introna, F. (2004) A case of *Megaselia scalaris* (Loew) (Dipt., Phoridae) breeding in a human corpse. *Anil Aggrawal's Internet Journal of Forensic Medicine and Toxicology*, **5**: 3–5.

Couri, M.S., Mallemont Cunha, A., Mendonça de Souza, S.M.F. and Laeta, M. (2009) *Ophyra capensis* (Wiedemann) (Diptera, Muscidae) found inside the esophagus of a mummy in Lisbon (Portugal). *Papéis Avulsos de Zoologia*, **49**: 87–91.

Couri, M.S., Mendonça de Souza, S.M.F., Mallemont Cunha, A., Pinheiro, J. and Cunha, E. (2008) Diptera Brachycera found inside the esophagus of a mummified adult male from the early XIX century, Lisbon, Portugal. *Memórias do Instituto Oswaldo Cruz*, **103**: 211–213.

De Carvalho, L.M.L. (2010) Toxicology and forensic entomology, Chapter 9. In: Amendt, J., Campobasso, C.P., Goff, M.L. and Grassberger, M. (eds), *Current Concepts in Forensic Entomology*. Springer: Dordrecht, pp. 163–178.

Dirrigl, F.J. and Greenberg, B. (1995) The utility of insect remains to assessing human burials: a Connecticut case study. *Archaeology of Eastern North America*, **23**: 1–7.

Durdle, A., van Oorschot, R.A. and Mitchell, R.J. (2013) The morphology of fecal and regurgitation artifacts deposited by the blow fly *Lucilia cuprina* fed a diet of human blood. *Journal of Forensic Sciences*, **58**: 897–903.

Faulkner, D.K. (1986) The mass burial: an entomological perspective. In: Donnon, C.B. and Cock, G.A. (eds), *The Pacatnamu Papers*, vol. **1**. Fowler Museum of Cultural History, University of California: Los Angeles, pp. 145–150.

Fenoglio, S., Merritt, R.W. and Cummins, K.W. (2014) Why do no specialized necrophagous species exist among aquatic insects. *Freshwater Science*, **33**: 711–715.

Fowler, K.D., Greenfield, H.J. and Van Schalkwyk, L.O. (2004) The effects of burrowing activity on archaeological sites: Ndondondwane, South Africa. *Geoarchaeology*, **19**: 441–470.

Gaudry, E. (2010) The insects colonisation of buried remains. In: Amendt, J., Goff, M.L, Campobasso, C.P. and Grassberger, M. (eds), *Current Concepts in Forensic Entomology*. Springer: Dordrecht, pp. 273–312.

Gautier, A. and Schumann, H. (1973) Puparia of the subarctic or black blowfly *Protophormia terraenovae* (Robineau-Desvoidy, 1830) in a skull of late Eemian(?) bison at Zemst, Brabant (Belgium). *Palaeogeography, Palaeoclimatology, Palaeoecology*, **14**: 119–125.

Gilbert, B.M. and Bass, W.M. (1967) Seasonal dating of burials from the presence of fly pupae. *American Antiquity*, **32**: 534–535.

Gilbert, R.M. (1966) Seasonal dating of burials at the Leavenworth site (39CO9), with the use of fly pupae. *Plains Anthropologist*, **11**: 172.

Gładykowska-Rzeczycka, J.J. and Parafiniuk, M. (2001) Atypical cranial vault and cervical vertebrae lesions caused by insects. *Journal of Paleopathology*, **13**: 75–78.

Gunn, A. and Bird, J. (2011) The ability of the blowflies *Calliphora vomitoria* (Linnaeus), *Calliphora vicina* (Rob-Desvoidy) and *Lucilia sericata* (Meigen) (Diptera: Calliphoridae) and the muscid flies *Muscina stabulans* (Fallén) and *Muscina prolapsa* (Harris) (Diptera: Muscidae) to colonise buried remains. *Forensic Science International*, **207**: 198–204.

Henssge, C., Madea, B., Krompecher, T., Knight, B. and Nokes, L. (2002) *The Estimation of the Time since Death in the Early Post Mortem Period*. Edward Arnold: London.

Holzer, F.J. (1939) Zerstorung an wasserleichen durch larvaen des kocherfliege. *Deutsche Zeitschrift für die gesamte gerichtliche Medizin*, **31**: 223–228.

Huchet, J.-B. (1996) L'archéoentomologie funéraire: Une approche originale dans l'interprétation des sépultures. *Bulletins et mémoires de la Société d'anthropologie de Paris*, **8**: 289–302.

Huchet, J.-B. (2010) Archaeoentomological study of the insect remains found within the mummy of Namenkhet Amon, San Lazzaro Armenian Monastery, Venice/Italy). *Advances in Egyptology*, **1**: 58–80.

Huchet, J.-B. (2013) L'archéo-entomologie: les insectes nécrophages associés aux soldats de Carspach. In: Schnitzler, B. and Landolt, M. (eds), *A l'est du nouveau! Archéologie de la Grande Guerre en Alsace et en Lorraine. Les approches méthodologiques*. Musée de Strasbourg, collection Archéologie: Strasbourg, pp. 109–110.

Huchet, J.-B. (2014a) L'archéoentomologie funéraire. In: Charabidze, D. and Gosselin, M. (eds), *Insectes, cadavres et scènes de crime, Principes et applications de l'entomologie médico-légale*. Editions De Boeck: Bruxelles, pp. 201–224.

Huchet, J.-B. (2014b) Approche ichnologique et taphonomique des altérations ostéolytiques dues aux insectes en contexte archéologique. In: Denys, C. and Patou-Mathis, M. (eds), *Manuel de Taphonomie*, Actes Sud – Errance, collection 'Archéologiques', Muséum National d'Histoire naturelle and CNRS: Paris, pp. 185–207.

Huchet, J.-B. (2014c) Insect remains and their traces: relevant fossil witnesses in the reconstruction of past funerary practices. *Anthropologie (Brno)*, **52**: 329–346.

Huchet, J.-B., Deverly, D., Gutierrez, B. and Chauchat, C. (2011) Taphonomic evidence of a human skeleton gnawed by termites in a Moche-civilisation Grave at Huaca De La Luna, Peru. *International Journal of Osteoarchaeology*, **21**: 92–102.

Huchet, J.-B. and Greenberg, B. (2010) Flies, Mochicas and burial practices: a case study from Huaca de la Luna, Peru. *Journal of Archaeological Science*, **37**: 2846–2856.

Huchet, J.-B., Le Mort, F., Rabinovich, R., Blau, S., Coqueugniot, H. and Arensburg, B. (2013a) Identification of dermestid pupal chambers on Southern Levant human bones: inference for reconstruction of Middle Bronze Age mortuary practices. *Journal of Archaeological Science*, **40**: 3793–3803.

Huchet, J.-B., Pereira, G., Gomy, Y., Phillips, T.K., Alatorre-Bracamontes, C.E. *et al.* (2013b) Archaeoentomological study of a pre-Columbian funerary bundle mortuary cave of Candelaria, Coahuila, Mexico. *Annales de la Société entomologique de France*, **49**: 277–290.

Introna, F., Campobasso, C.P. and Goff, M.L. (2001) Entomotoxicology. *Forensic Science International*, **120**: 42–47.

Manelli, L., Vanin, S. and Maistrello, L. (2014) Postmortem injuries caused by the freshwater crayfish (Girard, 1852). Abstract book. *11th Meeting of the European Association for Forensic Entomology*, Lille; p. 57.

Marchetti, D., Arena, E., Boschi, I. and Vanin, S. (2013) Human DNA extraction from empty puparia. *Forensic Science International*, **229**: e26–e29.

Martín-Vega, D., Gómez-Gómez, A. and Baz, A. (2011) The 'Coffin Fly' *Conicera tibialis* (Diptera: Phoridae) breeding on buried human remains after a postmortem interval of 18 years. *Journal of Forensic Sciences*, **56**: 1654–1656.

Masetti, M., Gabrielli, S., Menconi, M. and Fornaciari, G. (2008) Insect remains associated with the mummy of Cardinal Giulio della Rovere, Archbishop of Ravenna (1533–1578). In: Atoche, P., Peña , Rodríguez Martín, C., Ramírez Rodríguez, M.A. (eds), *Mummies and Science: World Mummies Research*. Proceedings of the VI World Congress on Mummy Studies, Teguise, Lanzarote, Islas Canarias, Academia Canaria de la Historia: Santa Cruz de Tenerife, pp. 379–385.

Mazzarelli, D., Vanin, S., Gibelli, D., Maistrello, L., Porta, D. *et al.* (2014) Splitting hairs: differentiating between entomological activity, taphonomy, and sharp force trauma on hair. *Forensic Science, Medicine and Pathology*, **11**: 104–110.

McBrearty, S. (1990) Consider the humble termite: termites as agents of post-deposition disturbance at African archaeological sites. *Journal of Archaeological Science*, **17**: 111–143.

McCaulay, R., Bostock, E., Elrington, P., Natale, G., Lenzi, P. and Vanin, S. (2014) Insects from Pre-Colombian Peruvian mummies: a funerary archaeoentomological approach. Abstract book. *11th Meeting of the European Association for Forensic Entomology*, Lille; p. 73.

Mégnin, P. (1887) La faune des tombeaux. *Compte Rendu Hebdomadaire des Séances de l'Académie des Sciences, Paris*, **105**: 948–951.

Miller, M., Lord, W., Goff, M.L. and Donnelly, B. (1994) Isolation of amitriptyline and nortriptyline from fly puparia (Phoridae) and beetle exuviae (Dermestidae) associated with mummified human remains. *Journal of Forensic Sciences*, **39**: 1305–1313.

Nystrom, K.C., Goff, A. and Goff, M.L. (2005) Mortuary behaviour reconstruction through palaeoentomology: a case study from Chachapoya, Peru. *International Journal of Osteoarchaeology*, **15**: 175–185.

Pittoni, E. (2009) Necropoli of Pill'e Matta Quartucciu (Cagliari, Sardinia): wild bee and solitary wasp activity and bone diagenetic factors. *International Journal of Osteoarchaeology*, **19**: 386–396.

Raoult, D., Reed, D.L., Dittmar, K., Kirchman, J.J., Rolain, J.-M. *et al.* (2008) Molecular identification of lice from pre-Columbian mummies. *The Journal of Infectious Diseases*, **197**: 535–543.

Richards, C.S., Paterson, I.D. and Villet, M.H. (2008) Estimating the age of immature *Chrysomya albiceps* (Diptera: Calliphoridae), correcting for temperature and geographical latitude. *International Journal of Legal Medicine*, **122**: 271–279.

Scharrer-Liska, G. and Grassberger, M. (2005) Archäoentomologische Untersuchungen von Grab 34 des awarischen Gräberfeldes von Frohsdorf, Niederösterreich. *Archäologisches Korrespondenzblatt*, **35**: 531–544.

Smith, K.G.V. (1986) *A Manual of Forensic Entomology*. The Trustees of the British Museum (Natural History): London.

Speight, M. (1974) Potential contributions to archaeology from animal remains, with special reference to insects. In: Scott, B.G. (ed.), *Perspectives in Irish Archaeology*. Association of Young Irish Archaeologists: Dublin, pp. 24–34.

Teskey, H.H. and Turnbull, C. (1979) Diptera puparia from prehistoric graves. *The Canadian Entomologist*, **111**: 527–528.

Thorne, B.L. and Kimsey, R.B. (1983) Attraction of neotropical *Nasutitermes* termites to carrion. *Biotropica*, **15**: 295–296.

Thorpe, W.H. (1931) The biology of the petroleum fly. *Science*, **73**: 101–103.

Turchetto, M. and Vanin, S. (2010) Climate change and forensic entomology. In: Amendt, J., Goff, M.L, Campobasso, C.P. and Grassberger, M. (eds), *Current Concepts in Forensic Entomology*, Springer: Dordrecht, pp. 327–351.

Turner-Walker, G. and Scull, C. (1997) Microfauna in Anglo Saxon graves: entomological evidence at Boss Hall and the Butter Market, Ipswich. In: Sinclair, A., Slater, E. and Gowlett, J. (eds), *Archaeological Sciences*. Oxbow Monograph 64: Oxford, pp. 320–327.

Ururahy-Rodrigues, A., Rafael, J.A., Wanderley, R.F., Marques, H. and Pujol-Luz, J.R. (2008) *Coprophanaeus lancifer* (Linnaeus, 1767) (Coleoptera, Scarabaeidae) activity moves a man-size pig carcass: Relevant data for forensic taphonomy. *Forensic Science International*, **182**: 19–22.

Vanin, S., Tasinato, P., Ducolin, G., Terranova, C., Zancaner, S. *et al.* (2008) Use of *Lucilia* species (Diptera: Calliphoridae) for forensic investigations in Southern Europe. *Forensic Science International*, **177**: 37–41.

Vanin, S., Turchetto, M., Galassi, A. and Cattaneo, C. (2009) Forensic entomology and the archaeology of war. *Journal of Conflict Archaeology*, **5**: 127–139.

Vanin, S. and Zancaner, S. (2011) Post-mortal lesions in freshwater environment. *Forensic Science International*, **212**: e18–20.

Vanin, S., Zanotti, E., Gibelli, D., Taborelli, A., Andreola, S. and Cattaneo, C. (2013) Decomposition and entomological colonization of charred bodies – a pilot study. *Croatian Medical Journal*, **54**: 387–393.

Wells, J.D. and Stevens, J.R. (2008) Application of DNA-based methods in forensic entomology. *Annual Review of Entomology*, **53**: 103–120.

Wood, W.R. and Johnson, D.L. (1978) A survey of disturbance processes in archaeological site. *Advances in Archaeological Method and Theory*, **1**: 315–381.

Wyss, C. and Cherix, D. (2006) *Traité d'Entomologie Forensique*. Press polytechnique et Universitaires Romandes: Lausanne.

14

Forensic Botany and Stomach Contents Analysis: Established Practice and Innovation

Jennifer Miller

14.1 Introduction

Forensic botany can be invaluable in legal investigation (Bock and Norris 2005). With cellulose-based cell walls and recognisable anatomies, plant fragments can often be identified, at least to tissue type (Esau 1965, 1977), but frequently to family, genus or species. Familial characteristics assist in identification of seeds, pollen and spores or vegetative parts, especially wood (e.g. Cappers *et al.* 2006; Gale and Cutler 2000; Moore *et al.* 1991; Schweingruber 1990). Habitat tolerances, ranges and plant community associations are also well understood (e.g. Gurevitch *et al.* 2006). These criteria are used by archaeobotanists to recreate previous environments and economies from archaeological samples and sediment cores (e.g. Dickson and Dickson 2000). Similarly, plant fragments on the clothing of a body can locate an attack site, link a suspect to a scene or provide evidence of seasonality, whilst diatoms within a drowned person's internal organs might, not may identify where they went into a river. The last meal in the stomach of a body missing for days, weeks or longer may also help narrow the window of death.

This chapter will outline briefly the range of established and crucial roles that whole plants and fragments now play in the interpretation of taphonomy. However, the main focus of this text is given to pioneering techniques including genetics, but especially stomach contents analysis, which has now played an invaluable role in the investigation of unexplained death on numerous occasions in recent years. A great deal of our food is plant-based and remains identifiable within the stomach, analysis of which can provide crucial information to criminal investigation, helping explain timings and events surrounding death. Illustrative case examples are given where appropriate to illustrate or help clarify relevant points. All cases cited have been tried under Crown or Scots Law and are in the public domain. Crime reference numbers or operation names are given to allow further details to be obtained by application to the relevant authority.

14.2 Forensic Applications of Botany

Various authors (e.g. Hall 1997; Hall and Byrd 2012; Miller-Coyle 2005) have discussed the wide spectrum of ways in which plants can assist in criminal investigation, detailing considerations for recording and collection. Plants provide evidence of contact and/or duration, for which the range of species, time of year and nature of the landscape are integral to the interpretation. For a body deposited outdoors, the surroundings can be a key source of evidence (Pokines and Symes 2013).

Taphonomy of Human Remains: Forensic Analysis of the Dead and the Depositional Environment, First Edition.
Edited by Eline M.J. Schotsmans, Nicholas Márquez-Grant and Shari L. Forbes.

Sample collection methods used will differ according to the environment and reasons for collection, with common sense prevailing. Clearly vegetative remains for anatomical analysis need to be prepared like herbarium specimens on card or paper and dried flat, whilst sediment samples for pollen or diatom studies would be collected into poly pots or bags and stored in a fridge or freezer. Accurate recording, sketched plans and detailed written notes are crucial in all cases, as is the photographic record, using scales of appropriate size. Surface samples should be recovered before the site is disturbed; the top 2 mm only may contain pollen relevant to the current season of growth. The authors cited above provide further details on specific sampling methods.

14.2.1 Impact of Decomposition upon Vegetation

Seasonal variations in temperature, day length and habitat help define the natural vegetation in any location, with many UK species dormant or practically so between November and February. Vegetation surrounding, overlying or below decomposing remains is subjected to those natural dictates in addition to stresses caused by the deceased. As such, plants may grow past a body overlying them, or die. Vegetation broken at the scene may or may not recover, dependent upon damage and the seasonal growth norm, whilst newly exposed soil may become populated by pioneer annual weeds, but only within the growing season. An understanding of the expected situation at any place or time of year can highlight anthropogenic change, helping to find human remains or determine duration on countless occasions.

During a search for a body missing between October and March (Miller 2005a), large areas of an overgrown cemetery with prolific growth of tall perennial weeds were excluded by examination of the upright dead stems from last season's growth, the undamaged status of which confirmed that no disturbance had occurred since the previous summer. In a similar case, the height differential between damaged perennial weeds adjacent to a grave dug in early April and undisturbed plants nearby helped assign duration when the remains were found in May (Miller 2013). Elsewhere, bud scales underneath a bag containing body parts at the edge of a seasonally fluctuating flood pond in September provided evidence of deposition in April to early May (Miller 2003). Autumn leaves from similar trees were stratigraphically below the bud scales. The uncrumpled leaves overlaid a moss common in shallow fluctuating water. to suggest deposition into standing water for concealment.

Roots can help assign deposition time in remains of several years duration. Growth rings on perennial roots can be counted like tree rings, helping to assign a minimum duration (Willey and Heilman 1987). Figure 14.1 shows root growth through the sleeping bag of a homeless man that helped to confirm death soon after the last sighting four years previously (Miller 2006). In that case and in many similar situations, algae staining and moss overgrowth on exposed bones also helped assign duration. Polkines and Symes (2013) discuss the relevance of colour staining and also root etching on bones.

14.2.2 Palynology

Palynology is a long-established area of archaeobotany used to investigate landscape change over time to study anthropogenic and/or climatic impact. By extrapolation, forensic palynology is the study of pollen and spores for legal investigation. Their forensic application relates to the habitat characteristics implied, thereby enabling a person or object to be linked to a particular locality (Mildenhall *et al.* 2006). Pollen is produced by higher plants and spores from algae, bryophytes and ferns. Fungi also produce spores, although they are not plants, and the palynological profile of any particular area will reflect the range of taxa growing there, the frequency of individuals of any given species and their mode of propagation. Flowering plants can be wind, vector or self pollinated, with resultant wide variation in the numbers of grains produced. Lower plants require water to complete their life cycles. The topography is also relevant, the wind transporting palynomorphs long distances across flat open

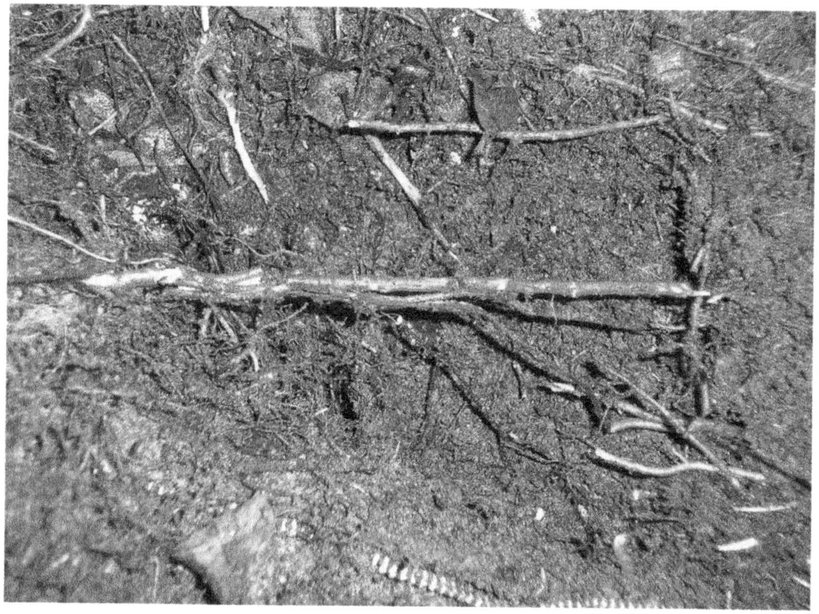

Figure 14.1 Roots growing through the sleeping bag of a homeless man.

areas, whilst the 'pollen rain' within a steep sided valley will be very local. Whether or not a species is mature enough to propagate, or is actually flowering, is also important. For example, attempts to link a suspect to a conifer plantation planted seven years ago via pollen would be futile as the trees would not be old enough to flower.

In recent years, palynology has been revealed as a versatile forensic technique (Adams-Groom 2012; Brown 2006; Wiltshire 2006a, 2009, 2010; Wiltshire and Black 2006), if not an absolute science. In an overview of forensic palynology, Wiltshire (2006b) outlines the range of applications, highlighting the impact of taphonomic variability upon the potential for valid palynological results in legal investigation. Issues include the fact that numbers of palynomorphs recovered from forensic samples are often too low to give an accurate picture of a particular location. However, local areas of similar vegetation types can have very different assemblages (Horrocks and Walsh 1998) and statistical modelling can further improve the forensic application (Dawson and Mayes 2015; Horrocks *et al.* 1999). Significant assemblages of palynomorphs are picked up from soil, sediment and other materials. Entirely uncontaminated samples on suspect footwear are rare, so most palynological profiles will have mixed origins. This must be taken into consideration, with corroboration from other areas of forensic geoscience consolidating the evidential value of palynology (Dawson and Mayes 2015).

Forensic palynology is labour intensive and requires significant experience, skill and appropriate sampling strategies. However, under such circumstances, it can provide excellent trace evidence (Walsh and Horrocks 2008), fulfilling the relevant criteria for transfer, persistence and detection (Morgan *et al.* 2010). The authors named above cite case examples that have yielded good results when taphonomy and other factors are given due consideration, a situation relevant for all areas of forensic botany.

14.2.3 Fungi

Although belonging to a different taxonomic kingdom, fungi have certain similarities to primitive plants and have a long history of study by botanists. Species can be saprophytic (i.e. feed on dead organic matter) or parasitic (feed on live material) and range from single-celled yeasts to the extensive mycelia (mat of fungal threads) that form familiar toadstools within woodland leaf litter. Forensic mycology has only recently become a regular addition to the toolkit for criminal investigation and has potential for various applications. These include contact trace evidence, determination of post-mortem interval or certain causes of death, location of buried remains or biological warfare (Hawksworth and Wiltshire 2011).

14.2.4 Diatoms and Phytoliths

Diatoms are silica-bodied algae found in habitats ranging from fast flowing rivers, ephemeral puddles or wet soil to marine environments. With silica frustules ('coats'), they are identifiable and durable, enabling ecologists and geoscientists to utilise diatoms to observe change in water levels or eutrophication over time. They also have forensic application in cases of drowning. Diatoms within the lung and kidney tissue of a person whose motorbike plunged around 9 m (30 ft) into water following a crash helped this author assist the pathologist to confirm that he had drowned, not died during impact (Figure 14.2). Diatoms have also helped estimate time or location of death (Cameron 2004). Certain clothing types retain them better than others, but collection and sampling methods have been investigated (Scott *et al.* 2014) and this valuable technique is now becoming better utilised, whether to confirm drowning, link a suspect to a scene or to aid the search for a deposition site.

Phytoliths are silica structures that accumulate in the tissues of some plants. They persist and accumulate over time within the soil, and they may be produced in abundance and can be identifiable. Phytolith analysis has recently become more widely practised within archaeobotany but also forensic geoscience, where it can help differentiate soils with similar mineralogy (Marumo and Yanai 1986).

14.2.5 Plant Genetics

Seeds are generally closely identifiable. However, tiny vegetative fragments are often recognisable only in terms of tissue type or family, with specific identification using traditional morphological methods

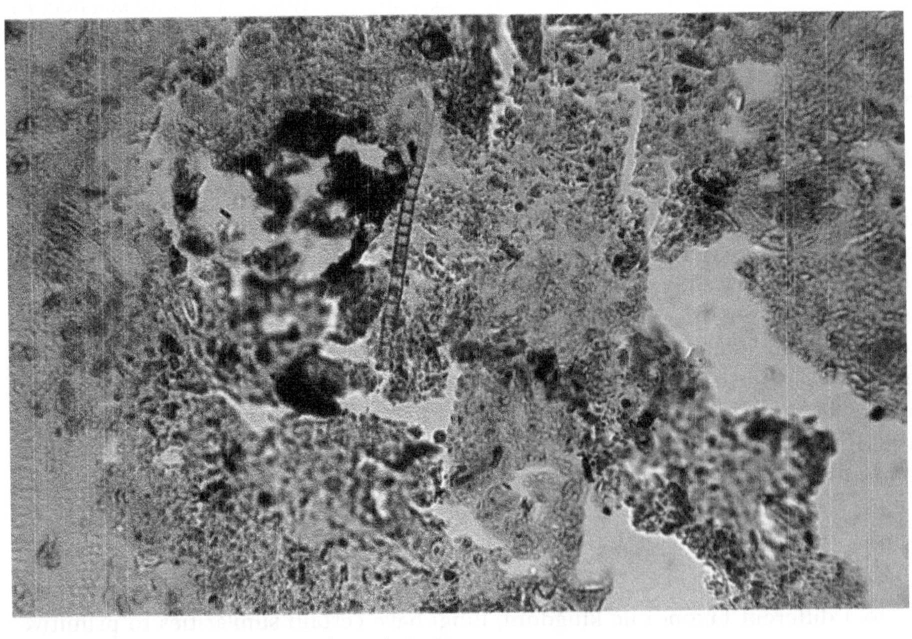

Figure 14.2 Lung tissue showing long chain diatom.

proving difficult (Miller-Coyle *et al.* 2001). Consequently, recent research has focused on strategies for understanding the potential for plant DNA characteristics to help link a specific fragment to a crime scene. Targeting selected loci on the genome of 25 genera of common grasses, Ward *et al.* (2005) correctly recognised 24 of them in a blind study, revealing the potential for DNA evidence to identify at least grasses to genus or closer.

Virtanen *et al.* (2007) reported that moss leaves can still be recovered from footwear after several hours of wear. Mosses are often specifically identifiable (Smith 2004; Dickson *et al.* 2009), but habitat ranges can be wide. The authors recovered intact DNA from mosses stored adversely for 18 months and since bryophytes are clonal, argue the potential for linking particular specimens to a scene. Craft *et al.* (2007) reported that recovering DNA from a dead leaf of sand live oak (*Quercus germinata*) within a suspect vehicle was more difficult than from comparative fresh material. However, once achieved, the authors used the information to exclude the suspect leaf from trees around a grave.

The potential and strategies for linking a plant fragment to any locus via DNA will vary with methods of reproduction. Clearly clonal and inbreeding taxa, or large individuals with thousands of genetically identical leaves, have greater potential to become trace evidence than small sexually reproduced species growing within vegetation stands of sexually unique individuals. Koopman *et al.* (2012) cite knotgrass (*Polygonum aviculare*) as an ideal study model in this respect. Knotgrass produces local populations of similar genetic composition, has widespread distribution, local abundance and is easily processed. Using DNA fingerprinting, the authors managed to distinguish the knotgrass population at a crime scene from others.

Discrepancy and disagreement between research groups regarding selection of universally applicable marker systems, led geneticists within the Consortium for the Barcode of Life (CBOL) to form the CBOL-Plant Working Group. Initial results gave 70–75% discrimination to species using a multilocus system based on plastid gene markers (Hollingsworth *et al.* 2009). Although lower than the cytochrome c oxidase I (COI) markers used for animal identification, this was a good starting point, given there are some known 380,000–400,000 plant species, and would still have forensic application (Ferri *et al.* 2015). Those authors' further research has now refined results to agree a multilocus solution focused upon two of the four chloroplast loci studied (rbcL + trnH-psbA); this best satisfies current forensic needs for species identification. The task of producing a global reference database is immense, and research groups vary in their strengths and focus within different plant groups. However, as databanks grow, DNA recognition of species should become more straightforward, leading to more widespread application of forensic plant DNA recognition.

14.2.6 Stomach Contents Analysis

In the same way that the last meal of an Iron Age bog body can be determined from analysis of food in their stomach (e.g. Helbaek 1950, 1958; Holden 1995), microscopic analysis of the gastric contents of a recently deceased person or of a pool of vomit at a crime scene can have significant forensic application (Bock *et al.* 1988; Lane *et al.* 1990; Hall 1997; Robertson 2013). Plant foods can often be identified rigorously, even to the shapes of starch grains within cells (Winton 1916), enabling the last foods consumed to be interpreted. Animal proteins can also be classified by visual examination, with specific confirmation achieved by chemical analysis. Fungi can also be recognised. Differing methods of preparation, cooking styles and fragment sizes/shapes help to make individual meals recognisable. Non-food items in the stomach, whether eaten intentionally or ingested accidentally, may also provide useful intelligence.

When the last meal is known, confirmation that similar food remains within the stomach may narrow the time span upon which enquiries should be focused. Alternatively, when movements are unknown, identification of the last foods consumed may reveal movements in the hours preceding death. Analysis of ingested food is now recognised as making a significant and valuable contribution to criminal investigation in relevant cases across the UK.

The author has examined in excess of 350 stomach contents of deceased persons in a variety of circumstances, of which a great many cases have aided the investigative process significantly. The technique has been tried and defended successfully under Crown or Scots jurisprudence on numerous occasions.

14.2.6.1 Processes of Digestion

Most of the digestive process occurs within the small intestines. Other than to retain ingested foods, the two main functions of the stomach are the initial enzymatic digestion of proteins and maceration of foods via rhythmic churning (peristalsis). Hydrolysis of starches into disaccharide sugars is initiated in the stomach through the actions of ptyalin from saliva, although enzyme function within the stomach is focused primarily on the breakdown of proteins, with rennin coagulating liquid milk proteins and pepsin breaking down solid proteins into short polypeptide chains for further digestion within the small intestine. Pepsin requires an acidic environment to activate it from the inactive precursor pepsinogen, to which end, hydrochloric acid secreted by the stomach maintains a pH generally lower than 2.0. The acidic environment of the stomach also helps to break plant cell walls to release nutrients. Conversely, bile salts from the liver help to make the pH of the small intestine distinctly alkaline to support the actions of various enzymes produced by the liver, pancreas and intestinal wall itself.

The other main role of the stomach in digestion is peristalsis, or stomach churning, causing mechanical disaggregation of large food items into fragments small enough to pass through the pyloric sphincter into the intestines. There, gastric transit becomes subject to numerous variables. Semi-digested foods may remain for hours to days or more, with diet, lifestyle and health playing a significant role in duration. A healthy individual with good diet may have a bowel movement daily; whilst someone with illness, poor diet, psychological concern, habituation or addiction may do so much less frequently. This variability in frequency of bowel emptying and co-mingling of semi-digested foods mean that particular meals are not generally recognisable within the intestines. Digestive processes within the stomach are also subject to extrinsic influences, although the intrinsic chemical and mechanical actions are less complex. Consequently, there is greater potential for analysis of foods within the stomach to have forensic application.

14.2.6.2 Methodology

Stomach contents samples should be frozen immediately upon seizure; in such cases they will remain preserved for months or potentially even years until required. The entire contents of the stomach should be analysed, noting any volume removed for toxicology.

Clear photographic record should be taken at all stages of analysis. The total volume should be ascertained and colour and viscosity of the matrix described. This volume is then drained gently through a sterile calibrated sieve (the author uses 72 μm mesh) and the volume of liquid recorded. Small subsamples of liquid are retained for closer detailed analysis and the rest returned to the original container. The solid volume is described, volume recorded and split into three parts. One-third is retained intact (with a one-third volume of liquid base matrix) pending subsequent analyses. The other two parts are examined separately and consecutively, thereby ensuring that any problems encountered during the initial analysis can be addressed for the second replicate. Small volumes are studied at low magnification and component parts separated. Care should be taken to avoid disaggregation of fragile foods, with minimal flushing water used; this should also be retained. Lugol's Iodine is used on subsamples as a presumptive test for starch. As with any forensic examination, detailed notes, attention to detail and good a photographic record of all stages of analysis are critical to ensure clarity of analysis for court purposes.

14.2.6.3 Passage of Different Foods

Medical examiners in the past attempted to use naked eye examination of foods in the stomach to determine the exact time of death (Knight 2002). However, this has been discredited and it is now widely recognised that estimations involving a spectrum of hours are more appropriate.

Water can pass almost unaided from the stomach, and low calorie liquids often leave before solid foods (Madea 2002). Different solid foods are disaggregated to a greater or lesser extent by peristalsis and maceration (Knight 2002). Size and 'digestibility' of individual fragments help determine how long a meal remains in the stomach, including which components remain longer than others (Horowitz and Pounder 1985). Proteins, soft carbohydrates and well cooked vegetables are disaggregated fairly rapidly by the combination of peristalsis, digestive juices and fluid imbibed, whilst nuts, seeds, raw vegetables, vegetable/fruit skins and cereal testa (bran) are barely broken down if at all, and pass through the stomach with little or no change. In usual circumstances, digestive transit commences with low calorie liquids, proteins such as milk and semi-digested meats, then soft carbohydrates and well cooked vegetable material (potato, carrot, etc.) before lipid-based or fat-rich foods, although not exclusively. Passage of foods into the duodenum is consequently a result of a variable combination of enzyme activity, the acidic environment and mechanical processes. Small volumes of semi-fluid, disaggregated and/or semi-digested foods and digestive juices (chyme) pass progressively from the stomach into the duodenum for further digestion in the hours following consumption, the composition of the chyme changing as digestion progresses. Some large or indigestible items such as leaves, seeds or fruit/vegetable skins are little affected by maceration and pass into the small intestine between periods of digestion (Madea 2002; Tröger *et al.* 1987).

14.2.6.4 Determining Duration

Determining duration of mixed foods from a single meal within the stomach is a complicated matter with many variables and cannot be done with critical accuracy (Brophy *et al.* 1986; Knight 2002). However, experimental studies have provided arbitrary time ranges for different meals to pass into the duodenum (Brophy *et al.* 1986; DiMaio and DiMaio 2001; Madea 2002; Moore *et al.* 1984; Tröger *et al.* 1987). There is variability between authors and subjects, although inclusive parameters of duration can be assigned to guide lines of enquiry on those terms. Madea reported a period of one to three hours for a small, light meal to leave the stomach, three to five hours for a moderate meal and five to eight hours for a large, heavy meal. DiMaio and DiMaio discuss half-emptying times, which may be more useful in many situations, and Moore *et al.* and Tröger *et al.* both produced graphs to estimate the percentage of food remaining over time. Using results from post-mortem stomach contents collection from 47 sudden, unexpected deaths and known last meals of mixed foods, Tröger *et al.* reported that if 90% of an original large meal of mixed foods was present, then consumption was usually within an hour before death, with 98% confidence limits of up to three to four hours. If 50% was present, then last food intake was around three to four hours before death, with 98% confidence of between one to ten hours. When only 30% food remains, last intake was four to five hours before death, with a 98% confidence range of two to ten hours.

The width of the confidence ranges reported, when only small volumes of food remained within the stomach, relates to variation in the components and calorific content of meals consumed. Consequently, if consideration is given to the types, digestibility and calorific value of foods present within the stomach as well as the total volume, this information can help narrow the timescale for the enquiry team to investigate from days to hours; most accurately when almost the entire meal is present, but also to within a moderate time range (hours) when stomach emptying is more advanced.

The calorific content of a meal is at least as important as size and 'digestibility' of individual food fragments, and has a greater bearing on duration than the volume of foods consumed. A smaller, fat-rich meal of mixed foods will remain longer than a larger volume of low calorie mixed items (Brophy *et al.* 1986; DiMaio and DiMaio 2001; Moore *et al.* 1984). There may also be a short lag in the onset of stomach emptying, especially where fat-rich meals are concerned. High calorie foods persist longer because fats can delay the triggering of gastric stretch receptors that initiate emptying or speed up the emptying rate of a large meal (DiMaio and DiMaio 2001). However, this does not always occur and any lag in gastric emptying due to high fat content will not generally delay transit substantially.

Alcohol can also induce a similar lag, caused by irritation of the stomach mucosa (Knight 2002). The effects are generally greater with wine and spirits than average beers, reflecting lower alcohol content and the increased volume of beer stimulating the gastric stretch receptors to speed up transit. Gastric emptying rate does not necessarily reflect blood alcohol content (BAC), although high BAC suggests potential for lag in transit. Delays in gastric transit mean that food consumed will stay within the stomach longer than might otherwise be expected. This phenomenon must always be considered, taking specific case details into account. In some circumstances it may only be feasible to identify the last meal without commenting on duration.

Various drugs including sedatives, especially opiate derivatives, can also affect digestive transit rates, causing slowing or temporary gastric stasis (Chan 2008; DiMaio and DiMaio 2001; Petring and Blake 1993). Other commonly prescribed medications do not affect transit, including Paracetamol and Diazepam (Petring and Blake 1993), whilst certain serotonergic antidepressants can actively assist transit in individuals where it is otherwise delayed (Grover and Camilleri 2013; Yin *et al.* 2014). The actions of synthetic cannabinoids, including so-called 'legal highs' upon digestive transit are not well reported within published literature, although cannabis itself can delay it somewhat (McCallum *et al.* 1999).

14.2.6.5 Individual Variation

Individual digestion rates vary and health, activity rates and mental state are also relevant to digestive transit (Knight 2002). Consequently, ascribing a definitive time range for the processes of gastric transit can only be done with caveats and margins that consider both the extrinsic and intrinsic factors affecting the subject's digestive system as well as types of foods and calorific content. Medical and toxicology records with regard to lifestyle and medication or other drugs ingested must always be considered with regard to their potential to impact upon digestive transit.

14.2.6.6 Trauma and Death

Great fear or stress may engender psychogenic hypermobility of the bowels, resulting in diarrhoea (Knight 2002). It can also effectively halt the digestive processes occurring within the stomach, by causing psychogenic spasm of the pyloric sphincter muscle between the stomach and duodenum. Normally, this alternately contracts and relaxes to allow small amounts of food to pass from the stomach into the small intestine, but in spasm it remains closed. Peristalsis also ceases, with cumulative effect that transit of food from the stomach into the intestine effectively ceases. Knight (2002) cites the case of a motorcycle accident where the victim remained in a coma for a week before death. At post-mortem the stomach contained the entire last meal eaten prior to the accident. Madea (2002) narrates similar findings. In such circumstances, stomach contents analysis can help determine the time frame for gastric transit up to the point of onset of an attack or stressful situation, even if the assault or stress continued for some time before death ensued. Pylorospasm may not always occur, but the potential should be considered in each case. Regardless, the passage of food from the stomach into the small intestine (gastric transit) and digestive enzyme production cease immediately upon death (Madea 2002).

The types and volume of foods consumed, presence of alcohol and additional extraneous factors including lifestyle, health and stress can all affect how long different components of a meal will remain within the stomach. These factors must be taken into account in any forensic examination, but although they mean that stomach contents analysis may not be applicable universally, in circumstances where due consideration is given to the relevant caveats, it can strengthen greatly the evidential value of the results obtained.

14.2.6.7 Case Examples

Since gastric transport of food into the duodenum ceases at death, this gives a discrete cut-off period in cases of sudden, unexpected death, such as in a drive-by shooting or unprovoked attack. Furthermore, although protein breakdown may continue somewhat, other foods within the undamaged stomach of a deceased person will remain identifiable until the organ decays, so the technique may still be applicable days or weeks after death has occurred. If a body has been frozen, contents can still be identified even thousands of years after death (Oeggl *et al.* 2007). The Chinese meal that a woman ate with her brother before she disappeared remained intact after she had lain for four years in a household freezer; this helped to convict her husband (Miller 2009). Also, the stomach contents of a woman missing for four days pointed to a particular type of burger having been ingested shortly prior to death. This led the enquiry team to examine CCTV footage of the branch of that restaurant closest to where she disappeared, placing the deceased and perpetrator together, thus helping to convict him for her shooting (Miller 2003). Similarly, the stomach contents of a homeless man found dead several weeks after the last sighting at a drop-in centre, contained the same food as he had eaten at the centre immediately prior to a violent disagreement with two others upon leaving (Miller 2004a). Despite ongoing decomposition, the food was still identifiable within the stomach, which gave the enquiry a positive direction to follow.

When the last meal of a man missing for four days was identified, it led the enquiry team to a particular restaurant where the waitress remembered him eating similar food with two others whom she was able to describe (Miller 1998a). Other than helping guide the enquiry, the results also corroborated the pathologist's findings, which were in dispute.

The efficiency of mastication affects the size of fragments arriving in the stomach; some people chew their food more thoroughly than others. Segments of orange in the stomach of a murdered girl and in the vomit of the man who killed her were chewed totally differently (Miller 1998b). Segments in the vomit had been swallowed almost whole, whilst those in the stomach of the girl were carefully chewed. The variation in chew patterns and presence of differing foods confirmed that the vomit was not from the deceased, helping to provide another line of enquiry. By contrast, vomit found beside a murdered man was entirely similar to the food still within his stomach (Miller 2005b). This enabled both pathologist and enquiry team to interpret peri-mortem events in greater detail.

Since foods leave the stomach at varying times, observations on specific items remaining following a known meal can guide the interpretation of time since consumption and death or attack to within a range of hours. When a man who had been witnessed eating a 230 g (8 oz) steak with mixed peppercorn sauce, thick cut chips, mushrooms, onions and salad was found dead two weeks later, the presence of numerous mushrooms, onions, salad and peppercorns in his stomach, but only microscopic strands of meat protein and small, almost indigestible end-pieces of chip (Miller 2005c) were strongly indicative of last consumption within a guide range of some six to ten hours prior to death. By contrast, the entire volume of half a white bread roll and raspberry jam (with a cup of tea) given to an elderly bedridden lady by her carer was still in her stomach when she was found dead that evening (Miller 2003). Highly processed bread products disaggregate very rapidly when ingested with liquid, but the roll was still in pieces large enough to imply ingestion shortly before onset of the attack that killed her. This was potentially just after the carer left, even considering the likelihood that her gastric activity may have been slowed due to poor health and mobility. This concurred with witness sightings of two men seen acting suspiciously at that time.

Almost the entire volume of a known, low calorie Chinese meal of vegetables, chicken and noodle soup with boiled rice remained within the stomach of a young girl found dead after five days. She was healthy and seemingly untroubled prior to disappearance. The chicken in the soup was cubed and friable, yet remained practically intact (Miller 2008a). Rice grains were abundant and primarily entire. A large volume of low calorie foods such as this meal would be expected to display increased gastric emptying as a result of the triggering of stretch receptors. However, the foods in the stomach were in the same proportions as the last known meal, with relative volume of components also similar. Consequently, it was possible to estimate that the attack commenced within around four hours and quite feasibly within two hours of consumption. The timescale criteria reflected the presence of practically the entire original volume of chicken and rice, relatively intact as consumed, interpreted with reference to data for mixed meals reported by Tröger *et al.* (1987) and Madea (2002). These results helped the enquiry team focus upon a four hours window of opportunity rather than a four days one, helping to focus resources considerably.

14.2.6.8 Other Facts to Consider

The modern habit of 'grazing' means that the potential for snacking between meals must be considered, especially when the last meal is unknown. Consequently, it will not always be feasible to determine what the last meal had been, although snack foods are often highly processed or obviously different to a constructed meal and hence generally remain recognisable. Grazed foods eaten over a period will be subject individually to the same digestive processes as a full meal, so the condition and volume of them within the stomach may also guide indications of duration, although, again, to an estimated window rather than definitively. If grazing is notable, it would be more appropriate to concentrate upon identification of foods to enable corroboration with witness accounts or evidence of purchase. However, regardless of grazing habits, analysis of stomach contents may still provide significant information by expanding the intelligence known regarding movements and actions of the deceased in the hours preceding death.

The potential also exists for the deceased to have eaten the same meal more than once, especially if a person has been absent for days or weeks. Nevertheless, corroboration of findings from the stomach contents with witness intelligence forms a positive line of enquiry to follow, and with this caveat the technique has yielded invaluable results.

An empty stomach can also be a useful indication of time since consumption. The absence of food but significant volume of blood within the stomach of a girl who was badly beaten supported intelligence that she had experienced prolonged violence for more than 24 hours prior to death (Miller 2014). Deceased addicts have often barely eaten, so when only tiny indigestible fried egg protein was recovered from the stomach of a known heroin user found a week after last sighting, it suggested that she probably died on the same evening or following day as she had been given a fried egg roll (Miller 2002). Since the entire digestive system of a substance abuser may function erratically, estimations of timing since last consumption must be a wider window than would be expected for a non-abuser. However, by contrast, the absence of food within the stomach of a healthy man of regular, good eating habits found beaten to death in his pyjamas after four days absence indicated that the assailant arrived before he ate breakfast, his girlfriend having already left for work (Miller 2008b). The girl returned and was also found dead, her last meal at work helping to estimate time of death, as discussed above (Miller 2008a). In this double homicide, stomach contents analysis played a significant part in directing the investigation.

Non-food items also regularly provide intelligence to assist the enquiry. A fragment of golden privet (*Ligustrum ovalifolium* 'Aureum') hedge within the stomach of a girl beaten and left within it to die, indicated that she was still alive when dragged into it following attack elsewhere (Miller 2008c). This was the only hedge of that sort within the surrounding parkland. Vegetation in her hair also located the original attack site some distance away. The presence of a particular undigested meal within the stomach of a drowned man missing for five days helped convict his wife and friend of his murder (Miller 2008d) by determining that digestive transit ceased within a very short period of eating a meal of the same sort. Small quantities of riverbank liverworts, leaf litter and gravel within the stomach also supported the pathologist's interpretation that he was held face down in the banking to drown him. Hairs, fibres, fragments of plastic and other small evidence have also been recovered from the stomachs of victims held face down on carpets or in vehicles; consideration must always be given to the potential significance of such items found.

Stomach contents analysis is greatly under-utilised as a forensic technique, but is now recognised as a valuable source of information. Every case must be assessed individually in terms of both the intelligence to hand and the anticipated results. The technique is not universally applicable, but should always be at least considered in cases of suspicious death, with the entire stomach contents seized for analysis. When frozen, the sample will remain undamaged pending decision for analysis, whether immediately or months later. Estimations on the window of opportunity for attack must err on the side of caution, with due consideration given to the caveats outlined to ensure that valid interpretations of results are obtained. Nevertheless, working within these criteria, stomach contents analysis can have immense value to forensic science and has assisted significantly in numerous situations.

14.3 Conclusion

Forensic botany draws upon established processes utilised by botanists since antiquarian times to interpret past environments, diet and anthropogenic impact. There has been excellent progress within molecular botany in the past few years and there is now a far greater clarity of the potential for plant DNA to have substantial evidential value. The plant kingdom is immense, so there is clearly a long way to go with this, but nevertheless, the future for plant genetics as an established forensic science appears very positive. Elsewhere, the discipline of forensic botany includes a range of very familiar and more recent techniques, all of which require significant identification skills. However, as in every branch of forensic science, the crucial factor in forensic terms is in the interpretation of results, which requires considerable experience and a rounded appreciation of when any particular technique may or may not be valid. For techniques involving contact trace evidence, for example palynology or diatoms, sample size and duration since the crime are critical in determining the usefulness of these analyses. Stomach contents analysis will also not always be feasible, or may require significant caveats, especially when alcohol or drugs misuse are contributing factors. Nevertheless, when relevant, these techniques can provide invaluable information and should never be dismissed out of hand.

Until only 15 years ago, forensic botany was a very under-utilised discipline, primarily due to a lack of understanding on the part of investigating officers. However, practitioners, academics and police scientific advisors have worked hard to increase awareness, which has resulted in a far wider appreciation of value. Now recognised and utilised effectively, the discipline has provided invaluable results to criminal investigation on countless occasions across the entire world. Furthermore, as focused research continues, the applicability and value of plants to forensic science can only increase.

References

Adams-Groom, B. (2012) Forensic palynology. In: Roberts, J. and Marquez-Grant, N. (eds), *Forensic Ecology Handbook: From crime scene to court*. Wiley-Blackwell: West Sussex, pp. 153–168.

Bock, J.H., Lane, M.A. and Norris, D.O. (1988) *Identifying Plant Food Cells in Gastric Contents for Use in Forensic Investigations: A laboratory manual*. National Institute of Justice US Department of Justice: Washington DC.

Bock, J.H. and Norris, D.O. (2005) Forensic botany. In: Byard, R.W., Corey, T., Henderson, C. and Payne-James, J. (eds), *Encyclopaedia of Forensic and Legal Medicine*. Academic Press: Waltham, pp. 332–334.

Brophy, C.M., Moore, J.G., Christian, P.E., Egger, M.J. and Taylor, A.T. (1986) Variability of gastric emptying measurements in man employing standardised radiolabelled meals. *Digestive Diseases and Sciences*, **31**: 799–806.

Brown, A.G. (2006) The use of forensic botany and geology in war crimes investigations in NE Bosnia. *Forensic Science International*, **163**: 204–210.

Burnett, J.H. (1964) (ed.) *The Vegetation of Scotland*. Oliver and Boyd: Edinburgh.

Cameron, N.G. (2004) The use of diatom analysis in forensic geoscience. In: Pye, K. and Croft, D.J. (eds), *Forensic Geoscience: Principles, techniques and applications*. Geological Society: London, pp. 277–280.

Cappers, R.T.J., Bekker, R.M. and Jans, J.E. (2006) *Digital Seed Atlas of The Netherlands*. Barkhuis Publishing: Groningen.

Chan, L.-N. (2008) Opioid analgesics and the gastrointestinal tract. *Practical Gasteroenterology*, **54**; 37–50.

Craft, K.J., Owens, J.D. and Ashley, M.V. (2007) Application of plant DNA markers in forensic botany: genetic comparison of *Quercus* evidence leaves to crime scene trees using microsatellites. *Forensic Science International*, **165**: 64–70.

Dawson, L.A. and Mayes, R.W. (2015) Criminal and environmental soil forensics: soil as physical evidence in forensic investigations. In: Murphy, B.L. and Morrison, R.D. (eds), *Introduction to Environmental Forensics*. Academic Press: Waltham, pp. 457–486.

Dickson, C.A. and Dickson, J.H. (2000) *Plants and People in Ancient Scotland*. Tempus: Stroud.

Dickson, J.H., Hofbauer, W., Porley, R., Schmidl, A, Kofler, W. and Oeggl, K. (2009) Six mosses from the Tyrolean Iceman's alimentary tract and their significance for his ethnobotany and events of his last days. *Vegetation History and Archaeobotany*, **18**: 13–22.

DiMaio, V.J. and DiMaio, D. (2001) *Forensic Pathology*. CRC Press: London.

Esau, K. (1965) *Plant Anatomy*. Wiley & Sons Inc: London.

Esau, K. (1977) *Anatomy of Seed Plants*. Wiley & Sons Inc: London.

Ferri, G., Corradini, B., Ferrari F., Santunione, A.L., Palazzoli, F. and Alu, M. (2015) Forensic botany II, DNA barcode for land plants: which markers after the international agreement? *Forensic Science International Genetics*, **15**: 131–136.

Gale, R. and Cutler, D. (2000) *Plants in Archaeology*. Westbury Publishing: Otley.

Grover, M. and Camilleri, M. (2013) Effects on gastrointestinal functions and symptoms of serotonergic psychoactive agents used in functional gastrointestinal diseases. *Journal of Gastroenterology*, **48**: 177–181.

Gurevitch, J., Scheiner, S.M. and Fox, G.A. (2006) *The Ecology of Plants*. Sinauer, Sunderland MA.

Hall, D.W. (1997) Forensic botany. In: Haglund, W.D. and Sorg, M.H. (eds), *Forensic Taphonomy and the Post-Mortem Fate of Human Remains*. CRC Press: New York, pp. 353–366.

Hall, D.W. and Byrd, J.H. (2012) *Forensic Botany: A practical guide*. Wiley-Blackwell: Oxford.

Hawksworth, D.L. and Wiltshire, P.E. (2011) Forensic mycology: the use of fungi in criminal investigations. *Forensic Science International*, **206**: 1–11.

Helbaek, H. (1950) Botanical study of the stomach contents of the Tollund Man. *Aarbøger for Nordisk Oldkyndighed og Historie*, pp. 329–341.

Helbaek, H. (1958) The last meal of Grauballe Man: an analysis of food remains in the stomach. *Kuml*, pp. 83–116.

Holden, T.G. (1995) The last meals of the Lindow Bog Man. In: Turner, R.C. and Scaife, R.G. (eds), *Bog Bodies. New Discoveries and New Perspectives*. British Museum: London, pp. 76–82.

Hollingsworth, P.M., Forrest, L.L., Spouge, J.L., Hajibabaei, M., Ratnasingham, S. *et al.* (2009) A DNA barcode for land plants. *National Academy of Sciences of the USA*, **106**: 12794–12797.

Horowitz, M. and Pounder, D.J. (1985) Gastric emptying – forensic implications of current concepts. *Medicine, Science and the Law*, **25**: 201–214.

Horrocks, M.J. and Walsh, K.A.J. (1998) Forensic palynology: assessing the value of the evidence. *Review of Palaeobotany and Palynology*, **103**: 69–74.

Horrocks, M.J., Coulson, S.A. and Walsh, K.A.J. (1999) Forensic palynology variation in the pollen content of soil on shoes and in shoe prints in soil. *Journal of Forensic Science*, **44**: 119–122.

Knight, B. (2002) The use of gastric contents in estimating time since death. In: Knight, B. (ed.), *The Estimation of the Time since Death in the Early Postmortem Period*. Arnold: London, pp. 209–215.

Koopman, W.J.M., Kuiper, I., Klein-Geltink, D.J.A., Sabatino, G.J.H. and Smulders, M.J.M. (2012) Botanical DNA evidence in criminal cases: knotgrass (*Polygonum aviculare* L.) as a model species. *Forensic Science International Genetics*, **6**: 366–374.

Lane, M.A., Anderson, L.C., Barkley, T.M., Bock, J.H., Gifford, E.M. *et al.* (1990) Forensic botany. Plants, perpetrators, pests, poisons and pot. *BioScience*, **40**: 34–39.

Madea, B. (2002) Gastric contents and time since death. In: Knight, B. (ed.), *The Estimation of the Time since Death in the Early Postmortem Period*, Arnold: London, pp. 215–225.

Marumo, Y. and Yanai, H.J. (1986) Morphological analysis of opal phytoliths for soil discrimination in forensic science investigation. *Journal of Forensic Sciences*, **31**: 1039–1049.

McCallum, R.W., Soykan, I., Srindhar, K.R., Ricci, D.A., Lange, R.C. and Plankey, M.W. (1999) Delta-9-tetrahydrocannabinol delays the gastric emptying of solid food in humans: a double-blind, randomized study. *Alimentary Pharmacology & Therapeutics*, **13**: 77–80.

Mildenhall, D.C., Wiltshire, P.E.J. and Bryant, V.M. (2006) Forensic palynology: why do it and how it works. *Forensic Science International*, **163**: 163–172.

Miller, J. (1998a) GUARD 1501198 Murder of Manus O'Donnell PFR: T981048 Strathclyde Police.

Miller, J. (1998b) GUARD 1500398 Murder of Margot Lafferty PFR: T98211 Strathclyde Police.

Miller, J. (2002) GUARD 1502902 Murder of Amy Anderson CR: LA01670502 Strathclyde Police.

Miller, J. (2003) GUARD 1505703 Murder of Vicki Elliot CR: KA02390603 Strathclyde Police.

Miller, J. (2004) GUARD 1508604 Murder of Darren Manders CR: 300166160 Cleveland Police.

Miller, J. (2005a) GUARD 1514105 Death of Scott McMinn CR: KA99990205 Strathclyde Police.

Miller, J. (2005b) GUARD 1513205 Murder of Courtney Davies CR: 300363118 Gloucestershire Constabulary.

Miller, J. (2005c) GUARD 1515205 Murder of Brian Diver CR: QA05070505 Strathclyde Police.

Miller, J. (2006) GUARD 1517506 Body Recovery, Westering Gailes Golf Course, Irvine 0106 Strathclyde Police.

Miller, J. (2008a) GUARD 1524108 Croydon Road Murders, Northumbria Constabulary.

Miller, J. (2008b) GUARD 1524308 Croydon Road Murders, Northumbria Constabulary.

Miller, J. (2008c) GUARD 1523608 Murder of Moira Jones CR: GE05880508 Strathclyde Police.

Miller, J. (2008d) GUARD 1523308 Operation Tower, West Mercia Constabulary.

Miller, J. (2009) GUARD 1526509 Operation Nepal, Surrey Constabulary.

Miller, J. (2013) Northlight Heritage NHF4350161 Operation Sandpiper, Police Scotland.

Miller, J. (2014) York Archaeological Trust DLF5000171 Operation Cabrini, Police Scotland.

Miller-Coyle, H., Ladd, C., Palmbach, T. and Lee, H.C. (2001) The green revolution: botanical contributions to forensics and drug enforcement *Croation Medical Journal*, **42**: 340–345.
Miller-Coyle, H. (2005) (ed.) *Forensic Botany: Principles and applications to criminal casework*. CRC Press: Bota Racon.
Moore, J.G., Christian, P.E., Brown, J.A., Brophy, C. *et al.* (1984) Influence of meal weight and calorific content on gastric emptying of meals in man. *Digestive Diseases and Sciences*, **29**: 513–519.
Moore, P.D., Webb, J.A. and Collinson, M.E. (1991) *Pollen Analysis*. Blackwell Scientific Publications: Oxford.
Morgan, R.M., French, J., O'Donnell. L. and Bull, P.A. (2010) The re-incorporation and redistribution of trace geoforensic particulates on clothing. *Science and Justice*, **50**: 195–199.
Oeggl, K., Kofler, W., Schmidl, A., Dickson, J.H. *et al.* (2007) The reconstruction of the last itinerary of Ötzi, the Neolithic iceman by pollen analyses from sequentially sampled gut contents. *Quaternary Science Reviews*, **26**: 853–861.
Petring, O.U. and Blake, D.W. (1993) Gastric emptying in adults: an overview related to anaesthesia. *Anaesthesia and Intensive Care*, **21**: 774–781.
Pokines, J. and Symes, S.A. (2013) *Manual of Forensic Taphonomy*. CRC Press: Boca Raton.
Robertson, J. (2013) Botany. In: Segal, J.A. and Saukko, P.J. (eds), *Encyclopaedia of Forensic Sciences*. Elsevier Science Publishing: London, pp. 217–221.
Schweingruber, F.H. (1990) *Anatomy of European Woods*. Haupt: Berne and Stuttgart.
Scott, K.R., Morgan, R.M., Jones, V.J. and Cameron, N.G. (2014) The transferability of diatoms to clothing and the methods appropriate for their collection and analysis in forensic geoscience. *Forensic Science International*, **241**:.127–137.
Smith, A.J.E. (2004) *The Moss Flora of Britain and Ireland*. Cambridge University Press: Cambridge.
Tröger, H.D., Baur, C. and Spann, K.W. (1987) *Mageninhalt und Todeszeitbestimmung*. Schmidt-Römhild.
Virtanen, V., Korpelainen, H. and Kostamo, K. (2007) Forensic botany: usability of bryophyte material in forensic studies. *Forensic Science International*, **172**: 161–163.
Walsh, K.W. and Horrocks, M.J. (2008) Palynology: it's position in the field of forensic science. *Forensic Science*. **53**: 1053–1060.
Ward, J., Peakall, R., Gilmore, S.R. and Robertson, J. (2005) A molecular identification system for grasses: a novel technology for forensic botany. *Forensic Science International*, **152**: 121–131.
Willey, P. and Heilman, A. (1987) Estimating time since death using plant roots and stems. *Journal of Forensic Sciences*, **32**: 1264–1270.
Wiltshire, P.E.J. (2006a) Hair as a source of forensic evidence in murder investigations. *Forensic Science International*, **162**: 241–248.
Wiltshire, P.E.J. (2006b) Consideration of some taphonomic variables of relevance to forensic palynological investigation in the United Kingdom. *Forensic Science International*, **163**: 173–182.
Wiltshire, P.E.J. (2009) Forensic ecology, botany and palynology: some aspects of their role in criminal investigation. In: Ritz, K., Dawson, L.A. and Miller, D. (eds), *Criminal and Environmental Soil Forensics*. Springer: London, pp. 129–149.
Wiltshire, P.E.J. (2010) Forensic ecology. In: White, P.C. (ed.), *Crime Scene to Court: The essentials of forensic science*. RSC Publishing: Cambridge, pp. 54–85.
Wiltshire, P.E.J. and Black, S. (2006) The cribriform approach to the retrieval of palynological evidence from the turbinates of murder victims. *Forensic Science International*, **163**: 224–230.
Winton, A.L. (1916) *The Microscopy of Vegetable Food*., Chapman & Hall Ltd: London.
Yin, J., Song, J., Lei, Y., Xu, X. and Chen, J.D.Z. (2014) Prokinetic effects of Mirtazapine on gastrointestinal transit. *American Journal of Physiology: Gastrointestinal Liver Physiology*, **306**: 796–801.

15

The Effects of Weathering on Bone Preservation

Soren Blau

15.1 Introduction

When a report on skeletal remains is being prepared, whether by an osteologist, zooarchaeologist, palaeontologist or forensic anthropologist, the initial part of the report typically includes a description of the preservation of the bones. In addition to commenting on how much of the skeleton survives (complete or partial), descriptions of modifications that may be determined by cultural (e.g. burial) and/or natural taphonomic (e.g. exposure) factors are provided (Henderson 1987). Such descriptions of preservation are vital as they define the framework for understanding the types of questions that can be addressed and justify the level of detail provided in a report. For example, the amount of information about a case involving a complete and well-preserved human skeleton will be different from one that only includes a fragmentary burnt human cranium.

Processes that modify skeletal remains include burning, animal activity (e.g. digestion, scavenging, trampling), trauma, chemical alterations, burial, excavation, laboratory procedures and weathering (Dirkmaat and Adovasio 1997; Manifold 2012). The latter process is the focus of this chapter. The term 'weathering' was first used in the disciplines of geology and geomorphology to describe the breakdown of rocks, soils and minerals through various forces including physical/mechanical (e.g. expanses of water when it freezes, exfoliation, thermal, etc.), chemical (water and gases) and/or biological (roots, fungi, lichens etc.). Some of the earliest studies of weathering by geologists date back to the late 19th century (Burt *et al.* 2008; Chorley *et al.* 2009). More recently, the term has been employed by palaeontologists, archaeologists (specifically zooarchaeologists) and forensic anthropologists interested in taphonomy to describe the post-mortem processes that alter the chemical (Gill-King 1997; White and Hannus 1983) or physical nature (Haglund and Sorg 2002) of human or non-human skeletal remains and/or teeth. Because the term applies to the hard tissue, weathering is distinguished from decomposition, which refers to the degeneration of soft tissues (Beary and Lyman 2012). While some practitioners (particularly archaeologists) refer to weathering as applying to skeletal remains when exposed at the surface (Haglund *et al.* 2002), others discuss the degradation resulting from subaerial or subsurface contexts (Beary and Lyman 2012; Junod and Pokines 2013).

15.2 A Brief History of Weathering Studies

The majority of research on bone weathering has been experimental and conducted using animal models (e.g. Bertrand and Oxenham 2014; Cunningham *et al.* 2011; Janjua and Rogers 2008;

Taphonomy of Human Remains: Forensic Analysis of the Dead and the Depositional Environment, First Edition.
Edited by Eline M.J. Schotsmans, Nicholas Márquez-Grant and Shari L. Forbes.

Miller 1975). Much of the work has been undertaken within the discipline of palaeontology and despite the macroscopic and microscopic differences between human and non-human remains (e.g. Adams and Crabtree 2008; Harsanyi 1992) the results were subsequently extrapolated to apply to human skeletal remains. Miller (1975) undertook a study of cattle and horses after they died in the Tierra Blanca Mountains of the Colorado Desert in California. Miller (1975) provided one of the first descriptions of the effects on bone from exposure in a desert environment equating the changes with time (Table 15.1).

However, it was the palaeobiologist Anna Kay Behrensmeyer whose study on bone weathering and the development of weathering stages has become seminal. Behrensmeyer (1978) used known times and seasons of death of large mammals (>11 lbs) from a number of habitats (including swamp, dense woodland, open woodland, plains, bush and lakebed) in the Amboseli Basin in southern Kenya to develop a six-stage key to facilitate the description of weathering of bone over time (Table 15.2). The aim of this work was to be able to utilise the stages to comment on time since death (see below). However, climatic and environmental differences mean Behrensmeyer's stages are not always applicable worldwide (see below, Table 15.2).

Despite the development of weathering stages (Behrensmeyer 1978), White's study of prehistoric cannibalism at Mancos in Colorado (1992) identified problems distinguishing heated, cooked and burned bone from weathered bone in an archaeological sample. More recent research has focused on the effects of weathering on specific age ranges (e.g. foetal bones; Huxley 1998) and anatomical areas such as teeth (Hughes and White 2009).

15.3 Variables that Influence Weathering

The potential effects of weathering on the physical and/or chemical nature of the cortical and/or trabecular bone are numerous. The changes may take the form or cracking/fracturing, flaking, shrinkage, warping, exfoliation, desiccation, polishing and/or grooving (caused by root and/or animal actions). Colour changes may also occur as a result of fungal growth, thermal effects and/or oxidation as a

Table 15.1 Description of bone weathering in a desert environment as provided by Miller (1975).

Time since death	Description
<1 year	<5% of the periosteum has been completely removed from the articulated bones; not more than one small longitudinal crack per long bone.
1 year	c. 25% of the periosteum is gone; exposed parts of the bone are bleached white; 2–3 longitudinal cracks have appeared and go right through the compact bone and into the marrow cavity.
? 2 years	Transverse cracks appear.
>4 years	Expect for some places where the bone is covered by sand, all the periosteum is gone; some long bones are still articulated; all exposed bone is thoroughly bleached white; exfoliation is just beginning and the surfaces of the bones are slightly powdery.
>18 years	Most of the organic material is gone, although parts of the bones that are covered with sand retain a brownish colour. The bone begins to lose the brilliant white colour of freshly bleached bone and starts to change to a dull greyish colour; exfoliation rapidly increases and many cracks and splinters are produced.
31–34 years	Severe deterioration, a dull grey colour with many cracks and splinters. The bone is so badly weathered that it is doubtful if fossilisation can take place.

Table 15.2 Stages of bone weathering as developed by Behrensmeyer 1978: p. 151 and adapted by Ross and Cunningham 2011, Table 1: p. 127.

Stage	Range in Years Since Death	Description
0	0–1	Fresh, de-fleshed bone which is still greasy and the bone surface shows no sign of cracking or flaking due to weathering. Marrow cavities contain tissue; skin and muscle/ligament may cover part or the entire bone surface.
1	0–3 or 4	Bone shows cracking, normally along the length of the bone; some soft tissue may still be present. Articular surfaces may show mosaic cracking of covering tissue as well as in the bone itself.
2a	2–6 or 7	Outermost concentric thin layers of bone show flaking, usually associated with cracks. Long thin flakes, with one or more sides still attached to the bone, are common; soft tissue may still be present.
2b	2–6 or 7	Deeper and more extensive flaking follows, until most of the outermost bone is gone. Crack edges are usually angular in cross-section. Remnants of ligaments, cartilage and skin may be present.
3	4–15+	Bone surface is characterised by patches of rough, homogeneously weathered compact bone resulting in a fibrous texture. Top-most layer of bone has almost completely flaked off. Weathering does not penetrate deeper than 1.0–1.5 mm at this stage, and bone fibres are still firmly attached to each other. Crack edges usually are rounded in cross-section. Soft tissue rarely present at this stage.
4	6–15+	The bone surface is coarsely fibrous and rough in texture; large and small splinters occur and may be loose enough to fall away from the bone when it is moved. Weathering penetrates into inner cavities. Cracks are open and have splintered or rounded edges.
5	6–15+	Inner, trabecular bone is exposed and bone is falling apart. Original bone shape may be difficult to determine.

result of contact with metals (Oller *et al.* 2012) or minerals such as manganese in the burial matrix (Junod and Pokines 2013).

While it has been argued that sunlight is the weathering force that 'causes the greatest post-mortem changes to the skeleton' (Byers 2011), in reality, there are a number of intrinsic (biological factors) and extrinsic variables (environmental and human actions) that may influence weathering processes. The interaction of these variables and the subsequent effects on bone is complex.

Intrinsic variables include:

- *Taxon*: determining whether the remains are human or non-human is important because weathering rates vary across taxa (Lyman and Fox 1997), predominantly related to the size of different species (see below);
- *Bone type and size*: the shape of the specific skeletal element may influence the degree of weathering which typically proceeds along lines of structural weakness in the bone (Brehensmeyer 1978). Stodder's 2008 study showed for example, that larger, denser bones illustrate differential weathering patterns because of their increased bone density (see also Willey *et al.* 1997). A large bone with greater surface area also provides an increased interface with ion solutions in soils and therefore, potentially increased chemical weathering (Gill-King 1997). The size of the skeletal element, either as a result of anatomical difference or age of the individual, is also an influencing factor (Janjua and Rogers 2008). Research undertaken on short-term changes (those occurring within a year) to juvenile domestic pigs as a proxy for human children found that '[l]ong tubular bones, including

long bones, metacarpals, metatarsals and phalanges, were more prone to flaking of the outer layers of cortical bone, while long bones, vertebrae, and ribs were more likely to have loss of bone at the articular facets, leading to exposure of interior trabecular bone' (Cunningham *et al.* 2011).

Extrinsic variables that may affect the weathering process include:

- *Environment*: soil type and pH levels, water (humidity, annual precipitation and groundwater), temperature, flora and fauna potentially play a role in the rate, sequence and appearance of the bone weathering process (Marden *et al.* 2013). The effects of different environments and climatic zones on weathering and bone preservation have been widely discussed in the literature, for example arid (Andrews and Whybrow 2005); semi-arid (Littleton 2000); cold (Marceau 2007; Passalacqua and Rainwater 2006); warm temperate (Andrews 1995; Andrews and Cook 1985); and tropical (Behrensmeyer 1978; Ross and Cunningham 2011) (Table 15.3).
- *Time and events that occurred between death and recovery*: In addition to environmental variables, the method of disposing of a deceased individual (e.g. burying, entombing, leaving on the surface, submerging, cremating, etc. or a combination of methods) will also influence the effects of weathering on bone. For example, disarticulated surface skeletal remains (Haglund 1997) or remains that are washed ashore (Nawrocki *et al.* 1997) or onto higher ground (Littleton 2000) are more exposed to weathering than the remains of individuals who are buried. If a deceased individual is deposited on the surface and the remains are exposed to the sun and heat, skeletal remains lose their collagen content and become dry and bleached, often resulting in the creation of small fractures. Once small fractures occur, moisture can seep into the crevices and expand as the temperatures decrease, often resulting in exfoliation of the bone surface (Haglund *et al.* 2002).

15.4 The Value of Bone Weathering Analyses in Forensic Investigations

In forensic investigations involving human skeletal remains, the examination of bone weathering can be of value, as outlined below.

15.4.1 Estimating Time Since Death

It has been argued that weathering, in association with awareness of decomposition and entomological data, forms part of the study of forensic taphonomy and is important in attempting to estimate a time since death or post-mortem interval (PMI) (Haglund and Sorg 1997). Although Behrensmeyer's (1978) stages have been employed by archaeologists (specifically zooarchaeologists) and palaeontologists, the ability to extrapolate an estimate of time since death from a description of weathering in prehistoric contexts has been questioned. This is predominantly because of variables that influence weathering such as dispositional microenvironment, exposure duration and accumulation history being generally unknown. Consequently, in contemporary contexts where variables such as environmental data are more accessible, relating weathering stages to a time since death estimate may be less difficult (Beary and Lyman 2012). Often however, the time span between death, discovery and recovery of remains in a forensic context is relatively short which, it has been argued, may result in limited effects of weathering on skeletal remains (Beary and Lyman 2012).

With the exception of Bielenstein's (1990 cited in Ubelaker 1997) research that demonstrated that Behrensmeyer's (1978) stages of bone weathering could be applied to modern forensic cases, very little research in weathering has actually been undertaken in forensic contexts. This is because weathering studies take time and often those involved in one to two year Masters or three to four year

Table 15.3 Summary of the effects of different environments and climatic zones on weathering and bone preservation.

Place	Environment	Climatic zone	Years since death (in years unless otherwise stated)	Length of Observations	Exposed (years)	Summary of Bone scores (after Behrensmeyer 1978)	Comment	Reference
Amboseli National park, Kenya	Various: swamp, dense woodland, open woodland, plains, bush and seasonally dry lakebed.	Tropical	Several	Over a 2 year period	3 or less	0-2	35 large animals; surface remains	Behrensmeyer 1978
					1	1		
					4–6	3–5		
					7–9	3–4		
					10-12	5		
Isla de Coiba, off the coast of Panama	Not described	Tropical	<10	3 years	N/A	1	14 burials; buried	Ross and Cunningham 2011
			10–15	3 years	N/A	1		
			15–20	3 years	N/A	2		
			20–30	3 years	N/A	3		
			30+	3 years	N/A	4		
Parc National des Virunga, Democratic Republic of the Congo	Grassy savannah	Equatorial	?	?	2–4	1–2	6000 surface remains; surface remains	Tappen 1994
			2	?	2	1-2	Recently skeletonised buffalo; surface remains	
			4	?	4	2		
Ituri, Democratic Republic of the Congo	Rainforest	Equatorial	?	?	>7	0	118 elephant bones; surface remains	
			?	?	16	0		
			?	?	>15	1–3		
	Large granite rock exposed to sunlight	Equatorial	?	?	1.3	1	Juvenile elephant; surface remains	
Somerset, England	Limestone, outcrop in woodland area	Warm temperate	8	Observed annually for 8 years	?	0	1 juvenile cow; surface remains	Andrews and Cook 1985

(*continued*)

Table 15.3 *(continued)*

Place	Environment	Climatic zone	Years since death (in years unless otherwise stated)	Length of Observations	Exposed (years)	Summary of Bone scores (after Behrensmeyer 1978)	Comment	Reference
Rhulen, Wales	Various (woodland, moorland, hill tops, valley floor)	Warm temperate	10–12	?	?	1	150 large and small animals; surface remains	Andrews and Cook 1985
			19	?	?	2		
Abu Dhabi, United Arab Emirates	Coastal	Arid	2	Every few years for 15 years		0–1	Adult camel; surface remains	Andrews and Whybrow 2005
			4–8	?		1		
			10–15	?		2–3		
Western New South Wales, Australia	River basin and associated tributaries	Semi-arid	?	3	?	Various	200 human burials in four different sites	Littleton 2000
Southern Ontario, Canada	Clearings in a mixed coniferous and deciduous tree forest	0-25° C	0–1 months	Often	Over 291 days	1	24 defleshed pig femora, 1 defleshed humerus and 25 metatarsals; surface remains	Janjua and Rogers 2008
			1–2 months			2		
			2–6 months			3		
			6–9.5 months			4		

doctoral research do not have the time span necessary to fully understand and complete detailed weathering studies (Beary and Lyman 2012). Furthermore, it has been argued that time since death estimates based on weathering studies will not provide the detail that is required in a forensic context (Beary and Lyman 2012).

In summary, the study of weathering is part of a suite of tools that is used to estimate the post-mortem interval (PMI) or time since death. However, compared to entomology and chemical-physical tests, weathering together with the assessment of floral and faunal evidence is considered less accurate (Dirkmaat and Adovasio 1997). While some authors suggest weathering can provide time since death intervals from months to years (Forbes 2008), Beary and Lyman (2012) concluded that 'the degree to which weathering can be used as an estimator of PMI prior to degradation remains largely unknown.'

15.4.2 Differentiating Peri- and Post-Mortem Trauma

In the same way that understanding the effects of weathering on non-human (animal) skeletal remains has been important in differentiating bones that have been altered by natural causes compared to animal bones that have been intentionally modified into human tools and artefacts (Miller 1975), understanding weathering assists the forensic anthropologist (and forensic pathologist) to differentiate post-mortem damage from peri-mortem trauma (Cale and Rogers 2007; Symes *et al.* 2012). While 'weathering cracks can resemble those produced by blunt force trauma' (Ubelaker 1997; see also Nawrocki 2009), and 'spiral fractures are found to occur as a result of natural weathering' (Hill 1976), typically, post-mortem fractures can be differentiated from those that occurred peri-mortem. Because the skeleton responds to force differently when it is covered with soft tissue (i.e. the bone is 'green') compared to when it is old and dry, there are a number of characteristics that facilitate differentiating peri- from post-mortem trauma. In addition to differences in colour and sharpness of the breaks, the rate of weathering of the edges of the fracture and exposed internal surfaces will be more extreme if the fractures occur post-mortem (Crist *et al.* 1997).

15.4.3 Interpreting Treatment of the Deceased around the Time of Burial

Understanding different weathering patterns has also been useful in providing information for reconstructing how the deceased was treated around the time of burial, that is, the sequence of events leading to burial or deposition. For example, in their work on the American Battle of Little Bighorn, Scott and Conner (1997) described how the left side of many of the skeletal remains showed different weathering patterns to the rest of the body. This pattern suggested that the left side of the body had been exposed after the soft tissue had decomposed and before reburial (Scott and Connor 1997).

Ubelaker (1997) summarises a forensic case presented by Mann and Owsley (1992), in which a human skeleton associated with a shotgun was discovered in a farmer's field. An examination of the weathering of the bones of the pelvis in conjunction with an analysis of the skeletal defects facilitated an interpretation of the sequence of post-mortem events: the individual had been lying in the field for some time before the perforations made by pellets occurred.

15.4.4 Assessing the Potential for DNA Analysis

Forensic anthropologists are often asked to take samples for DNA analysis. Although weathering may significantly alter the physical appearance of bone, Misner *et al.*'s (2009) work showed that despite the bone's appearance (e.g. fragmentary with erosion of the cortical bone), the quality and quantity of DNA was not influenced by general skeletal weathering or the individual bone weathering state

(Misner *et al.* 2009). Similar findings have been documented by Quincey *et al.* (2013) during their work on DNA sex determination from degraded bone samples.

15.5 Conclusion

The effects of weathering on the preservation of skeletal remains and teeth have been widely discussed in the literature as part of the suite of post-mortem taphonomic changes. However, a review of forensic taphonomy research listed in the *Proceedings of the American Academy of Forensic Sciences* between 2002 and 2009 showed that studies of weathering were the least represented (Beary and Lyman 2012). Beary and Lyman (2012) suggested these results indicate that researchers see little benefit in conducting weathering studies. This is more than likely because the number of factors potentially involved and their interaction in the weathering process is complex (Christensen *et al.* 2014). Although there has been an attempt to develop a set of descriptions of weathering stages to facilitate understanding time since death intervals (Behrensmeyer 1978), the complexity of the weathering process is highlighted by the fact that there are extreme differences between sites located within the same geographic region (Ross and Cunningham 2011). Nonetheless, experimental research on the effects of weathering on bone continues to be undertaken in different environments around the world (e.g. Australia – Menzies 2016; New Zealand – Dudley 2016). Due to the increase in access to forensic research facilities which use donated bodies such research will inevitably shift away from using animal models to understand the effects of weathering on human skeletal remains.

Acknowledgements

I am grateful for the comments provided on a draft of this chapter by Jillian Garvey and the reviewers.

References

Adams, B.J. and Crabtree, P.J. (2008) (eds) *Comparative Skeletal Anatomy: A photographic atlas for medical examiners, coroners, forensic anthropologists and archaeologists.* Humana Press: Totowa.

Andrews, P. and Cook, J. (1985) Natural modifications to bones in a temperate setting. *Man*, **20**: 675–691.

Andrews, P. (1995) Experiments in taphonomy. *Journal of Archaeological Science*, **22**: 147–153.

Andrews, P. and Whybrow, P. (2005) Taphonomic observations on a camel skeleton in a desert environment in Abu Dhabi. *Palaeontologia Electronica*, **8**: 1–17.

Beary, M.O. and Lyman, R.L. (2012) The use of taphonomy in forensic anthropology: Past trends and future prospects. In: Dirkmaat, D.C. (ed.), *A Companion to Forensic Anthropology.* Wiley-Blackwell: Chichester, pp. 499–527.

Behrensmeyer, A.K. (1978) Taphonomic and ecological information from bone weathering. *Paleobiology.* **4**: 150–162.

Bertrand, J. and Oxenham, M.F. (2014) Low-temperature-induced bone shrinkage: a controlled study using kangaroo femora. *Australian Journal of Forensic Sciences*, **47**: 1–9.

Bielenstein, D.E.M. (1990) *Forensic Taphonomy: Definitions and applications to forensic anthropology and paleoanthropology.* Unpublished Master's Thesis, George Washington University, Washington DC.

Burt, T.P., Chorley, R.J., Brunsden, D., Cox, N.J. and Goudie, A.S. (2008) *The History of the Study of Landforms of the Development of Geomorphology.* The Geological Society Publishing House: Bath.

Byers, S.N. (2011) *Introduction to Forensic Anthropology.* Pearson: Boston.

Cale, S. and Rogers, T. (2007) Taphonomic changes to blunt force trauma: a preliminary study. *Journal of Forensic Sciences*, **48**: 717–724.

Chorley, R.J., Dunn, A.J. and Beckinsale, R.P. (2009) *The History of the Study of Landforms or the Development of Geomorphology*. Routledge: Oxford.

Christensen, A.M., Passalacqua, N.V. and Bartelink, E.J. (2014) *Forensic Anthropology: Current Methods and Practice*. Academic Press: Oxford.

Crist, T.A.J., Washburn, A., Park, H., Hood, I. and Hickey, M.A. (1997) Cranial bones displacement as a taphonomic process in potential child abuse cases. In: Haglund, W.D. and Sorg, M.C. (eds), *Forensic Taphonomy: The postmortem fate of human remains*. CRC Press: Boca Raton, pp. 331–348.

Cunningham, S.L., Kirkland, S.A. and Ross, A.H. (2011) Bone weathering of juvenile-sized remains in the North Carolina Piedmont. In: Ross, A.H. and Abel, S.M. (eds), *The Juvenile Skeleton in Forensic Abuse Investigations*. Springer: New York, pp. 179–196.

Dirkmaat, D.C. and Adovasio, J.M. (1997) The role of archaeology in the recovery and interpretation of human remains from an outdoor forensic setting. In: Haglund, W.D. and Sorg, M.H. (eds), *Forensic Taphonomy: The postmortem fate of human remains*. CRC Press: Boca Raton, pp. 53–78.

Dudley, J.M. (2016) Post-mortem interval of skeletal remains in New Zealand. Paper presented at the Australian and New Zealand Forensic Science Society 23rd International Symposium on the Forensic Sciences. Auckland, New Zealand.

Forbes, S.L. (2008) Potential determinants of postmortem and postburial interval of buried remains. In: Tibbett, M. and Carter, D.O. (eds), *Soil Analysis in Forensic Taphonomy: Chemical and biological effects of buried human remains*. CRC Press: Boca Raton, pp. 225–246.

Gill-King, H. (1997) Chemical and ultastructural aspects of decomposition. In: Haglund, W.D. and Sorg, M.H. (eds), *Forensic Taphonomy: The postmortem fate of human remains*. CRC Press: Boca Raton, pp. 105–120.

Haglund, W.D. and Sorg, M.C. (1997) Method and theory of forensic taphonomy research. In: Haglund, W.D. and Sorg, M.H. (eds), *Forensic Taphonomy: The postmortem fate of human remains*. CRC Press: Boca Raton, pp. 27–40.

Haglund, W.D. (1997) Dogs and coyotes: Postmortem involvement with human remains. In: Haglund, W.D. and Sorg, M.H. (eds), *Forensic Taphonomy: The postmortem fate of human remains*. CRC Press: Boca Raton, pp. 376–390.

Haglund, W.D. and Sorg, M.H. (eds), (2002) *Advances in Forensic Taphonomy: Method, theory and archaeological perspective*. CRC Press: London, pp. 133–150.

Haglund, W.D., Connor, M. and Scott, D.D. (2002) The effect of cultivation on buried human remains. In: Haglund, W.D. and Sorg, M.H. (eds), *Advances in Forensic Taphonomy: Method, theory and archaeological perspective*. CRC Press: London, pp. 133–150.

Harsanyi, L. (1992) Differential diagnosis of human and animal bone. In: Grupe, G. and Garland, E.N. (eds), *Histology of Ancient Human Bone: Methods and diagnosis*. Springer-Verlag: Berlin, pp. 79–94.

Henderson, J. (1987) Factors determining the state of preservation of human remains. In: Boddington, A., Garland, A.N. and Janaway, R.C. (eds), *Death, Decay and Reconstruction: Approaches to archaeology and forensic science*. Manchester University Press: Manchester, pp. 43–54.

Hill, A.P. (1976) On carnivore and weathering damage to bone. *Current Anthropology*, **17**: 335–336.

Hughes, C.E. and White, C.A. (2009) Crack propagation in teeth: A comparison of perimortem and postmortem behaviour of dental material and cracks. *Journal of Forensic Sciences*, **54**: 263–266.

Huxley, A.K. (1998) Analysis of shrinkage in human fatal diaphysis lengths from fresh to dry bone using Peterson and Kohler's data. *Journal of Forensic Sciences*, **43**: 423–426.

Janjua, M.A. and Rogers, T..L (2008) Bone weathering patterns of metatarsal v. femur and the post-mortem interval in Southern Ontario. *Forensic Science International*, **178**: 16–23.

Junod, C.A. and Pokines, J.T. (2013) Subaerial weathering. In: Pokines, J. and Symes, S.A. (eds), *Manual of Forensic Taphonomy*. CRC Press: Boca Raton, pp. 287–314.

Littleton, J. (2000) Taphonomic effects of erosion on deliberately buried bodies. *Journal of Archaeological Science*, **27**: 5–18.

Lyme, R.L. and Fox, G.L. (1997) A critical review of bone weathering as an indication of bone assemblage formation. In: Haglund, W.D. and Sorg, M.H. (eds), *Forensic Taphonomy: The postmortem fate of human remains*. CRC Press: Boca Raton, pp. 223–247.

Manifold, B.M. (2012) Intrinsic and extrinsic factors involved in the preservation of non-adult skeletal remains in archaeology and forensic science. *Bulletin of the International Association for Paleodontology*, **6**: 51–69.

Mann, R.W. and Owsley, D.W. (1992) Human osteology: Key to the sequence of events in postmortem shooting. *Journal of Forensic Sciences*, **37**: 1386–1392.

Marceau, C.M. (2007) *Bone Weathering in a Cold Climate: Forensic applications of a field experiment using animal models*. Unpublished MA Thesis, University of Alberta.

Marden, K., Sorg, M.H. and Haglund, W.D. (2013) Taphonomy. In: Di Gangi, E.A. and Moore, M.K. (eds), *Research Methods in Human Skeletal Biology*. Elsevier: London, pp. 241–262.

Menzies, J. (2016) A taphonomic experiment near Belanglo State Forest seeks to improve the estimation of time since death for skeletal remains in Australia. Paper presented at the Australian and New Zealand Forensic Science Society 23rd International Symposium on the Forensic Sciences. Auckland, New Zealand.

Miller, G.J. (1975) A study of cuts, grooves, and other marks on recent and fossil bone. II: Weathering, cracks, fractures, splinters, and other similar natural phenomena. In: Swanson, E. (ed.), *Lithic Technology*. Mouton Publishers: Paris, pp. 211–226.

Misner, L.M., Halvorson, A.C., Dreier, J..L, Ubelaker, D.H. and Foran, D.R. (2009) The correlation between skeletal weathering and DNA quality and quantity. *Journal of Forensic Sciences*, **54**: 822–828.

Nawrocki, S.P., Pless, J.E., Wahley, D.A. and Wagner, S.A. (1997) Fluvial transport of human crania. In: Haglund, W.D. and Sorg, M.H. (eds), *Forensic Taphonomy: The postmortem fate of human remains*. CRC Press: Boca Raton, pp. 531–554.

Nawrocki, S.P. (2009) Forensic taphonomy. In: Blau, S. and Ubelaker, D.H. (eds), *Handbook of Forensic Archaeology and Anthropology*. Left Coast Press: Walnut Creek, pp. 284–294.

Oller, N.A., Gràcia, X.E., Nociarová, D. and Morera, A.M. (2012) Taphonomical study of the anthropological remains from Cova des Pas (Minorca). *Quaternary International*, **275**: 112–119.

Passalacqua, N.V. and Rainwater, C.W. (2006) The effect of freeze and thaw cycles on bone. *Presented at the Annual Meeting, Mountain, Swamp and Beach (MSB)*, Radford VA.

Quincey, D., Carle, G., Alunni, V. and Quatrehomme, G. (2013) Difficulties of sex determination from forensic bone degraded DNA: a comparison of three methods. *Science and Justice*, **53**: 253–260.

Ross, A.H. and Cunningham, S.L, (2011) Time-since-death and bone weathering in a tropical environment. *Forensic Science International*, **204**: 126–133.

Scott, D.D. and Conner, M. (1997) Context delicit: archaeological context in forensic work. In: Haglund, W.D. and Sorg, M.H. (eds), *Forensic Taphonomy: The post-mortem fate of human remains*. CRC Press: Boca Raton, pp. 27–38.

Schultz, J.J. (2012) Determining the forensic significance of skeletal remains. In: Dirkmaat, D.C. (ed.), *A Companion to Forensic Anthropology*. Wiley-Blackwell: London, pp. 66–84.

Stodder, A.L.W. (2008) Taphonomy and the nature of archaeological assemblages. In: Katzenberg, M.A. and Saunders, S.R. (eds), *Biological Anthropology of the Human Skeleton*. John Wiley & Sons: Hoboken, pp. 71–114.

Symes, S.A., L'Abbé, E.N., Chapman, E.N., Wolff, I. and Dirkmaat, D.C. (2012) Interpreting traumatic injury to bone in medicolegal investigations. In: Dirkmaat, D.C. (ed.), *A Companion to Forensic Anthropology*. Wiley-Blackwell: London, pp. 340–389.

Tappen, M. (1994) Bone weathering in the tropical rain forest. *Journal of Archaeological Science*, **21**: 667–673.

Ubelaker, D.H. (1997) Taphonomic applications in forensic anthropology. In: Haglund, W.D. and Sorg, M.H. (eds), *Forensic Taphonomy: The postmortem fate of human remains*. CRC Press: Boca Raton, pp. 90–103.

White, E.M. and Hannus, L.A. (1983) Chemical weathering of bone in archaeological soils. *American Antiquity*, **48**: 316–322.

White, T.D. (1992) *Prehistoric Cannibalism at Mancos 5MTUMR-2346*. Princeton University: Princeton.

Willey, P., Galloway, A. and Snyder, L. (1997) Bone mineral density and survival of elements and element portions in the bones of the Crow Creek massacre victims. *American Journal of Physical Anthropology*, **104**: 513–528.

16

The Effects of Terrestrial Mammalian Scavenging and Avian Scavenging on the Body

Alexandria Young

16.1 Introduction

Buried and surface deposited human remains, whether deposited indoors or outdoors, have the potential to be scavenged by animal scavengers. The taphonomic process of scavenging involves an animal using their dentition or mandibles to tear, remove, disarticulate, gnaw, masticate, fracture or consume soft tissue and/or bone. Scavenging can modify, scatter and remove soft tissue and bone, potentially hindering the search, recovery, identification and interpretation of human remains. Scavenging can also obscure, modify, remove and mimic sites of trauma in soft tissue and bone (Byard *et al.* 2002; Janjua and Rogers 2008; Mann *et al.* 1990; Rothschild and Schneider 1997; Tsokos and Schulz 1999). Scavenger-inflicted bone modifications most frequently include bone fragments, fractures and bite marks (Buschmann *et al.* 2011; Domínguez-Solera and Domínguez-Rodrigo 2009; Haglund *et al.* 1988, 1989; Haynes 1980, 1983a, 1983b; Hill 1979; Johnson 1985; Moran and O'Connor 1992). Bite mark types include pits, punctures, scores and furrows (Andrés *et al.* 2012; Andrews and Fernández-Jalvo 1997; Binford 1981; Coard 2007; Delaney-Rivera *et al.* 2009; Haglund *et al.* 1988; Haynes 1983a; Milner and Smith 1989; Pickering *et al.* 2004). Pits are depressions in bone surfaces caused by the tip of a tooth cusp and do not include the collapse of the bone surface (Binford 1981; Coard 2007; Delaney-Rivera *et al.* 2009; Haglund *et al.* 1988; Haynes 1983a; Milner and Smith 1989; Pickering *et al.* 2004). Unlike pits, punctures are perforations in the bone surface wherein the bone surface collapses (Binford 1981; Coard 2007; Delaney-Rivera *et al.* 2009; Haglund *et al.* 1988; Haynes 1983a; Milner and Smith 1989; Pickering *et al.* 2004). A score is typically caused by a tooth dragging across the bone surface and has a length that is three times greater than its breadth (Coard 2007; Delaney-Rivera *et al.* 2009). Furrows are longitudinal features located at the ends of long bone shafts and are created by scavengers using their molars to access the bone marrow cavity (Binford 1981; Coard 2007; Delaney-Rivera *et al.* 2009; Haglund *et al.* 1988; Haynes 1983a; Milner and Smith 1989; Pickering *et al.* 2004).

During scavenging, damage to human remains can also occur as scratch marks, 'scooping', licking, trampling and digestion. Scooping can create thinned compact bone where scavengers have accessed the bone marrow cavity (Binford 1981; Haglund *et al.* 1988; Johnson 1985). Licking of bone can round and polish bone surfaces (Lyman 1994). Trampling can scatter and fracture bones, which may mimic human-inflicted cut marks (Behrensmeyer 1978; Behrensmeyer *et al.* 1986; Haynes 1980, 1983b). The gastric acids involved in digestion can corrode and smooth bone surfaces (Andrews and Evans 1983; Cruz-Uribe 1991; Pickering 2001; Stiner *et al.* 2012). Scavenging also exposes soft tissue and bone to weathering and insect activity, which can increase the rate of decomposition and contribute to an

Taphonomy of Human Remains: Forensic Analysis of the Dead and the Depositional Environment, First Edition.
Edited by Eline M.J. Schotsmans, Nicholas Márquez-Grant and Shari L. Forbes.

uneven pattern of decomposition in a set of human remains. Scavengers can also damage and remove hair, personal effects, clothing and other evidence associated with a set of human remains (Bass 1997; Komar and Beattie 1998; Komar 2003; Rippley *et al.* 2012; Rodriguez 1997).

Forensic taphonomic research seeks to interpret scavenging and its effects on human remains in different scenarios in order to improve forensic investigations, because all scavengers do not share the same scavenging behaviour and scatter patterns. Likewise, species-typical scavenging behaviours and scatter patterns will be affected by different crime scene scenarios. Scavenging behaviours and scatter patterns are influenced by factors pertaining to the deposit site (region, environment, topography, weather, season), human remains (carcass size, bone morphology, condition and deposition, length of exposure) and the scavenger species (body size, jaw size, dental or beak morphology, bite force, territoriality, home range size, hunting and foraging behaviour, sociality, trophic resources, prey-switching behaviour) (Byard *et al.* 2002; DeVault *et al.* 2004; Gittleman and Harvey 1982; McNab 2000; Moreno-Opo *et al.* 2010; O'Brien *et al.* 2007; Rothschild and Schneider 1997; Spradley *et al.* 2012; Wroe *et al.* 2005; Young 2013). The aforementioned factors can influence the following: if and when a scavenger will access a set of human remains; whether a scavenger is able to remove a whole body from a deposition site; the areas on a body it can access to scavenge and/or disarticulate; the elements it can disarticulate and transport from the deposition site; the locations to which remains are transported; and the types of modifications it makes to soft tissue and bone surfaces. Incorporating varying factors of different crime scene scenarios assists in the search and recovery of scavenged and scattered human remains and the more accurate interpretations of scavenger-induced trauma, minimum number of individuals (MNI) and length of exposure.

This chapter focuses on the most common terrestrial mammalian and avian scavengers found in forensic cases in North America and Europe. The class and species of scavengers affecting forensic cases will vary depending on the region and environment, amongst other factors, relating to the crime scene scenario. Nevertheless, focusing on mammalian and avian scavengers provides a wide array of potential scavengers of human remains. Each section of this chapter presents the general characteristics of scavenger species' scavenging behaviours and patterns, as well as damage and modifications to soft tissue and bones. Additionally, if applicable, the disarticulation, transportation and scattering of remains are discussed.

16.2 Terrestrial Mammalian Scavengers

16.2.1 Canid

Canid scavengers are widely discussed in the forensic literature as scavengers of human remains, in particular coyote (*Canis latrans*), wolf (*C. lupus*) and domestic dog (*C. familiaris*) (Binford 1981; D'Andrea and Gotthardt 1984; Haglund *et al.* 1988, 1989; Haglund 1997a, 1997b; Haynes 1980, 1983a, 1983b; Kjorlien *et al.* 2009; Komar 1998; Lyman 1994; Milner and Smith 1989; Steadman and Worne 2007; Tsokos and Schulz 1999; Vanlaerhoven and Hughes 2008; Willey and Snyder 1989). The red fox (*Vulpes vulpes*) is also a canid scavenger of human remains but tends to be overshadowed by the scavenging activities of larger-sized scavengers (Haglund *et al.* 1988, 1989; Young *et al.* 2014a, 2015a). Canid scavenging typically produces uneven, crenulated, wound margins with V-shaped punctures in soft tissue (Buschmann *et al.* 2011; Haglund 1997b; Rippley *et al.* 2012; Tsokos and Schulz 1999). However, canid-inflicted soft tissue damage can mimic sharp force trauma, for instance, Tsokos and Schulz (1999) noted soft tissue modifications by a pit bull terrier that resembled scalping trauma and Buschmann *et al.* (2011) recorded cases of scavenging by German Shepherds that resulted in decapitation. The incisor, canine and carnassial teeth can produce punctures in scavenged soft tissue.

Lacerations in soft tissue are caused by the canine and carnassial teeth shearing soft tissue from bone (Haglund *et al.* 1989; Rippley *et al.* 2012; Tsokos and Schulz 1999). The claw morphology of canids can produce linear scratch marks in soft tissue when scavenging and steadying remains (Tsokos and Schulz 1999).

Haynes (1982), Willey and Snyder (1989) and Haglund *et al.* (1989) found wolf, coyote and outdoor domestic dog scavenging to be similar, such that scavenging begins with the removal of soft tissue at either the site of trauma and/or face and neck, followed by concentration at the thoracic cavity. In comparison, Young *et al.* (2015a) found that the red fox initiates and concentrates scavenging deer at extremities and not at the site of trauma, head or neck. Domestic dogs found in indoor settings are known to scavenge human remains in various situations wherein the owner died suddenly or the owner died and there was no other food source (Buschmann *et al.* 2011; Rothschild and Schneider 1997; Steadman and Worne 2007; Tsokos and Schulz 1999). Soft tissue modifications by domestic dogs indoors are typically focused at the face and neck, but can also occur at any exposed areas of soft tissue (Buschmann *et al.* 2011; Rothschild and Schneider 1997).

Scavenging by canids is not limited to soft tissue consumption but includes bone modifications through disarticulation, removal, gnawing and fracturing of bones. Haglund *et al.* (1989) stated five stages of canid scavenging of human remains, as based on coyote and dog, beginning with the removal of soft tissue (0), then the scavenging, disarticulation and removal of remaining soft tissue and skeletal elements in the following order: the thorax and upper limbs (1), the lower limbs (2), a partially to completely articulated vertebral column (3) and finally, total disarticulation and heavily gnawed bones (4). Young *et al.* (2015a) found that scavenging and disarticulation by the red fox is not precluded by the removal of only soft tissue such as larger canids. Red fox scavenging begins with the removal of a set of remains, if possible, from the deposit site to a location where a fox can then scavenge and consume soft tissue without competition from other scavengers (Young *et al.* 2015a). If a set of remains cannot be removed from the site, then scavenging and disarticulation will occur at the site and disarticulated elements will be removed (Young *et al.* 2015a). In comparison, scavenging and consumption of soft tissue by wolves, coyotes and dogs predominantly occur at the deposition site (Haglund 1997b; Willey and Snyder 1989). Scavenging, disarticulation and removal by the red fox are initially focused at the extremities, then continue to the thorax and eventually to the cervical vertebrae and skull (Young *et al.* 2015a).

Bite marks on bone surfaces produced by canids include pits, punctures, furrows and scores (Haglund *et al.* 1988; Lyman 1994). Bite mark size will depend on the scavenger size, dental morphology, jaw size and bite force, as well as the carcass size, condition of remains and bone morphology. Pits and scores can potentially be created by any tooth from the canid dentition (Figure 16.1). Punctures are produced by the canine and carnassial teeth, whilst the premolars and molars are attributed with furrows (Coard 2007; Haglund *et al.* 1988; Milner and Smith 1989; Pickering *et al.* 2004) (Figures 16.2 and 16.3). The scavenging of the head can cause pits and scores on areas of the cranium where soft tissue was removed and where the scavenger held the head for transportation. Haglund *et al.* (1988) recorded a lack of bite marks on the atlas and axis from canid scavenged human remains. Scores and punctures are found on the mandible, but ramii are often chewed off (Haglund *et al.* 1988; Haynes 1980).

Scavenging and disarticulation of the head, neck and thoracic cavity can modify the sternum, clavicles, ribs and vertebrae. The sternum and clavicles are often destroyed and removed (Buschmann *et al.* 2011; Haynes 1982). Scavenging of ribs commonly results in many fragments. The sternal ends of ribs are most frequently destroyed, fractured (i.e. curvilinear), or heavily gnawed and display pits and scores (D'Andrea and Gotthardt 1984; Haglund *et al.* 1988; Haynes 1980, 1982) (Figure 16.4). Vertebral processes tend to be gnawed and splintered with pits, punctures and scores occurring on the body of vertebrae and remaining processes (Buschmann *et al.* 2011; D'Andrea and Gotthardt 1984;

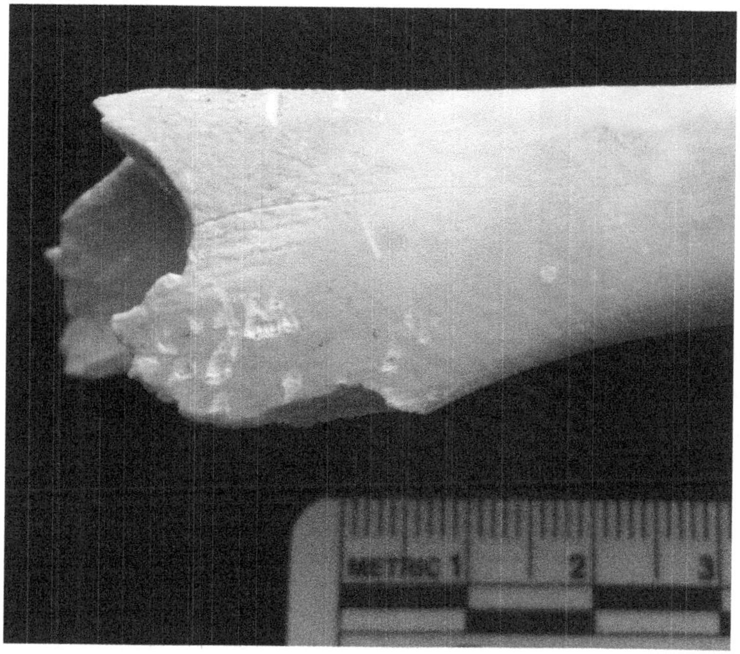

Figure 16.1 Pits and scores produced by foxes whilst scavenging a deer tibia.

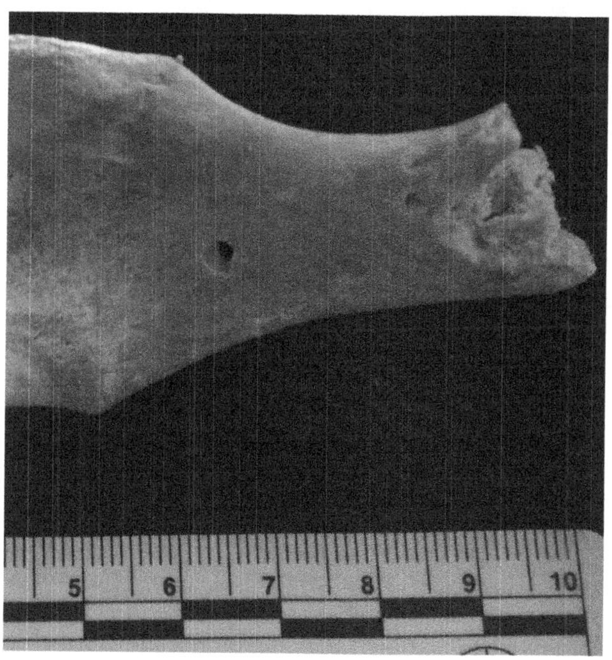

Figure 16.2 Fox-inflicted punctures located on the shaft of the ilium of deer innominate bones.

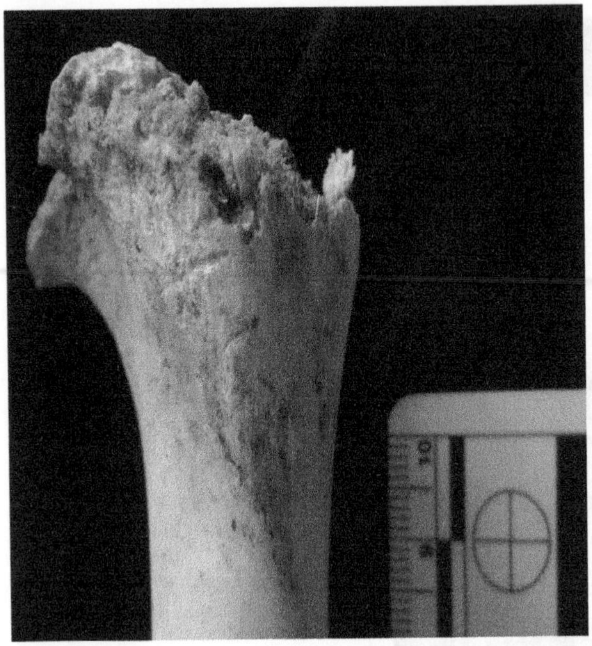

Figure 16.3 Damage and gnawing of the epiphyseal ends of long bones by foxes can produce numerous furrows.

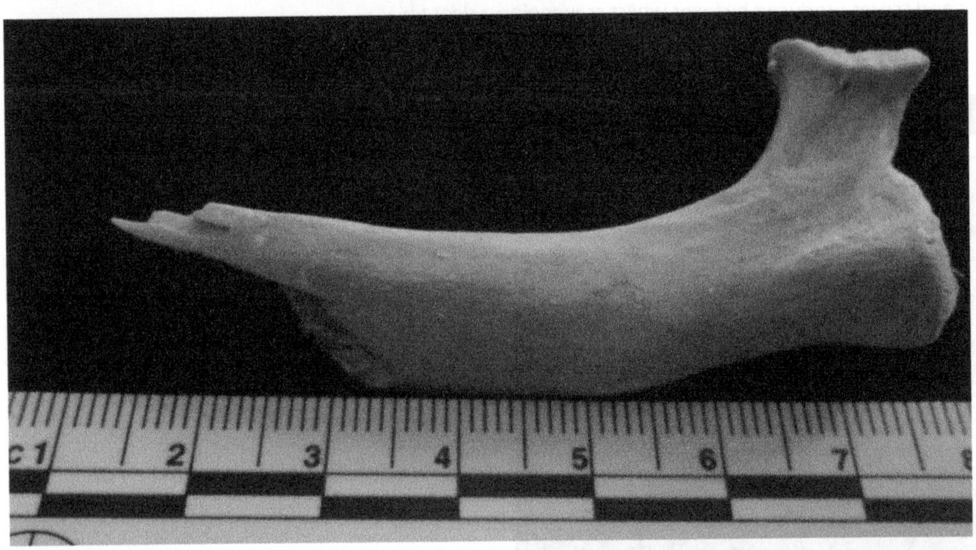

Figure 16.4 Foxes commonly fracture the sternal ends of deer ribs and produce additional bite marks such as pits.

Haglund *et al.* 1988; Haynes 1980, 1982; Lyman 1994; Lord *et al.* 2007; Shipman 1981) (Figure 16.5). Extensive gnawing and marks are common at the borders of scapulae, as well as pits and punctures at the spine, coracoid process, acromion and margins of the glenoid cavity (D'Andrea and Gotthardt 1984; Haglund *et al.* 1988; Haynes 1980, 1982; Shipman 1981) (Figure 16.6).

Scavenging and disarticulation of the lower limbs can cause gnawing damage to the innominate bones, typically observed as pits, punctures and furrows at the iliac crest, ischial tuberosities and

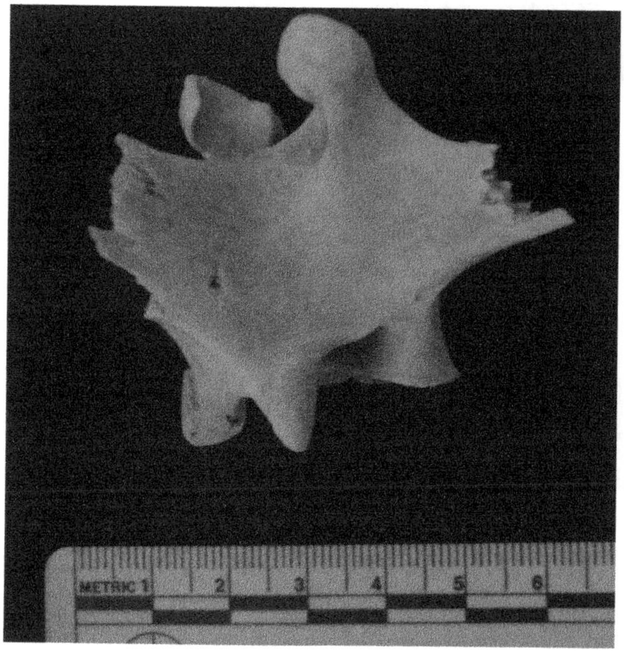

Figure 16.5 Scavenging of deer lumbar vertebrae created punctures and fractured the spinous and transverse processes.

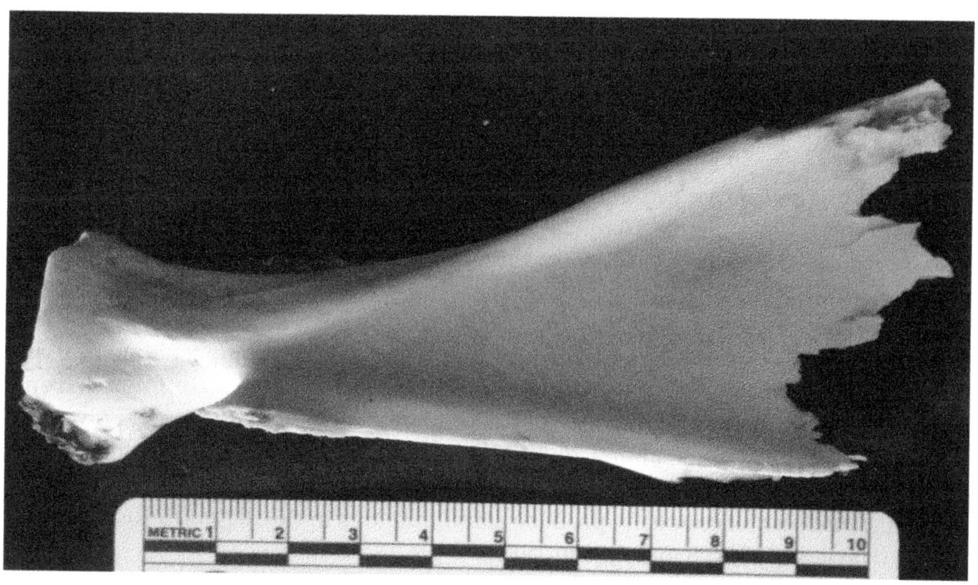

Figure 16.6 Scavenging of deer scapulae by canids, especially foxes, is often seen along the medial border.

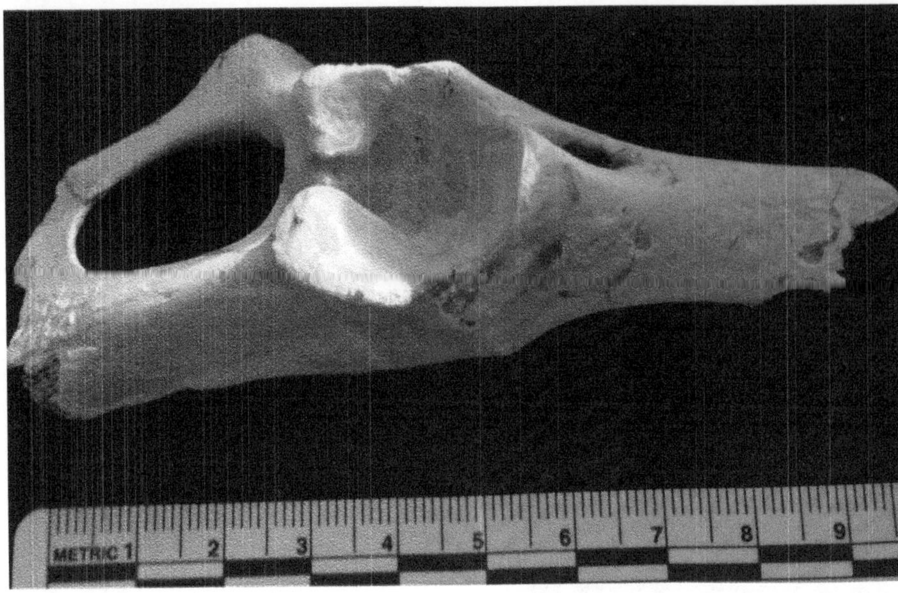

Figure 16.7 Foxes caused damage to deer innominate bones, in particular to the ischium, pubis and ilium with pits and scores located on the pubis, ischium and shaft of the ilium. Punctures are common at the acetabulum or in this case on the shaft of the ilium.

pubic symphysis (D'Andrea and Gotthardt 1984; Haglund *et al.* 1988; Haynes 1980, 1982; Shipman 1981) (Figure 16.7). A main characteristic of canid-inflicted bone modifications is the scavenging of cancellous bones for the removal of cancellous tissue and access to bone marrow, especially at the epiphyseal ends of long bones (Binford 1981; D'Andrea and Gotthardt 1984; Haglund *et al.* 1988; Haynes 1980, 1982; Lyman 1994; Lord *et al.* 2007; Shipman 1981). Pits and scores are also produced on the diaphyses and epiphyses of long bones when canids scavenge and remove soft tissue, disarticulate, gnaw and transport long bones (D'Andrea and Gotthardt 1984; Haglund *et al.* 1988; Lord *et al.* 2007). The gnawing of cancellous bones with cheek teeth creates furrows at epiphyseal ends and uneven, crenulated margins (D'Andrea and Gotthardt 1984; Haglund *et al.* 1988; Haynes 1980, 1982; Lyman 1994; Shipman 1981) (Figure 16.8). Epiphyseal ends tend to be completely gnawed and removed through furrowing (D'Andrea and Gotthardt 1984; Haglund *et al.* 1988; Haynes 1980, 1982; Lyman 1994; Shipman 1981).

Canids can produce a 'scooping' effect, in which gnawing and furrowing removes the epiphyseal end and continued licking of cancellous tissue and bone marrow creates thinned compact bone (Binford 1981; Haglund *et al.* 1988; Johnson 1985). The licking of bone surfaces can also create a rounded and polished edge to bones (Lyman 1994). After the removal of epiphyseal ends, canids can apply static pressure with their cheek teeth to the remaining long bone shaft and cause splintering, flaking and/or longitudinal fractures of the diaphysis (Haynes 1983b; Johnson 1985; Young 2013). If the epiphyseal ends are still present, canids can occasionally produce spiral fractures in the diaphysis to access the bone marrow cavity (Haynes 1980, 1983b; Johnson 1985).

Binford (1981) and Haynes (1982) documented extensive gnawing and pits on bones scavenged by domestic dogs and bones recovered from wolf dens. Binford (1981) interpreted the extended gnawing of bones by these canids as 'boredom chewing'. Wolves, coyotes and dogs scavenge, disarticulate and consume soft tissue and bones mainly at deposit sites but can scatter, cache and transport soft tissue and bones (D'Andrea and Gotthardt 1984; Haglund 1997b; Haglund *et al.* 1988, 1989;

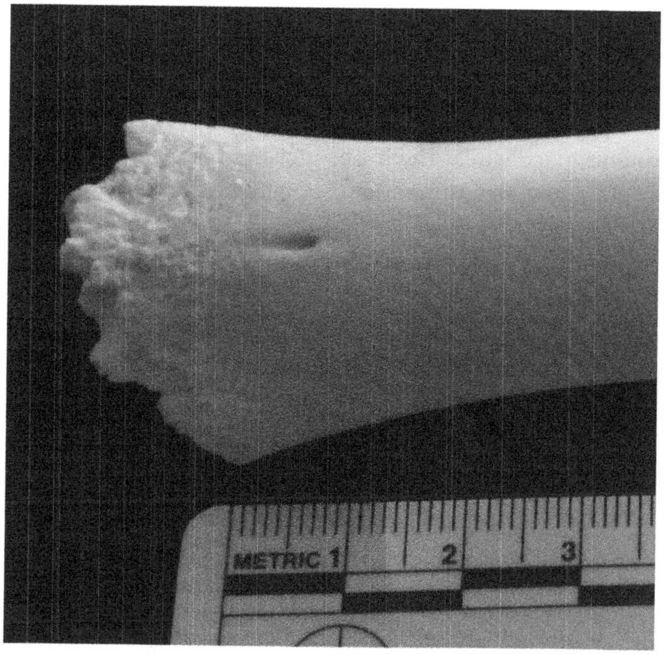

Figure 16.8 Fox scavenging of the proximal end of the deer long bone created a canid-typical uneven wound margin.

Harrington 1981, 1982; Haynes 1982, 1983a; Hill 1979; Lord *et al.* 2007; Phillips *et al.* 1991). Wolves and coyotes transport scavenged and disarticulated skeletal elements back to dens, thus allowing more time for gnawing of bones by adults and offspring (D'Andrea and Gotthardt 1984; Haglund 1997b; Haglund *et al.* 1988, 1989). Domestic dogs have also been documented with transporting bones back to their homes (Haglund 1997b; Mann *et al.* 1990). Young *et al.* (2015a) observed that foxes will not only scavenge, disarticulate, cache, transport and scatter soft tissue and bones from deposit sites but will also re-scavenge and re-scatter skeletal remains and any remaining soft tissue. Foxes transport soft tissue and bones to dens and setts for further scavenging and gnawing of bones, as well as to scavenging and caching locations (Doncaster and Macdonald 1991; Doncaster *et al.* 1990; Young *et al.* 2015a).

16.2.2 Rodent

Rodent scavengers of varying sizes, from the small wood mouse (*Apodemus sylvaticus*) (Young *et al.* 2014a) and domestic hamster (Ropohl *et al.* 1995) to larger common rats (*Rattus norvegicus*) (Haglund 1992; O'Brien *et al.* 2007), have been documented as scavengers of soft tissue from human remains and large carrion. These scavengers are not restricted to scavenging soft tissue but are also capable of modifying bone surfaces if skeletal elements are accessible. Rodents have been observed to scavenge both fresh and greasy bones to remove soft tissue and access bone marrow (Haglund 1992, 1997; Patel 1994; Ropohl *et al.* 1995; Tsokos and Schulz 1999), as well as to gnaw dry bones in order to wear down their continuously growing incisors (Andrews 1995; Brain 1981; Haglund 1992, 1997c; Klippel and Synstelien 2007). Additional rodent scavengers, more often associated with the scavenging of bones, include squirrels (*Sciuridae*) (Haglund 1992; Klippel and Synstelien 2007) and African porcupine (*Hysterix africaeustralis*) (Brain 1981).

Scavenging of soft tissue by rodents is generally concentrated at exposed areas on a body, such as the lips, nose, ears, eyes and hands, as well as sites of trauma (Haglund 1992; Mann *et al.* 1990; Patel

1994; Rippley *et al.* 2012; Ropohl *et al.* 1995; Schulz *et al.* 2006; Tsokos and Schulz 1999). The incisors of rodents produce wounds in soft tissue and bone surfaces that have even margins characterised by serrated edges and parallel striations or furrows (Haglund 1992; Haglund *et al.* 1988; Klippel and Synstelien 2007; Patel 1994; Potmesil 2005; Ropohl *et al.* 1995; Tsokos and Schulz 1999) (Table 16.1). The upper incisors of rodents hold the bone in place whilst the lower incisors repeatedly gnaw at the bone surface, thus producing an overlay of parallel striations and scalloped grooves or 'windows' (Johnson 1985; Klippel and Synstelien 2007) (Figure 16.9). Rodent gnaw marks can occur on all surface areas of a bone, dependent on bone morphology, rodent size and condition of the bone. Gnawing

Table 16.1 The different characteristics of the soft tissue and bone modifications typically produced by canids, rodents, felids, ursids, suids, mustelids, procyonids, phalangerids, peramelids, artiodactyls and avians whilst scavenging a body.

	General Characteristics of Scavenger-Inflicted Modifications[a]	
Scavenger	**Soft Tissue**	**Bone**
Canid	Uneven wound margin; V-shaped punctures	Uneven wound margin; Pit, score, puncture, and furrow bite marks; Fractures and fragmentation; Gnawing and/or removal of epiphyseal ends; Scooping of epiphyseal ends caused by licking
Rodent	Even wound margins with serrated edges and parallel striations	Even wound margins with serrated edges and parallel striations; Overlay of parallel striations producing scoops or windows typically at diaphyses
Felid	Even wound margins with layered tissue; Punctures; Tearing with even margins	Pit, score, puncture, and furrow bite marks; Fractures and fragmentation; Lack of scooping or crushing
Ursid	Punctures; Lacerations	Uneven wound margin; Produce less pit, score, puncture, and furrow bite marks than canids and fields; Furrows are the most frequent mark; Scores appear as groups with uneven margins; Gnawing can cause crushing and scooping
Suid	Punctures	Pit, score, puncture, and furrow marks; Wide and shallow furrows and scores (multiple); L-shaped punctures; Fractures and fragmentation; Gnawing and/or removal of epiphyseal ends
Mustelid	Punctures; Tearing	Uneven wound margin; Pit, score, puncture, and furrow bite marks; Fractures and fragmentation; Gnawing and/or removal of epiphyseal ends; Scooping of epiphyseal ends caused by licking
Procyonid	Punctures; Lacerations	Pit and score bite marks
Didelphid	Punctures; Lacerations	Pit and score bite marks
Phalangerid	Punctures; Lacerations	Pit and score bite marks
Peramelid	Punctures; Lacerations	Pit and score bite marks
Artiodactyl		Multiple transverse grooves as marks; Forked or pronged ends
Avian	Serrated wound margins; String-like effect	Conical punctures; V- or L-shaped score marks; Circular pit marks

a) The sizes and types of modifications are dependent on the following: scavenger species; scavengers' hunting behaviours, scavenging behaviours, disarticulation and scattering patterns, body size, dental morphology, claw morphology, jaw size and bite force; carcass size; condition and deposition of human remains.

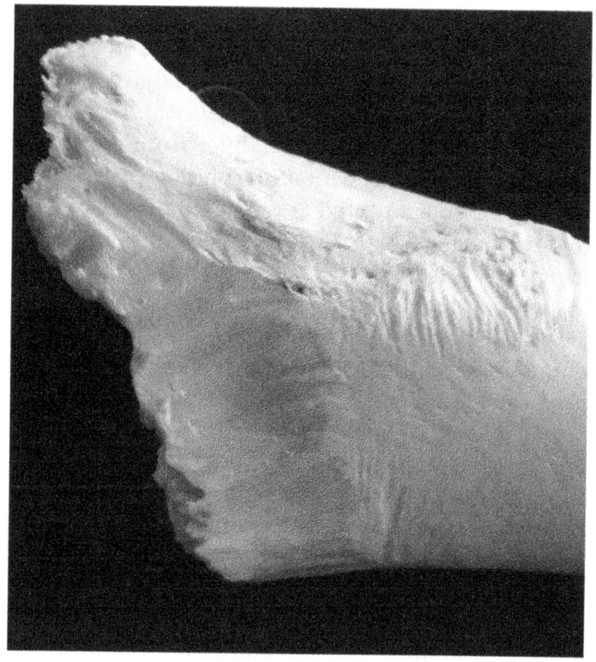

Figure 16.9 Rodent scavenging of the ends of deer long bones produced rodent-typical parallel striations in the bone surfaces.

at epiphyseal ends of long bones can result in only a small portion of the gnawed end remaining attached to the shaft via a thin piece of bone (Haglund 1997c; Klippel and Synstelien 2007). Gnawing and furrowing at cancellous bone to access the bone marrow cavity can also cause the bone surface to be thinned and have a 'fanned' appearance which slightly mimics canid scavenger scooping. However, the key distinguishing factors of rodent gnaw marks are even wound margins and parallel striations created by the incisors (Figure 16.9).

In addition to scavenging bones, rodents are also known to scatter and collect bones for further gnawing (e.g. porcupine, rat, mouse and squirrel), depending on bone morphology and rodent size (Brain 1981; Haglund 1997c; Klippel and Synstelien 2007; Lyman 1994; Mann *et al.* 1990). Rodents are also capable of damaging textiles whilst accessing human remains (Haglund 1992). Haglund (1992) noted cases in which rats damaged textiles (i.e. clothing, a plastic bag) in order to access the thoracic cavity of a body, wherein nests were built and soft tissue was scavenged.

16.2.3 Felid

Scavenging of human remains by domestic cats (*Felis catus*) has been identified in situations where an owner has died indoors and the cat has been left without access to other food sources (Bury *et al.* 2012; Komar 2003; Patel 1994; Rossi *et al.* 1994; Schulz *et al.* 2006). Domestic cats typically scavenge soft tissue from exposed areas of a body, such as the face, neck and upper extremities (Bury *et al.* 2012; Rossi *et al.* 1994). Domestic cats are capable of producing layered soft tissue damage with even wound margins similar to those produced by rodents, despite their different dentitions (Hillson 2005; Patel 1994; Rippley *et al.* 2012) (Table 16.1). Punctures can also be present in soft tissue scavenged by felids because of the canine teeth. Domestic cats can produce pit, puncture, score and furrow bite marks on bone surfaces. The majority of bone modifications occur on cancellous bones. Unlike larger felids, domestic cats are limited by their dental morphology, jaw size and bite force in the complete destruction of skeletal elements (Moran and O'Connor 1992). Moreover, domestic cats appear less likely to partake in 'boredom chewing' at epiphyseal ends like domestic dogs and other canids (Binford 1981; Domínguez-Rodrigo 1999; Moran and O'Connor 1992).

Scavenging of human remains and large prey or carrion by large felids, such as lynx (*Lynx rufus, L. lynx, L. pardinus*), leopard (*Panthera pardus*), cheetah (*Acinonyx jubatus*), mountain lion (*Puma concolor*) and lion (*P. leo*), can differ from that of domestic cats because of hunting and scavenging behaviour, body size, dental morphology, jaw size and bite force. Soft tissue damage by large felids is generally concentrated at the neck, the thoracic cavity to gain access to viscera, areas of high fat content and muscle tissue (i.e. upper arms, hips, thighs) and joints (Mondini and Muñoz 2008; Pickering and Carlson 2004; Ray *et al.* 2014; Virchow and Hogeland 1994). Leopards and lions have been observed to fully remove and consume flesh from medium- to large-sized prey except for the head (Brain 1981; Domínguez-Rodrigo 1999). Large felids can produce large tears in soft tissue with even wound margins that resemble sharp force trauma (e.g. knife wounds) (Rippley *et al.* 2012). Likewise, large scratch marks can also be present in soft tissue as a single scratch or multiple parallel lines caused by claws (Rippley *et al.* 2012).

Gnawing, fragmentation and ingestion of bones by large felids are a result of the scavenging and removal of soft tissue (Domínguez-Rodrigo 1999; Pickering and Carlson 2004; Stiner *et al.* 2012). In contrast to canids, felids are not interested in accessing bone marrow, thus evidence of scooping and crushing damage to bones is unusual (Domínguez-Rodrigo 1999; Pickering *et al.* 2004; Stiner *et al.* 2012). For instance, Pickering and Carlson (2004) observed leopards disarticulating and consuming the soft tissue and whole bones of phalanges, carpals and tarsals of baboons (*Papio ursinus*). Stiner *et al.* (2012) found that immature bones of prey consumed by mountain lions were not chewed or crushed but sheared in a similar method to soft tissue. The fracturing of bones is possible during the scavenging and disarticulation process (Borrero and Martín 1996). Borrero and Martín (1996) noted the fracturing of sheep (*Ovies aries*) femora and humerii by pumas (*P. concolor*) during the disarticulation of front limbs.

Bite marks on bone surfaces caused by large felids can include punctures, scores, furrows and pits, with the punctures being the most common type of mark produced. Ribs are most frequently found with extensive gnawing and fragmentation because felids have accessed and scavenged the thoracic cavity (Domínguez-Rodrigo 1999; Stiner *et al.* 2012). Scavenging of the thoracic cavity, upper limbs and neck also produces punctures and furrows on vertebrae, clavicles and the borders of scapulae (Brain 1981; Domínguez-Rodrigo 1999; Pickering and Carlson 2004; Stiner *et al.* 2012). Punctures, scores and furrows are often found on innominate bones, especially the external borders of the ischium and iliac crest (Brain 1981; Domínguez-Rodrigo 1999; Pickering and Carlson 2004; Stiner *et al.* 2012).

Large felids tend to remove carcasses to areas of shelter, dense vegetation, or even up trees (i.e. leopard) to commence scavenging and disarticulation (Brain 1981; Mondini and Muñoz 2008; Ray *et al.* 2014). However, Stiner *et al.* (2012) observed mountain lions scavenging and discarding deer where they were killed. Scattered skeletal elements and soft tissue by large felids are usually recovered in close proximity to the remainder of the skeleton (Domínguez-Rodrigo 1999; Stiner *et al.* 2012). The kill or deposition site where the felid scavenges is kept tidy by using their claws to scrape the soil surface and any debris surrounding a set of remains (Rippley *et al.* 2012). Felid scavengers will often remove human hair from the body it is scavenging and possibly ingest hair but will primarily use it, along with debris, loose vegetation and soil to cover the body (Rippley *et al.* 2012).

16.2.4 Ursid

Bears (*Ursus arctos; U. americanus; U. maritimus*) have been recorded as scavengers of human remains (Komar 2003; Merbs 1997; Murad and Boddy 1987) and small- to large-sized animals

(D'Andrea and Gotthardt 1984; Elgmork 1982; French and French 1990; Green *et al.* 1997; Haynes 1980, 1983a; Sala and Arsuaga 2013; Saladié *et al.* 2013). Scavenging of soft tissue is concentrated at the thoracic cavity and the removal of viscera (Elgmork 1982). Bear dentition and claw morphology can produce punctures and lacerations of varying size in soft tissue (Cardall and Rosen 2003). Bears typically do not fully scavenge and consume a carcass, but will partially scavenge or consume and then transport, cache or abandon a carcass (Elgmork 1982; French and French 1990; Green *et al.* 1997; Sala and Arsuaga 2013; Saladié *et al.* 2013). Sala and Arsuaga (2013) and Saladié *et al.* (2013) found that brown bears do not transport remains to caves or dens for further scavenging. Carcasses are transported to an area (e.g. denser woodland) to be further scavenged, cached or covered with soil and plant materials (Sala and Arsuaga 2013). Bear caching activity differs to the caching activity of canids in the following ways:

1) the burying of whole and half-consumed carcasses in peat bogs and other water environments; and
2) remaining with their cache for an extended period of time (Elgmork 1982).

Bear scavenging of soft tissue can cause the disarticulation, scattering and modification of skeletal elements (Haynes 1980, 1983a; Sala and Arsuaga 2013; Saladié *et al.* 2013). Bite marks produced on bone surfaces include pits, punctures, scores and furrows. In comparison to canids and felids, ursids produce a lower quantity of bite marks on bones (Andrews and Fernández-Jalvo 1997; Haynes 1980, 1983a; Saladié *et al.* 2013). The most frequent type of mark produced on bones is furrow and the least frequent are puncture and pit (Sala and Arsuaga 2013; Saladié *et al.* 2013). Haynes (1980) attributes the broad occlusal surface of bunodont teeth with producing small to large pits on epiphyses and diaphyses of long bones. Scores can occur in groups as short and wide, similar to rodent scores but with irregular margins, or as long and thin striations (Saladié *et al.* 2013) (Table 16.1). Marks are mainly located at the cancellous bone of ribs, scapulae, vertebrae, innominate bones and the epiphyseal ends of long bones (Sala and Arsuaga 2013; Saladié *et al.* 2013). Sala and Arsuaga (2013) recorded that there was a distinct lack of bite marks on the carpals, tarsals, metapodials and phalanges of ungulates scavenged by brown bear. Likewise, Merbs (1997) noted unmarked whole human fingers recovered from polar bear scat.

Crushing, as a result of gnawing and scooping damage to bones are also common with bear scavenging (Haynes 1980, 1983a; Sala and Arsuaga 2013; Saladié *et al.* 2013). In comparison to canids, the bite force, jaw size and broad bunodont teeth of bears contribute to the gnawing and crushing of cancellous bone (Haynes 1980, 1983a; Sala and Arsuaga 2013; Saladié *et al.* 2013). Bears are not commonly characterised with the fracturing of bones (Saladié *et al.* 2013). However, fractures that do occur are present with irregular margins at the ends, processes and borders of flat bones, such as ribs, vertebrae and scapulae (Sala and Arsuaga 2013). Fracturing and crushing of additional skeletal elements is possible by bears but is dependent on the size of the bear, carcass size and age (i.e. immature bones) and the condition and deposition of remains.

16.2.5 Suid

Wild and domestic pigs (*Sus scrofa, S. scrofa domesticus*) can scavenge and modify both soft tissue and skeletal remains from small- to large-sized animal carcasses and human remains (Berryman 2002; DeVault *et al.* 2004; Domínguez-Solera and Domínguez-Rodrigo 2009; Frederick 1998; Galdikas 1978; Greenfield 1988; Jedrzejewski *et al.* 1993; Ray *et al.* 2014). Suid scavenging focuses on the removal of soft tissue from the head, neck and viscera within the thoracic cavity (Berryman 2002; Frederick 1998; Möttönen and Nuutila 1977; Wade and Browns 1985). The incisors and canines can produce small to large punctures in soft tissue. Suids tend to completely deflesh a set of remains and can disarticulate limbs (Domínguez-Solera and Domínguez-Rodrigo 2009; Wade and Browns 1985). Scavenged remains are often scattered in close proximity of the deposit or scavenging site and are a by-product of scavenging and disarticulation. Unlike canids and felids, which use their carnassials and molars to remove and shear soft tissue, suids use their mandibular incisors to scrape soft tissue from bones, which can cause bone modifications (Domínguez-Solera and Domínguez-Rodrigo 2009) (Table 16.1).

Suid-inflicted bite marks include scores, pits, punctures and furrows. In contrast to canids, the incisors create wide and shallow furrows and scores, the latter often appearing as multiple parallel striations (Berryman 2002; Domínguez-Solera and Domínguez-Rodrigo 2009; Greenfield 1988). The incisors also create pits and occasional punctures in bone surfaces. There is extensive furrowing and destruction of epiphyseal ends and cancellous bone of scapulae, vertebrae, sacrum, long bones and innominate bones scavenged by suids (Berryman 2002; Domínguez-Solera and Domínguez-Rodrigo 2009; Greenfield 1988). Berryman (2002) found scores on the cranium, clavicles, ribs, innominate bones and tibia of a set of human remains scavenged by domestic pigs in the southeastern USA. (Greenfield 1988) and attributed the production of scores on flat bones as a characteristic of suid scavenging. Punctures, caused by the premolars, display an L-shape in bones (Domínguez-Solera and Domínguez-Rodrigo 2009). Suids can heavily fragment skeletal remains with the aid of their molars; most notably the cranium, vertebrae, sacrum, innominate bones, long bones and tarsals (Domínguez-Solera and Domínguez-Rodrigo 2009; Galdikas 1978; Greenfield 1988). Suids have also been observed to return to previously scavenged or fragmented bones and consume fragments or partake in 'boredom chewing' (Binford 1981; Domínguez-Solera and Domínguez-Rodrigo 2009).

16.2.6 Mustelid, Procyonid, Didelphid, Phalangerid and Peramelid

In addition to the more readily researched scavengers in forensic and taphonomic studies (e.g. canids, felids, rodents), mustelid, procyonid, didelphid, phalangerid and peramelid have been documented as scavengers of small- to medium-sized animal analogues. Recent studies have discussed the scavenging activities of mustelids and their potential to be scavengers of human remains. The Eurasian badger (*Meles meles*) has not been recorded directly scavenging on human remains but has been observed as active (e.g. scat, latrine, sett) within crime scene areas where scavenged and scattered human remains were recovered (Young *et al.* 2014a). The Eurasian badger has been identified in ecological studies as a scavenger of carrion and small mammals, depending greatly on seasonal changes and trophic resources (Kauhala *et al.* 1998; Kruuk and Parish 1981, 1985; Revilla and Palomares 2002). The dentition and claw morphologies of the Eurasian badger allow for the tearing of soft tissue. Claws are used to both steady the item being scavenged and assist in tearing soft tissue. The incisors and canines can tear, remove and puncture soft tissue. The broad multi-cusp morphology of the molars, especially the upper molar, aid in chewing and gnawing soft tissue and bone (Lüps and Roper 1988; Young *et al.* 2015b). Bite marks produced on bone surfaces include pits, scores, furrows and punctures, the most common being pits. Similar to canids, there is extensive damage to epiphyseal ends and scooping (Young *et al.* 2015b) (Table 16.1). The ends also tend to have uneven margins like those gnawed by canids. In general, the Eurasian badger produces larger pits than the red fox, due to the dentition, jaw muscle morphology and stronger bite force of the badger (Lee and Mill 2004; Wroe *et al.* 2005). The scattering and removal of a set of remains by badgers is dependent on carcass size and bone morphology. The Eurasian badger has been observed to scavenge and consume small mammals at deposition sites, as well as to transport fresh and greasy bones down into setts for further scavenging (Young *et al.* 2015a).

The mink (*Neovison vison*) is another potential mustelid scavenger of human remains that has appeared in forensic studies in North America using animal analogues. Hobischak (1997) and MacDonell and Anderson (1997) recorded mink scavenging soft tissue from unclothed areas of pigs submerged in pond and stream environments. Hobischak (1997) noted that mink were more attracted to bloated rather than fresh pigs and did not scavenge skeletal remains.

Procyonid, didelphid, phalangerid and peramelid scavengers have also been recognised in forensic and taphonomic studies as scavengers of small- to medium-sized animal carrion. In a study by O'Brien *et al.* (2007), brush-tailed possum (*Trichosurus vulpecul*) and bandicoot (*Isoodon obesulus*) in Western Australia were documented as scavenging the soft tissue from pig carcasses but not skeletal remains. DeVault *et al.* (2004) recorded the scavenging of soft tissue by raccoon (*Procyon lotor*) and Virginia opossum (*Didelphis marsupialis*) in southeastern USA. Morton and Lord (2006) also observed opossum scavenging and disarticulating small pig carcasses, including the gnawing of skeletal remains. Although there is limited literature on the scavenging effects of mink, raccoon, brush-tail possum, opossum and bandicoot, their dental morphologies suggest the potential to produce small lacerations and punctures in soft tissue, as well as small pits and scores in bone, depending on carcass size and bone morphology.

16.2.7 Artiodactyl

Artiodactyls (e.g. deer) are known to occasionally chew dry bones because of a nutritional dysfunction that causes the animal to be deficient in phosphorous (Cáceres *et al.* 2011). Artiodactyls use their cheek teeth, especially molars, to chew bones in a side-to-side motion that can produce multiple transverse grooves, similar in appearance to scores or furrows, in cortical bone surfaces (Brothwell 1976; Cáceres *et al.* 2011; Johnson 1985; Sutcliffe 1973) (Table 16.1). In comparison to bite marks produced by carnivores, artiodactyls create grooves that are 'flat in section and smooth bottom with cracking and micro-striations' (Cáceres *et al.* 2011). Artiodactyl chewing can eventually remove cancellous bone and create a forked or pronged shape modification (Cáceres *et al.* 2011; Johnson 1985; Sutcliffe 1973). Additional bone modifications by artiodactyls include rounded and polished bone surfaces where licking has occurred (Cáceres *et al.* 2011).

16.3 Avian Scavengers

Avian scavenger species commonly discussed in forensic and taphonomic studies include carrion crow (*Corvus corone*), raven (*C. corax*), vulture (*Cathartidae, Accipitridae*) and magpie (*Pica pica*) (Asamura *et al.* 2004; Bass 1997; Domínguez-Solera and Domínguez-Rodrigo 2011; Kendall 2014; Komar and Beattie 1998; Mann *et al.* 1990; O'Brien *et al.* 2007; Ray *et al.* 2014; Reeves 2009; Spradley *et al.* 2012; Young *et al.* 2014b). Additional avian scavengers known to scavenge medium- to large-size carrion and potentially human remains include the common buzzard (*Buteo buteo*) and Eurasian jay (*Garrulus glandarius*) (Ray *et al.* 2014; Selva 2004; Young *et al.* 2014b). In addition to the aforementioned factors that can affect the scavenging behaviour and patterns of all scavengers, avian scavenger-induced soft tissue modifications are influenced by beak and talon morphologies (Fowler *et al.* 2009; Kendall 2014; Simmons *et al.* 2010). Beak and talon morphologies may impact the areas on a body that an avian scavenger can access and remove soft tissue (Fowler *et al.* 2009; Kendall 2014; Simmons *et al.* 2010). For example, the carrion crow focuses its scavenging efforts on removing the tongue, eye and soft tissue from sites of trauma (e.g. gunshot wound) (Young *et al.* 2014b). Similarly, the common buzzard removes soft tissue mainly from the site of trauma on a carcass (Young *et al.* 2014b).

Carrion crow, raven, magpie and common buzzard remove soft tissue from a carcass through a pecking action in which soft tissue is clasped by the beak and pulled away from the body. The result of this pecking action is a string-like effect on soft tissue and serrated wound margins (Asamura *et al.* 2004). The pecking action not only modifies and removes soft tissue but can also produce conical punctures in bone surfaces (Komar and Beattie 1998). In contrast, the removal of soft tissue by vultures follows a tearing method (Kendall 2014). Scavenging by vultures can be extensive and result in the complete skeletonisation, disarticulation and scattering of human remains (Domínguez-Solera and Domínguez-Rodrigo 2011; Kendall 2014; Lyman 1994; Reeves 2009; Spradley *et al.* 2012). Bone surface modifications produced by vultures tend to be more varied than other avian scavengers (Domínguez-Solera and Domínguez-Rodrigo 2011; Fetner and Soltysiak 2013). Scavenging by vultures can produce puncture, pit and score marks on bone surfaces (Domínguez-Solera and Domínguez-Rodrigo 2011; Fetner and Soltysiak 2013). Scores and pits can potentially be found on all areas of a body scavenged by vultures, but with regard to long bones, marks are concentrated at diaphyses (Domínguez-Solera and Domínguez-Rodrigo 2011). Domínguez-Solera and Domínguez-Rodrigo (2011) found punctures to be limited to bones with flat surfaces such as innominate bones, cranium and scapula. Scores are the most common types of mark produced by vultures and can be seen as multiple linear striations forming shallow V- or L-shape (tick-shape) marks (Domínguez-Solera and Domínguez-Rodrigo 2011; Fetner and Soltysiak 2013). Domínguez-Solera and Domínguez-Rodrigo (2011) also found that within a vulture-produced score there are 'parallel microstriations' caused by the irregular edge of the vulture beak morphology. Pits show characteristics similar to pits caused by mammalian carnivores, such that pits are circular or oval in shape and do not penetrate the bone cortex (Binford 1981; Coard 2007; Domínguez-Solera and Domínguez-Rodrigo 2011; Haglund *et al.* 1988; Haynes 1983a; Milner and Smith 1989) (Table 16.1). The shape of punctures is greatly variable and not limited to the conical-shaped punctures produced by smaller avian scavengers.

Avian scavenging is not limited to soft tissue and bone modifications but can extend to the removal of hair and personal effects. Through scavenging and accessing different areas of soft tissue, scavengers can remove and ingest hair, textiles and personal effects as a by-product of scavenging. However, carrion crows and magpies have been documented as removing hair from bodies for nesting (Bass 1997; Komar 2003; Rodriguez 1997) and personal effects, such as credit cards (Komar and Beattie 1998).

16.4 Applications to Crime Scene Investigation

Crime scene investigations have been aided by the use of actualistic methods in forensic taphonomic research into the scavenging of human remains (Bass 1997; Kjorlien *et al.* 2009; Komar and Beattie 1998; Morton and Lord 2006; Reeves 2009; Willey and Snyder 1989; Young *et al.* 2014b, 2015a, 2015b). For example, the misinterpretation of scavenging by domestic dogs as scalping (Tsokos and Schulz 1999), decapitation (Buschmann *et al.* 2011) or attacks (Rothschild and Schneider 1997) and by rodents as sexual offences (Ropohl *et al.* 1995). Actualistic methods drawn from taphonomy, zooarchaeology and archaeology (Andrews 1995; Bartosiewicz 2008; Behrensmeyer 1978; Fernández-Jalvo *et al.* 2002; Shipman 1981) allow for the recreation of different crime scene scenarios. In general, forensic taphonomic experiments in scavenging use actualistic methods to compare the effects scavengers (taphonomic agent) and scavenging (taphonomic processes) have on human remains and/or animal analogues in the present to those in the past (i.e. crime scene scenario), in order to better understand the conditions surrounding past events. Actualistic methods coupled with qualitative and quantitative analyses of bite marks in soft tissue and bones of scavenged human and faunal remains have also assisted crime scene investigations and the interpretation of peri- and post-mortem trauma (Blumenschine *et al.* 1996; Buschmann *et al.* 2011; Byard *et al.* 2002; Coard 2007; Domínguez-Solera and Domínguez-Rodrigo 2009; Domínguez-Rodrigo and Piqueras 2003; Gidna *et al.* 2013; Haglund *et al.* 1988; Haynes 1983b; Klippel and Synstelien 2007; Murmann *et al.* 2006; Patel 1994; Ropohl *et al.* 1995; Tsokos and Schulz 1999; Young *et al.* 2015b). Care must always be taken in the interpretation of any type of trauma, especially with peri-mortem trauma. There is the potential for difficulties in accurate interpretations of peri-mortem trauma in forensic cases where, for example, an individual was attacked by a dog or an individual died indoors and the dog bit their owner in an attempt to awake them (Buschmann *et al.* 2011; Byard *et al.* 2002; Rothschild and Schneider 1997; Tsokos and Schulz 1999; Steadman and Worne 2007).

Actualistic methods and bite mark analyses have been utilised in research and crime scene investigations in order to identify scavengers, interpret species-typical scavenging behaviour and scatter patterns (Kjorlien *et al.* 2009; Morton and Lord 2006; Spradley *et al.* 2012; Vanlaerhoven and Hughes 2008; Young *et al.* 2014b, 2015a, 2015b), distinguish between scavenger-inflicted trauma and foul play (Asamura *et al.* 2004; Buschmann *et al.* 2011; Byard *et al.* 2002; Ropohl *et al.* 1995) and interpret MNI (Haglund and Reay 1993; Haglund *et al.* 1988; Marean and Spencer 1991). Accurate identification and interpretation of scavengers active within the crime scene and surrounding areas and their species-typical scavenging behaviour and scatter patterns can divulge information pertaining to how and what areas of a body different scavenger species will scavenge, disarticulate and remove. Analyses of the areas scavenged, disarticulated and removed from a set of human remains, along with information on species-typical scavenging behaviour and scatter patterns, can provide further interpretations. For instance, the following: was the body deposited as whole or dismembered; was there clothing or other materials present that only exposed certain areas to scavengers or that prohibited or permitted different scavenger species; was the body in a certain stage of decomposition that was favoured or disliked by a scavenger species; and was the body deposited somewhere accessible or favoured by certain scavenger species or even none (e.g. indoors or outdoors; urban or rural environment)?

Applying scavenging information to the interpretation of the post-mortem interval (PMI) is still a debated topic, because scavenging exposes areas of soft tissue to insect activity and weathering which, in turn, contribute to increased rates and uneven patterns of decomposition (Janjua and Rogers 2008; Mann *et al.* 1990; Spradley *et al.* 2012). Additionally, scavenging intensity may be increased or decreased due to varying factors (e.g. season, insect activity, trophic resources), some scavenger species will re-scavenge human remains, and remains may not be exposed to scavengers until the later stages of the PMI. Scavenging information can be better applied to interpretations pertaining to the length of exposure of human remains in a crime scene scenario (Morton and Lord 2006; Spradley *et al.* 2012; Willey and Snyder 1989). Estimations in length of exposure are assisted by forensic taphonomic studies, such as Morton and Lord (2006), Reeves (2009) and Spradley *et al.* (2012), in which the PMI and length of exposure are known and compared to observations of the sequence of scavengers at a carcass, the time required by each scavenger to utilise a carcass and the effects of different scavenging behaviours. Understanding how scavenger species and their scavenging behaviours and scatter patterns are affected by different factors also aids in adapting search methods, delineating search perimeters and locating deposit sites (Kjorlien *et al.* 2009; Owsley *et al.* 1992; Vanlaerhoven and Hughes 2008).

16.5 Conclusion and Future Research

Crime scene investigations will benefit from continued use of actualistic methods and bite mark analyses in forensic studies. The vast majority of forensic taphonomic studies of scavenging have stemmed from research based in North America (Haglund *et al.* 1988, 1989; Kjorlien *et al.* 2009; Komar 1998; Milner and Smith 1989; Morton and Lord 2006; Reeves 2009; Spradley *et al.* 2012; Vanlaerhoven and Hughes 2008; Willey and Snyder 1989) with limited forensic taphonomic research from other regions, such as Australia (Brown *et al.* 2006; Byard *et al.* 2002; O'Brien *et al.* 2007) and

Northwestern Europe (Coard 2007; Moraitis and Spiliopoulou 2010; Ruffell and Murphy 2011; Young *et al.* 2014b, 2015a, 2015b). Additionally, previous scavenging research has tended to generalise scavengers either by their dietary habits or taxon and thus overlook species-typical scavenging behaviours and the effects of different crime scene scenarios on behaviours. Forensic taphonomy needs more species-typical, region-specific and environment-specific research and analyses of the effects of different crime scene scenarios on scavenging behaviours, in order to aid search and recovery efforts and enable more accurate identifications and interpretations of scavenged human remains, deposit sites and associated evidence.

References

Andrés, M., Gidna, A.O., Yravedra, J. and Domínguez-Rodrigo, M. (2012) A study of dimensional differences of tooth marks (pits and scores) on bones modified by small and large carnivores. *Archaeological and Anthropological Sciences*, **4**: 209–219.

Andrews, P. (1995) Experiments in taphonomy. *Journal of Archaeological Science*, **22**: 147–153.

Andrews, P. and Evans, E.M.N. (1983) Small mammal bone accumulations produced by mammalian carnivores. *Paleobiology*, **9**: 289–307.

Andrews, P. and Fernández-Jalvo, Y. (1997) Surface modifications of the Sima de los Huesos fossil humans. *Journal of Human Evolution*, **33**: 191–217.

Asamura, H., Takayanagi, K., Ota, M., Kobayashi, K. and Fukushima, H. (2004) Unusual characteristic patterns of post-mortem injuries. *Journal of Forensic Sciences*, **49**: 1–3.

Bartosiewicz, L. (2008) Taphonomy and palaeopathology in archaeology. *Geobios*, **41**: 69–77.

Bass, W.M. (1997) Outdoor decomposition rates in Tennessee. In: Haglund, W.D. and Sorg, M.H. (eds), *Forensic Taphonomy. The post-mortem fate of human remains.* CRC Press: Boca Raton, pp. 181–186.

Behrensmeyer, A.K. (1978) Taphonomic and ecologic information from bone weathering. *Paleobiology*, **4**: 150–162.

Behrensmeyer, A.K., Gordon, K.D. and Yanagi, G.T. (1986) Trampling as a cause of bone surface damage and pseudo-cutmarks. *Nature*, **319**: 768–771.

Berryman, H.E. (2002) Disarticulation pattern and tooth mark artifacts associated with pig scavenging of human remains: a case study. In: Haglund, W.D. and Sorg, M.H. (eds), *Advances in Forensic Taphonomy. Method, theory, and archaeological perspectives.* CRC Press: Boca Raton, pp. 487–496.

Binford, L.R. (1981) *Bones: Ancient Men and Modern Myths.* Academic Press: New York.

Blumenschine, R.J., Marean, C.W. and Capaldo, S.D. (1996) Blind tests of inter-analyst correspondence and accuracy in the identification of cut marks, percussion marks, and carnivore tooth marks on bone surfaces. *Journal of Archaeological Science*, **23**: 493–507.

Borrero, L.A. and Martín, F.M. (1996) Tafonomía de carnívoros: un enfoque regional. In: Gómez Otero, J. (ed.), Arqueología, Sólo Patagonia, CENPAT (CONICET): Puerto Madryn, pp. 189–206.

Brain, C.K. (1981) *The Hunters or the Hunted? An introduction to African cave taphonomy.* The University of Chicago Press: Chicago.

Brothwell, D. (1976) Further evidence of bone chewing by ungulates: the sheep of North Ronaldsay, Orkney. *Journal of Archaeological Science*, **3**: 179–182.

Brown, O.J.F., Field, J. and Letnic, M. (2006) Variation in the taphonomic effect of scavengers in semi-arid Australia linked to rainfall and the El Niño Southern Oscillation. *International Journal of Osteoarchaeology*, **16**: 165–176.

Bury, D., Langlois, N. and Byard, R. (2012) Animal-related fatalities. Part I: Characteristic autopsy findings and variable causes of death associated with blunt and sharp trauma. *Journal of Forensic Sciences*, **57**: 375–380.

Buschmann, C., Solarino, B., Püschel, K., Czubaiko, F., Heinze, S. and Tsokos, M. (2011) Post-mortem decapitation by domestic dogs: three case reports and review of the literature. *Forensic Science, Medicine, and Pathology*, **7**: 344–349.

Byard, R., James, R. and Gilbert, J. (2002) Diagnostic problems associated with cadaveric trauma from animal activity. *The American Journal of Forensic Medicine and Pathology*, **23**: 238–244.

Cáceres, I., Esteban-Nadal, M., Bennàsar, M. and Fernández-Jalvo, Y. (2011) Was it the deer or the fox? *Journal of Archaeological Science*, **38**: 2767–2774.

Cardall, T.Y. and Rosen, P. (2003) Grizzly bear attack. *The Journal of Emergency Medicine*, **24**: 331–333.

Coard, R. (2007) Ascertaining an agent: using tooth pit data to determine the carnivores responsible for predation in cases of suspected big cat kills in an upland area of Britain. *Journal of Archaeological Science*, **34**: 1677–1684.

Cruz-Uribe, K. (1991) Distinguishing hyena from hominid bone accumulations. *Journal of Field Archaeology*, **18**: 467–486.

D'Andrea, A.C. and Gotthardt, R.M. (1984) Predator and scavenger modification of recent equid skeletal assemblages. *Arctic*, **37**: 276–283.

Delaney-Rivera, C., Plummer, T.W., Hodgson, J.A., Forrest, F., Hertel, F. and Oliver, J.S. (2009) Pits and pitfalls: taxonomic variability and patterning in tooth mark dimensions. *Journal of Archaeological Science*, **36**: 2597–2608.

DeVault, T..L, Brisbin, I.L, and Rhodes, O.E. (2004) Factors influencing the acquisition of rodent carrion by vertebrate scavengers and decomposers. *Canadian Journal of Zoology*, **82**: 502–509.

Domínguez-Rodrigo, M. (1999) Flesh availability and bone modifications in carcasses consumed by lions: palaeoecological relevance in hominid foraging patterns. *Palaeogeography, Palaeoclimatology, Palaeoecology*, **149**: 373–388.

Domínguez-Rodrigo, M. and Piqueras, A. (2003) The use of tooth pits to identify carnivore taxa in tooth-marked archaeofaunas and their relevance to reconstruct hominid carcass processing behaviours. *Journal of Archaeological Science*, **30**: 1385–1391.

Domínguez-Solera, S.D. and Domínguez-Rodrigo, M. (2009) A taphonomic study of bone modification and of tooth-mark patterns on long limb bone portions by suids. *International Journal of Osteoarchaeology*, **19**: 345–363.

Domínguez-Solera, S.D. and Domínguez-Rodrigo, M. (2011) A taphonomic study of a carcass consumed by griffon vultures (*Gyps fulvus*) and its relevance for the interpretation of bone surface modifications. *Archaeological and Anthropological Sciences*, **3**: 385–392.

Doncaster, C.P. and Macdonald, D.W. (1991) Drifting territoriality in the red fox *Vulpes vulpes*. *Journal of Animal Ecology*, **60**: 423–439.

Doncaster, C.P., Dickman, C.R. and Macdonald, D.W. (1990) Feeding ecology of red foxes (*Vulpes vulpes*) in the city of Oxford, England. *Journal of Mammalogy*, **71**: 188–194.

Elgmork, K. (1982) Caching behavior of brown bears (*U. arctos*). *Journal of Mammalogy*, **63**: 607–612.

Fernández-Jalvo, Y., Sánchez-Chillón, B., Andrews, P., Fernández-Lopéz, S. and Alcalá Martinéz, L. (2002) Morphological taphonomic transformations of fossil bones in continental environments, and repercussions on their chemical composition. *Archaeometry*, **44**: 353–361.

Fetner, R. and Soltysiak, A. (2013) Shape and distribution of Griffon vulture (*Gyps fulvas*) scavenging marks on a bovine skull. *Journal of Taphonomy*, **11**: 41–47.

Fowler, D.W., Freedman, E.A, and Scannella, J.B. (2009) Predatory functional morphology in raptors: interdigital variation in talon size is related to prey restraint and immobilisation technique. *PLoS One*, **4**: e7999.

Frederick, J.M. (1998) Overview of wild pig damage in California. *Proceedings of the Vertebrate Pest Conference*, **18**: 82–86.

French, S.P, and French, M.G. (1990) Predatory behavior of grizzly bears feeding on elk calves in Yellowstone National Park. *Bears: Their Biology and Management*, **8**: 335–341.

Galdikas, B. (1978) Orangutan death and scavenging by pigs. *Science*, **4337**: 68–70.

Gidna, A., Yravedra, J. and Domínguez-Rodrigo, M. (2013) A cautionary note on the use of captive carnivores to model wild predator behavior: a comparison of bone modification patterns on long bones by captive and wild lions. *Journal of Archaeological Science*, **40**: 1903–1910.

Gittleman, J.L. and Harvey, P.H. (1982) Carnivore home-range size, metabolic needs and Ecology. *Behavioral Ecology and Sociobiology*, **10**: 57–63.

Green, G., Mattson, D. and Peek, J. (1997) Spring feeding on ungulate carcasses by grizzly bears in Yellowstone National Park. *The Journal of Wildlife Management*, **61**: 1040–1055.

Greenfield HJ (1988) Bone consumption by pigs in a contemporary Serbian village: implications for the interpretation of prehistoric faunal assemblages. *Journal of Field Archaeology*, **15**: 473–479.

Haglund, W.D. (1992) Contribution of rodents to post-mortem artifacts of bone and soft tissue. *Journal of Forensic Sciences*, **37**: 1459–1465.

Haglund, W.D. (1997a) Scattered skeletal human remains: search strategy considerations for locating missing teeth. In: Haglund, W.D, and Sorg, M.H. (eds), *Forensic Taphonomy. The post-mortem fate of human remains*. CRC Press: Boca Raton, pp. 383–394.

Haglund, W.D. (1997b) Dogs and coyotes: post-mortem involvement with human remains. In: Haglund, W.D. and Sorg, M.H. (eds), *Forensic Taphonomy. The post-mortem fate of human remains*. CRC Press: Boca Raton, pp. 365–382.

Haglund, W.D. (1997c) Rodents and human remains. In: Haglund, W.D. and Sorg, M.H. (eds), *Forensic Taphonomy. The post-mortem fate of human remain*. CRC Press: Boca Raton, pp. 405–414.

Haglund, W.D. and Reay, D.T. (1993) Problems of recovering partial human remains at different times and locations: concerns for death investigators. *Journal of Forensic Sciences*, **38**: 69–80.

Haglund, W.D., Reay, D.T. and Swindler, D.R. (1988) Tooth mark artifacts and survival of bones in animal scavenged human skeletons. *Journal of Forensic Sciences*, **33**: 985–997.

Haglund, W.D., Reay, D.T, and Swindler, D.R. (1989) Canid scavenging/disarticulation sequence of human remains in the Pacific Northwest. *Journal of Forensic Sciences*, **34**: 587–606.

Harrington, F.H. (1981) Urine-marking and caching behavior in the wolf. *Behaviour*, **76**: 280–288.

Harrington, F.H. (1982) Urine marking at food and caches in captive coyotes. *Canadian Journal of Zoology*, **60**: 776–782.

Haynes, G. (1980) Evidence of carnivore gnawing on Pleistocene and recent mammalian bones. *Paleobiology*, **6**: 341–351.

Haynes, G. (1982) Utilisation and skeletal disturbances of North American prey carcasses. *Arctic*, **35**: 266–281.

Haynes, G. (1983a) A guide for differentiating mammalian carnivore taxa responsible for gnaw damage to herbivore limb bones. *Paleobiology*, **9**: 164–172.

Haynes, G. (1983b) Frequencies of spiral and green-bone fractures on ungulate limb bones in modern surface assemblages. *American Antiquity*, **48**: 102–114.

Hill, A. (1979) Disarticulation and scattering of mammal skeletons. *Paleobiology*, **5**: 261– 274.

Hillson, S. (2005) *Teeth*, 2nd edition. Cambridge University Press: Cambridge.

Hobischak, N.R. (1997) Freshwater invertebrate succession and decompositional studies on carrion in British Columbia. Unpublished MSc thesis, Simon Fraser University.

Janjua, M.A. and Rogers, T.L. (2008) Bone weathering patterns of metatarsal v. femur and the post-mortem interval in Southern Ontario. *Forensic Science International*, **178**: 16–23.

Jedrzejewski, W., Schmidt, K., Milkowski, L., Jedrzejewska, B. and Okarma, H. (1993) Foraging by lynx and its role in ungulate mortality: the local (Bialowieza Forest) and the Palaearctic viewpoints. *Acta Theriologica*, **38**: 385–403.

Johnson, E. (1985) Current developments in bone technology. *Advances in Archaeological Method and Theory*, **8**: 157–230.

Kauhala, K., Laukkanen, P. and von Rége, I. (1998) Summer food composition and food niche overlap of the raccoon dog, red fox and badger in Finland. *Ecography*, **21**: 457–463.

Kendall, C. (2014) The early bird gets the carcass: temporal segregation and its effects on foraging success in avian scavengers. *The Auk: Ornithological Advances*, **131**: 12–19.

Kjorlien, Y.P., Beattie, O.B. and Peterson, A.E. (2009) Scavenging activity can produce predictable patterns in surface skeletal remains scattering: observations and comments from two experiments. *Forensic Science International*, **188**: 103–106.

Klippel, W.E. and Synstelien, M.A. (2007) Rodents as taphonomic agents: bone gnawing by brown rats and gray squirrels. *Journal of Forensic Science*, **52**: 765–773.

Komar, D. (1998) Decay rates in a cold climate region: a review of cases involving advanced decomposition from the medical examiner's office in Edmonton, Alberta. *Journal of Forensic Sciences*, **43**: 57–61.

Komar, D, (2003) Twenty-seven years of forensic anthropology casework in New Mexico. *Journal of Forensic Sciences*, **48**: 1–4.

Komar, D. and Beattie, O. (1998) Identifying bird scavenging in fleshed and dry remains. *Canadian Society of Forensic Science Journal*, **31**: 177–188.

Kruuk, H. and Parish, T. (1981) Feeding specialization of the European badger *Meles meles* in Scotland. *Journal of Animal Ecology*, **50**: 773–788.

Kruuk, H. and Parish, T. (1985) Food, food availability and weight of badgers (*Meles meles*) in relation to agricultural changes. *Journal of Applied Ecology*, **22**: 705–715.

Lee, S. and Mill, P.J. (2004) Cranial variation in British mustelids. *Journal of Morphology*, **260**: 57–64.

Lord, T.C., O'Connor, T.P., Siebrandt, D.C. and Jacobi, R.M. (2007) People and large carnivores as biostrationomic agents in late glacial cave assemblages. *Journal of Quartenary Science*, **22**: 681–694.

Lüps, P. and Roper, T.J. (1988) Tooth size in the European badger (*Meles meles*) with special reference to sexual dimorphism, diet and intraspecific aggression. *Acta Theriologica*, **33**: 21–33.

Lyman, R.L. (1994) *Vertebrate Taphonomy*. Cambridge University Press: Cambridge.

MacDonell, N. and Anderson, G. (1997) Aquatic forensics determination of time since submergence using aquatic invertebrates. Unpublished Report 09-97, Canadian Police Research Centre.

Mann, R.W., Bass, W.M. and Meadows, L. (1990) Time since death and decomposition of the human body variables and observations in case and experimental field studies. *Journal of Forensic Sciences*, **35**: 103–111.

Marean, C.W. and Spencer, L.M. (1991) Impact of carnivore ravaging on zooarchaeological measures of element abundance. *American Antiquity*, **56**: 645–658.

McNab, B.K. (2000) Energy constraints on carnivore diet. *Nature*, **407**: 584.

Merbs, C.F. (1997) Eskimo skeleton taphonomy with identification of possible polar bear victims. In: Haglund, W.D. and Sorg, M.H. (eds), *Forensic Taphonomy. The post-mortem fate of human remains*. CRC Press: Boca Raton, pp. 249–260.

Milner, G.R. and Smith, V.G. (1989) Carnivore alteration of human bone from a late prehistoric site in Illinois. *American Journal of Physical Anthropology*, **79**: 43–49.

Mondini, M. and Sebastián Muñoz, A. (2008) Pumas as taphonomic agents: a comparative analysis of actualistic studies in the Neotropics. *Quaternary International*, **180**: 52–62.

Moraitis, K. and Spiliopoulou, C. (2010) Forensic implications of carnivore scavenging on human remains recovered from outdoor locations in Greece. *Journal of Forensic and Legal Medicine*, **17**: 298–303.

Moran, N.C. and O'Connor, T.P. (1992) Bones that cats gnawed upon: a case study in bone modification. *Circaea*, **9**: 27–34.

Moreno-Opo, R., Margalida, A., Arredondo, Á., Guil, F., Martín, M. *et al.* (2010) Factors influencing the presence of the cinereous vulture *Aegypius monachus* at carcasses: food preferences and implications for the management of supplementary feeding sites. *Wildlife Biology*, **16**: 25–34.

Morton, R.J. and Lord, W.D. (2006) Taphonomy of child-sized remains: a study of scattering and scavenging in Virginia, USA. *Journal of Forensic Sciences*, **51**: 475–479.

Möttönen, M. and Nuutila, M. (1977) Post-mortem injury caused by domestic animals, crustaceans, and fish. In: Tedeschi, C., Eckert, W. and Tedeschi, L. (eds), *Forensic medicine: A study in trauma and environmental hazards*. Saunders: Philadelphia, pp. 1096–1098.

Murad, T.A. and Boddy, M.A. (1987) A case with bear facts. *Journal of Forensic Sciences*, **32**: 1819–1826.

Murmann, D.C., Brumit, P.C., Schrader, B.A. and Senn, D.R. (2006) A comparison of animal jaws and bite mark patterns. *Journal of Forensic Sciences*, **51**: 846–860.

O'Brien, R.C., Forbes, S.L., Meyer, J. and Dadour, I.R, (2007) A preliminary investigation into the scavenging activity on pig carcasses in Western Australia. *Forensic Science, Medicine, and Pathology*, **3**: 194–199.

Owsley, D.W., Roberts, E.D. and Manning, E.M. (1992) Field recovery and analysis of horse skeletal remains. *Journal of Forensic Sciences*, **37**: 163–175.

Patel, F. (1994) Artefact in forensic medicine: post-mortem rodent activity. *Journal of Forensic Sciences*, **39**: 257–260.

Phillips, D.P., Ryon, J., Danilchuk, W. and Fentress, J.C. (1991) Food caching in captive coyotes: stereotypy of action sequence and spatial distribution of cache sites. *Canadian Journal of Psychology*, **45**: 83–91.

Pickering, T.R. (2001) Carnivore voiding: a taphonomic process with the potential for the deposition of forensic evidence. *Journal of Forensic Sciences*, **46**: 406–411.

Pickering, T.R. and Carlson, K.J. (2004) Baboon taphonomy and its relevance to the investigation of large felid involvement in human forensic cases. *Forensic Science International*, **144**: 37–44.

Pickering, T.R., Domínguez-Rodrigo, M., Egeland, C.P. and Brain, C.K. (2004) Beyond leopards: tooth marks and the contribution of multiple carnivore taxa to the accumulation of the Swartkrans Member 3 fossil assemblage. *Journal of Human Evolution*, **46**: 595–604.

Potmesil, M. (2005) Bone dispersion, weathering, and scavenging of cattle bones. *Nebraska Anthropologist*, **6**: 26–32.

Ray, R.R., Seibold, H. and Heurich, M. (2014) Invertebrates outcompete vertebrate facultative scavengers in simulated lynx kills in the Bavarian Forest National Park, Germany. *Animal Biodiversity and Conservation*, **37**: 77–88.

Reeves, N. (2009) Taphonomic effects of vulture scavenging. *Journal of Forensic Sciences*, **54**: 523–528.

Revilla, E. and Palomares, F. (2002) Spatial organization, group living and ecological correlates in low-density populations of Eurasian badgers, *Meles meles*. *Journal of Animal Ecology*, **71**: 497–512.

Rippley, A., Larison, N.C., Moss, K.E., Kelly, J.D. and Bytheway, J.A. (2012) Scavenging behavior of *Lynx rufus* on human remains during the winter months of Southeast Texas. *Journal of Forensic Sciences*, **57**: 699–705.

Rodriguez, W.C. (1997) Decomposition of buried and submerged bodies. In: Haglund, W.D. and Sorg, M.H. (eds), *Forensic Taphonomy. The post-mortem fate of human remains*. CRC Press: Boca Raton, pp. 459–468.

Ropohl, D., Scheithauer, R. and Pollak, S. (1995) Post-mortem injuries inflicted by domestic golden hamster: morphological aspects and evidence by DNA typing. *Forensic Science International*, **72**: 81–90.

Rossi, M.L., Shahrom, A.W., Chapman, R.C. and Vanezis, P. (1994) Post-mortem injuries by indoor pets. *The American Journal of Forensic Medicine and Pathology*, **15**: 105–109.

Rothschild, M.A. and Schneider, V. (1997) On the temporal onset of post-mortem animal scavenging 'motivation' of the animal. *Forensic Science International*, **89**: 57–64.

Ruffell, A. and Murphy, E. (2011) An apparently jawless cadaver: a case of post-mortem slippage. *Science and Justice*, **51**: 150–153.

Sala, N. and Arsuaga, J.L. (2013) Taphonomic studies with wild brown bears (*Ursus arctos*) in the mountains of northern Spain. *Journal of Archaeological Science*, **40**: 1389–1396.

Saladié, P., Huguet, R., Díez, C., Rodríguez-Hidalgo, A. and Carbonell, E. (2013) Taphonomic modifications produced by modern brown bears (*Ursus arctos*). *International Journal of Osteoarchaeology*, **23**: 13–33.

Schulz, I., Schneider, P.M., Olek, K., Rothschild, M.A. and Tsokos, M. (2006) Examination of post-mortem animal interference to human remains using cross-species multiplex PCR. *Forensic Science, Medicine, and Pathology*, **2**: 95–101.

Selva, N. (2004) The role of scavenging in the predator community of Bialowieza Primeval Forest (E. Poland). Unpublished PhD Thesis, University of Sevilla.

Shipman, P. (1981) *Life History of a Fossil: An introduction to taphonomy and paleoecology*. Harvard University Press: Cambridge, MA.

Simmons, T., Adlam, R. and Moffatt, C. (2010) Debugging decomposition data-comparative taphonomic studies and the influence of insects and carcass size on decomposition rate. *Journal of Forensic Sciences*, **55**: 8–13.

Spradley, M., Hamilton, M. and Giordano, A. (2012) Spatial patterning of vulture scavenged human remains. *Forensic Science International*, **219**: 57–63.

Steadman, D.W. and Worne, H. (2007) Canine scavenging of human remains in an indoor setting. *Forensic Science International*, **173**: 78–82.

Stiner, M.C., Munro, N.D. and Sanz, M. (2012) Carcass damage and digested bone from mountain lions (*Felis concolor*): implications for carcass persistence on landscapes as a function of prey age. *Journal of Archaeological Science*, **39**: 896–907.

Sutcliffe, A.J. (1973) Similarity of bones and antlers gnawed by deer to human artefacts. *Nature*, **246**: 428–430.

Tsokos, M. and Schulz, F. (1999) Indoor post-mortem animal interference by carnivores and rodents: report of two cases and review of the literature. *International Journal of Legal Medicine*, **112**: 115–119.

Vanlaerhoven, S.L. and Hughes, C. (2008) Testing different search methods for recovering scattered and scavenged remains. *Canadian Society of Forensic Science Journal*, **41**: 209–213.

Virchow, D. and Hogeland, D. (1994) Bobcat. In: Hyngstrom, S.E., Timm, R.M. and Larson, G.E. (eds), *Prevention and Control of Wildlife Damage*. University of Nebraska Cooperative Extension: Lincoln, Nebraska, pp. 35–43.

Wade, D.A. and Browns, J.E. (1985) *Procedures for Evaluating Predation on Livestock and Wildlife*. Bulletin Number B-1429 Texas Agricultural Extension Service, Texas A and M University: San Angelo, Texas.

Willey, P. and Snyder, L.M. (1989) Canid modification of human remains: implications for time-since-death estimations. *Journal of Forensic Sciences*, **34**: 894–901.

Wroe, S., McHenry, C. and Thomason, J. (2005) Bite club: comparative bite force in big biting mammals and the prediction of predatory behaviour in fossil taxa. *Proceedings of the Royal Society B*, **272**: 619–625.

Young, A. (2013) An investigation of patterns of mammalian scavenging in relation to vertebrate skeletal remains in a Northwest European context: forensic applications. Unpublished PhD thesis, Bournemouth University.

Young, A., Stillman, R., Smith, M.J. and Korstjens, A. (2014a) Scavenging in Northwestern Europe: a survey of UK police specialist search officers. *Policing*, **8**: 156–164.

Young, A., Stillman, R., Smith, M.J. and Korstjens, A. (2014b) An experimental study of vertebrate scavenging behavior in a Northwest European woodland context. *Journal of Forensic Sciences*, **59**: 1333–1342.

Young, A., Márquez-Grant, N., Stillman, R., Smith, M.J. and Korstjens, A. (2015a) An investigation of red fox (*Vulpes vulpes*) and Eurasian badger (*Meles meles*) scavenging, scattering and removal of deer remains: forensic implications and applications. *Journal of Forensic Sciences*, **60**: S39–55.

Young, A., Stillman, R., Smith, M.J. and Korstjens, A. (2015b) Scavenger species-typical alteration to bone: using bite mark dimensions to identify scavengers. *Journal of Forensic Sciences*, **60**: 1426–1435.

17

Decomposition in Aquatic Environments

Barbara H. Stuart and Maiken Ueland

17.1 Introduction

Each year, many thousands of individuals lose their lives in water-related deaths. Many of the deaths are the result of accidents or disasters, including recreational boating accidents, ferry sinkings, plane crashes or natural disasters. The management of drowning deaths on a large scale is very much in the public eye at the current time, with world attention focused on the movement of large numbers of migrants into Europe, many of whom attempt a perilous journey across the Mediterranean Sea. With the many thousands of deaths at sea to date in 2016 alone, pathologists face an enormous task of investigating such drowning deaths. Some other examples of high profile incidents include the 2004 Indian Ocean Tsunami that killed at least 230,000 people, Hurricane Katrina that devastated New Orleans during 2005 (killing at least 1,833), the Air France Flight 447 crash in the Atlantic Ocean during 2009 (killing 228), the ferry disasters involving the *MS Herald of Free Enterprise* from Zeebrugge in 1987 (killing 193) and the *MV Sewol* in South Korea in 2014 (killing at least 295 on board). And, of course, *RMS Titanic* sank on her maiden voyage in 1912, with 1,517 people dying in the North Atlantic Ocean. Other water-related deaths are the result of suicide and, less frequently, the result of criminal activity where the bodies are deposited in water after death.

The process of decomposition of human remains begins soon after immersion in a water environment (Boyle *et al.* 1997; Haglund and Sorg 2002; Sorg *et al.* 1997). The types and rates of decomposition processes are dependent on the nature of the water environment, as well as on the condition of the remains themselves. Potential water sources include rivers, lakes, oceans and man-made swimming pools. Each environment will possess specific characteristics that will influence decomposition processes and there is a great deal of variability in environments. Significantly, the taphonomic processes observed in aquatic systems will behave differently to the well-established processes reported for terrestrial environments. This chapter provides an overview of the decomposition stages observed in aquatic environments. Central to death investigation is a determination of the time since death. There are established strategies applied in terrestrial environments for such estimations, but these approaches do not automatically apply for bodies recovered from water. A discussion of the methodology for determining post-mortem times for aquatic remains is also provided in this chapter.

In order to understand aquatic decomposition, knowledge of environmental factors including temperature, the types of flora and fauna present, water chemistry and flow, the presence of clothing and the nature of the waterbed are required. Specifically how these factors enhance or inhibit the decomposition process is described.

Taphonomy of Human Remains: Forensic Analysis of the Dead and the Depositional Environment, First Edition.
Edited by Eline M.J. Schotsmans, Nicholas Márquez-Grant and Shari L. Forbes.

Much of the current knowledge regarding taphonomic processes in water environments is derived from casework. Examples of case reports and studies are presented in this chapter to demonstrate the development of current practices. There are particular challenges associated with the collection of a body from an aquatic environment and an overview of the protocols for the collection of human remains and associated evidence is provided.

17.2 Decomposition Processes in Aquatic Environments

17.2.1 Stages of Decomposition

The concept of decomposition stages for bodies submerged in aquatic environments is based on a modification of the well-established stages identified for decomposition in terrestrial environments (fresh, bloat, active decay, advanced decay, dry stage) (Merritt and Wallace 2010). Studies of immersed pigs (*Sus scrofa*) were originally used to divide aquatic decomposition into six stages: submerged fresh, early floating, floating decay, bloated deterioration, floating remains and sunken remains (Payne and King 1972). The findings of subsequent investigations have reduced aquatic decomposition to five stages resulting from the difficulty that exists in distinguishing between the two stages of decay (Haefner *et al.* 2004; Hobischak and Anderson 2002). Table 17.1 provides an overview of the five recognised stages of decomposition in water environments.

In order to semi-quantitatively assess the stages of decomposition, decompositional scoring systems (DSSs) have been developed and applied to aquatic systems (De Donno *et al.* 2014; Heaton *et al.* 2010; Introna *et al.* 2013). Post-mortem changes are visually assessed based on case reports and photographs. The body is usually divided into three regions (head, limbs and torso) to take into account any variation of the decomposition rate. An example of a scoring system used to evaluate bone exposure in human remains recovered from aquatic environments is presented in Table 17.2 (Haglund 1993; Introna *et al.* 2013).

The general rate of decomposition of remains in water is slower than that observed in terrestrial environments (Rodriguez 1997; Sorg *et al.* 1997). Although one of the main determining factors for this overall reduction in decay is the cooler temperature and the absence or reduction in insect activity, the duration of decomposition can depend on a number of environmental factors. These factors, which will be discussed later in this chapter, include the nature of the flora and fauna, water chemistry and flow, as well as the presence of body.

17.2.2 Flotation

When a carcass enters a body of water it will either float or sink (Haglund and Sorg 2002; Higgs and Pokines 2013; Rodriguez 1997). The buoyancy will depend on the presence of air in the lungs,

Table 17.1 Decomposition phases in aquatic environments (Haefner *et al.* 2004; Merritt and Wallace 2010).

Decomposition stage	Description of stage
1. fresh submerged	fresh; sunken remains
2. early floating	bloated; floating at water surface
3. early floating decay	minor decay apparent; disarticulation of soft tissue
4. advanced floating decay	major decay apparent; exposure of skeleton
5. sunken remains	remains sink; bones remaining at stage end

Table 17.2 Scoring system for the evaluation of bone exposure of human remains in aquatic environments (Haglund 1993; Introna *et al.* 2013).

Score	Description
0	soft tissue intact
1	partial exposure of bone due to loss of soft tissue in some regions
2	total exposure of bone with articulation maintained by ligament
3	disarticulation and total exposure of remaining bones
4	absence of body parts

decomposition gases, body fat content and the presence and type of clothing. When a body is floating at the surface, the limbs and head hang beneath the water surface, potentially producing more lividity in these regions compared to the torso. A body is more likely to float in seawater compared to fresh water, due to the higher density associated with the mineral content. If water has entered the lungs, buoyancy decreases and the body is more likely to sink. As a body sinks, there is increasing pressure from the surrounding water on the remaining gas pockets in the body and this causes a further decrease in buoyancy. The body will resurface with the onset of autolysis and putrefaction: the buoyancy is changed by gas production and the resulting bloating. Once the gas is released, the remains will sink once again as the decomposition process continues.

17.2.3 Soft Tissue Changes

As with decomposition in air, the process of autolysis occurs in a body underwater (Boyle *et al.* 1997; Erskine and Armstrong 2010). At an early stage, often within minutes after immersion in water, the appearance of wrinkled skin on hands and feet will be observed (see Figure 1.6 in Chapter 1). Such wrinkling is caused by the narrowing of blood vessels under the epidermis (vasoconstriction) – the nervous system restricts blood flow in response to the environmental change, and the loss of volume causes the skin to shrink inwards. With increased immersion time, partial or complete detachment of the skin can occur and within days skin slippage may result, due to the outer layer of skin becoming detached as a result of autolysis and putrefaction. During putrefaction, a notably slower rate of loss of soft tissue is observed in an underwater decomposition environment. This is largely associated with the lack of a maggot mass that is observed during putrefaction, the stage where most of the soft tissue is usually destroyed in terrestrial remains (Higgs and Pokines 2013).

Adipocere is a decomposition product known to be formed in moist or wet environments and has been widely observed in cases where remains have been recovered from aquatic environments (Dix 1987; Kahana *et al.* 1999; Lawler 1992; Lucas *et al.* 2002). The appearance of adipocere can slow the decomposition process and even preserve remains (Haglund and Sorg 2002; Sorg *et al.* 1997). This product is usually grey-white in appearance, and its consistency varies from waxy to friable, depending on its composition. Figure 17.1 shows the appearance of adipocere formed in a cadaver recovered from Lake Brienz, Switzerland in 1996 (Thali *et al.* 2011). In this case, only the torso remained and all the soft tissue and remaining internal organs had transformed into adipocere. Dating of the cadaver revealed that it belonged to a drowning victim from the 18th century, but the remains had been buried in the lake sediment for several hundred years.

Adipocere is comprised of a mixture of fatty acids, and its formation results from the degradation of triglycerides into the component fatty acids through the action of intrinsic lipases (Forbes *et al.* 2004, O'Brien and Kuehner 2007). When the cells break down, the resulting fatty acids are released

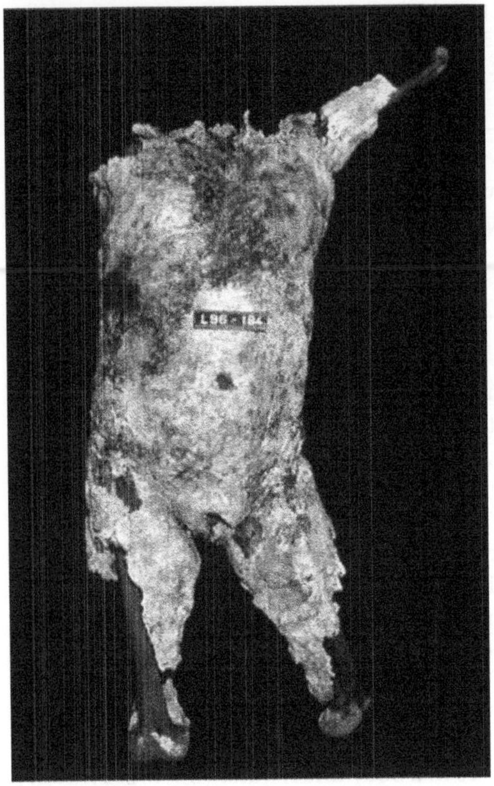

Figure 17.1 Adipocere formation on human remains recovered from the Lake Brienz, Switzerland (Source: Thali 2011. Reproduced with permission of Elsevier).

and can undergo hydrolysis and/or hydrogenation due to the presence of anaerobes such as *clostridium perfringens*. The major components of adipocere include saturated fatty acids, such as palmitic, stearic and myristic acids, along with the 10-hydroxy versions of these fatty acids. Unsaturated fatty acids, including oleic, palmitoleic and linoleic acids, may also be present, depending on the stage of adipocere formation.

17.2.4 Disarticulation

With the initial disappearance of soft tissue, the underlying bones begin to become exposed and are susceptible to separation (Haglund 1993; Haglund and Sorg 2002). Disarticulation of body parts usually follows a general sequence, beginning with the bones of the hands and wrists, then the feet and ankles. This is followed by the mandible and the cranium. The lower legs, forearms and upper arms separate next, leaving the torso and pelvic bones. As body parts may separate from the torso, particularly in environments with significant currents, they are frequently separated from the remaining body, thus complicating the recovery of remains (Haglund 1993; Haglund and Sorg 2002).

17.2.5 Skeletal Stage

When a body reaches the skeletal stage, the bones are susceptible to modifying factors such as abrasion, encrustation and erosion (Haglund and Sorg 2002; Higgs and Pokines 2013; Sorg *et al.* 1997). Bones can be abraded by sediment and objects such as rocks and reefs, particularly in active environments such as waves near a shoreline. In a forensic context, such action can modify evidence of trauma, such as bone damage caused by stab wounds. Abrasion effects can also provide information about the history of archaeological remains (Brooks and Brooks 1997).

A variety of marine organisms can adhere to skeletal remains, either to feed on or to use the bones as a support. Such species, including barnacles, molluscs, worms and algae, can erode the bone surface features or deposit hard growths on the bone surface. However, there is potential to exploit the changes to bone associated with microorganisms, as the appearance produced by certain species may be connected to a particular location or time since death (Sorg *et al.* 1997). Bones also undergo bleaching in a seawater environment, due to the dissolution of the organic component of bone via the reaction with salt ions.

17.2.6 Fluvial Transport

It is possible that a body or body parts recovered from a flowing water environment, such as rivers and oceans, may have travelled some distance from the point of entry. There are three recognised phases of fluvial transport (Evans 2006, 2013; Haglund and Sorg 2002; Nawrocki *et al.* 1997). First, there may be movement of the complete body prior to disarticulation. The impact associated with such movement due to tidal activity or interaction with objects such as boats, can affect the interpretation of *livor mortis*. Second, once disarticulation occurs, there can be movement of individual body parts. Most studies have focused on the third phase – the movement of isolated bones. The shape, size, density and initial orientation, all contribute to the transport properties of bones. This has been a source of information for palaeontologists and archaeologists due to the significance of fossil bone accumulation.

17.3 Post-Mortem Submersion Interval

A knowledge of the time between a death and the recovery of the body – the post-mortem interval (PMI) or the time since death – is central to an investigation of a death. In an aquatic environment, the time since death is also known as the post-mortem submersion interval (PMSI) (Henssge and Madea 2007, Saukko and Knight 2004). As already established, the nature of aquatic decomposition differs from terrestrial decomposition. Importantly, an estimation of the PMSI is challenging due to the variety of environmental conditions that will influence this time.

The lack of a validated means of measuring PMSI has limited its use in practice. However, in recent years, attempts have been made to develop a more quantitative methodology for PMSI estimation (De Donno *et al.* 2014; Heaton *et al.* 2010; Humphreys *et al.* 2013). The use of accumulated degree days (ADDs), the summation of the average daily temperature to which a body is exposed, in combination with a measurement of total aquatic decomposition (TAD) has been demonstrated as an approach to estimate the PMSI. TAD is a scoring system that is a combination of facial, body and limb aquatic decomposition points (Heaton *et al.* 2010). For example, descriptive decomposition stages have been established based on 125 cases of bodies recovered from waterways in the UK and the assigned DSS scores used in that study are listed in Table 17.3. The monitoring of TAD scores as a function of the ADD value for human cases allowed a quantitative relationship to be established using the regression equation:

$$\text{TAD} = -3.706 + 7.778 \log_{10}\text{ADD}$$

Thus, with a determination of the TAD and knowledge of the average daily temperature, the PMSI may be estimated. However, it is recognised that caution should be exercised when utilising such an approach. The formation of adipocere will delay or inhibit the appearance of late decompositional changes, leading to inaccuracy in the model (De Donno *et al.* 2014).

Table 17.3 Total aquatic decomposition scoring system.

Score	Head/Neck	Torso	Limbs
1	no visible changes	no visible changes	no visible changes
2	slight pink discolouration; darkened lips; horripilation	slight pink discolouration; horripilation	mild wrinkling of skin on hands and/or feet; possible horripilation
3	reddening and marbling of face/neck; possible early signs of animal activity on nose, ears, lips	yellow/green discolouration of abdomen and chest; marbling; early autolysis/decomposition of internal organs	skin on palms of hands and/or soles of feet becoming white, wrinkled and thickened; slight pink discolouration of arms and legs
4	bloating of face; green discoloration; sloughing of skin	dark green discolouration of abdomen; mild abdominal bloating; initial skin slippage	skin on palms of hands becomes soggy and loose; marbling, predominantly on upper arms and legs
5	sloughing of head hair; brain softening and liquefaction; exposure of tissue on face and neck; green black discolouration	green/purple discolouration; extensive abdominal bloating; tense to touch; swollen scrotum in males; exposure of underlying fat and tissues	sloughing of skin on hands/feet; tallow/green to green/black discolouration on arms and/or legs; initial skin slippage in arms and/or legs
6	bone becoming exposed, mainly in orbital, frontal and parietal regions but also some on mandible and maxilla; early adipocere formation	black discolouration; bloating becomes softer; initial exposure of internal organs and bones	degloving of hands and/or feet-exposing large areas of underlying muscles and tendons; patchy skin sloughing on arms and/or legs
7	more extensive skeletonisation on the cranium; disarticulation of mandible	further loss of tissues and organs; more bone exposed; initial adipocere formation	exposure of hand and/or feet bones; muscles, tendons and areas of exposed in lower arms and/or legs
8	complete disarticulation of skull from torso; extensive adipocere formation	complete skeletonisation and disarticulation	hand/feet bones begin to disarticulate; bones of upper arms and/or legs becoming exposed
9			complete skeletonisation and disarticulation

(Source: Heaton *et al.* 2010, reproduced with premission of John Wiley & Sons).

17.4 Factors Influencing Aquatic Decomposition Processes

Bodies found in water environments will likely be exposed to diverse and possibly changing environmental conditions. This history makes the interpretation of the taphonomy of human remains recovered from such conditions particularly challenging. Factors that will influence the rate of decomposition include flora and fauna, temperature, water chemistry, water flow and the presence of body coverings. As such factors can change the time at which the markers that are traditionally used to monitor the decomposition occur, it is important to have a clear understanding of how these parameters influence decomposition rate. For instance, if the decomposition process is inhibited then an incorrect short time since death may be predicted. The principal environmental influences on decomposition processes are described here.

17.4.1 Flora and Fauna

Microorganisms, including bacteria, algae and fungi, contribute to the natural decomposition of human remains in an aquatic environment. Such microorganisms can already be present on the body, injected with an intake of water on death, or in the water environment at various decomposition stages. Their presence has been recognised as a potential means of estimating the time since death or an indication of whether drowning has occurred. A number of studies have investigated the potential of utilising microorganism growth, but a reliable method for determining the time since the submergence of a body has yet to be established (Dickson *et al.* 2011; Haefner *et al.* 2004; Heaton *et al.* 2010).

Diatoms (unicellular algae) have been widely employed to establish if drowning is the cause of death (Ludes 2013; Peabody 1989, 1997). Diatoms show unique cell structures and are found in fresh water and seawater. The 'diatom test' relies on the fact that the composition of diatoms in a water environment is unique and can be visually distinguished from the composition reported for any other environment. The diatom test is used to determine if the cause of death was drowning. If a person is alive when they enter the water, diatoms can enter the lungs when that person inhales water. The diatoms are then circulated to other parts of the body, including the brain, kidneys and bone marrow. If a person is dead when they enter the water, diatoms are unable to gain entry into the body. However, it should be noted that the absence of diatoms does not exclude drowning as a cause of death. There continues to be debate about the effectiveness of the diatom test due to the common occurrence of diatoms and the potential for contamination.

The use of insects in determining the time since death in the aquatic environment is not as widespread as the application of terrestrial insects for such purposes, due to the lack of sarcophagous aquatic insects (Haskell *et al.* 1989; Merritt and Wallace 2010). It is difficult to develop a successional insect model for aquatic environments, such as that which exists with blow flies (*calliphoridae*) in terrestrial environments, as many aquatic insects are drifters. Thus, the presence of such an insect on a corpse may be the result of an accidental encounter rather than a deliberate colonisation. Many aquatic insects are dipterans (flies) and midges are common freshwater insects. The presence of maggots on a submerged body is more likely an indication that the body has been exposed to air long enough after death for flies to lay eggs. Their appearance indicates that death occurred in a terrestrial environment before disposal in water, or that the body refloated long enough for the maggots to hatch. Although such maggots cannot be used for the estimation of the time elapsed since death, they may be useful for toxicological analysis.

Animal activity accelerates the decomposition process of immersed bodies due to soft tissue consumption and dismemberment. Importantly, such activity can damage a body such that identifying features and wounds are lost. Scavenging by fish, arthropods and molluscs will particularly hasten the decomposition process and can potentially cause skeletonisation within weeks. Scavenger activity has been described by three phases (Anderson and Hobischak 2004). Initially there is a mobile scavenger phase, where large numbers of vertebrates and invertebrate scavengers remove most of the soft tissue. This is followed by a second phase where there is a sizeable population of arthropods, such as crustaceans, and colonisation of the bones by marine worms (polychaetes). During a third stage, anaerobic microorganisms will feed on the remaining skeleton. This final stage may endure for decades, while the first stages may occur within months or several years.

Crustaceans, such as crabs and crayfish, can cause considerable damage to remains (Anderson 2010; Becker 2006; Rodriquez 1997; Sorg *et al.* 1997). They are active in shallow warm water and are very common in both seawater and freshwater environments. Crabs feed on the most exposed regions of the body and the damage they inflict to remains can be mistaken for cutting injuries. Saltwater and freshwater fish may scavenge an immersed body, but the damage will be less extensive than that inflicted by crustaceans. Small fish tend to be observed feeding on the flesh on the finger, toes and lips and ears. The influence of fauna on the rate of decomposition will be affected by how long a body remains afloat, as floating remains are only available to fauna that swim or float (Anderson and Hobischak 2004). Many scavengers inhabit sediment and, therefore, are only able to feed on a sunken body. Figure 17.2 illustrates an example of the type and progression of scavenger activity on a pig carcass located in a deep coastal marine environment in Canada (Anderson and Bell 2014).

17.4.2 Temperature

The rate of decomposition will be affected by water temperature (Becker 2006). Temperatures decrease as water depth increases, so decomposition rates are expected to be slower at greater depths. Thus, the temperature at the depth at which remains are recovered, as well as the temperature at the water's surface, need to be considered when observing post-mortem changes. Gas formation, and therefore the time for reappearance of a body at the water surface, will be affected by water temperature. In cold water, gas formation will be suppressed.

Temperature is an influential factor for the formation of adipocere in aquatic environments. Earlier investigations indicated that adipocere is more likely to be formed in aquatic environments at temperatures in the range 21–45°C, as this correlates with the conditions suitable for bacterial growth and survival (Cotton *et al.* 1987; O'Brien and Kuehner 2007; Payne and King 1972). However, other studies and case reports have demonstrated that adipocere can form at cooler temperatures (Dumser and Turkay 2008; Forbes *et al.* 2011; Kahana *et al.* 1999). A study involving submerged pig carcasses in Lake Ontario, Canada, confirmed that adipocere can form in cooler temperatures (4–20°C) after one month, but the product does form at a slower rate compared to the rate observed for warmer temperatures. Although *Clostridium perfringens* does not grow below 21°C, it is known that the enzymes that this bacterium produces are active at lower temperatures (Cotton *et al.* 1987).

17.4.3 Water Chemistry

The decomposition process is affected by the salinity and bacterial content of an aquatic environment (Boyle *et al.* 1997; Davis 1986; Rodriguez 1997). In freshwater environments, such as rivers or lakes, an increase in blood volume can occur such that tissues, such as the lungs, are damaged. Freshwater is taken into the lungs by osmosis and the resulting blood dilution causes haemolysis. By comparison, as a result of the higher salt concentration in seawater, osmosis will cause water from the blood to move into the lungs and results in blood thickening. There will be resulting differences in the autolysis rates and bacterial activity due to the differing salt concentrations. The decomposition of a body in a saltwater environment is slower than that observed for a body in fresh water, due to the modification of bacterial activity. There will also be variation in decomposition rates within different freshwater environments, depending on the bacterial content. For instance, a body submerged in a body of water containing a high quantity of organic waste will decompose at a higher rate than if located in cleaner fresh water with a lower bacterial content. Additionally, due to the differences in density between seawater (more dense) and fresh water, the rate at which a body moves through water will be affected.

As for decomposition occurring in terrestrial situations, the decomposition of a body in an aquatic environment is affected by the level of environmental oxygen available (Gill-King 1997). The decomposition process is inhibited by a lack of oxygen due to a decline in microbiological activity. Oxygen levels generally decline as water depth increases. Also, where a body is exposed to underwater burial conditions where oxygen is excluded, preservation of the remains is possible. For instance, in waterlogged anaerobic conditions buried under alkaline silt, preservation of bones is possible because the bacteria responsible for the breakdown of organic material cannot survive

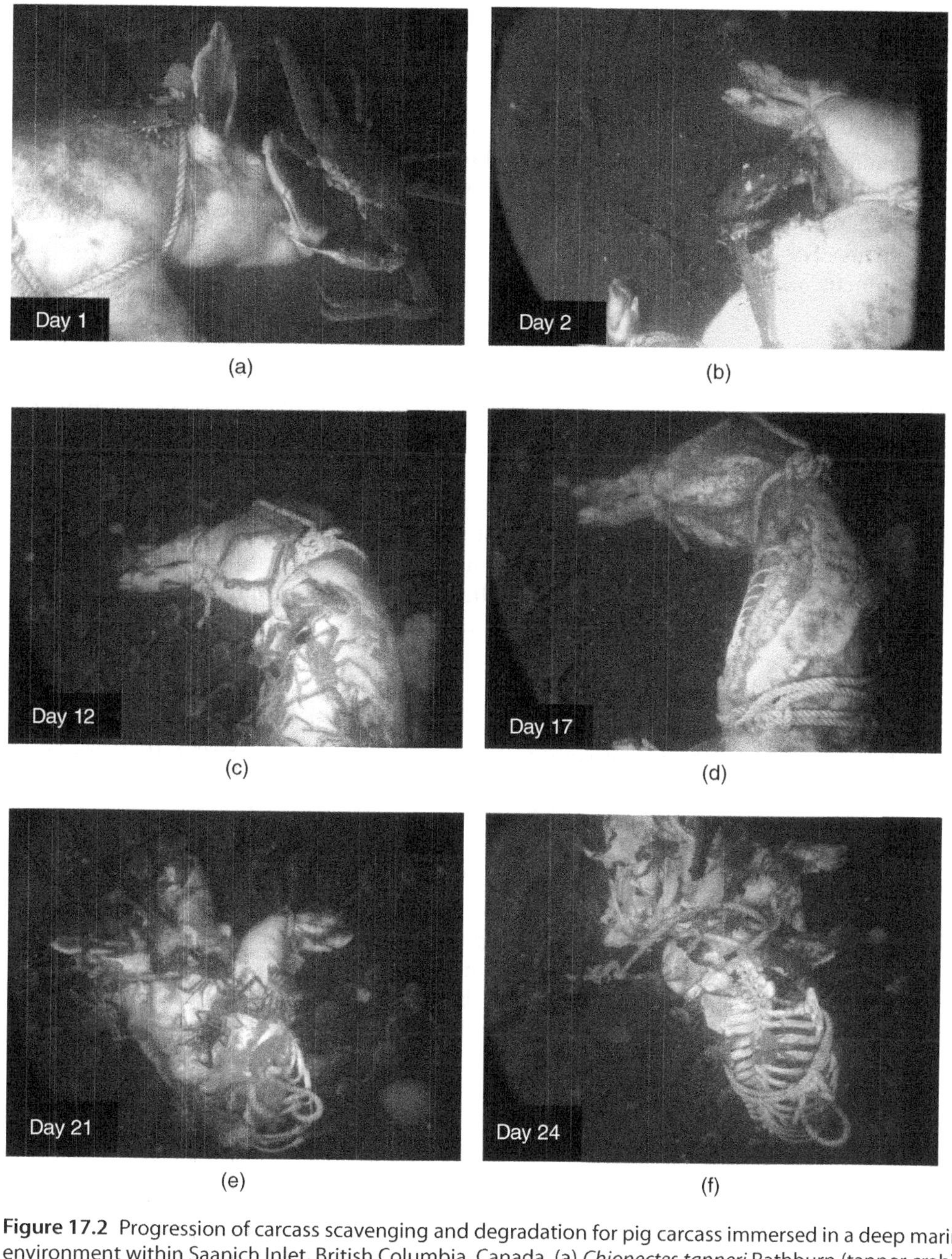

Figure 17.2 Progression of carcass scavenging and degradation for pig carcass immersed in a deep marine coastal environment within Saanich Inlet, British Columbia, Canada. (a) *Chionectes tanneri* Rathburn (tanner crab) attracted to the face. (b) *Metacarcinus magister* Dana (Dungeness crab) reaching into abdominal area and consuming internal tissues with *Munida quadrispina* Benedict (squat lobster) and *Pandalus platyceros* Brandt (three spot shrimp) waiting nearby. (c) Rib ends exposed and large numbers of *M. quadrispina* dominate the carcass. (d) *Orchomenella obtusa* Sars cover the exposed tissue. (e) Half of carcass removed by shark, carcass being skeletonised from inside out by *O. obtusa* with *M. quadrispina* feeding on skin. (f) Skin pulled over torso and cranium by *M. quadrispina* exposing skeleton (Source: Anderson & Bell 2014, http://journals.plos.org/plosone/article?id=10.1371/journal.pone.0110710. Used under CC BY 4.0 https://creativecommons.org/licenses/by/4.0/).

in the absence of oxygen (such as in the case of the hard well-preserved bones recovered from the *Mary Rose* shipwreck) (Stirland 2005).

Changes in pH in an aquatic environment are associated with both the nature of the environment in which the body is immersed and the body itself (Christensen and Myers 2011; Gill-King 1997). Generally bodies of water have a pH in the range 6–8, but this can vary, with some environments being quite acidic (pH 4) or alkaline (pH 10). The environmental pH will influence the rate of decomposition by, for example, inhibiting bacterial activity or providing a more reactive environment for pH dependent decay processes. The biological activity associated with decomposition processes is responsible for pH changes on remains. For example, the bacteria that promote the formation of adipocere produce an alkaline environment, which inhibits bacterial growth and so slows the decomposition (Forbes *et al.* 2011).

17.4.4 Water Flow

The degree of flow in a water environment is a factor that needs to be considered when examining the state of a recovered body or body parts (Haglund and Sorg 2002; Nawrocki *et al.* 1997). The movement of a body has a significant effect on the soft tissue decay process. Impact with a river or sea bed or with objects within the environment can damage tissue and so accelerate disintegration. Likewise, the removal of decomposition products in a flowing system, such as a river, will result in a different decay rate when compared to a standing body of water, such as a lake. In a fast flowing environment, decomposition products will quickly be removed from the immediate environment and so will affect the microbial activity (Haglund and Sorg 2002; Nawrocki *et al.* 1997).

17.4.5 Body Coverings

As observed for terrestrial decomposition, the processes in an underwater environment are affected by the presence of clothing or other body coverings (De Donno *et al.* 2014; Mann *et al.* 1990; Haglund and Sorg 2002; Notter and Stuart 2012; Pakosh and Rogers 2009). When a body is well protected by clothing, the overall putrefactive processes are delayed, as access to the body is limited. However, it is possible for clothing to initially accelerate the decomposition process by maintaining the body temperature and, therefore, the conditions that are suitable for the microorganisms that are involved in the decay process. The nature of the body coverings will also produce varying effects on the rate of decomposition with, for instance, heavier clothing having a more insulating effect. Likewise, synthetic clothing materials are generally less water absorbent than natural textiles and this has consequences for the underlying decomposition processes. The normal bacterial behaviour associated with decomposition is also considerably inhibited when a body is tightly wrapped in plastic due to a lack of oxygen and disruption to microbiological activity (De Donno *et al.* 2014; Haglund and Sorg 2002; Mann *et al.* 1990; Notter and Stuart 2012; Pakosh and Rogers 2009).

17.5 Case Reports and Studies

Much of the current knowledge of taphonomic processes in aquatic environments is based on case reports. Provided in this section are examples of how such cases have been able to provide data to develop the methodology for reporting the stage of decomposition of aquatic remains, and to an understanding of how environmental factors influence the decomposition process. Although more limited, a number of experimental studies have been carried out to develop the understanding of the role that specific environmental factors play in the rate of decomposition in an aquatic system. An example of how the use of model systems can be used to develop knowledge of the role of individual parameters is also discussed.

17.5.1 Decompositional Scoring Systems

DSSs have been applied as part of a marine taphonomy study of victims of a shipwreck (De Donno *et al.* 2014; Introna *et al.* 2013). In 1997, the *Kater Radez I*, a boat containing Albanian refugees collided with an Italian naval ship in the Adriatic Sea. The *Kater Radez I* sank quickly and settled at the bottom of the sea, with 52 people trapped in the hold and drowning. The bodies of those who drowned were recovered after seven months, when the boat could be lifted from the seabed. The heavily clothed remains exhibited varying stages of decomposition and partial skeletonisation. In the first report of the taphonomic investigation, a semi-quantitative evaluation of the 52 victims was made using the skeletonisation scoring system introduced in Table 17.2 (Introna *et al.* 2013). Table 17.4 lists the scores obtained for the 52 *Kater Radez I* victims. Despite the long PMI, the remains were in a surprisingly preserved condition. Table 17.4 shows a high frequency of 0 scores. Soft tissues are significantly preserved, particularly in the upper arms, pelvic girdle and feet, due to the presence of heavy multilayers of clothing. The hands, wrists, head and neck regions show high scores due to the exposure of these regions. A further study of the *Kater Radez I* using a different DSS has been reported (De Donno *et al.* 2014). This study used the scoring system outlined in Table 17.3, a system that includes nine stages rather than five. Scoring was also applied to three anatomical regions: head and neck, trunk and limbs. For this approach, scores 6 and 7 were mostly assigned to the head/neck and limbs compared to mostly scores of 5 and 6 for the torso.

17.5.2 Adipocere

Most case studies reporting the formation of adipocere in aquatic environments have dealt with individual cadavers. However, one case report has examined the taphonomy of a series of bodies recovered from a shipwreck, a Belgian flag cargo ship, the *MV Mineral Dampier*, which sank after a collision off the Japanese coast in 1995 (Kahana *et al.* 1999). In the accident, 27 seamen perished and 15 victims were recovered as part of an Israeli repatriation process. As the recovery process was logistically difficult, bodies were recovered gradually over a period of 433 days. The bodies recovered were located in the middle ship deck at a depth of 65 m with a water temperature of 10–12°C. As the bodies were recovered periodically, a longitudinal study of adipocere formation within human remains

Table 17.4 Decompositional scoring for 52 bodies recovered from a shipwreck using the scoring system provided in Table 17.2.

	Scores				
Region	**0**	**1**	**2**	**3**	**4**
Cranium and mandible	3	20	24	5	–
Neck	11	23	11	7	–
Hands and wrists	7	14	19	10	2
Forearm	46	1	3	2	–
Upper arm	51	–	1	–	–
Foot	51	1	–	–	–
Leg	45	4	2	1	–
Pelvic girdle	52	–	–	–	–
Torso	39	11	2	–	–

(Source: Introna 2013. Reproduced with permission of Springer).

Table 17.5 Adipocere formation in bodies recovered from the *MV Mineral Dampier* shipwreck.

Time since death (days)	Number of bodies	Adipocere observation
2	2	no adipocere
25	3	no adipocere
38	1	focal adipocere
68	2	extensive subcutaneous adipocere
109	3	total saponification covered by thin friable crust
433	4	total saponification covered by thick friable crust

(Source: Kahana 1999. Reproduced with permission of ASTM International).

in a cold marine environment could be made and Table 17.5 summarises the reported observations. Notably, the observations made in this case are at odds with investigations of adipocere formation in cold water, where the product was only observed at much later submersion times (12–18 months) (Mellen *et al.* 1993).

17.5.3 Scavenger Activity

A comparison of two case studies of fatal aircraft accidents at deep-sea depths (540–580 m) provides evidence of the influence of local fauna on the rate of decomposition of human remains (Dumser and Turkay 2008). In the first case, skeletonised and disarticulated human remains from a German military aircraft crash site off the Namibian coast were recovered, three months after the accident. A comparison with a second case involving human remains recovered from a helicopter crash site in the Mediterranean Sea near Sicily one month after the accident, demonstrated a significant difference in the preservation state of the remains. These remains were largely intact with evidence of adipocere formation. These two studies demonstrated that at this depth the nature of the fauna was the dominant factor causing the considerable difference in decomposition rates. Specifically, it was the activity of crustaceans (*Lysianassoid amphipods*) that were present in the waters off Namibia that was responsible for the advanced stage of decomposition of the remains found in this location. There was an absence of such fauna in the Mediterranean, where the recovered remains were well preserved.

17.5.4 Body Coverings

A study of the rate of formation of adipocere for pig adipose tissue, covered in various clothing and carpet types in an aquatic environment, has been used to demonstrate that adipocere forms faster when covered with all clothing and carpet materials (Notter and Stuart 2012). Coverings made of natural fibres were shown to accelerate the formation of adipocere compared with the coverings produced from the synthetic fibres examined. The thicker carpet coverings were also shown to have an accelerating effect, but this factor does not appear to be as significant as the effect of fibre type. The findings were associated with the water absorbency of the fibres and the removal of decomposition products adjacent to the adipose tissue.

17.6 Recovery Protocols

The recovery of human remains from an aquatic environment can be challenging (Boyle *et al.* 1997; Haglund and Sorg 2002; Sorg *et al.* 1997). Submerged, floating or beached remains are commonly discovered by accident. If, for instance, a submerged body is discovered accidently by a fishing net, it can be difficult to collect comprehensive information about the recovery location. If a recovery can be carried out under controlled conditions as part of a forensic investigation, then data about the immediate surroundings of the remains can be established. Information about location, water depth, water bottom type (e.g. sandy, rocky, etc.), water current, temperature, water chemistry, flora and fauna should be gathered where possible to provide a comprehensive view of the scene.

Prior to removal of a body, a record should be made of the position (e.g. submerged, floating, face up, face down, etc.), wounds and a description of any clothing (Houck *et al.* 2012). The body should be placed in a body bag that allows water to be drained without losing any debris associated with the remains. It is recommended that the hands and feet should be protected with plastic bags to protect for fingerprinting and to retain potential trace evidence. Clothing stained with biological fluids should be allowed to dry at room temperature prior to analysis, such as deoxyribonucleic analysis (DNA) testing. Associated materials, such as documents, are best stored in plastic and then frozen immediately after collection so that they can be freeze-dried in order to retain detail. Skeletal remains create a different challenge, as bones will often be located over a large area, particularly with fast moving fluvial systems and where there is a high level of scavenger activity.

17.7 Conclusion and Future Research

Despite the number of water-related deaths that occur worldwide each year, less is known about the decomposition processes that occur in water relative to the volume of knowledge about terrestrial decomposition. The challenge with understanding death in aquatic environments lies with the great variation in the environmental factors from scene to scene. Much of the existing knowledge of taphonomic processes in water is derived from casework. While there has been work in recent years into an understanding of the individual factors that affect the rate and nature of decomposition processes that occur to human remains in aquatic environments, further studies to understand the influence of all environmental parameters are required. As the decomposition process is a complex interplay of variables, investigations into how factors influence each other are required. There have also been some attempts to develop a quantitative means of determining the PMI. Further work is required to provide a validated quantitative approach that can be adopted for forensic purposes to match terrestrial interpretation.

References

Anderson, G.S. (2010) Decomposition and invertebrate colonisation of cadavers in coastal marine environments. In: Amendt, J., Goff, M.L., Campobasso, C.P. and Grassberger, M. (eds), *Current Concepts in Forensic Entomology*. Springer, Dordrecht, pp. 223–272.

Anderson, G.S. and Hobischak, N.R. (2004) Decomposition of carrion in the marine environment in British Columbia, Canada. *International Journal of Legal Medicine*, **118**: 206–209.

Anderson, G.S. and Bell, L.S. (2014) Deep coastal marine taphonomy: investigation into carcass decomposition in the Saanich Inlet, British Columbia using a baited camera. *PLOS One*, **9**: e110710.

Becker, R.F. (2006) *Underwater Forensic Investigation*. Prentice Hall: Upper Saddle River.

Boyle, S., Galloway, A. and Mason, R.T. (1997) Human aquatic taphonomy in the Monterey Bay Area. In: Haglund, W.D. and Sorg, M.H. (eds), *Forensic Taphonomy: The postmortem fate of human remains*. CRC Press: Boca Raton, pp. 605–614.

Brooks, S. and Brooks, R.H. (1997) The taphonomic effects of flood waters on bone. In: Haglund, W.D. and Sorg, M.H. (eds), *Forensic Taphonomy: The postmortem fate of human remains*. CRC Press: Boca Raton, pp. 553–558.

Christensen, A.M. and Myers, S.W. (2011) Macroscopic observations of the effects of varying fresh water pH on bone. *Journal of Forensic Sciences*, **56**: 475–479.

Cotton, G.E., Aufderheide, A.C. and Goldschmidt, V.G. (1987) Preservation of human tissues immersed for five years in fresh water of known temperature. *Journal of Forensic Sciences*, **32**: 1125–1130.

Davis, J.H. (1986) Bodies found in water: an investigative approach. *American Journal of Forensic Medicine and Pathology*, **7**: 291–297.

De Donno, A., Campobasso, C.P., Santoro, V., Leonardi, S., Tafuri, S. and Introna, F. (2014) Bodies in sequestered and non-sequestered aquatic environments: a comparative taphonomic study using decompositional scoring system. *Science and Justice*, **54**: 439–446.

Dickson, G.C., Poulter, R.T.M., Maas, E.W., Probert, P.K. and Kieser, J.A. (2011) Marine bacterial succession as a potential indicator of post-mortem submersion interval. *Forensic Science International*, **209**: 1–10.

Dix, J.D. (1987) Missouri's lakes and the disposal of homicide victims. *Journal of Forensic Sciences*, **32**: 806–809.

Dumser, T.K. and Turkay, M. (2008) Post-mortem changes of human bodies on the Bathyal Sea floor – two cases of aircraft accidents above the open sea. *Journal of Forensic Sciences*, **53**: 1049–1052.

Erskine, K.L. and Armstrong, E.J. (2010) On-scene body assessment. In: Armstrong, E.J. and Erskine, K.L. (eds), *Water-related Death Investigation: Practical methods and forensic applications*. CRC Press: Boca Raton, pp. 109–131.

Evans, T. (2006) Fluvial transport of bones: our state of knowledge and future direction. *Proceedings of the American Academy of Forensic Sciences*, **12**: 173–173.

Evans, T. (2013) Fluvial taphonomy. In: Pokines, J.T. and Symes, S.A. (eds), *Manual of Forensic Taphonomy*. CRC Press: Boca Raton, pp. 115–141.

Forbes, S.L., Stuart, B..H, Dadour, I.R. and Dent, B.B. (2004) A preliminary investigation of the stages of adipocere formation. *Journal of Forensic Sciences*, **49**: 1–9.

Forbes, S.L., Wilson, M.E.A. and Stuart, B.H. (2011) Examination of adipocere formation in a cold water environment. *International Journal of Legal Medicine*, **125**: 643–650.

Gill-King, H. (1997) Chemical and ultrastructural aspects of decomposition. In: Haglund, W.D. and Sorg, M.H. (eds), *Forensic Taphonomy: The postmortem fate of human remains*. CRC Press: Boca Raton, pp. 93–108.

Haefner, J.N., Wallace, J.R. and Merritt, R.W. (2004) Pig decomposition in lotic aquatic systems: the potential use of algal growth in establishing a post-mortem submersion interval (PMSI). *Journal of Forensic Sciences*, **49**: 330–336.

Haglund, W.D. (1993) Disappearance of soft tissue and the disarticulation of human remains from aqueous environments. *Journal of Forensic Sciences*, **38**: 806–815.

Haglund, W.D. and Sorg, M.H. (2002) Human remains in water environments. In: Haglund, W.D. and Sorg, M.H. (eds), *Advances in Forensic Taphonomy: Method, theory and archaeological perspectives*. CRC Press: Boca Raton, pp. 201–218.

Haskell, N.H., McShaffrey, D.G., Hawley, D.A., Williams, R.E. and Pless, J.E. (1989) Use of aquatic insects in determining submersion interval. *Journal of Forensic Sciences*, **34**: 622–632.

Heaton, V., Lagden, A., Moffatt, C. and Simmons, T. (2010) Predicting the post-mortem submersion interval for human remains recovered from UK waterways. *Journal of Forensic Sciences*, **55**: 302–307.

Henssge, C. and Madea, B. (2007) Estimation of the time since death. *Forensic Science International*, **165**: 182–184.

Higgs, N.D. and Pokines, J.T. (2013) Marine environmental alterations to bone. In: Pokines, J.T. and Symes, S.A. (eds), *Manual of Forensic Taphonomy*. CRC Press: Boca Raton, pp. 143–180.

Hobischak, N.R. and Anderson, G.S. (2002) Time of submergence using aquatic invertebrate succession and decompositional changes. *Journal of Forensic Sciences*, **47**: 142–151.

Houck, M., Crispino, F. and McAdam, T. (2012) *The Science of Crime Scenes*. Elsevier: Amsterdam.

Humphreys, M.K., Panacek, E., Green, W. and Albers, E. (2013) Comparison of protocols for measuring and calculating post-mortem submersion intervals for human analogs in fresh water. *Journal of Forensic Sciences*, **58**: 513–517.

Introna, F., Di Vella, G. and Campobasso, C.P. (2013) Migrant deaths and the *Kater Radez I* wreck: from recovery of the relict to marine taphonomic findings and identification of the victims. *International Journal of Legal Medicine*, **127**: 871–879.

Kahana, T., Almog, J., Levy, J., Shmeltzer, E., Spier, Y. and Hiss, J. (1999) Marine taphonomy: adipocere formation in a series of bodies recovered from a single shipwreck. *Journal of Forensic Science*, **44**: 897–901.

Lawler, W. (1992) Bodies recovered from water: a personal approach and consideration of difficulties. *Journal of Clinical Pathology*, **45**: 654–659.

Lucas, J., Goldfelder, L.B. and Gill, J.R. (2002) Bodies found in the waterways of New York City. *Journal of Forensic Sciences*, **47**: 137–141.

Ludes, B. (2013) *Immersion deaths*. In: Siegel, J.A. and Saukko, P.J. (eds), *Encyclopedia of Forensic Sciences*, vol. **2**. Academic Press: Waltham, pp. 11–15.

Mann, R.W., Bass, W.M. and Meadows, L. (1990) Time since death and decomposition of the human body: variables and observations in case and experimental field studies. *Journal of Forensic Sciences*, **35**: 103–111.

Mellen, P.F.M., Lowry, M.A. and Micozzi, M.S. (1993) Experimental observations on adipocere formation. *Journal of Forensic Sciences*, **38**: 91–93.

Merritt, R.W. and Wallace, J.R. (2010) The role of aquatic insects in forensic investigations. In: Byrd, J.H. and Castner, J.L. (eds), *Forensic Entomology: The utility of arthropods in legal investigations*. CRC Press: Boca Raton, pp. 271–319.

Nawrocki, S.P., Pless, J.E., Hawley, D.A. and Wagner, S.A. (1997) Fluvial transport of human crania. In: Haglund, W.D. and Sorg, M.H. (eds), *Forensic Taphonomy: The post-mortem fate of human remains*. CRC Press: Boca Raton, pp. 529–552.

Notter, S.J. and Stuart, B.H. (2012) The effect of body coverings on the formation of adipocere in an aqueous environment. *Journal of Forensic Sciences*, **57**: 120–125.

O'Brien, T.G. and Kuehner, A.C. (2007) Waxing grave about adipocere: soft tissue changes in an aquatic environment. *Journal of Forensic Sciences*, **52**: 294–301.

Pakosh, C.M. and Rogers, T.L. (2009) Soft tissue decomposition of submerged, dismembered pig limbs enclosed in plastic bags. *Journal of Forensic Sciences*, **54**: 1223–1228.

Payne, J.A. and King, E.W. (1972) Insect succession and decomposition of pig carcasses in water. *Journal of the Georgia Entomological Society*, **7**: 153–162.

Peabody, A.J. (1989) Diatoms and drowning: a review. *Forensic Science*, **1**: 397–407.

Peabody, A.J. (1997) Diatoms in forensic science. *Journal of the Forensic Science Society*, **17**: 81–87.

Rodriguez, W.C. (1997) Decomposition of buried and submerged bodies. In: Haglund, W.D. and Sorg, M.H. (eds), *Forensic Taphonomy: The postmortem fate of human remains*. CRC Press: Boca Raton, pp. 459–468.

Saukko, P. and Knight, B. (2004) *Knight's Forensic Pathology*. CRC Press: Boca Raton.

Sorg, M.H., Dearborn, J.H., Monahan, E.I., Ryan, H.F., Sweeney, K.G. and David, E. (1997) Forensic taphonomy in marine contexts. In: Haglund, W.D. and Sorg, M.H. (eds), *Forensic Taphonomy: The postmortem fate of human remains*. CRC Press: Boca Raton, pp. 567–604.

Stirland, A. (2005) The crew of the *Mary Rose.* In: Gardiner, J. and Allen, M.J. (eds), Before the Mast, Life and Death Aboard the *Mary Rose*: The archaeology of the *Mary Rose*. *Mary Rose* Trust: Portsmouth, pp. 515–563.

Thali, M.J., Lux, B., Lösch, S., Rösing, F.W., Hurlimann, J. *et al.* (2001) 'Brienzi' – the blue Vivianite man of Switzerland: time since death estimation of an adipocere body. *Forensic Science International*, **211**: 34–40.

18

Post-Mortem Differential Preservation and its Utility in Interpreting Forensic and Archaeological Mass Burials

Caroline Barker, Esma Alicehajic and Javier Naranjo Santana

18.1 Introduction

Taphonomic profiling of depositional contexts containing buried human remains and artefacts is of interest to archaeological and forensic science researchers and practitioners alike. Both seek to understand the processes responsible for the post-mortem modification (macro- and microscopic) of the deposit and its contents and the significance of these changes to their respective investigations.

Among other things, developing a taphonomic profile for a particular context can: elucidate whether remains are of archaeological or forensic significance; assist in the development of estimations of time since death or burial; help reconstruct past or palaeoenvironments; determine any actions taken to conceal the victims' identity or the crime; identify patterns of behaviours; explain the factors and agents responsible for the survival, destruction and differential preservation of physical remains and macromolecules (proteins, lipids, DNA); and help establish the relative timing of peri-mortem versus post-mortem fractures and defects (e.g. Barker *et al.* in press; Beary and Lyman 2012; Carter and Tibbet 2008; Dautartas 2009; Dirkmaat and Passalacqua 2012; Dupras *et al.* 2012; Haglund 2002; Haglund and Sorg 1997, 2002; Janaway *et al.* 2009; Pokines and Symes 2014; Stein 2001; Troutman *et al.* 2014).

This chapter will look at the status of research into differential preservation in mass burials of forensic and archaeological timescales. Two case study examples will demonstrate that differential preservation in mass burials (between burials and within burials) can elucidate localised depositional circumstances and identify patterns of human behaviour, but is of limited use as a primary indicator of the post-mortem interval (PMI).

18.2 Assessment of Taphonomic Change in Forensic and Archaeological Contexts

18.2.1 Assessment of Taphonomic Change

Comparisons have been made between the similarities of carrying out an archaeological excavation and investigating a crime scene because, in principle, they both aspire to reconstruct past events through the analysis and interpretation of physical evidence (Dilley 2005; Gardner and Bevel 2009; Saul and Saul 2002). However, as noted by Hunter (2002), there are differences in how the physical evidence is interrogated between these two contexts, not least of which is the need to establish the personal identity of the deceased and the legal context of any findings in forensic casework.

Taphonomy of Human Remains: Forensic Analysis of the Dead and the Depositional Environment, First Edition.
Edited by Eline M.J. Schotsmans, Nicholas Márquez-Grant and Shari L. Forbes.

However, questions central to the discovery of any mass burial must include: are the remains of forensic or archaeological interest (PMI) and has there been any alteration or tampering with the grave (Dirkmaat and Passalacqua 2012)?

The tipping point between what is deemed to be of forensic, as opposed to archaeological concern, can be somewhat vague. In the UK for example, any buried remains believed to be older than 70 years are not routinely investigated by the police, the presumption being that any perpetrator(s) involved in the clandestine burial of a body is likely to be deceased (Hunter and Cox 2005). If the PMI of buried remains falls within the forensic window of interest, further refinement is needed to determine whether the PMI is a matter of hours, days, months or years.

18.2.2 The Relationship Between PMI and Decomposition

Estimating PMI is challenging, with a decrease in accuracy over increasing timescales (Pounder 2000; Rogers 2010) (see Chapter 10). Often PMI is based on the status of soft tissue decomposition (Fitzgerald and Oxenham 2009; Swift 2006; Swift *et al.* 2001; Troutman *et al.* 2014; Tumer *et al.* 2013), and it is generally accepted that the shorter the time since death, the more soft tissue preservation there will be (Janaway *et al.* 2009). The accumulated degree day model (ADD) proposed by Megyesi *et al.* (2005) for measuring soft tissue changes over time refined the approach to PMI estimates, having shown that decomposition is best modelled on accumulated temperature and not just time. However, the reliability of the ADD model has had limited success in other contexts (Myburgh *et al.* 2013), as more research is typically carried out on surface, as opposed to buried, remains (e.g. Dautartas 2009; Michaud and Moreau 2011; Myburgh *et al.* 2013).

In burial environments, soft tissue decomposition is generally retarded and skeletonisation occurs much later, but the precise timing is highly variable (Breitmeier *et al.* 2005; Janaway *et al.* 2009; Troutman 2014). Environmental factors such as moisture content have, on occasion (Carter *et al.* 2010), been shown to be the dominant factor in soft tissue decomposition in burial deposits. The introduction of cadaver-derived nutrients into soils will influence the prevailing biological and chemical attributes of the burial matrix (Carter *et al.* 2007; Hopkins *et al.* 2000). Initial studies using rat cadavers and investigating soil chemistry indicate that different substances peak at different times and may be useful to estimate PMI, particularly for intervals over 30 days (Benninger *et al.* 2008). Once remains are skeletonised, Piepenbrink (1986) maintains that the principle decay mechanism is the biological action of soil bacteria; however, it has also been asserted that groundwater has the greatest impact on diagenesis (Nielsen-Marsh *et al.* 2000).

The burial of multiple bodies in mass graves as part of the same depositional event adds an additional layer of taphonomic complexity that needs to be considered. Differential preservation of human remains (between bodies and on a single body) and artefacts in mass graves with the same post-mortem and post-burial interval have been observed in forensic (authors' own experience, Mant 1950, 1987), archaeological (Loe *et al.* 2014a) and experimental contexts (Troutman 2014). Some of the factors attributed to this phenomenon are a direct consequence of whether a particular body is within the mass or on the periphery (feather edge effect, see Section 18.5), the presence or absence of clothing, the grave hydrological regime (diffusive, recharge and flow; Hedges and Millard 1995) and contact with other materials such as metals (Janaway 1996).

Developing reliable or functional estimates of the PMI based on the degree of soft tissue preservation is fraught with difficulty, an issue that can only be amplified when dealing with mass graves contexts where, according to Haglund (2002), the mass grave creates its own microenvironment. Further work is needed, in particular controlled experiments (e.g. Jessee 2003), if our knowledge of the relationship between PMI and decomposition in mass graves is to be meaningfully enhanced. Other experimental work over the last two decades has added to the suite of available techniques to estimate

PMI, and is indicative of the level of importance associated with the search for reliable indicators (e.g. Introna *et al.* 1999; Kanz *et al.* 2014; McLaughlin and Lednev 2011; Schwarcz *et al.* 2010). Nevertheless, little is known about the effects of decay processes, in particular bone diagenesis, within a mass of bodies where the burial medium of a body within the mass is adjacent and overlapping decomposing remains, rather than soil.

Fortunately, the broad categorisation of whether buried remains are of forensic or archaeological significance can often be established using other indicators. For example, the dated stratigraphic context (Figure 18.1) or the grave contents (Figures 18.2, 18.3 and 18.4).

18.3 The Study of Taphonomy in Forensic and Archaeological Contexts

The historical development of the study of taphonomy, from its palaeontological origins (Efremov 1940) to its more recent application to forensic contexts, is comprehensively covered in a multitude of texts (e.g. Beary and Lyman 2012; Behrensmeyer 1978; Boddington *et al.* 1987; Bristow *et al.* 2011; Dirkmaat *et al.* 2008; Haglund and Sorg 1997, 2002; Pokines 2014; Pope 2010; Rogers 2010; Simmons and Cross 2013; Sorg *et al.* 2012; Tibbett and Carter 2008;. Also, the relevance of this area of study to the interpretation of forensic contexts is widely acknowledged by many scientific researchers and practitioners (e.g. Bristow *et al.* 2011; Carter and Tibbett 2008; Dirkmaat and Passalacqua 2012; Mant 1987; Nawrocki 1996).

18.3.1 Forensic Taphonomy

Forensic taphonomy is concerned with determining which post-mortem changes are of interest to the law and any criminal investigation. In cases of mass burials, this interest will cover the legal requirement to account for the dead (Hunter and Cox 2005), by establishing the identity of the deceased,

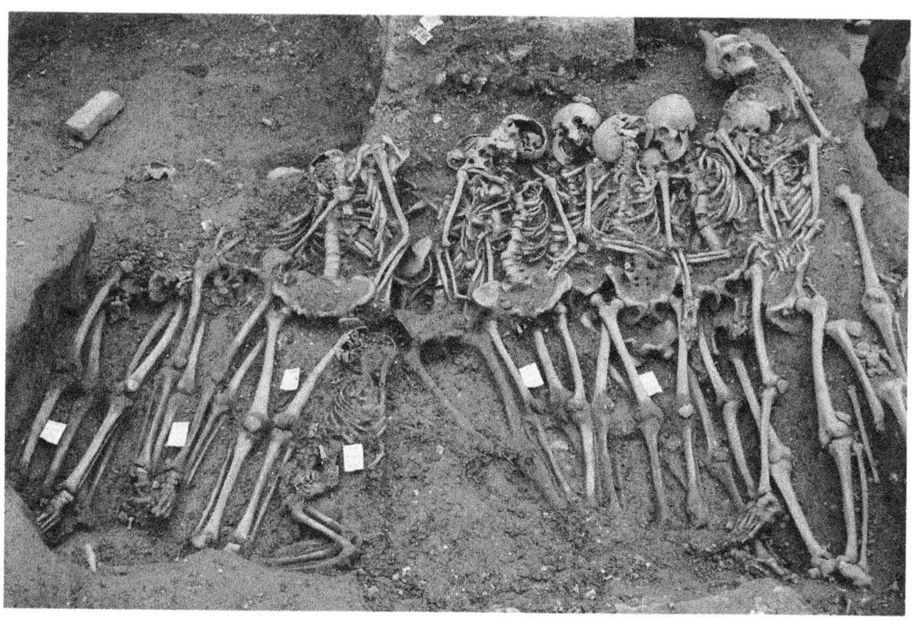

Figure 18.1 Mass burial contemporaneous with 13th- to 14th-century deposits associated with the priory and hospital of St Mary's Spital without Bishopsgate, London (photo: C. Barker).

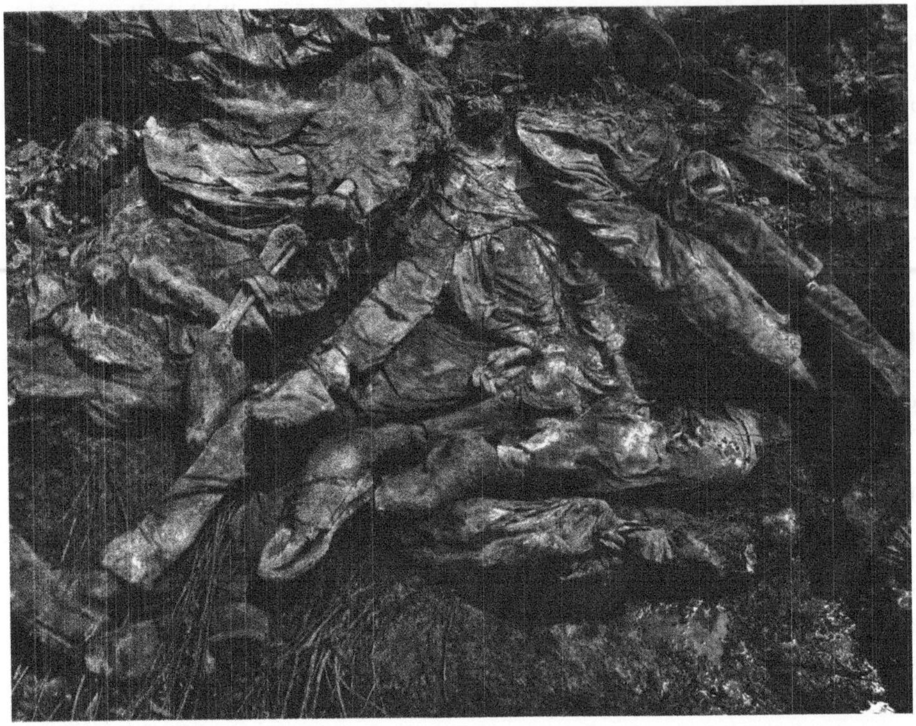

Figure 18.2 Undisturbed primary grave (Kozluk 3 exhumed in 1999) containing a disorganised mass of bodies. The human remains are predominantly saponified wearing well-preserved modern civilian clothing and footwear, also *in-situ* fabric ligatures binding the wrists are visible on the body in centre of the photograph (photo: T. Loveless).

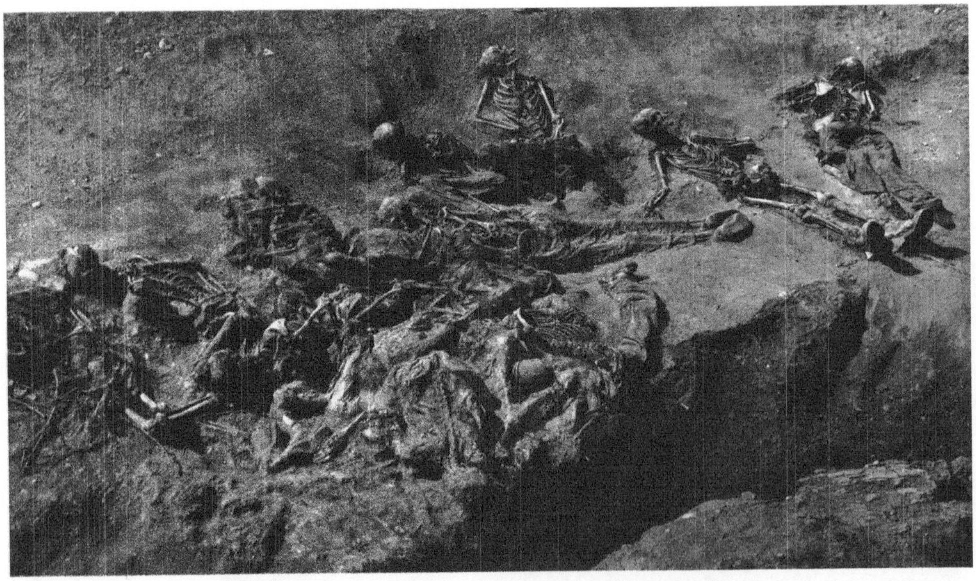

Figure 18.3 Partially robbed primary grave (Kozluk 2 exhumed in 1999) containing a disorganised mass of bodies. The human remains are predominantly skeletonised and associated with partial preservation of modern civilian clothing and footwear. *In-situ* fabric ligatures on the wrists of one body and the robbing of the grave by mechanical excavator are also visible in the photograph (photo: T. Loveless).

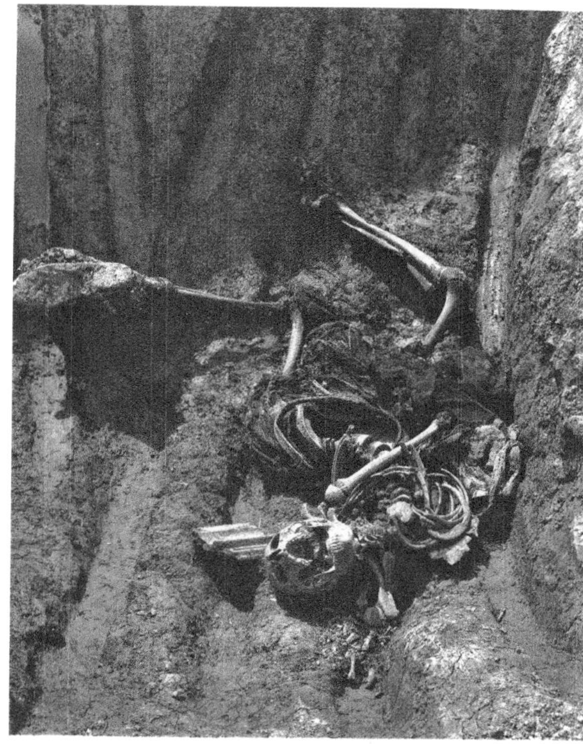

Figure 18.4 Robbed primary grave (Glogova exhumed in 2000) containing a partly disarticulated set of skeletonised human remains disturbed or re-deposited on the base of the grave during the robbing event. The body is associated with fragments of modern civilian clothing and footwear and mechanical excavator marks from the robbing event are visible in the photograph (photo: T. Loveless).

cause and manner of death and circumstances around the time of death (peri-mortem) and deposition. The investigative steps taken and ancillary disciplines employed will revolve around these central questions.

Forensic taphonomy however is, to some extent, regarded as an emerging sub-discipline within forensic archaeology and anthropology. The development and implementation of standards and best practices still needs to catch up with other areas of basic analysis, such as pathology or trauma (Jessee 2003; Pokines and Symes 2014) and, according to Simmons and Cross (2013), forensic taphonomy needs to receive the same amount of research attention as other areas of forensic archaeology and anthropology. Experimental studies on the decomposition of human remains have tended to concentrate on soft tissues; once remains are skeletonised they are collected for other research and teaching purposes (Pokines 2014). Thus, experimental research into the highly destructive processes influencing the preservation and condition of bone and teeth is often excluded. Troutman *et al.* (2014) contend that there has been little additional quantitative work on decomposition processes in mass graves since Mant's early work in the mid-20th century (Mant 1950).

18.3.2 Taphonomy in Archaeological Contexts

Taphonomy is a routine consideration in the interpretation of the site and human remains in ancient burials (archaeological timescales). However, this area of study is more often referred to as *site formation processes*, with archaeologists drawing the distinction between the cultural and non-cultural (natural) processes (C and N transforms) at play in the alteration of the site, terrain and any remains (human and non-human) (e.g. Bristow *et al.* 2011; Duhig 2003; Grant *et al.* 2008; Holliday 2004; Jessee and Skinner 2005; Schiffer 1987; Stein 2001).

Often, all that remains of buried bodies recovered from archaeological contexts is bone and/or teeth. The degree to which osseous and dental tissue survives and its gross macroscopic condition is highly variable, between contemporaneous burial environments and across different archaeological epochs (e.g. Kjellström 2005; Loe *et al.* 2014a; Manifold 2012; Nielson-March *et al.* 2000; Stojanowski *et al.* 2001; authors' own experience).

18.4 Taphonomic Assessment in Mass Burial Deposits

18.4.1 The Context and Anatomy of Mass Burials

The deliberate and legal burial of single cadavers in designated cemeteries is commonplace, whereas mass burials, as a means of disposal, tend to occur under extraordinary circumstances, for example mass burial sites due to tragedies such as famine, disease, disaster or war (Rugg 2000). According to Varas and Leiva (2012) however, there are examples of mass burials in Europe during the Palaeolithic period, (e.g. the Predmosti mass grave in the Czech Republic of the upper Palaeolithic Gravettian culture, ca. 28,000–22,000 BP) and post-depositional human intervention has been documented since the Neolithic (ca. 7000–2500 BC).

Mainly within the forensic literature, there is much scholarly debate about what constitutes a mass grave or burial (e.g. Congram 2010; Connor 2009; Haglund 2002; Haglund *et al.* 2000; Jaeger 2013; Jessee 2003; Jessee and Skinner 2005; Juhl 2005; Mant 1987; Schmitt 2002; Sinamati *et al.* 2011;Skinner 1987). Much of the discussion revolves around the minimum number of bodies, their organisation and motive for their disposal. Often, the context of the mass burial or grave is behavioural, which will underpin any definition or typology proposed (Haglund 2002; Jessee and Skinner 2005), for example, whether a grave is criminal or non-criminal in nature, indicative of a surface execution site, primary or secondary grave or past burial and funerary practices.

The United Nations (UN), for example, developed a legal definition to describe criminal disposal methods of multiple bodies of civilian victims in the war in the former Yugoslavia:

> ...locations where three or more victims of extrajudicial, summary or arbitrary executions were buried, not having died in combat or armed confrontations.
>
> (UN 1993: Annex 1, paragraph 5)

With 'locations' taken to mean any mass disposal site, ranging from purpose dug graves to existing cavities or spaces such as ravines, wells, disused mineshafts and caves.

Large-scale death assemblages due to natural catastrophes may also result in organised mass graves. While the origin of such graves carries no criminal intent, there is a forensic dimension with the need to identify the dead. In the Philippines for example, many hundreds of bodies, the victims of typhoon Haiyan in 2013, were interred in individual body bags and/or coffins in mass graves as part of a dead body management approach (Aljazeera 2013; IRIN 2013).

In archaeological contexts, the emphasis is often on site formation processes (Jessee and Skinner 2005; Stein 2001), and the determination of taphonomic patterns created by past behaviours that are distinct from patterns created by later cultural and natural processes. For example, there are differences in the context and taphonomic profiles of mass burials of battlefield dead (e.g. Fiorato *et al.* 2007; Kjellström 2005; Loe *et al.* 2014a, b; Lougas 1991; Signoli *et al.* 2004), 14th century plague pits (Antoine 2008; Callaway 2011) and medieval hospital cemeteries (Symonds 2012) (Figure 18.1).

Additional confusion on what constitutes a 'mass grave' arises from differences in terminology between different schools of traditional archaeology. French archaeologists and anthropologists tend to distinguish between plural, multiple and collective burials, while the Anglo-Saxon archaeological community uses those terms interchangeably. French authors define a 'plural burial' as the remains of several bodies within the same structure, also known as mass burial or mass grave. However, to elucidate further, any temporal component in the disposal of the dead, 'multiple burial' refers to the simultaneous deposition of several cadavers, whereas 'collective burial' means that the deposition of several cadavers took place over a period of time (Castex *et al.* 2014).

Throughout this chapter, the terms mass burial and mass grave will be used interchangeably, and correspond to Haglund's (2002) broad definition of a mass of bodies (organised or disorganised) in intimate contact with each other and deposited in the same grave.

18.4.2 The Sequence of Decomposition in Human Cadavers

The decomposition sequence of a human cadaver is more or less divided into two phases (Carter and Tibbett 2008; Fiedler and Graw 2003; Payne 1965; Swift 2006). The destruction of the soft tissues (autolysis, putrefaction, liquefaction, disintegration) leading to skeletonisation occurs in the earlier phase and, the degradation of bone and teeth (diagenesis) in the later phase; with each advancing and transformative stage associated with a loss in cadaver mass (Carter and Tibbett 2008; Fiedler and Graw 2003).

However, post-mortem decay processes are by no means sequential. For example, Brown and Brown (2011) determined that the degradation of biomolecules in bone and teeth, including DNA, commences immediately after death during autolysis, due to the biological action of a cadaver's own enzymes. Also, the effects of these enzymes on nuclear and mitochondrial DNA are different, due to the intrinsic properties of the molecules and how they are packaged within the cell (Allentoft *et al.* 2012; Andra-Sorina *et al.* 2014; Collins *et al.* 2002).

Mummification and adipocere formation may halt or temporarily sidestep the usual decay sequence and retard other decomposition processes (Fiedler and Graw 2003). Mummification is the preservation of the soft tissues due to the rapid drying (desiccation) of a body and inhibition of the destructive putrefactive processes of microorganisms (Forbes *et al.* 2005a), and has been observed in dry, well-drained soils (Mant 1987). Adipocere formation is the post-mortem conversion of neutral fats into a lipid mixture with the water content of the burial environment seemingly one of the most crucial factors in its formation (Connor 2007; Durães *et al.* 2010; Forbes *et al.* 2005a, b; Stuart *et al.* 2000; Takatori 1996, 2001). The persistence of adipocere in mass graves tends to last longer than in single graves, due to the increased likelihood of water being retained within the mass grave from the bodies, groundwater and rain (Connor 2007; Froentjes 1965).

18.4.3 In-Soil Human Decomposition and the Taphonomic Processes at Work

A burial deposit containing human remains and associated death scene materials is a complex environment, characterised by its physical, biological and chemical properties and their interdependence (Bristow *et al.* 2011; Fitzpatrick 2008; Janaway *et al.* 2009; Troutman *et al.* 2014). The soft tissue decomposition of buried body/bodies is influenced by the intrinsic properties of the cadaver(s) and extrinsic factors of the particular context (e.g. Benninger *et al.* 2008; Campobasso *et al.* 2001; Carter and Tibbett 2008; Carter *et al.* 2007, 2008, 2010; Christensen *et al.* 2014; Cross and Simmons 2010; Damann and Carter 2014; Dent *et al.* 2004; Fitzgerald and Oxenham 2009; Goff 2009; Haglund and Sorg 2002; Jaggers and Rodgers 2009; Janaway *et al.* 2009; Janjua and Rodgers, 2008; Jessee 2003; Jessee and Skinner 2005; Payne 1965; Pope 2010; Prieto *et al.* 2004; Rogers 2010; Swift 2006). Buried bone is vulnerable to diagenetic change, a consequence of the isotopic, molecular, biochemical and structural attributes of the bone (intrinsic properties) and its environmentally determined behaviours in the burial deposit (extrinsic factors) (e.g. Andra-Sorina *et al.* 2014; Bell *et al.* 1996; Behrensmeyer and Kidwell 1985; Berna *et al.* 2003; Brown and Brown 2011; Collins *et al.* 1995; Galloway *et al.* 1997; Hedges 2002; Jans *et al.* 2004; King *et al.* 2011; Lindahl 1993; Manifold 2012; Muller *et al.* 2011; Nieslen-Marsh and Hedges 2000; Rogers *et al.* 2010; Somadeva 2013; Trueman *et al.* 2004; Weiner 2010; Weiner and Bar-Yousef 1990; Wright and Schwarcz 1996). At any one time, a multitude of taphonomic processes will influence (promote or retard) human decomposition processes in soil, with environmental shifts throughout the interment period (Wilson *et al.* 2007). The dynamism, complexity and interaction of these processes is perhaps exemplified in mass graves, where differential preservation can be seen both between individuals and on the remains of a single individual (e.g. Loe *et al.* 2014a; Radanov 1992; Wright 1999; Zychowski 2011; Figures 18.2 and 18.3).

The principle intrinsic and extrinsic biological, chemical and physical taphonomic factors affecting in-soil human decomposition can be seen in Tables 18.1 and 18.2 (adapted from Benninger *et al.* 2008; Campobasso *et al.* 2001; Carter *et al.* 2008, 2010; Christensen *et al.* 2014; Cross and Simmons 2010; Dautartas *et al.* 2014; Dent *et al.* 2004; Fiedler and Graw 2003; Haglund 2002; Haglund and Sorg 2002; Henderson 1987; Jaggers and Rogers 2009; Janaway 1987; Janjua and Rogers 2008; 1996; Jessee 2003; Jessee and Skinner 2005; Manifold 2012; Mann *et al.* 1990; Mant 1987; Micozzi 1991, 1997; Miloš *et al.* 2007; Perper 2006; Pope 2010; Rodriguez and Bass 1983; Schotsmans *et al.* 2012; Surabian 2012; Turner and Wiltshire 1999; Vass *et al.* 1992; Von Endt and Ortner 1984).

18.5 Taphonomic Processes and Differential Preservation in Mass Burials: Current Research and Application

Mant's pioneering work in the 1950s (Mant 1950) on European WWII graves was the first occasion to consider the variables at work in the decomposition of human remains in mass graves (Haglund 2002; Troutman *et al.* 2014). Mant's work (1950, 1987) clearly demonstrated that mass graves create their own unique depositional environment and that they differ from single burials as the result of the interactions between the intrinsic properties of the bodies, among other things. Moreover, Mant was the first to document the feather edge effect, noting that bodies at the edges of a mass grave tended to exhibit accelerated decomposition in comparison with bodies in the centre of the mass. Bodies at the centre are in intimate contact with one another and exposed to the interaction of taphonomic factors and agents within the cluster of bodies. In contrast, bodies on the periphery are exposed to the factors and agents at the interface between it, the deposit and the grave cut.

According to Troutman *et al.* (2014), there has been little additional experimental work since Mant's early observations on the taphonomic effects of multiple bodies within the same deposit. To remedy this deficit, Troutman *et al.* (2014) set up a series of experimental mass graves using human body analogues (rabbits), to test the effects of carcass position within the mass and along the periphery. The results indicate that temperature was the main driver of decomposition, with carcasses closer to the surface decomposing more rapidly. However, the effect of other variables, such as oxygen availability and compaction of carcasses, requires additional experimentation to understand their significance in differential decomposition.

Generally, there is a reliance on case-based, somewhat anecdotal literature, to enhance our understanding of differential preservation in mass burials of both archaeological and forensic significance (e.g. Ferllini and Croft 2009; ICTY 2000, 2001, 2011; Kjellström 2005; Loe *et al.* 2014; Radanov 1992; Wright 1999; Zychowski 2011). The taphonomic profiling and interpretation of actual mass grave contexts has tended to take the inductive and/or deductive approach consistent with Quinney's (Bristow *et al.* 2011; Quinney 2000) palaeotaphonomy model. Whereby deposits and the condition and preservation of remains and artefacts are interpreted contextually, for example, consideration is given

Table 18.1 Intrinsic biological, chemical and physical taphonomic factors affecting in-soil human decomposition

Characteristics		Variables	Taphonomic Effects & Processes
Intrinsic	Physical, chemical & biological attributes of a Body	***Biological profile*** *(age, sex, body mass/physique)*	• **Body mass may influence initial gut microbial biomass and development of adipocere** • Bodies with higher fat content have a greater tendency to form adipocere • On average female bodies are more likely to develop adipocere than males due to higher fat content and fat distribution • **Age and sex can affect bone density as well as pathology and consequently DNA quantity** • Generally male bones are more dense than female
		Bone chemistry, morphology and density	• Rates of decay and bone diagenesis have been proven to be inversely proportional to the bone size • Bones of children more vulnerable due to their smaller size and higher collagen content (less mineralised) • Collagen and hydroxyapatite vulnerable to dissolution in water • **The protective mineral and protein matrix of bone serves as a mechanical barrier to micro-organism** attack and isolates the DNA from detrimental conditions of the environment
		Peri-mortem trauma	• Trauma can alter the usual speed and pattern of decomposition, e.g. access by other micro and meso organisms, exsanguination impeding putrefactive processes, though studies have also shown it to **have little to no effect on the state of decomposition**
		Health & cause of death	• **Health of the body at the time of death will influence body biochemistry and subsequent decay** processes, e.g. sepsis associated with increased micro-organism load, higher levels of sugars in diabetics accelerates putrefactive changes • Presence of antibiotics, poisons, alcohol and other drugs may inhibit decomposition processes • Pathological changes to bone may weaken bone structure and mineral density, e.g. osteoporosis
		State of decomposition at time of burial	• **Time between death and burial will influence the decomposition stage reached at the time of burial, varying states of decomposition behave differently once buried**

Table 18.2 Extrinsic biological, chemical and physical taphonomic factors affecting in soil human decomposition

Characteristics		Variables	Taphonomic Effects & Processes
Extrinsic	Grave Attributes	*Compaction of sediment*	• **Can act as a physical barrier from other taphonomic agents, limiting or increasing their effects e.g. the capacity to transmit fluids and** accessibility to insects and other animals • May cause plastic deformation and breakage of skeletal remains
		Depth of burial	• **An increase in depth decreases and stabilises temperature due to the insulating effect of soil, with cooler temperatures** inhibiting decay • An increase in depth acts as a physical barrier to animal and insect activity with shallower graves more susceptible to disturbance by human, animal and insect activity • An increase in depth increases the likelihood of adipocere formation due to the retention of water in a grave
		Inclusions	• Dependent on their characteristics, inclusions can retard or accelerate decomposition e.g. hydrated lime or quicklime can retard early **decomposition processes by restricting the release of volatile organic compounds and negating the effects of the grave soils**
		Intervening fill	• **The fill serves as a barrier between multiple body deposits and can cause changes in decomposition between the deposits**
		Typology of grave	• **Mass burials in primary, robbed, secondary graves will have different taphonomic factors influencing decomposition processes**
	Temporal	*PMI prior to burial*	• **The duration of the PMI prior to deposition in a burial will affect the stage of decomposition reached at the time of burial e.g. amount** of insect colonisation and destruction of the soft tissues prior to burial
		Duration of burial	• **The amount of time specific taphonomic agents have had to act on a body/bodies will affect preservation of macromolecules such as** DNA e.g. amount of DNA decreases with increasing PMI
		Season	• **Temperature, moisture, animal and insect activity are influenced by the season**
	Physical, chemical & biological attributes of Soil	*pH*	• **Changes in the pH can alter microbial activity which will affect the decomposition rates.** Soil pH can be affected by secretions from roots • A neutral pH leads to slower bone dissolution, while low pH (acidic) accelerates bone dissolution • Acidic conditions also negatively impact on DNA preservation • Metals and bone are better preserved in neutral to slightly alkaline burial environments
		Drainage	• Water can retard or accelerate decomposition as well as bone diagenesis • **Excess water, in the case of waterlogged remains, leads to anoxia which can retard some bacterial degradation e.g. preservation of hair, finger/** toe nails, woolen textiles and brain matter due to inhibition of proteolytic bacteria and enzymatic action of proteolysis
		Compaction	• **Reduced compaction decreases the capacity to transmit fluids, and increases accessibility to insects and animals. Can also account for** distortion of skeletal remains
		Coarseness	• **Will affect compaction of soil, fluid transmission and physical weathering, e.g. clays are highly impermeable and sands are abrasive**
		Chemistry	• **Ion content in soils will affect conductivity of ions produced by decomposition and leached into the soil** • Certain chemical elements within soil, such as mercury, copper and lead ,help maintain low microbial populations
		Oxygen Content	• Aerobic microbes are dependent on oxygen to create enzymes which increase decomposition. Denser soils may act as a barrier between bodies and oxygen. • Essential for aerobic microbial activity, a key factor in early stages of decomposition

Extrinsic	Physical, chemical & biological attributes of Soil	*Water/Moisture*	• Water volume and movement is a key taphonomic agent in decomposition as water is the medium for many processes including microbial activity and ion exchange. • **Moist environments promote decomposition, arid environments retard decomposition and rapid drying promote mummification of** soft issues • **Leaching due to water removes organic bone substrates previously broken down by bacterial enzymes and decalcifies the inorganic** component of bone
		Contaminants	• Toxic heavy metals, such as lead and mercury, will impact the composition of the microbial community of the soil and function of **specific pathways e.g. micro-organism enzyme inactivation**
		Botany	• **Plant roots within soil can affect its chemical composition e.g. hydrological regime, and cause mychorrhizal root etchings on bone and** physical destruction of bone (breakage and separation of bone tissue)
		Soil history	• **Influences the size and nature of the population of dormant microorganisms and may be of particular importance during the later** stages of decomposition • Soil bacteria becomes the principle decay mechanism once remains are skeletonised, the protein-mineral bonds of the organic collagen matrix are broken down by bacterial enzymes (collagenases) into their amino acids
	Body assemblage	*Thickness & extent*	• **Increased surface area and contact with surrounding factors, such as the soil will influence what taphonomic agents are at play at any** one time
		Body position In the grave	• **Differential decomposition rates in core of body mass relative to the perimeter resulting in the 'feathering effect'** • **The burial environment of bodies in an aggregate or disorganised mass may exclude intimate contact between bodies and soil and the** taphonomic processes associated with in-soil human burials • Organised mass burials where all bodies are in contact with the soil and adjacent bodies may show more uniform decomposition across the assemblage
	Other characteristics	*Temperature*	• Temperature can accelerate or retard decomposition as most chemical (e.g. cell breakdown) and biological (e.g. bacterial growth) reactions speed up as temperature rises. Temperature is one of the most important drivers of decomposition • Extreme high temperatures can inhibit bacterial growth and replication • Freezing can completely halt bacterial activity
		Post burial exposure of remains to atmosphere	• **Once remains have been exposed to the atmosphere, different taphonomic agents will act upon them. In the example of an excavated** buried mass grave, removing the physical barrier can restart the decomposition process
		Human activity	• Can include disturbance of the burial location, the attempt to destroy the bodies by means of burning, accidental mutilation done during excavation, etc.
		Clothing or other wrappings	• **Clothing and other wrappings can act as a physical barrier to extrinsic factors affecting the body and can retard decomposition**
		Animal & insect activity	• Animal and inset activity can lead to disarticulation and destruction of remains • Microbes digest bone collagen but they are not able to penetrate the mineral frame
		Fungal activity	• Focal destruction – soil water content and temperature are important factors in focal destruction and favoured in soils with moderate moisture in summer weather. Focal destruction less likely to occur in wet, water-logged or dry soils • **The preliminary biological breakdown of hair is through fungal keratinolysis (action of enzymes that break down keratin)** • **Fungus can affect soil pH and consequently microbial activity and decomposition**
		Gravity	• Movement of skeletal remains and small bones as soft tissue decomposes, e.g. thoracic and cranial cavities vulnerable to breakage and crushing, small bones of hands and feet vulnerable to movement
		Geological & topological features	• **Slope and erosion may influence the hydrological regime and exposure to weathering of the human remains**

to temporo-spatial patterning to explain the anatomy and architecture of graves (see Case Study 2 below). However, interpretation will also draw upon modern environmental analogies to interpret results and findings, in addition to the wealth of applicable literature available in areas such as soil science (e.g. Benninger *et al.* 2008; Carter *et al.* 2007; Damann and Carter 2014; Hopkins *et al.* 2000; Tibbett and Carter 2008; Tumer *et al.* 2013; Wilson *et al.* 2007; Zychowski 2011) and human decomposition and decay of death scene materials (e.g. Boddington *et al.* 1987; Dautartas 2009; Janaway *et al.* 1996, 2009; Matuszewski *et al.* 2014; Miller 2002).

Lyman (2002) contends there is a divergence of the study of taphonomy between the two contexts of forensics and archaeology. Stating that forensic taphonomy uses the data as evidence, in contrast, archaeology seeks to identify taphonomic changes to discount them from obscuring the truth. The caveat is that Lyman was not specifically referring to the study of mass burials. Nevertheless, this observation has some standing if we consider one of the frequently cited rationales for taphonomic profiling throughout the forensic taphonomy literature (e.g. Fitzgerald and Oxenham 2009; Swift *et al.* 2001; Swift 2006; Tumer *et al.* 2013), namely, to assist in the development of PMI estimations based on the identifiable stages of soft tissue alteration and decomposition. Yet differential soft tissue preservation in mass burials, where there is a cluster of bodies, is recognised as a phenomenon that would seem to preclude this potential (e.g. Mant 1950, 1987; Troutman *et al.* 2014; Wright 1999).

While those within the respective disciplines are mindful of the limits and capacity of PMI estimations based on the status of preservation of buried remains (Chapter 10), it is incumbent upon forensic practitioners and researchers to also raise awareness of these limitations to other non-specialists (law enforcement officials, lawyers). A defence argument in the trial of Radovan Karadžić, for example, attempted to infer different PMIs for bodies interred in a particular mass grave (Glogova) due to differences in preservation (skeletonised and saponified), asserting that some of the remains were those of soldiers killed in combat in May 1992, and not the civilian victims of the Srebrenica genocide from July 1995 (see Case Study 2 below).

There are shortcomings in the level of research, and thus our understanding, of the principle drivers of post-depositional changes over time in mass burials. Nonetheless, as the following two case studies will show, an inductive or deductive approach on a case-by-case basis has merit, and both examples illustrate how efforts to understand differences in preservation can assist in the overall interpretation of mass graves. The first case study is an example of spatial differences in the preservation of remains and artefacts between mass graves of the same PMI. It is argued that these differences are the result of variation in the prevailing hydrological regime over time, a consequence of the adjacency of some of the graves to woodland. The second case study is an example of the probative value of taphonomic profiling in forensic contexts. Here, the differential preservation of physical remains and artefacts and, evidence of the agents and factors responsible for their survival and destruction, was used to deduce relative chronologies between mass graves and infer patterns of behaviours and actions taken to conceal the crime of genocide.

18.6 Case Study 1: Differential Preservation of Human Remains and Artefacts in Archaeological Mass Graves of the Same PMI and its Utility to Establish Differences in Burial Environments over Time

18.6.1 Background and Archaeological Profile of the Pheasant Wood Mass Graves

The mass graves at the site of Pheasant Wood in northern France are of an archaeological timescale (PMI of 93 years) and constitute the mainly organised burial, by German soldiers, of 250 WWI Commonwealth soldiers killed in action at the Battle of Fromelles (1916) (Loe *et al.* 2014a).

The site presented as 8 rectangular pits of similar dimensions (10 × 1.5 m and a depth of 1 – 1.5 m) in two parallel rows (~10 m apart), 6 of the features were found to be graves and contained between 3 and 52 skeletonised individuals interred in 2 layers. The graves were dug into poorly draining blue Ypresian clay and clayey silty sub-soils, located at the bottom of a gentle slope, with three of the graves adjacent to the trees of Pheasant Wood. Over 5,000 artefacts were recovered, comprising of military and personal items, such as textile fragments of the soldiers' woollen uniforms, metals (ballistics, badges and insignia) and organic materials (wood, leather, paper). Fly pupae indicated that the soldiers had been buried or the graves backfilled five to ten days post-mortem. Peri-mortem trauma was observed in 237 of the individuals, ranging from smaller penetrating injuries to gross anatomical disruption of the hard tissues due to blast related trauma (Barker *et al.* in press; Loe *et al.* 2014b).

18.6.2 Taphonomic Profiling of the Graves

The majority of the skeletons (84.4%) were classified as complete (>95%) and two principle bone textures and conditions were observed. Approximately 60% of the skeletal remains presented as wet/green (survival of some organic component, collagen) and the remainder presenting as dry/crumbly (none or minimal organic component remaining). Preserved brain tissue was recovered from some of the remains, but only from those graves with remains classified as wet/green. In addition to woollen uniform fragments, other keratinaceous proteins in the form of hair, finger and toenails also survived.

The survival in the burial deposits of metals and sensitive organic materials (paper, leather, collagen in bone) coupled with the relative differences between neighbouring graves was used to determine the environmental history of the graves. Using prior research findings (e.g. Boddington *et al.* 1987; Dent *et al.* 2004; Hedges 2002; Janaway 1996, 2008, 2009; Rodriguez 1997) and testing of the soils (Pollard *et al.* 2008), Loe *et al.* (2014a) established that overall the preservation of remains and associated death scene materials indicate anaerobic environmental conditions, due to sustained waterlogging, with a neutral to slightly alkaline pH. However, it was also noted that there was differential preservation of both bone and other materials between the two parallel rows of graves. Greater preservation was observed in those graves located further away from the wood and up the slope, and it was asserted that the proximity of the wood had a detrimental effect on the hydrology of the graves at the base of the slope; inducing periodic drier periods of short duration throughout the post-mortem period.

The study of the archaeological mass graves at Pheasant Wood took a formation processes approach and sought to identify taphonomic changes to discount them from obscuring the truth. Consequently, the taphonomic findings underpinned the interpretation of the timing of peri-mortem trauma (Barker *et al.* in press), with more conservative estimates for the timing of fractures and defects in those less well preserved skeletons recovered from graves closer to the wood.

The work at Pheasant Wood had a forensic element, to identify the individual remains (to the name by which an individual was known in life) and adhere to forensic protocols such as chain of custody procedures. Inherited DNA markers from the maternal (mitochondrial DNA) and paternal lines (Y profile, nuclear DNA) formed part of the individual soldiers' post-mortem profile for comparison with ante-mortem data. To date, DNA typing has contributed to the successful identification of 144 of the 250 soldiers recovered (Loe *et al.* 2014a). The preservation of macromolecules (DNA) across the assemblage and all graves suggests that the macroscopic appearance of the hard tissues (dry/crumbly versus wet/green) is not a reliable indicator of microscopic preservation and/or the potential for DNA yields to be present in sufficient quantities to be able to contribute towards personal identification.

18.7 Case Study 2: Differential Preservation of Human Remains in Forensic Mass Graves and its Use as an Evidentiary Tool

18.7.1 Background and Forensic Profile of the Srebrenica Genocide

In the summer (July) of 1995, the United Nations' (UN) safe area of Srebrenica in Eastern Bosnia fell to the Bosnian Serb forces of the Army of Republika Srpska (Vojska Republike Srpske – VRS). Over several days (11–19 July 1995), the VRS and other forces forcibly detained an estimated 7,000–8,000 civilian men and boys, many of whom were bound and blindfolded. Subsequently, over 7,000 were executed using automatic weapons and hand grenades, and their bodies disposed of in mass graves (ICTY 2000). Heavy earth moving machinery was used to dig the graves (e.g. at the Petkovići Dam and Hodžići road sites), or move soil to cover the bodies disposed of in existing features (e.g. at the Kozluk site).

The VRS was made aware that the international community had learned of the genocide and the presumed locations of the graves. Consequently, in the autumn of 1995 (September to October, some three months after the genocide), in an attempt to conceal these crimes, a number of the primary graves were robbed and the bodies reburied in secondary graves in more remote locations several kilometres away, with the longest distance between any primary and secondary grave being some 40 km (Branjevo Farm to Čančari Road) (ICTY 2001). Once again, heavy earth moving machinery was employed to uncover and exhume the bodies from the primary graves, dig the secondary graves and back fill both secondary and primary graves.

18.7.2 Legal Context: the Interpretation of Forensic Taphonomic Evidence

In 2001, the International Criminal Tribunal for the former Yugoslavia (ICTY) found Radislav Krstić guilty of the crimes of genocide, persecution and murder in the 1995 Srebrenica killings. The narrative Judgment neatly sets out the legal context for all evidence and level of proof required to sustain a conviction:

> ...**find, from the evidence presented** during the trial, what happened...and, ultimately, whether the defendant in this case...was criminally responsible, under the tenets of international law. [The] defendant, like all others, deserves individualised consideration and can be **convicted only if the evidence presented in court shows, beyond a reasonable doubt**, that he is guilty of acts that constitute crimes covered by the Statute of the Tribunal.
>
> (ICTY 2001: paragraph 2, emphasis added)

It stands to reason that any expert forensic archaeological evidence presented, including assessment of differential preservation, needs to be of probative value and capable of withstanding the level of legal scrutiny consistent with the requirement of 'beyond a reasonable doubt'.

Laroche and Baccard (2015) state that ICTY's *Rules of Procedures and Evidence* (RPE) offer limited guidance on the admissibility of scientific evidence, with the tribunal having adopted early on a flexible approach, not based on an overly proscriptive set of technical rules. However, it is likely that in the future, international tribunals will choose to adopt a model that more closely resembles that of the USA (e.g. Daubert 1993; Kumho 1999; Larocche and Baccard 2015), undoubtedly resulting in tougher standards for the admissibility of scientific evidence, including inferences based on taphonomic assessment of the grave and its contents (e.g. Grivas and Komar 2008). Consequently, the recommendations by Pokines and Symes (2014) and Simmons and Cross (2013) to develop accepted standards and best practices in forensic taphonomy and increase baseline research in this specialist sub-discipline, become increasingly urgent.

18.7.3 Taphonomic Profiling of Mass Graves

Forensic evidence supporting the assertion that the VRS committed genocide and human rights violations and, later attempted to hide the evidence and cover up the crimes, was essential to the criminal investigation and subsequent prosecutions. While the testimony of survivors and aerial imagery, among other things, helped define the evidentiary footprint for these crimes, there was also a clear forensic taphonomy dimension to unravelling the chronology and reconstructing peri- and post-mortem events.

The taphonomic profiling of the individual graves and consideration of the similarities and differences within and between them was a crucial component to explaining those factors and agents responsible for the survival, destruction and differential preservation of the physical remains. Furthermore, this evidence was also used to elucidate the patterns of behaviours and actions taken to conceal the crime.

Wright's expert witness report (1999) to the ICTY states that differences in condition of human remains between the different gravesites was a principal factor used to recognise or confirm a grave as primary or secondary in nature. Irrespective of whether the bodies were skeletonised, with soft tissue, or a combination of both, intact (not robbed) primary graves, or parts thereof, were represented by complete bodies, (Figures 18.2 and 18.3); robbed primary graves, or parts thereof, contained some grossly disarticulated body parts within the fill, with concentrations on the base of the grave and access ramp dug by machine during the robbing event (Figure 18.4); secondary graves were characterised by a commingled mass of bodies and body parts throughout the extent of the grave (Figure 18.5). Wright (1999) also asserted that the type and extent of breakage and disarticulation of those bodies robbed from primary graves was the result of putrefactive changes weakening the cohesion of the parts, coupled with the *modus operandi* employed to disinter the remains and dispose of them in secondary graves, namely mechanical excavators and heavy machinery. Corroborating physical evidence from within the graves, such as soil and pollen analysis, blindfolds and ligatures, shell cases and other inclusions, was also used to establish the linkages between the primary and secondary graves and timeline of events (see ICTY 2000, 2005).

It is not the purpose or scope of this chapter to detail the taphonomic properties of all of the secondary mass graves exhumed. However, it is worth noting that the types of body parts represented were often influenced by the clothing and footwear worn at the time of death. For example, a pattern

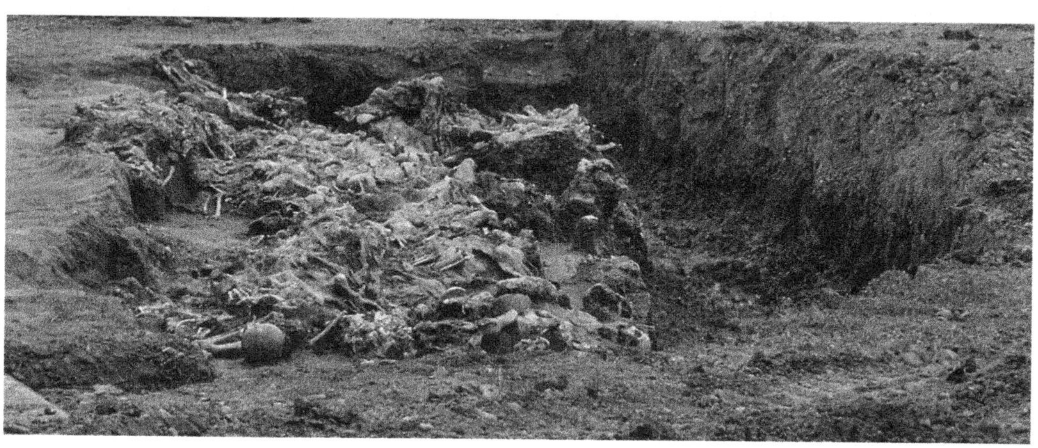

Figure 18.5 Mass of commingled, partially saponified and skeletonised bodies and body parts associated with modern civilian clothing fragments, deposited in a secondary grave (Čančari 12 exhumed in 1998) (photo: C. Barker).

of disarticulation and separation into upper (thorax and upper limbs with or without the head) and lower body parts (pelvis, lower limbs with or without feet) was often observed, with separation occurring in the region of the abdomen at the junction between the clothing of the upper and lower body. Noted exceptions to this general trend were seen in secondary graves exhibiting a high degree of disarticulation, commingling and skeletonisation. Here the nature of the primary burial deposit, looser fills and in some instances gravel and boulders (Petkovići Dam), impacted on the degree of soft tissue decomposition and, subsequently, the capacity of a set of remains to withstand the post-mortem assault of disinterment, carriage and secondary disposal using mechanical excavators and heavy machinery.

Less is known about the differential preservation of the remains from the mass graves at the microscopic level. Nevertheless, the observations and findings of Miloš *et al.* (2007) provide us with some insight into the factors responsible for differential preservation of DNA over time. The study included over 5,000 DNA profiles obtained from 13 different skeletal elements received from 2001–2007 belonging to victims of the 1995 Srebrenica genocide. The study found that the recovery of DNA is significantly linked to the intrinsic factors of hard tissue. Those elements with the highest degree of protection from within the body and greatest total amount of starting DNA provide the best yields over time. Less is known about the extrinsic agents responsible for DNA degradation in mass graves, access to relevant data covering environmental conditions over time, and during storage prior to testing were unknown. Also, there is an inherent difficulty in assessing the influence of environmental variables on DNA preservation; controlled experimentation using a large sample size over a significant period of time would be required to answer these complex research questions.

18.7.4 Forensic Taphonomy: Differential Preservation Presented in Evidence

The Krstić judgment (ICTY 2001) makes direct reference to the probative value of all the forensic evidence. The evidence presented demonstrated that primary graves had been robbed and the bodies removed to more remote locations in a concerted effort to conceal them and the crime and, that the graves had been dug using a mechanical excavator, all of which requires planning and organisation and therefore indicative of the intention to commit these crimes.

As stated previously, establishing the PMI of buried remains is of central importance and, in some forensic contexts, the status of gross soft tissue decomposition may add value to PMI estimations (e.g. Swift 2006; Tumer *et al.* 2013; Chapters 1 and 10). However, as Wright contends in his expert testimony at the trial of Radovan Karadžić (ICTY 2011:22306), differences in the state of preservation are not to be taken as indicating different periods of burial at the Glogova site. Differences in preservation were due to the location of a particular body within the grave, with those on the periphery more prone to putrefactive changes and skeletonisation in contrast to those within the mass of bodies.

The observations from the Srebrenica genocide case highlight the evidentiary potential of taphonomic assessment to reconstruct the past and relative chronologies, determine the actions taken to conceal the victims' identity and the crime and explain the factors and agents responsible for the survival, destruction and differential preservation of physical remains. However, on its own, the condition and preservation of the human remains does little to assist in the development of estimations of time since death or burial.

18.8 Conclusion and Future Research

It is clear that practitioners and researchers alike seek to provide sound, evidence-based conclusions to explain differential preservation of human remains and associated death scene materials in mass burials. Presently, there is limited empirical research specifically looking at the taphonomic processes responsible for differential preservation in mass graves. The implication, for forensic practitioners in particular, is how readily conclusions and findings from one site can be applied to the interpretation of another, especially in forensic casework where legal demands require a solid scientific basis for findings and conclusions. This is compounded by the absence of agreed criteria on what constitutes a mass grave and standards and best practices for recording the taphonomic properties of burial deposits. Therefore, the first step would be to develop standards and incorporate this framework into research methodologies, as well as organisational databases designed to record the findings and analyses of real forensic cases, for example the International Committee of the Red Cross (ICRC) and International Commission on Missing Persons (ICMP).

There are many avenues of potential and continuing research through controlled experimentation, for example, assessing the impact and interaction of specific taphonomic variables, as shown in Tables 18.1 and 18.2, within an aggregate of bodies in contrast to more organised mass graves, where bodies may be adjacent but not intertwined. Actual forensic mass graves, such as those discovered in post conflict areas, may provide some materials, such as soils, for researchers to sample and test; though ethical considerations, such as sampling of human tissue and issues of sub-judice would prevent certain lines of inquiry and/or the publication of results.

Acknowledgements

The authors would like to thank Mr Almir Olovcic for his invaluable help and input on the chemical process of mass graves, photographer Tim Loveless for permission to use his detailed images of the Srebrenica mass graves and Richard Wright for his valuable comments on the draft text of this chapter.

References

Alaeddini, R., Walsh, S.J. and Abbas, A. (2010) Forensic implications of genetic analyses from degraded DNA – a review. *Forensic Science International: Genetics*, **4**: 148–157.

Aljazeera, (2013) Philippines digs mass graves for typhoon victims at http://america.aljazeera.com/articles/2013/11/14/philippines-digsmassgravesfortyphoonvictims.html (Accessed 30 March 2015).

Allentoft, M.E., Collins, M., Harker, D., Haile, J., Oskam, C.L. *et al.* (2012) The half-life of DNA in bone: measuring decay kinetics in 158 dated fossils. *Proceedings of the Royal Society of Biological Sciences*, **279**: 4724–4733.

Alonso, A., Martin, P., Albarran, C., Garcia, P., Fernandez de Simon, L. *et al.* (2005) Challenges of DNA profiling in mass disaster investigations. *Croatian Medical Journal*, **46**: 540–548.

Andra-Sorina, T., Ponta, O. and Kelemen, B. (2014) Bone diagenesis and FTIR indices: a correlation. *Studia Universitatis Babes-Bolyai, Biologia*, **59**: 101–113.

Antoine, D. (2008) The archaeology of 'plague'. *Medical History, Supplement* **27**: 101–114.

Barker, C., Loe, L. and Flavel, A. (in press) Skeletal trauma resulting from explosive munitions: examples from WWI mass graves, Fromelles, Northern France. In: Kimmerle, E. and Baraybar, J.P. (eds), *Skeletal Trauma: Identification of injuries resulting from Human Rights abuse and armed conflict*, 2nd edition. Humana Press Inc: New York City.

Baxter, K. (2004) Extrinsic factors that effect the preservation of bone. *The Nebraska Anthropologist*, **19**: 38–45.

Beary, M.O. and Lyman R.L. (2012) The use of taphonomy in forensic anthropology: past trends and future prospects. In: Dirkmaat, D.C. (ed.), *A Companion to Forensic Anthropology.* Blackwell: Chichester, UK, pp. 499–527.

Behrensmeyer, A.K. (1978) Taphonomic and ecologic information from bone weathering. *Paleobiology,* **4**: 150–162.

Behrensmeyer, A.K. and Kidwell, S.M. (1985) Taphonomy's contributions to paleobiology. *Paleobiology,* **11**: 105–119.

Bell, L.S., Skinner, M.F. and Jones, S.J. (1996) The speed of post-mortem change to the human skeleton and its taphonomic significance. *Forensic Science International,* **82**. 129–140.

Benninger, L.A., Carter, D.O. and Forbes, S.L. (2008) The biochemical alteration of soil beneath a decomposing carcass. *Forensic Science International,* **180**: 70–75.

Berna, F., Matthews, A. and Weiner, S. (2003) Solubilities of bone mineral from archaeological sites: the recrystallization window. *Journal of Archaeological Science,* **31**: 867–882.

Boddington, A., Garland, A.N. and Janaway, R.C. (1987) *Death, Decay and Reconstruction: Approaches to archaeology and forensic science.* Manchester University: Manchester.

Breitmeier, D., Graefe-Kirci, U., Albrecht, K., Weber, M., Trögera, H.D. and Kleemann, W.J. (2005) Evaluation of the correlation between time corpses spent in in-ground graves and findings at exhumation. *Forensic Science International,* **154**: 218–223.

Bristow, J., Simms, Z. and Randolph-Quinney, P. (2011) Taphonomy. In: Black, S. and Ferguson, E. (eds), *Forensic Anthropology 2000 to 2010.* CRC Press: Boca Raton, pp. 279–317.

Brown, T. and Brown, K. (2011) *Biomolecular Archaeology – An Introduction.* John Wiley & Sons: Chichester, UK.

Buckley, M., Anderung, C., Penkman, K., Raney, B.J., Gotherstrom, A. *et al.* (2008) Comparing the survival of osteocalcin and mtDNA in archaeological bone from European sites. *Journal of Archaeological Sciences,* **35**: 1756–1764.

Callaway, E. (2011) Plague genome: the Black Death decoded. *Nature,* **478**: 444–446.

Campobasso, C.P., Di Vella, G. and Introna, F. (2001) Factors affecting decomposition and Diptera colonization. *Forensic Science International,* **120**: 18–27.

Carter, D.O. and Tibbet, M. (2008) Cadaver decomposition and soil: processes. In: Tibbet, M. and Carter, D.O. (eds), *Soil Analysis in Forensic Taphonomy: Chemical and biological effects of buried human remains.* CRC Press: Boca Raton. pp. 29–51.

Carter, D.O., Yellowlees, D. and Tibbett, M. (2007) Cadaver decomposition in terrestrial ecosystems. *Naturwissenschaften,* **94**: 12–24.

Carter, D.O., Yellowlees, D. and Tibbett, M. (2008) Temperature affects microbial decomposition of cadavers (*Rattus rattus*) in contrasting soils. *Applied Soil Ecology,* **40**: 129–137.

Carter, D.O., Yellowlees, D. and Tibbett, M. (2010) Moisture can be the dominant environmental parameter governing cadaver decomposition in soil. *Forensic Science International,* **200**: 60–66.

Castex, D., Kacki, S., Réveillas, H., Souquet-Leroy, Y., Sachau-Carcel, G. *et al.* (2014) Revealing of archaeological features linked to mortality increases, *Anthropologie: International Journal of the Science of Man,* **LII/3**: 299–318.

Christensen, A.M., Passalacqua, N.V. and Bartelink, E.J. (2014) *Forensic Anthropology: Current methods and practice.* Academic Press: Amsterdam.

Collins, M.J., Riley, M., Child, A.M. and Turner, W.G. (1995) A basic mathematical simulation of the chemical degradation of ancient collagen. *Journal of Archaeological Science,* **22**: 175 – 183.

Collins, M.J., Nielsen-Marsh, C.M., Hiller, J., Smith, C.I., Roberts, J.P. *et al.* (2002) The survival of organic matter in bone: a review. *Archaeometry,* **44**: 383–394.

Congram, D. (2010) *Spatial Analysis and Predictive Modelling of Clandestine Graves from Rearguard Repression of the Spanish Civil War.* PhD Dissertation, Simon Fraser University: Burnaby.

Connor, M.A. (2007) *Forensic Methods. Excavation for the archaeologist and investigator*. AltaMira Press: Lanham.

Connor, M.A. (2009) *Mass Grave Investigation*. Wiley Encyclopedia of Forensic Science: Chichester. UK.

Cross, P., Simmons, T., Cunliffe, R. and Chatfield, L. (2009) Establishing a taphonomic research facility in the United Kingdom. *Forensic Science Policy Management: An International Journal*, **1**: 187–191.

Cross, C. and Simmons, T. (2010) The influence of penetrative trauma on the rate of decomposition. *Journal of Forensic Science*, **55**: 295–301.

Damann, F.E. and Carter, D.O. (2014) Human decomposition ecology and postmortem microbiology. In: Pokines, J.T. and Symes, S.A. (eds), *Manual of Forensic Taphonomy*. CRC Press: Boca Raton, pp. 37–50.

Daubert (1993) Daubert v. Merrell Dow Pharmaceuticals, Inc., 509 US 579.

Dautartas, A.M. (2009) *The Effect of Various Coverings on the Rate of Human Decomposition*. Unpublished Masters thesis. University of Tennessee: Knoxville.

Dent, B.B., Forbes, S.L. and Stuart, B.H. (2004) Review of human decomposition processes in soil. *Environmental Geology*, **45**: 576–585.

Dilley, R. (2005) Legal matters. In: Hunter, J. and Cox, M. (eds), *Forensic Archaeology: Advances in Theory and Practice*. Routledge Taylor Francis Group: London, pp. 177–203.

Dirkmaat, D.C. and Passalacqua, N.V. (2012) Forensic taphonomy: introduction to part VI. In: Dirkmaat, D.C. (ed.), *A Companion to Forensic Anthropology*. Blackwell Publishing Ltd: Chichester, UK, pp. 473–476.

Dirkmaat, D.C., Cabo, L.L, Ousley, S.D. and Symes, S.A. (2008) New perspectives in forensic anthropology. *Yearbook of Physical Anthropology*, **51**: 33–52.

Dirrigl, F.J. (2001) Bone mineral density of wild turkey (*Meleagris gallopavo*) skeletal elements and its effect on differential survivorship. *Journal of Archaeological Science*, **28**: 817–832.

Duhig, C. (2003) Non-forensic remains: the use of forensic archaeology, anthropology and burial taphonomy. *Science and Justice*, **43**: 211–214.

Dupras, T.L., Schultz, J.J., Wheeler, S.M. and Williams, L.J. (2012) *Forensic Recovery of Human Remains: Archaeological approaches*, 2nd edition. CRC Press: Boca Raton.

Durães, N., Cortez, D., Algarra, M., Sánchez, F.G., Rodríguez-Borges, J.E. *et al.* (2010) Comparison of adipocere formation in four soil types of the Porto (Portugal) district. *Forensic Science International*, **195**: 168.e1–168.e6.

Edson, S.M., Ross, J.P., Michael, D., Coble, M.D., Parsons, T.J. and Barritt, S.M. (2004) Naming the dead: confronting the realities of the rapid identification of degraded skeletal remains, *Forensic Science Review*, **16**: 63–90.

Efremov, I.A. (1940) Taphonomy: a new branch of paleontology. *Pan-American Geologist*, **74**: 81–93.

Ferllini, R. and Croft, A.M. (2009) The case of an Armenian mass grave. *Journal of Human Rights*, **8**: 229–244.

Fiedler, S. and Graw, M. (2003) Decomposition of buried corpses, with special reference to the formation of adipocere. *Naturwissenschaften*, **90**: 291–300.

Fiorato, V., Boylston, A.. Knusel, C. and Erolin, C. (eds) (2007) *Blood Red Roses: The archaeology of a mass grave from the battle of Towton AD 1461*. Oxbow Books: Oxford.

Fitzgerald, C.M. and Oxenham, M. (2009) Modelling time-since-death in Australian temperate conditions. *Australian Journal of Forensic Sciences*, **41**: 27–41.

Fitzpatrick, R.W. (2008) Nature, distribution, and origin of soil materials. In: Carter, D.O. and Tibbet, M. (eds), *Analysis in Forensic Taphonomy. Chemical and biological effects of buried human remains*. CRC Press: Boca Raton, pp. 1–28.

Forbes, S.L., Stuart, B.H. and Dent, B.B. (2005a) The effect of the method of burial on adipocere formation. *Forensic Science International*, **154**: 44–52.

Forbes, S.L., Stuart, B.H. and Dent, B.B. (2005b) The effect of the burial environment on adipocere formation. *Forensic Science International*, **154**: 24–34.

Froentjes, W. (1965) Kurzer Bericht über unvollständige Leichenzersetzung auf Friedhöfen und die Adipocirebildung. *Deutsche Zeitschrift fur die Gesamte Gerichtliche Medizin*, **56**: 205–207.

Galloway, A., Willy, P. and Snyder, L. (1997) Human bone mineral densities and survival of bone elements: a contemporary sample. In: Haglund, W.D. and Sorg, M.H. (eds), *Forensic Taphonomy: The postmortem fate of human remains*. CRC Press: Boca Raton, pp. 295–317.

Gardner, R.M. and Bevel, T. (2009) *Practical Crime Scene Analysis and Reconstruction*. CRC Press: Boca Raton.

Ge, J., Budowle, B. and Chakrabotry, R. (2011) Choosing relatives for DNA identification of missing persons. *Journal of Forensic Sciences*, **56**: S23–S28.

Goff, M.L. (2009) Early post-mortem changes and stages of decomposition in exposed cadavers. *Experimental and Applied Archaeology*, **49**: 21–36.

Gotherstrom, A., Collins, M.J., Angerbjorn, A. and Liden, K. (2002) Bone preservation and DNA amplification. *Archaeometry*, **44**: 395–404.

Grant, J., Gorin, S. and Fleming, N. (2008) *The Archaeology Coursebook: An introduction to themes, sites, methods, and skills*. Routledge: London.

Graw, M., Weisser, H.J. and Lutz, S. (2000) DNA typing of human remains found in damp environments. *Forensic Science International*, **113**: 91–95.

Grivas, G.R. and Komar, D.A. (2008) Kumho, Daubert, and the nature of scientific inquiry: implications for forensic anthropology. *Journal of Forensic Sciences*, **53**: 771–776.

Hackett, C.J. (1981) Microscopical focal destruction (tunnels) in exhumed human bones. *Medicine Science and Law*, **21**: 243–265.

Haglund, W.D., Connor, M. and Scott, D.D. (2000) The archaeology of contemporary mass graves. *Historical Archaeology*, **35**: 57–69.

Haglund, W.D. and Sorg, M.H. (eds) (1997) *Forensic Taphonomy. The postmortem fate of human remains*. CRC Press: Boca Raton.

Haglund, W.D. and Sorg, M.H. (eds) (2002) *Advances in Forensic Taphonomy. Method, theory, and archaeological perspectives*. CRC Press: Boca Raton.

Haglund, W.D. (2002) Recent mass graves, an introduction. In: Haglund, W.D. and Sorg, M.H. (eds), *Advances in Forensic Taphonomy. Method, theory, and archaeological perspectives*. CRC Pres: Boca Raton, pp. 243–262.

Hedges, J.W. and Millard, A.R. (1995) Bones and groundwater: towards the modelling of diagenetic processes. *Journal of Archaeological Sciences*, **22**: 155–164.

Hedges, R.E.M. (2002) Bone diagenesis: an overview of processes. *Archaeometry*, **44**: 319–328.

Henderson, J. (1987) Factors determining the state of preservation of human remains. In: Boddington, A. and Garland, A.N. (eds), *Death, Decay and Reconstruction: Approaches to archaeology and forensic science*. Manchester University Press: Manchester, pp. 43–54.

Hochmeiser, M.N., Budowle, B., Borer, U.V., Eggmann, U., Comet, C.T. and Dirnhofer, R. (1991) Typing of deoxyribonucleic-acid (DNA) extracted from compact-bone from human remains. *Journal of Forensic Sciences*, **36**: 1649–1661.

Holliday, V.T. (2004) *Soils in Archaeological Research*. Oxford University Press: Oxford.

Hopkins, D.W., Wiltshire, P.E.J. and Turner, B.D. (2000) Microbial characteristics of soil from graves: an investigation at the interface of soil microbiology and forensic science. *Applied Soil Ecology*, **14**: 283–288.

Hunter, J.R. (2002). Foreward from archaeology: a pilgrim in forensic archaeology – personal view. In: Haglund, W.D. and Sorg, M.H. (eds), *Advances in Forensic Taphonomy. Method, theory, and archaeological perspectives*. CRC Press: Boca Raton, p. xxv.

Hunter, J.R. and Cox, M. (2005) *Forensic Archaeology: Advances in theory and practice*. Routledge: London.

ICTY (2000) Srebrenica Investigation: *Summary of forensic evidence execution points and mass graves by Dean Manning, ICTY Investigator*. http://abunodisceomnes.wellcomecollection.org/wp-content/uploads/2015/01/Manning-D.-24-August-2003-Srebrenica-investigation-Summary-of-forensic-evidence-Execution-points-and-mass-graves-2001-ICTY-Investigations-Team-Leader.pdf (Accessed 12 March 2015).

ICTY (2001) *Prosecutor v. Radislav Krstic (Trial Judgement)*, International Criminal Tribunal for the former Yugoslavia (ICTY), 2 August 2001, http://www.refworld.org/docid/414810d94.html (Accessed 16 March 2015).

ICTY (2005) Facts about Srebrenica. http://www.icty.org/x/file/Outreach/view_from_hague/jit_srebrenica_en.pdf. (Accessed 19 March 2015).

ICTY (2011) Trial transcript http://www.icty.org/x/cases/karadzic/trans/en/111201IT.htm (Accessed 19 March 2015).

Imaizumi, K., Miyasaka, S. and Yoshino, M. (2004) Quantitative analysis of amplifiable DNA in tissue exposed to various environments using competitive PCR assays. *Science and Justice*, **44**: 199–208.

Introna, F. Jr., Di Vella, G. and Campobasso, C.P. (1999) Determination of postmortem interval from old skeletal remains by image analysis of luminol test results. *Journal of Forensic Sciences*, **44**: 535–538.

IRIN (2013) *Why identifying typhoon Haiyan's dead matters to the living*, http://www.irinnews.org/printreport.aspx?reportid=99432 (Accessed 30 January 2015).

Jaeger, J.H. (2013) *Mass grave or communal burial? A discussion of terminology*, https://www.academia.edu/1276944/Mass_grave_or_communal_burial_A_discussion_of_terminology (Accessed March 2015).

Jaggers, K.A. and Rogers, T..L (2009) The effects of soil environment on postmortem interval: a macroscopic analysis. *Journal of Forensic Science*, **54**: 1217–1222.

Janaway, R.C. (1996) The decay of buried human remains and their associated materials. In: Hunter, J., Roberts, C. and Martin, A. (eds), *Studies in Crime: An introduction to forensic archaeology*. Batsford Ltd: London, pp. 58–85.

Janaway, R.C. (2008) The decomposition of materials associated with buried cadavers. In: Tibbet, M. and Carter, D.O. (eds), *Soil Analysis in Forensic Taphonomy: Chemical and biological effects of buried human remains*. CRC Press: Boca Raton. pp. 153–201.

Janaway, R.C., Percival, S.L. and Wilson, A.S. (2009) Decomposition of human remains. In: Percival, S.L. (ed.), *Microbiology and Aging*. Springer: New York, pp. 313–334.

Janjua, M.A. and Rogers, T.L. (2008) Bone weathering patterns of metatarsal v. femur and the postmortem interval in Southern Ontario. *Journal of Forensic Sciences*, **178**: 16–23.

Jans, M.M.E., Nielsen-Marsh, C.M., Smith, C.J., Collins, M.J. and Kars, H. (2004) Characterisation of microbial attack on archaeological bone. *Journal of Archaeological Science*, **31**: 87–95.

Jessee, E. (2003) *Some Recommendations for the Creation of a Series of Experimental Mass Grave and Mass Grave-related Test Sites*. Unpublished MA thesis, Simon Fraser University: Burnaby.

Jessee, E. and Skinner, M. (2005) A typology of mass grave and mass grave-related sites. *Forensic Science International*, **152**: 55–59.

Juhl, K. (2005) *The Contribution by (Forensic) Archaeologists to Human Rights Investigations of Mass Graves*. Museum of Archaeology: Stavanger.

Juhl, K. and Olsen, O.E. (2006) Societal safety, archaeology and the investigation of contemporary mass graves. *Journal of Genocide Research*, **8**: 411–435.

Kaestle, F.A. and Horsburgh, K.A. (2002) Ancient DNA in anthropology: methods, applications and ethics. *American Journal of Physical Anthropology*, **119**: 92–130.

Kanz, F., Reiter, C. and Risser, D.U. (2014) Citrate content of bone for time since death estimation: results from burials with different physical characteristics and known PMI. *Journal of Forensic Sciences*, **59**: 613–620.

King, C.L., Tayles, N. and Gordon, K.C. (2011) Re-examining the chemical evaluation of diagenesis in human bone apatite. *Journal of Archaeological Science*, **38**: 2222–2230.

Kjellström, A. (2005) A sixteenth-century warrior grave from Uppsala, Sweden: the Battle of Good Friday. *International Journal of Osteoarchaeology*, **15**: 23–50.

Kumho (1999) Kumho Tire Company, Ltd. v. Carmichael, 526 US 137.

Laroche, X. and Baccard, E. (2015) International courts and forensic science In: Houck, M.M. (ed.) *Professional Issues in Forensic Science: Advanced Forensic Science Series.* Academic Press: New York, pp. 303–312.

Lindahl, T. (1993) Instability and decay of the primary structure of DNA. *Nature*, **22**: 709–715.

Loe, L., Barker, C., Brady, K., Cox, M. and Webb, H. (2014a) *'Remember me to all': The archaeological recovery and identification of soldiers who fought and died in the Battle of Fromelles 1916*. Oxford Archaeology: Oxford.

Loe, L., Barker, C. and Wright, R.V. (2014b) An osteological profile of trench warfare: peri-mortem trauma sustained by soldiers who fought and died in the Battle of Fromelles. In: Smith, M. and Knüsel, C.J. (eds), *The Routledge Handbook of the Bioarchaeology of Human Conflict*. Routledge: London, pp. 575–601.

Lougas, V. (1991) The archaeology of terror. Archaeological excavations of mass murder sites in the Soviet Union. *Fennoscandia Archaeologica*, **7**: 77–84.

Lyman, R.L. (2002) Foreward from palaeontology. In: Haglund, W.D. and Sorg, M.H. (eds), *Advances in Forensic Taphonomy: Method, theory, and archaeological perspectives.* CRC Press: Boca Raton, p. xxiii.

Manifold, B.M. (2012) Intrinsic and extrinsic factors involved in the preservation of non adult skeletal remains in archaeology and forensic science. *Bulletin of the International Association of Paleodontolgy*, **6**: 51–69.

Mann, R.W., Bass, W.M. and Meadows, L. (1990) Time since death and decomposition of the human body: variables and observations in case and experimental field studies. *Journal of Forensic Sciences*, **35**: 103–111.

Mant, A.K. (1950) *A Study in Exhumation Data*. MD Thesis, University of London: London.

Mant, A.K. (1987) Knowledge acquired from Post-War exhumations. In: Boddington, A., Garland, A.N. and Janaway, R.C. (1987) *Death, Decay and Reconstruction: Approaches to Archaeology and Forensic Science*. Manchester University Press: Manchester, pp. 65–78.

Matuszewski, S., Konwerski, S., Fratczak, K. and Szafałowicz, M, (2014) Effect of body mass and clothing on decomposition of pig carcasses. *International Journal of Legal Medicine*, **128**: 1039–1048.

Megyesi. M.S., Nawrocki, S.P. and Haskell, N.H. (2005) Using accumulated degree-days to estimate the postmortem interval from decomposed human remains. *Journal of Forensic Sciences*, **50**: 618–626.

McLaughlin, G. and Lednev, I.K. (2011) Potential application of Raman spectroscopy for determining burial duration of skeletal remains. *Analytical and Bioanalytical Chemistry*, **401**: 2511–2518.

Michaud, J.P. and Moreau, G. (2011) A statistical approach based on accumulated degree days to predict decomposition related processes in forensic studies. *Journal of Forensic Sciences*, **56**: 229–232.

Micozzi, M.S. (1991) Postmortem Change in Human and Animal Remains: A systematic approach. *Charles C*. Thomas: Springfield.

Micozzi, M.S. (1997) Frozen environments and soft tissue preservation. In: Haglund, W.D. and Sorg, M.H. (eds), *Forensic Taphonomy. The postmortem fate of human remains*. CRC Press: Boca Raton, pp. 171–180.

Miller, R.A. (2002) *The Effects of Clothing on Human Decomposition: Implications for estimating time since death*. Unpublished Master's Thesis, University of Tennessee: Knoxville.

Miloš, A., Selmanović, A., Smajlović, L., Huel, R.L.M., Katzmarzyk, C. *et al.* (2007) Success rates of nuclear short tandem repeat typing from different skeletal elements. *Croatian Medical Journal*, **48**: 486–493.

Minser, L.M., Halvorson, A.C., Dreier, J.L., Ubelaker, D.H. and Foran, D.R. (2009) The correlation between skeletal weathering and DNA quality and quantity. *Journal of Forensic Sciences*, **54**: 822–828.

Muller, K., Chadefauxe, C., Thomas, N. and Reiche, I. (2011) Microbial attack and archaeological bones versus high concentration of heavy metals in the burial environment. A case study of animal bones from mediaeval copper workshop in Paris. *Palaeogeography, Palaeoclimatology and Palaeoecology*, **310**: 39–51.

Mundorff, A.Z., Bartelink, E.J. and Mar-Cash, E. (2009) DNA preservation in skeletal elements from the World Trade Center disaster: recommendations for mass fatality management. *Journal of Forensic Sciences*, **54**: 739–745.

Myburgh, J., L'Abbé, E.N., Steyn, M. and Becker, P.J. (2013) Estimating the postmortem interval (PMI) using accumulated degree-days (ADD) in a temperate region of South Africa. *Forensic Science International*, **229**: 165–e1.

Nawrocki, S. (1996) *An Outline of Forensic Taphonomy*. University of Indianapolis Archaeology and Forensics Laboratory: http://archlab.uindy.edu (Accessed 27 March 2015).

Nielsen-Marsh, C., Gernaey, A., Turner-Walker, G., Hedges, R., Pike, A. and Collins, M. (2000) The chemical degradation of bone. In: Cox, M. and Mays, S. (eds), *Human Osteology in Archaeology and Forensic Science*. Cambridge University Press: Cambridge, pp. 439–454.

Nielsen-Marsh, C.M. and Hedges, R.E.M. (2000) Patterns of diagenesis in bone. *I: The effects of site environments. Journal of Archaeological Science*, **27**: 1139–1150.

Payne, J.A. (1965) A summer carrion study of the baby pig *Sus Scrofa* Linnaeus. *Ecology*, **46**: 592–602.

Perper, J. (2006) Time of death and changes after death. Anatomical considerations. In: Spitz, W. and Fisher, D. (eds), *Medicolegal Investigation of Death*. Charles C. Thomas: Springfield, pp. 87–127.

Piepenbrink, H. (1986) Two examples of biogenous dead bone decomposition and their consequences for taphonomic interpretation. *Journal of Archaeological Science*, **13**: 417–430.

Pokines, J.T. and Symes, S.A. (eds) (2014) *Manual of Forensic Taphonomy*. CRC Press: Boca Raton.

Pokines, J.T. (2014) Collection of macroscopic osseous taphonomic data and the recognition of taphonomic suites of characteristics. In: Pokines, J.T. and Symes, S.A. (eds), *Manual of Forensic Taphonomy*. CRC Press: Boca Raton, pp. 1–17.

Pollard, T., Lelong O., MacKinnon, G., Banks, I. and Barton, P. (2008) *Pheasant Wood Fromelles: Data structure report*. Unpublished GUARD Report, University of Glasgow: Glasgow.

Pope, M.A. (2010) *Differential Decomposition Patterns of Human Remains in Variable Environments of the Midwest*. Unpublished Masters thesis, University of South Florida: USA.

Pounder, D.J. (2000) Postmortem interval. In: Siegel, J.A., Saukko, P.J. and Knupfer, G.C. (eds), *Encyclopedia of Forensic Sciences*. Academic: San Diego, pp. 1167–1172.

Prieto, J.L., Magana, C. and Ubelaker, D.H. (2004) Interpretation of post-mortem change in cadavers in Spain. *Journal of Forensic Sciences*, **49**: 918–923.

Primorac, D., Andelinovic, S., Definis-Gojanovic, M., Drmic, I., Rezic, B. *et al.* (1996) Identification of war victims from mass graves in Croatia, Bosnia and Herzegovina by use of standard forensic methods and DNA typing. *Journal of Forensic Sciences*, **41**: 891–894.

Quinney, P.S. (2000) Paradigms lost: changing interpretations of hominid behavioural patterns since ODK. In: Rowley-Conway, P. (ed.), *Animal Bones, Human Societies*. Oxbow Press: Oxford, pp. 12–19.

Radanov, S., Stoev, S., Davidov, M., Nachev, S., Stanchev, N. and Kirova, E. (1992) A unique case of naturally occurring mummification of human brain tissue. *International Journal of Legal Medicine*, **105**: 173–175.

Rodriguez, W.C. and Bass, W.M. (1983) Insect activity and its relationship to decay rates of human cadavers in East Tennessee. *Journal of Forensic Sciences*, **28**: 423–432.

Rodriguez, W.C. (1997) Decomposition of buried and submerged bodies. In: Haglund, W.D. and Sorg, M.H. (eds), *Forensic Taphonomy: The postmortem fate of human remains*. CRC Press: Boca Raton, pp. 459–467.

Rogers, C.J. (2010) *Dating Death: Forensic taphonomy and the postmortem interval*. Unpublished PhD thesis, University of Wolverhampton: Wolverhampton.

Rogers, K., Beckett, S., Samira, K., Chamberlain, A. and Clement, J. (2010) Contrasting the crystallinity indicators of heated and diagenetically altered bone mineral. *Palaeogeography, Palaeoclimatology and Palaeoecology*, **296**: 125–129.

Rugg, J. (2000) Defining the place of burial: what makes a cemetery a cemetery? *Mortality*, **5**: 259–275.

Salamon, M., Tuross, N., Arensburg, B. and Weiner, S. (2005) Relatively well preserved DNA in present in the crystal aggregates of fossil bones. *Proceedings of the National Academy of Sciences*, **102**: 13783–13788.

Saul, J.M. and Saul, F.P. (2002) Forensics, archaeology and taphonomy: the symbiotic relationship. In: Haglund, W.D. and Sorg, M.H. (eds), *Advances in Forensic Taphonomy. Method, theory and archaeological perspectives*. CRC Press: Boca Raton, pp. 71–98.

Schiffer, M.B. (1987) *Formation Processes of the Archaeological Record*. University of New Mexico Press: Albuquerque.

Schmitt, S. (2002) Mass graves and the collection of forensic evidence: genocide, war, crimes and crimes against humanity. In: Haglund, W.D. and Sorg, M.H. (eds), *Advances in Forensic Taphonomy. Method, theory and archaeological perspectives*. CRC Press: Boca Raton, pp. 277–292.

Schotsmans, E.M.J., Denton, J., Dekeirsschieter, J., Ivaneanu, T., Leentjes, S. *et al.* (2012) Effects of hydrated lime and quicklime on the decay of buried human remains using pig cadavers as human body analogues. *Forensic Science International*, **21**: 50–59.

Schwarcz, H.P., Agur, K. and Jantz, L.M. (2010) A new method for determination of postmortem interval: citrate content of bone. *Journal of Forensic Sciences*, **55**: 1516–1522.

Signoli, M., Ardagna, Y., Adalian, P., Devriendt, W., Lalys, L. *et al.* (2004) Discovery of a mass grave of Napoleonic period in Lithuania (1812, Vilnius). *Comptes Rendus Palevol*, **3**: 219–227.

Simmons, T. and Cross, P. (2013) Forensic taphonomy. In: Siegel, J.A. and Saukko, P.J. (eds), *Encyclopedia of Forensic Sciences*. Academic Press: London, pp. 12–17.

Sinamati, A., Tahiri, Y.I., Vyshka, G. and Çipi, B. (2011) Osteological proofs of torture and cruelty. Forensic findings form a secret cemetery in Tirana, Albania. *Torture*, **21**: 197–207.

Skinner, M.F. (1987) Planning the archaeological recovery of evidence from recent mass graves. *Forensic Science International*, **34**: 267–287.

Smith, C.J., Chamberlain, A.T., Riely, M.S., Stringer, C. and Collins, M.J. (2003) The thermal history of human fossils and the likelihood of successful DNA amplification. *Journal of Human Evolution*, **45**: 203–217.

Somadeva, R. (2013) Human and skeletal remains found at the District General Hospital Premise in Matale. The report on forensic anthropology submitted by author to Matale magistrate in March 2013.

Sorg, M.H., Haglund, W.D. and Wren, J.A. (2012) Current research in forensic taphonomy. In: Dirkmaat, D.C. (ed.), *A companion to Forensic Anthropology*. Blackwell Publishing: Chichester, UK, pp. 477–498.

Stein, J.K. (2001) A review of site formation processes and their relevance to geoarchaeology. In: Goldberg, P., Holliday, V.T. and Ferring, C.R, (eds). *Earth Sciences and Archaeology*. Kluwer Academic Plenum Publishers: New York, pp. 77–106.

Stojanowski, C.M., Seidemann, R.M. and Doran, G.H. (2002) Differential skeletal preservation at windover pond: causes and consequences. *American Journal of Physical Anthropology*, **119**: 15–26.

Stuart, B.H., Forbes, S., Dent, B.B. and Hodgson, G. (2000) Studies of adipocere using diffuse reflectance infrared spectroscopy. *Vibrational Spectroscopy*, **24**: 233–242.

Surabian, D. (2012) *Preservation of Buried Human Remains in Soil*. US Department of Agriculture, Natural Resources and Conservation Science: Connecticut.

Swift, B., Laudera, I., Black, S. and Norris, J. (2001) An estimation of the post-mortem interval in human skeletal remains: a radionuclide and trace element approach. *Forensic Science International*, **117**: 73–87.

Swift, B. (2006) The timing of death. In: Rutty, G.N. (ed.), *Essentials of Autopsy Practice Current Methods and Modern Trends*. Springer: New York, pp. 189–214.

Symonds, M. (2012) London's volcanic winter: Spitalfields cemetery and the famine of 1258. *Current Archaeology*, **270**: 12–19.

Takatori, T. (2001) The mechanism of human adipocere formation. *Legal Medicine*, **3**: 193–204.

Takatori, T. (1996) Investigations on the mechanism of adipocere formation and its relation to other biochemical reactions. *Forensic Science International*, **80**: 49–61.

Tibbet, M. and Carter, D.O. (eds) (2008) *Soil Analysis in Forensic Taphonomy: Chemical and biological effects of buried human remains*. CRC Press: Boca Raton.

Troutman, L., Moffatt, C. and Simmons, T. (2014) A preliminary examination of differential decomposition patterns in mass graves. *Journal of Forensic Science*, **59**: 621–626.

Trueman, C.N.G., Behrensmeyer, A.K., Tuross, N. and Weiner, S. (2004) Mineralogical and compositional changes in bones exposed on soil surfaces in Amboseli National Park, Kenya: diagenetic mechanisms and the role of sediment pore fluids. *Journal of Archaeological Science*, **31**: 721–739.

Turner, B. and Wiltshire, P. (1999) Experimental validation of forensic evidence: a study of the decomposition of buried pigs in a heavy clay soil. *Forensic Science International*, **101**: 113–122.

Turner-Walker, G. (2008) The chemical and microbial degradation of bones and teeth. In: Pinhasi, R. and Mays, S. (eds), *Advances in Human Palaeopathology*. Wiley and Sons Ltd: Chichester, UK, pp. 3–29.

Tumer, A.R., Karacaoglu, E., Namli, A., Keten, A., Farasat, S. *et al.* (2013) Effects of different types of soil on decomposition: an experimental study. *Legal Medicine*, **15**: 149–156.

UN (1993) *Report on the Situation of Human Rights in the Territory of the Former Yugoslavia submitted by Mr Tadeusz Mazowiecki, special sapporteur of the Commission on Human Rights, pursuant to commission resolution 1992/S-1/1 of 14 August 1992*. E/CN.4/1993/50, http://www.unhchr.ch/huridocda/huridoca.nsf/70ef163b25b2333fc1256991004de370/c0a6cfd5274508fd802567900036da9a?OpenDocument (Accessed 15 March 2015).

Varas, C.G. and Leiva, M.I. (2012) Managing commingled remains from mass graves: considerations, implications and recommendations from a human rights case in Chile. *Forensic Science International*, **219**: 19–24.

Vass, A.A., Bass, W.M., Wolt, J.D., Foss, J.E. and Ammons, J.T. (1992) Time since death determinations of human cadavers using soil solution. *Journal of Forensic Sciences*, **37**: 1236–1253.

Von Endt, D.W. and Ortner, D.J. (1984) Experimental effects of bone size and temperature on bone diagenesis. *Journal of Archaeological Sciences*, **11**: 247–253.

Weiner, S. and Bar-Yosef, O. (1990) States of preservation of bones from prehistoric sites in the Near East: a survey. *Journal of Archaeological Science*, **17**: 187–196.

Weiner, S. and Price, P.A. (1986) Disaggregation of bone into crystals. *Calcified Tissue International*, **39**: 365–375.

Weiner, S. (2010) *Microarchaeology: Beyond the visible archaeological record*. Cambridge University Press: Cambridge.

Wilson, A.S., Janaway, R.C., Holland, A.D., Dodson, H.I., Baran, E. *et al.* (2007) Modelling the buried human body environment in upland climes using three contrasting field sites. *Forensic Science International*, **169**: 6–18.

Wright, L.E. and Schwarcz, H.P. (1996) Infrared and isotopic evidence for diagenesis of the bone apatite at Dos Pilas, Guatemala: palaeodietary implications. *Journal of Archaeological Sciences*, **23**: 933–944.

Wright, R.V. (1999) *Exhumations in Eastern Bosnia Report to ICTY*. http://archive.forensicarchitecture.org/wpcontent/uploads/2012/10/ACE85181R0000340603.pdf (Accessed 12 March 2015).

Wright, R. and Sterenberg, J. (2005) The archaeology of mass graves. In: Hunter, J. and Cox, M. (eds), *Forensic Archaeology: Advances in theory and practice*. Routledge: London, pp. 137–158.

Ye, J., Ji, A.Q., Parra, E.J., Zheng, X.F., Jiang, C.T. and Zhao, X.C, (2004) A simple and efficient method for extracting DNA from old and burned bone. *Journal of Forensic Sciences*, **49**: 754–759.

Żychowski, J. (2011) Geological aspects of decomposition of corpses in mass graves from WWI and II, located in SE Poland. *Environmental Earth Sciences*, **64**: 437–448.

19

Reconstructing the Original Arrangement, Organisation and Architecture[1] of Burials in Archaeology

Dominique Castex and Frédérique Blaizot

19.1 Introduction

Developed in France over the last 30 years, archaeothanatology aims to reconstruct the funerary context of human remains in order to understand funerary treatments of the deceased. Grounded in the teaching of Henri Duday, archaeothanatology, previously called 'field anthropology', argues that the way in which the dead are buried has an effect on how the body decays or is preserved. The application of archaeothanatology makes it possible to reconstruct the original conditions of the deposit. Moreover, by analysing the taphonomic anomalies visible on the skeletal remains, it is possible to reconstruct the original deposition, including the degraded elements, which were once present. For example, the original burial architecture has an influence on the disarticulation of certain anatomical segments. Therefore, by analysing these disarticulations and movement of skeletal remains within the burial, it is possible to re-create the original burial architecture.

As such, archaeothanatology combines knowledge of human decomposition with detailed observations of the burial environment in order to explain the spatial configuration of the skeletal remains and, based on those observations, the original burial context. The method is based upon observation, recording and analysis of taphonomic anomalies and deviations from anatomical articulation of the skeleton, together with environmental characteristics within which the body decomposed. This information supplies a theoretical framework that can help with the interpretation, but is in no case a direct explanation of the original burial context. Interpretation depends on the quality of the field data and accurate records, since any information that is not observed and/or recorded in the field is lost forever. The methodological procedures and principles of analysis of archaeothanatology have been described in several English language publications and will not be repeated in detail here (Duday 2006; Duday *et al.* 2014). Instead, this chapter describes case studies to illustrate the analytical approach that leads to the interpretation of the original funerary context of several burials. The objective is to demonstrate the potential of archaeothanatological analysis in order to improve analysis and interpretation of buried forensic cases.

---

1 'l'appareil funéraire' or 'le dispositif funéraire' are the original words in French that cannot be translated by one word in English. Therefore, the translation became: 'Burial arrangement, organisation and architecture'.

Taphonomy of Human Remains: Forensic Analysis of the Dead and the Depositional Environment, First Edition.
Edited by Eline M.J. Schotsmans, Nicholas Márquez-Grant and Shari L. Forbes.

19.2 The Reconstruction of Perishable Funerary Architecture and its Arrangement

The easiest way to bury a dead body is to dig a pit and place the body into it, in direct contact with the bottom and walls of the pit. In an archaeological context, when the body is placed along its length, those graves are generally narrow and cut to the shape of the body, sometimes with a niche for the head. In most cases, the bottom of the pit rises slightly at both ends. In some cases, the rise is only present at one end of the grave, more often towards the feet. In graves with a niche, the cranium is often resting higher, caused by an intentionally created raised surface to support the head, comparable to a step in the grave (Figure 19.1). Furthermore, in graves with a niche, the pit narrows in the region of the neck, pushing the shoulders slightly above the torso (i.e. elevating and medially rotating). In cross-section, the shape of the bottom of these types of pits will frequently be that of a 'trough'[2] (i.e. the shape of a more or less rounded broader concavity) or occasionally have the shape of a 'gutter'[3] (i.e. with a more narrow base) (Figure 19.1).

Clearly, the different characteristics of the pits have an important effect on the final configuration of the skeletal remains within them (Blaizot 2008). The convergence of the walls, which follows the shape of the body, creates compression at the shoulders: scapulae are upright (i.e. in a protracted position), humeral heads project anteriorly and clavicles are verticalised with their lateral extremities moving upwards above the original volume of shoulders[4]. Another consequence of this type of pit is that the trunk becomes cone-shaped (Figure 19.2: grave 3042). Compression of the shoulders can be very marked, as seen in burial 609 (Figure 19.2), where the scapulae are vertical. The right clavicle is observed parallel to the spinal column and the left clavicle has moved anterior to the upper thoracic vertebrae. Furthermore, the right humerus is rotated to reveal its posterior surface and the left humerus has moved into a position posterior to the scapula (Figure 19.2: grave 609).

Similarly, when there is a step in front of the niche (Figure 19.1), generally only the cranium and the cervical region of the vertebral column are affected. When the side of the step is abrupt, such as in grave 609 (Figure 19.2), the cranium can slide downwards in between the shoulders. The depth and shape in cross-section of the niche also contribute to the final position of the cranium. If the bottom of the niche is flat or is cut so that it slopes away towards the head end of the grave, or if the bottom is as deeply excavated under the head as it is under the shoulders, the cranium will stay either in the standard anatomical position as seen in burial 561 (Figure 19.2) or roll posteriorly to the base of the cranium.

Constraints occur when the grave is very narrow: in the case of skeleton 561 (Figure 19.2), the shoulders are raised as they abut against the step. Furthermore, humeri and scapulae, constrained by the pit's walls, are rotated into a lateral position and compress the ribs.

When the humeri rest on the slanting walls of a slightly concave pit, the ribs will follow the rounded bottom. In grave 609, the ribs are collapsed into a V-shaped pattern[5] and the scapulae are tilted toward the mid-line of the body (Figure 19.2). If the concavity is a little more pronounced, the sternal ends of the ribs might be raised, in particular at mid-thorax (i.e. the 5th to 8th ribs), because of the lateral constraint of the burial pit, as observed in burial 3042 (Figure 19.2). Depending on the width of the grave, the ribs can be stacked one on top of another with an opening in the mid-line, as in grave 561 (Figure 19.2). These phenomena vary greatly, depending on how the body is placed in the pit and whether it is placed against the slanting wall of the grave-cut or in the centre of the grave pit.

2 In French: une auge
3 In French: une goutière
4 For the anatomical terminology, see Duday (2009): 16.
5 In French: en chevrons

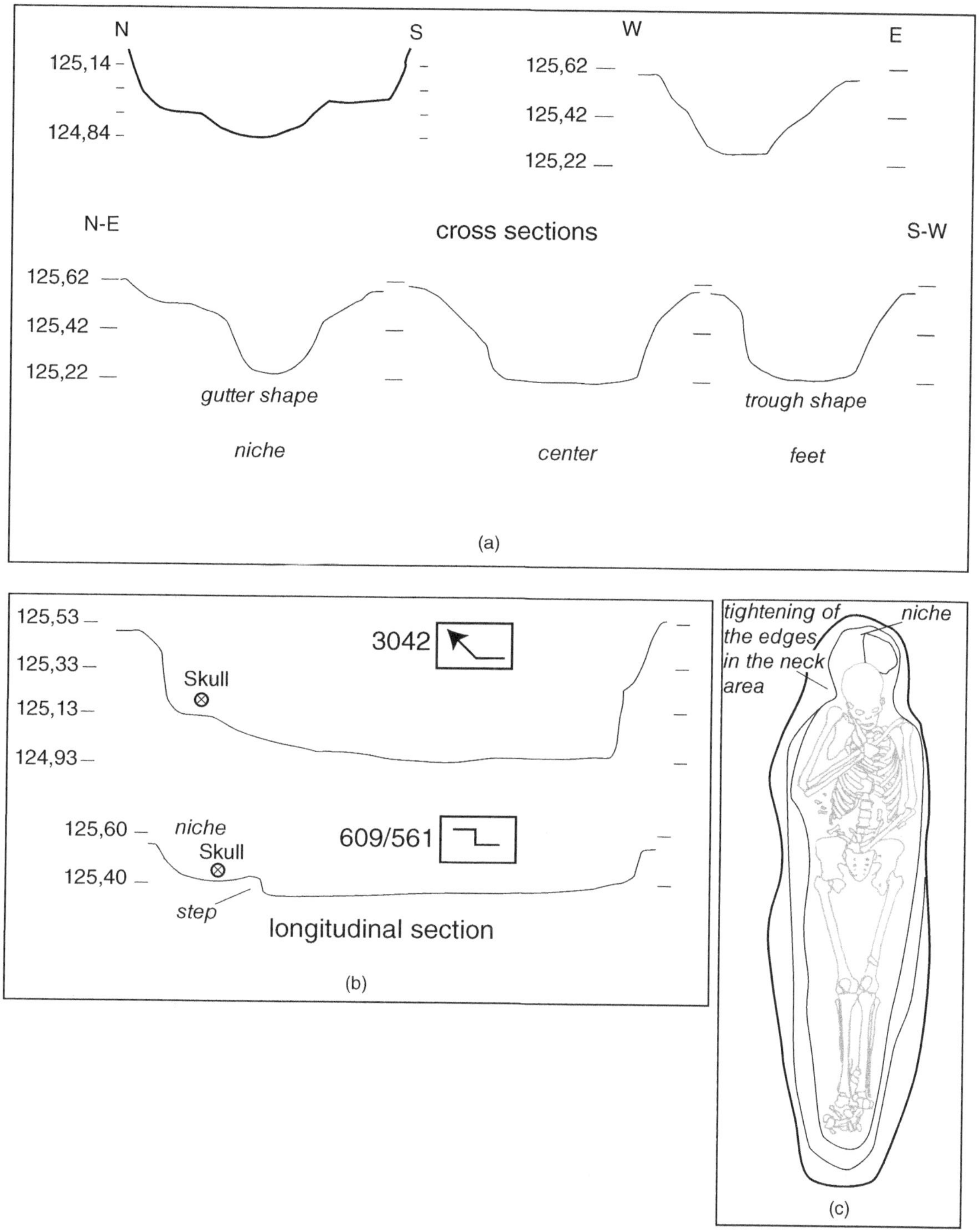

Figure 19.1 Cross-sections and longitudinal sections from burials 3042, 609 and 561 related to Figure 19.2 (drawings: F. Blaizot).

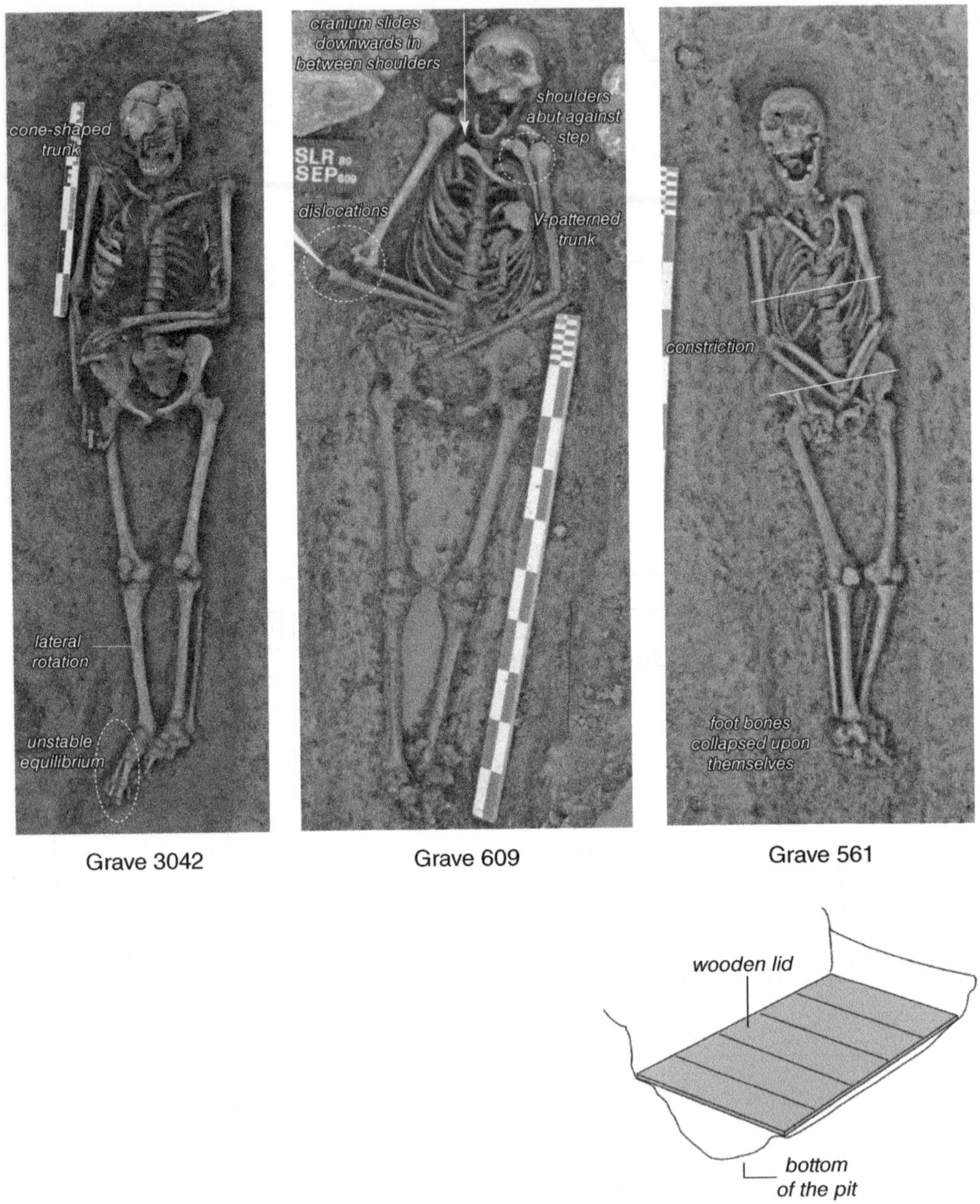

Figure 19.2 Early medieval burials showing various effects of burial pits on skeletons and their reconstruction in pits with a cover. Burial 3042 with convergence of the edges (Les Forgettes at Quincieux in Rhône, France). Burial 609 with a rounded bottom (Les Ruelles at Serris in Seine-et-Marne, France). Burial 561 with narrow pit (Les Ruelles at Serris in Seine-et-Marne, France) (photos and drawing: F. Blaizot).

The grave's shape in cross-section has a major influence on the position of the feet. When the feet are tightly laterally constrained, the foot bones will collapse upon themselves or they will fall down parallel to one another (Figure 19.2: burials 561 and 609). It is also possible that only one of the feet will fall laterally, taking the whole limb with it into a lateral position. The anterior aspect of the tarsal bones and metatarsals, if constrained by the grave wall, will be aligned with the leg (tibia and fibulae) or be positioned in an unstable equilibrium such that the medio-dorsal surface is uppermost (Figure 19.2). This is observed in the appearance of the right foot in grave 3042. All these observations of the skeletal remains are recorded in burials where the burial cut was visible and will aid with the reconstruction of the morphology of a burial without a visible burial cut.

The narrowness of the bottom of the grave prevents displacement of bones. The skeleton gradually sinks into the soil as the body decays, and the concavity of the burial produces constraints so that the illusion of the volume of the corpse is preserved. On the one hand, there is hardly any evidence of decomposition in a void[6] showing movement of elements away from the space originally occupied by the body, while on the other hand, the arguments in favour of decay in a filled space[7] cannot be maintained either, because of the characteristics of the pits. This problem may be increased by the nature of the sediment, for example in the case of a fine-grained loess soil, the walls of the pit might crumble and settle into the empty spaces, which were once occupied by decayed soft tissue. The effect of the grave cut on the disposition of elements mimics changes normally associated with decomposition in a filled space but if it is well observed, it should be noticed that this is not correct. For example, dislocated anatomical parts are an indication of decomposition in a void. In grave 609 (Figure 19.2), it is observable that the right elbow and left shoulder are disarticulated out of the initial volume of the body. However, because of the arguments presented above, the examples in Figure 19.2 belong to a burial pit, which was closed with a wooden cover.

The next example describes decomposition in a narrow coffin of which the bottom has a gutter shape. When skeletal remains are covered by sediment upon discovery, it is not always clear if decomposition took place in a void, such as a coffin. Normally, when a body decays in a void, disarticulation of joints progressively liberates elements that may move within the void. Some European proto-historic, late antique and early medieval societies used tree-trunk coffins to deposit the deceased (Blaizot 2014). In some cases, blocks of stone were placed beneath the corners of the coffin in order to stabilise them; these can be found in contact with and sometimes under bones of the skeleton (Figure 19.3). When a tree-trunk coffin decays, there is no physical evidence of its presence, but the U-shaped cross-section of the tree trunk is similar to a gutter and, as a result, this shape contributes to a slight descent of the cranium and sometimes elements of the torso towards the bottom of the grave. In the case of a deep and narrow gutter-like coffin, the skeleton presents a 'transverse narrowing' effect. For example, in Figure 19.3, the body was placed in a low trough, which caused the pelvic bones to open slightly. The humeri are pressed tightly against the ribs. They are slightly raised above the bottom of the grave because they abutted the slanted walls of the coffin. The left humerus has moved into a posterior position. The ribs follow the concavity of the bottom of the coffin and the scapulae rest on the once slanted wall of the coffin.

Furthermore, the clavicles have moved into a superior position above the shoulders. Both feet have moved towards the median longitudinal axis of the grave because of the concavity of the tree trunk. In this grave, additional evidence of a tree trunk can be gathered by looking at the position of the three ceramic vessels. They can be observed to obey a curved line, away from the left leg and foot of the skeleton, indicating a rounded angle and slanted walls. The fact that two vessels lie on their sides (Figure 19.3: 33 and 34) indicates that the pit was not filled by earth and closed by a lid. Before closing

6 For more details regarding decomposition in a void, see Duday 2009: 32–38.
7 For a detailed description of decomposition in a filled space see Duday 2009: 38–40.

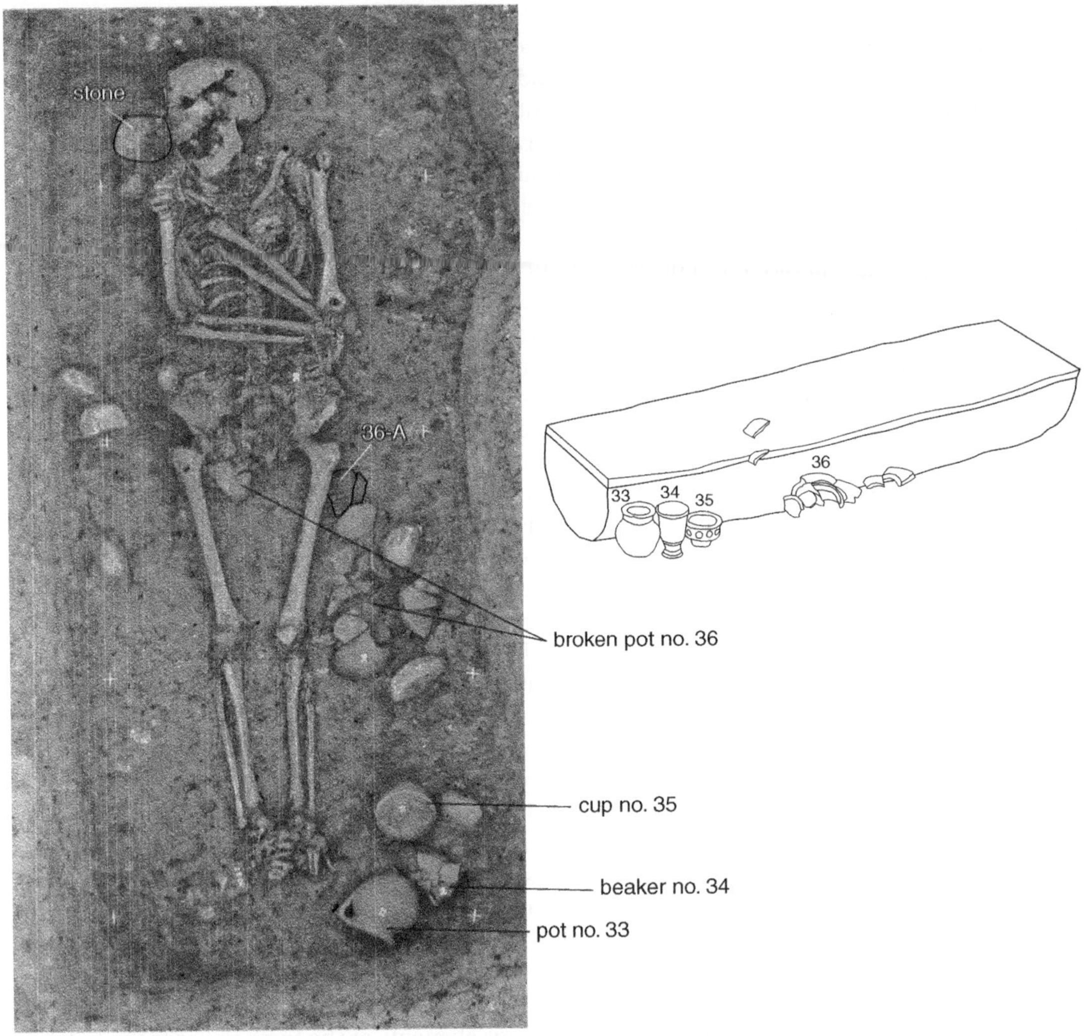

Figure 19.3 Burial from late antiquity in a hollowed tree trunk and placement of the vessels at Malbosc in Montpellier (Hérault, France) (photo and drawing: F. Blaizot).

the grave, a fourth vessel was intentionally broken and its pieces thrown into the pit (Figure 19.3: 36). Two sherds have fallen on the once coffin lid, while the other sherds lie along what had originally been the side of the coffin. The position of some of these sherds, close to the skeleton, especially one, which passes partly behind the left femur (Figure 19.3: 36A), is further evidence for the presence of the convex angle of the coffin.

For many archaeologists, the presence of nails is automatically synonymous with the use of a nailed coffin. It is important to look at other evidence and only accurate three-dimensional data recording of the nails permits such an interpretation. In fact, the side and bottom panels of a container might not be assembled with nails, but with wooden pegs, for example. Nails may only have been used to assemble the lid. In burial 1169 (Figure 19.4), evidence for a container is based on observations such as:

1) reduction of the initial volume of the body such that bones present a thin, flat layer due to gravity as the bones disarticulate in the empty space of the coffin;

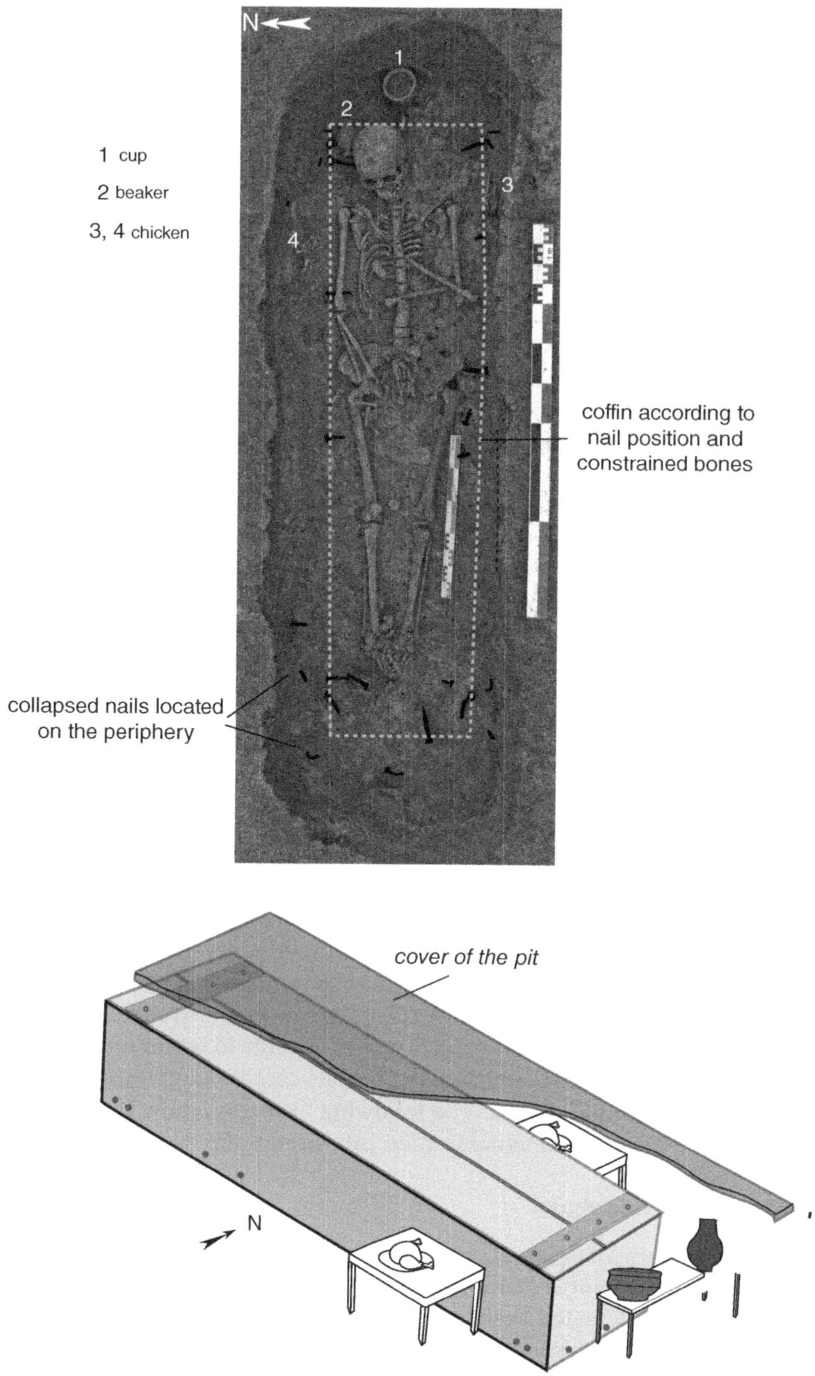

Figure 19.4 Late antiquity burial in a nailed coffin and reconstruction of coffin, cover and grave furniture at Les Forgettes in Quincieux (Rhône, France) (photo and drawing: F. Blaizot).

2) bone displacements away from the space originally occupied by the body;
3) several constraint effects that occur away from the edges of the grave-pit. One of those constraints can be observed at the cranium, which is oriented with the apex of the cranial vault uppermost, while the first cervical vertebra is oriented with its anterior aspect uppermost

Other constraints are observed on both sides of the skeleton. On the right side, the humerus has remained in lateral view, in spite of the collapse of the pelvis that should have rotated the upper limb. The upper limb did not turn because of the constraint of the coffin.

On the left side, the ulna has passed the humerus laterally out of the volume of the arm, but its proximal end has remained within the nail alignment. The distal end of the humerus, in anterior lateral view, lies 2.5 cm above the bottom of the pit, indicating that the elbow was resting against a wall (here, the side of the coffin) and explains the dislocation and movement of the elbow when the wall of the coffin collapsed. The biggest nails lie on the bottom of the pit. The tips of the nails are pointing towards the skeleton, indicating that they joined the base to the sideboards of the coffin. In contrast, other, smaller nails were observed between 7.5 and 18 cm above the bottom, with their tips pointing downwards to the base of the grave, and are located outside the alignment of the larger nails. This demonstrates that the smaller nails probably belonged to a lid, and their position suggests the use of wooden transversal boards to fasten the two parallel boards that comprised the lid to one another (Figure 19.4: reconstruction). Other nails, located outside the alignment of the larger nails, show that they do not belong to the lid of the coffin, but to a cover above the pit.

The four funerary deposits (two ceramic vessels and two parts of a chicken) were located outside the boundaries of the coffin based on the arguments of coffin alignment developed above, and were recorded as several centimetres above the bottom of the pit. Beaker number 2 (Figure 19.4) fell over and is covering one nail of the coffin. This shows that the beaker was probably put on a shelf, which was placed against the outer wall of the coffin. The shelf too had decayed and collapsed (Figure 19.4).

19.3 Analysis of Several Individuals in the Same Pit

While the previous section focuses on individual primary burials, the study of burials containing several individuals is more complex. Many forensic and conventional archaeologists do not distinguish between collective and multiple burials. Collective burials are formed by the deposition of bodies spread out over a long period and follow a natural pattern of deaths, while multiple burials result from the simultaneous deposition of several cadavers (Castex *et al.* 2014; Duday 2006). Archaeothanatological analysis helps to reconstruct these complex burials and provides insights to better understand the dynamics of the deposition, in order to conclude whether the burials contain individuals buried simultaneously or successively over an extended period. The following examples show that distinguishing between these two types of burial is fundamental to their interpretation.

19.3.1 Two Superimposed Coffins or a 'Double' Burial

The first example (Figure 19.5) derives from a late medieval parish cemetery where densely packed burials were found in front of the cathedral of Notre-Dame (Grenoble, France), resulting from burials made over several centuries. Two partly articulated individuals were identified amongst dislocated bones. The articulations between joints of the earlier deposit were maintained completely, in particular those of the right hand, in spite of their unstable equilibrium. Above this individual, partially articulated bones were observed. The largest skeletal elements such as the cranium, scapula and os coxa were found at the top, while the smaller bones, such as phalanges, epiphyses of long bones, ribs, a clavicle and some vertebrae lay in the lower part of the burial. The hand bones were found directly on

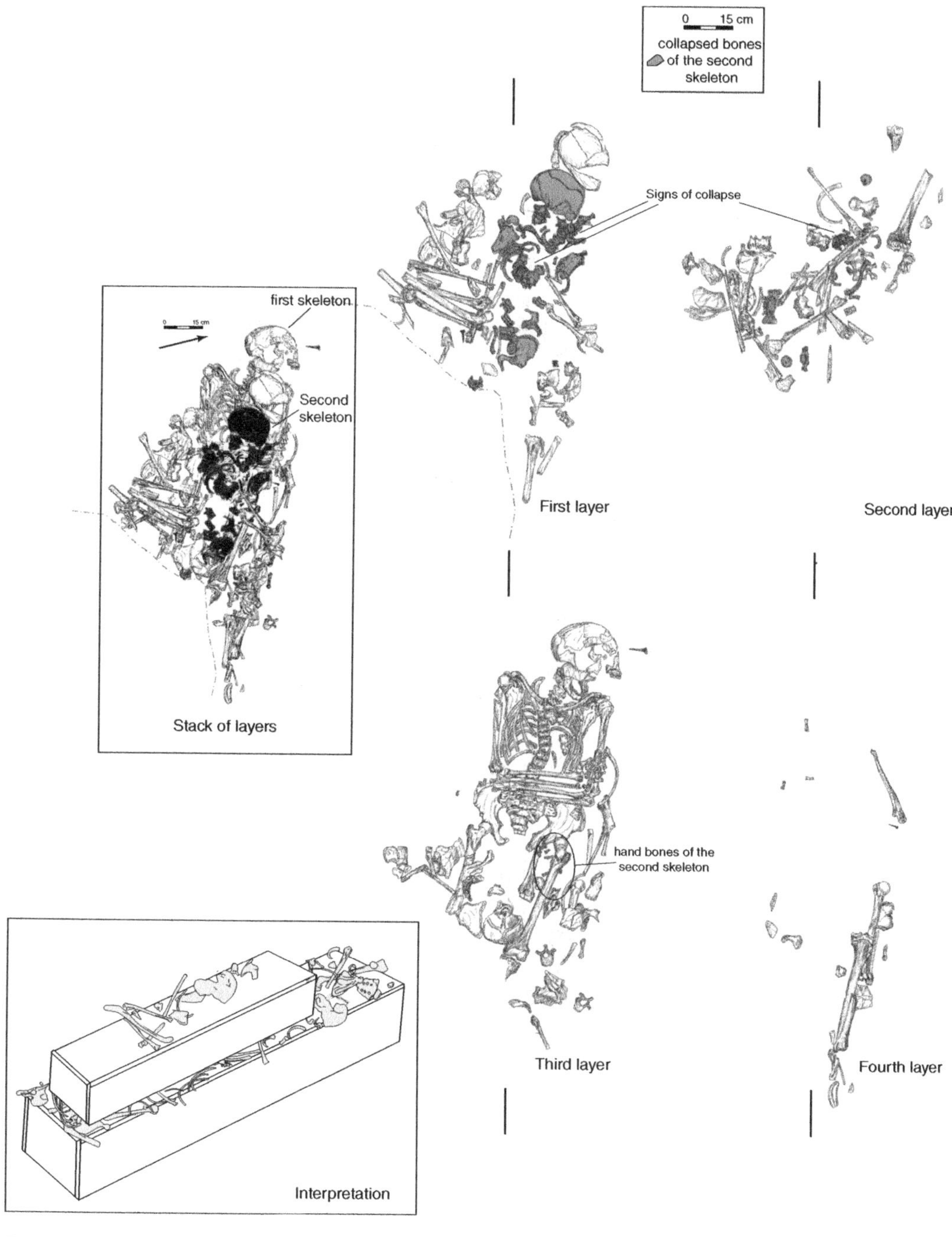

Figure 19.5 The skeletal remains from two stacked coffins from Notre-Dame at Grenoble (Isère, France) (drawings: F. Blaizot).

the left femur of the first skeleton. The many disarticulated elements reflect several collapses. A 'dive effect'[8] is characterised by steeply downward dips of bones, or groups of bones, and two significant gaps are noted in the neck and abdomen areas. The inferior aspect of the mandible was uppermost, vertebral segments lay upside down in an almost vertical position towards the bottom of the grave, and the upper part of the vertebral column could be observed above the shoulders in the form of two heaps of partially articulated bones. Based on these observations, two primary deposits could be identified.

On first sight, the preservation of the anatomical connections of the lower skeleton and the numerous collapses observed on the upper one, suggest the possibility that both deposits were made in a single coffin. In reality, these features can be interpreted as the result of a stack of two coffins, separated by a thin layer of earth containing disarticulated bones (Figure 19.5). The collapse of the first-placed coffin caused major disruptions within the joints of the decayed individual in the coffin placed second, resulting in a mix of bones of both individuals. The remains in the second placed coffin fell exactly within the boundaries of the previous coffin.

19.3.2 Successive versus Simultaneous Burials (Collective versus Multiple Burials)

While the following two examples might appear similar, they illustrate the difference between successive and simultaneous inhumations. Each grave contains three individuals whose skeletons are well preserved. At first sight, the only difference is the presence of a sarcophagus in one grave (Figure 19.6), whereas the other burial is represented by a pit, without an apparent container (Figure 19.7).

The first burial is part of a group of several sarcophagi from a Merovingian cemetery at Jau-Dignac-et-Loirac (France) situated close to a small church (Figure 19.6a). The lid of the sarcophagus was not present, but the container itself was well conserved. In order to understand the chronology of the different osseous deposits, it was necessary to dismantle the layers one by one. By observing the representation and distribution of the bones of the different individuals, conclusions could be drawn concerning the nature and arrangement of the deposits. Data gathered by precise recording during excavation (field notes, drawings and photographs) indicated a primary deposit, based on the preservation of anatomical relations between several bones of the same individual and on the presence of all of the phalanges in the sarcophagus; together these occurrences showed that decomposition of the bodies took place within the container. All three individuals were superimposed in the same direction, with heads to the west. The bones of the previous individuals were manipulated when the next body was added to the sarcophagus (Figure 19.6b). Initially, the container served for one individual (subject 1). Once skeletonised, the cranium and the pelvic bones of subject 1 were moved against the north side of the container and a second individual (subject 2) was added on top. After skeletonisation of the second individual, the container was used once again for a third individual (subject 3). The third subject was superimposed with hardly any manipulation of the skeletal remains of the previous individual, except for the bones of the pelvis and the right femur. These successive burials took place within an empty space, indicated by the displacement of crania, ribs, many vertebrae and the disarticulated state of the phalanges of the hands and feet.

The discovery of several individuals in the same tomb is observed in numerous early medieval burial grounds. This re-use of tombs gives archaeologists the chance to study the management and organisation of the funerary space. This sarcophagus is relatively unique because of the minimal manipulation of the previously buried individuals. It is important to realise that the evidence that supports the interpretation of these as primary successive deposits can be very subtle, and that these observations are important to be able to differentiate successive from simultaneous burials.

8 In French: effet de gouffre (Blaizot 2014: 276, Fig. 11).

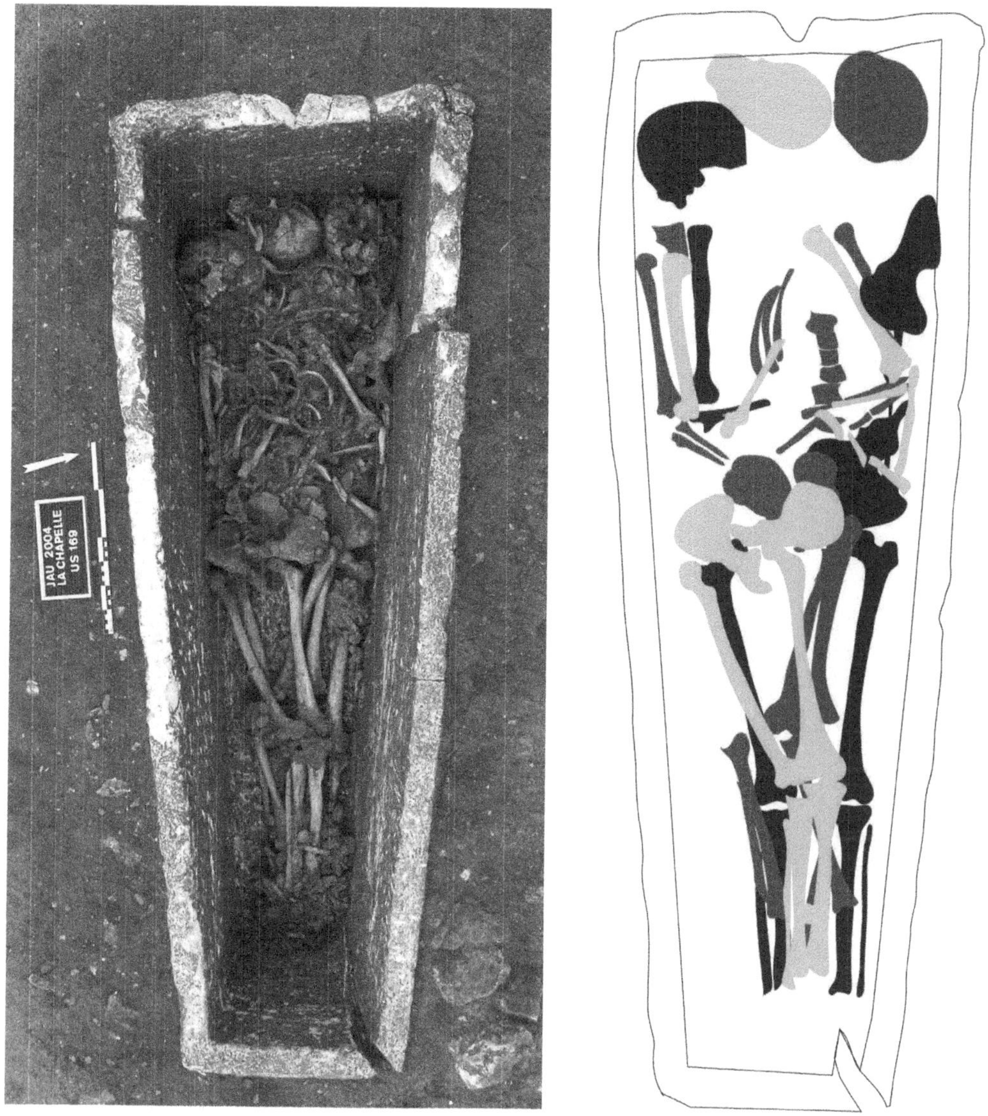

(a) (b)

Figure 19.6 Burial 169 from the Merovingian cemetery at Jau-Dignac-et-Loirac (Gironde, France). (a) General view of the stone sarcophagus (photo: H. Réveillas). (b) Illustration of the displacement of remains within the deposits: individual 1 (black), individual 2 (dark grey), individual 3 (light grey) (CAD drawing: G. Sachau-Carcel). Only the long bones, the pelvises and crania are depicted in order to highlight the most important bone displacements.

For comparison, Figure 19.7 shows a triple burial from Termonde in Belgium (15th century). In this tomb, three individuals are superimposed in various directions (Figure 19.7). There are several indications that demonstrate that this was a simultaneous deposit. First, the bones of the individuals are in direct contact with each other without soil or sediment in between them. For example, the lower limbs of subject 3 rest on the *ossa coxae* and thoraces of the underlying individuals (Figure 19.7b). Also noticeable are certain remaining anatomical connections such as that of the right acetabulo-femoral

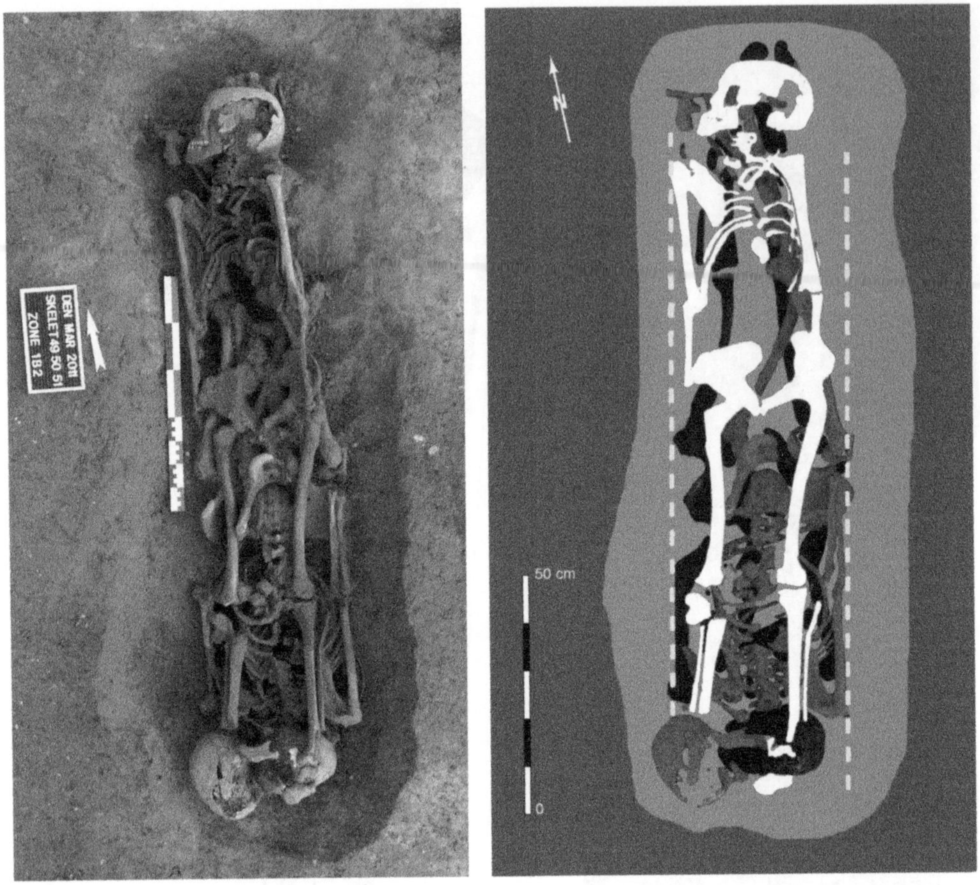

(a) (b)

Figure 19.7 Burial H from a 15th-century cemetery at Termonde (East Flanders, Belgium). (a) General view of the stone sarcophagus (photo: G. Gueguen). (b) Illustration of the movements within the deposits: subject 1 (black), subject 2 (grey), subject 3 (white) (reconstruction: G. Devilder).

joint of individual 2, which are supported by the left os coxae of individual 3. In contrast, other skeletal remains had been disarticulated due to the empty spaces created during the process of decompositions, into which bones could fall. For example, the majority of the thoracic vertebrae of individual 2 had become disarticulated and had migrated towards the thorax of individual 1.

There is also evidence of the internal arrangement of the burial (such as wooden boards/lids), although they can no longer be observed. The constraints of a container have visible effects on the remains, such as the verticality of the feet of individual 3 and the strict rectilinear alignment of the left upper limbs of individuals 2 and 3. Decomposition in an empty space is suggested by the displacement of certain skeletal remains. For example, the position of the cranium of individual 1 had been displaced by the disarticulation of the left shoulder of individual 1, which led to the posterior aspect of the proximal end of the humerus appearing uppermost.

Based on the previous observations, it could be concluded that this burial was very likely a simultaneous deposit of three individuals in wooden containers. Similar triple burials were identified at the same site in Termonde, Belgium. In terms of the interpretation of the organisation of burial space and the methods of deposition of the cadavers, this site demonstrates a fine example of the handling of bodies as a result of a mortality crisis (Castex 2009). The archaeological data showed the simultaneity of the deposit, and the epidemic nature of the deaths was precisely demonstrated by a biological study of the skeletal material. This is a relatively rare example of coffined burials attributed to an epidemic, because most often bodies related to epidemics are placed in plain soil and thus in an in-filled space (Castex *et al.* 2014).

19.3.3 Complex Simultaneous Deposits (Multiple Burials)

Large-scale death assemblages of a natural or criminal nature are often seen in forensic contexts (Chapter 18). Interpretation becomes more difficult when many bodies are grouped together. However, the analysis of the remains should be similar to the examples described above. Figure 19.8 shows a multiple burial from a cemetery at Issoudun (Indre, France) (Souquet-Leroy *et al.* 2015). This example is one of 14 mass graves, containing at least 22 individuals, dated from the late 17th to the early 18th centuries.

The grave pit is rectangular with more or less rounded corners, about 1 m wide and 2.1 m long. A portion of the pit walls appeared during manual clearing of the surface and the archaeologists were able to uncover them to a depth of 50 cm. At first sight, analysis of this burial appeared complex because of the great number of individuals and overlapping of skeletal remains interred within it (Figure 19.8). In a context of rescue archaeology, it was important to excavate the 14 mass burials fairly quickly, which required a specific protocol. As the excavation of the grave advanced, different layers could be observed (Figure 19.9). Scaled drawings of the pit and its limits were made on tracing paper and superimposed in order to detail the different layers of skeletons and/or skeletal parts that it contained. By taking into account anatomical relationships and articulations, a rapid recording

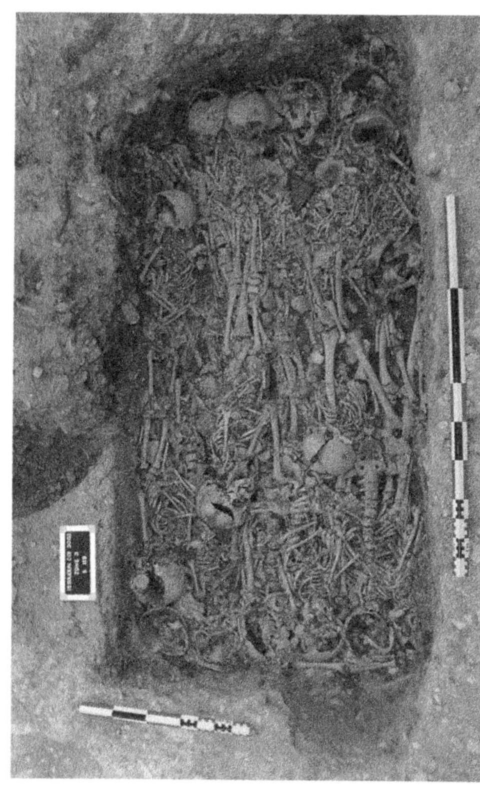

Figure 19.8 One of the 14 simultaneous burials from burial 119 at Issoudun (Indre, France), containing 22 individuals (photo: F. Porcell, Inrap).

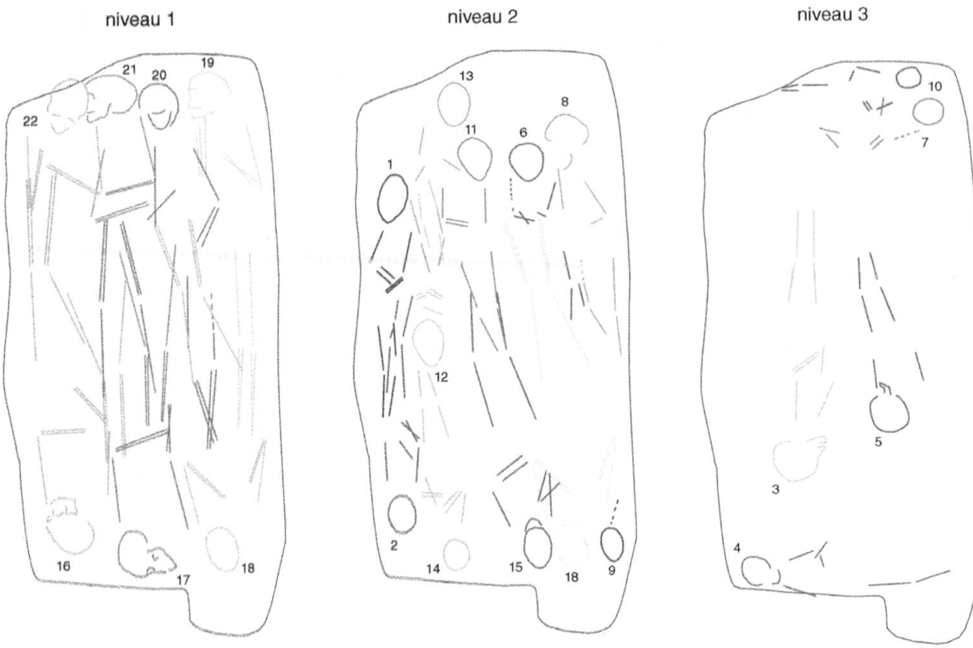

Figure 19.9 Diagram of the 3 layers of individuals and movement of skeletal elements within the deposit from burial 119 at Isssoudun (Indre, France) (drawing: I. Souquet-Leroy, Inrap).

of the position and orientation of each individual and the establishment of their relationships with the surrounding individuals was possible. This approach helped greatly in the reconstruction of the relative chronology of the deposits inferred from their organisation. Movement due to synchronous decay of piled cadavers was noted. In their decomposition, soft tissues of the individuals lying more inferiorly had created empty spaces. Small bones, in particular phalanges from the hands and feet, had migrated under the effect of gravity into the empty spaces created from the decomposition of individuals below. These elements were thus found among the lower layers and in contact with the skeletons below. This phenomenon, together with the maintenance of anatomical connections and the presence of certain articulations (especially the most labile ones, such as the phalanges of hands and feet) at the bottom of the pit, led to the conclusion that this was a primary deposit (i.e. they had not been moved to this location from another) (Figure 19.10).

In general, identification of the simultaneous or successive nature of deposits relies upon the observation of the proximity of the individuals, their superposition and contact between the bones. The maintenance of articulations between anatomical segments and the absence of manipulation leads to the conclusion that this burial represents a simultaneous primary deposit. Observations made it clear that all of the individuals were deposited in the pit before the onset of decomposition. When several bodies are deposited simultaneously into the same pit, they interact with each other and the previously described taphonomic observations, which apply to individual burials, are not always as immediately visible in simultaneous deposits.

In this example, those individuals at the bottom of the pit show well-preserved anatomical connections, including those most labile terminal phalanges of hands and feet. While these observations are usually indications of interment in a plain earth, this is caused, however, by spaces between densely packed bodies. The weight and density of the accumulated bodies above prevents migration of small

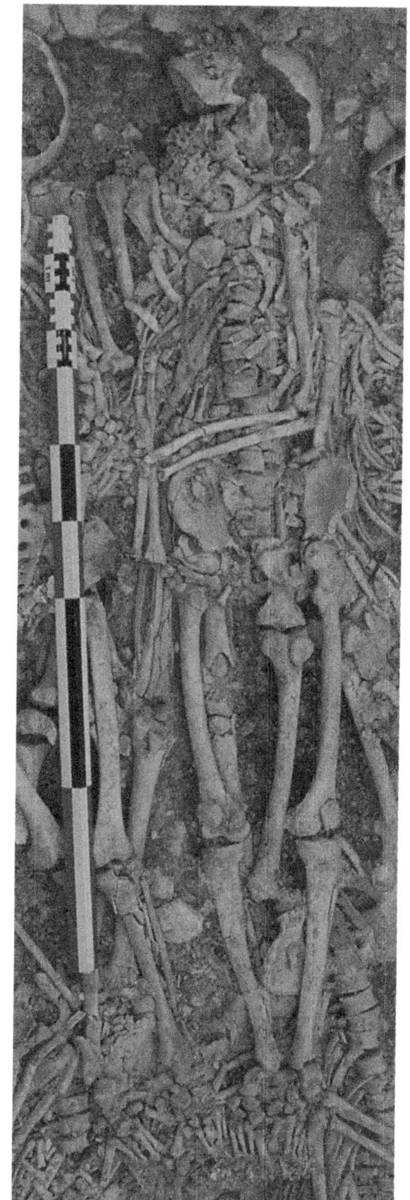

Figure 19.10 Primary deposit of individual 17 from layer 1 in burial 119 at Issoudun (Indre, France) (photo: F. Porcell, Inrap).

bones of those individuals placed beneath. In addition, evidence of empty spaces and migration of small bones towards the bottom of the grave demonstrates that there was no barrier to prevent their movement between bodies as they decomposed in the grave. Additional arguments in favour of simultaneous burial directly into the soil are based on direct contact between the skeletal remains and the sides of the pit (Figure 19.11). It was clear that all subjects found at the edges were in direct contact with the sides, and that no partition of perishable matter, such as wooden boards, could be identified.

The study of the relative chronology of the deposits showed that the burial was composed of several layers of individuals, which corresponded to the successive filling of the grave pit. Each layer was

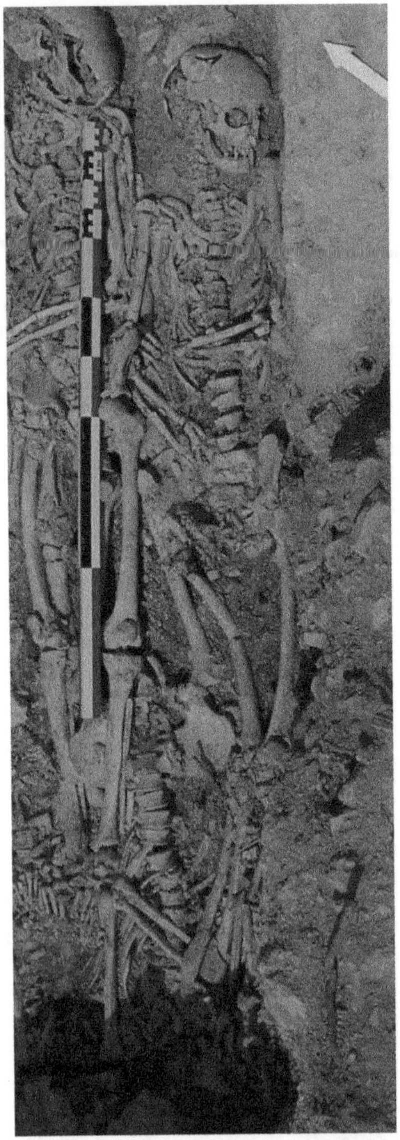

Figure 19.11 An example of primary deposits in an in-filled space; individual 16 from layer 1 in burial 119 at Issoudun (Indre, France) (photo: F. Porcell, Inrap).

composed of at least two, and often several, phases of filling. The entire pit contained at least 22 individuals in three layers. Individuals deposited in the first layer – the lowest at the bottom layer in the grave – were placed along the lengthwise axis of the pit, organised head to toe. A great majority lay supine with some variations due to restrictions in space because of the limited dimensions of the pit. Other individuals were deposited on their sides with their upper limbs overlapping. This first layer mainly contained the tallest individuals. This means that stature, rather than age, was the most important criterion for deposition by those responsible for the placement and organisation of the burial. In the second layer, it looked like the individuals were less restricted than in the first layer. There must have been enough space left for the remaining individuals so that they were all placed supine.

The most superior level contained the youngest individuals, with the majority aligned with the adults underneath and some deposited perpendicular, and squeezed against the side of the pit or into a remaining space.

In all layers, the lower limbs were mostly extended with the feet together (i.e. towards the mid-line of the body). The position of the forearms varied and was either extended, slightly flexed or flexed, with flexion more frequent in the lowest layer, probably related to the more extreme compression and constraint between individuals.

Archaeological observations indicated the presence of shrouds or winding sheets. Two fragments of iron pins were found, one close to the feet of an individual, the other near the mid-diaphysis of the humerus of another individual. Therefore, these observations should be interpreted as direct evidence for the presence of shrouds, because constraint and compression effects were not systematic and could be the result of the grave itself (such as the narrowness of the pit, the accumulation of the bodies and the interactions between them). A reconstruction of the deposit of the cadavers within the pit was created based on its estimated depth of 1.50 m (Figure 19.12).

The burial of several individuals within the same grave is less common and represents a particularly unusual example of funerary practice, adopted as a means to cope with abnormal mortality related to a particular event. After excavation of this burial and other burials of simultaneous deposits found nearby, it became clear that the deposits were related to at least one and probably several large-scale mortality crises of an epidemic nature (discussed in Castex 2009). This burial contradicts the notion that funerary traditions are abandoned and replaced by hasty burial activities during a mortality crisis, such as an epidemic. The deposition of the cadavers at Issoudun was carried out with attention and care: the bodies were handled and arranged rationally in accordance with the available space. This

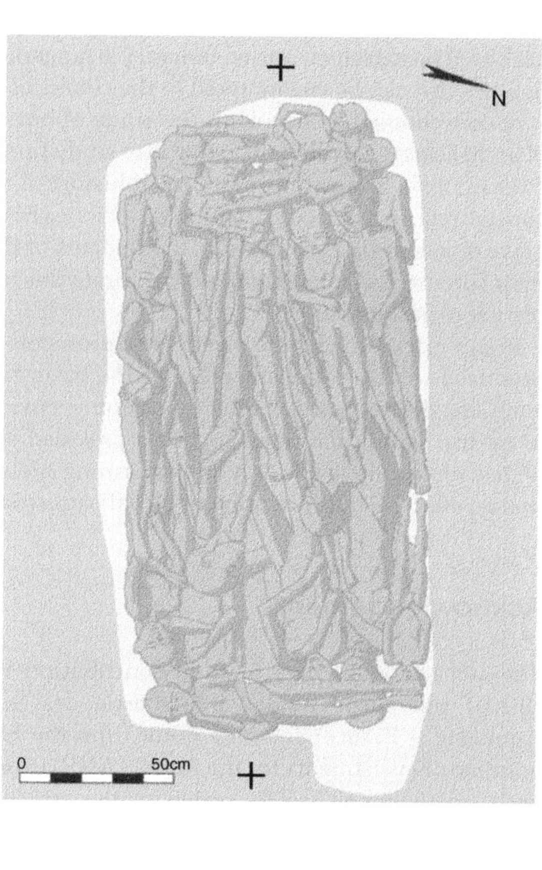

Figure 19.12 Reconstruction of the organisation of the deposits of simultaneous burial 119 at Issoudun (Indre, France) (CAD drawing: B. Ducourneau, Inrap).

case offers a detailed image of the treatment of the dead in a particular context, which lies far from a more generally held stereotype of chaos and loss of control in such situations.

19.4 Conclusion

Archaeothanatology is receiving more attention to date. At the present time, it is one of the best-suited methods to aid understanding of funerary practices. In the future, archaeothanatology should be applied to forensic analysis in order to identify the kinds of observations necessary for the resolution of diverse problems and questions that arise during an investigation. The conventional archaeological methods, such as those based on stratigraphy and dating, remain important, but the taphonomic observations and archaeo-anthropological data are indispensable.

The objective of the case studies above was to demonstrate the practical potential of archaeothanatological analysis to better interpret different forensic cases consisting of individual and multiple burials. The first, the individual case studies, are more closely related to historical cases. As not all forensic victims are buried in a supine position, the aim was to demonstrate this particular way of making observations in the field. Forensic anthropology is more than determining sex, age, stature, mode, manner and cause of death; it begins with observations that can only be made in the field.

This authors wish to highlight the importance of the methodology implemented during excavation and data recording. Moreover, this chapter demonstrates that archaeothanatology contributes an indispensable rationale to making interpretations that aid in the reconstruction of the funerary architecture and arrangement (i.e. identification, morphology and construction methods of wooden containers, grave furniture, and methods of depositing bodies). The examples in this contribution are based on extremely varied funerary arrangements and possible ambiguities of interpretation, difficulties that can be encountered in the course of analysis.

In conventional archaeology, the study of burial methods remains to a great extent in the hands of archaeologists, whose objective is to study funerary practices and social organisation of past societies in order to answer questions of historical importance. In contrast, forensic science does not concentrate on the reconstruction of societies but on individual events. In both situations, whether a grave or a depositional location, the remains of the deceased should be analysed in association with their context. It is important to incorporate this broader picture in order to achieve a more complete picture of past events.

In summary, funerary archaeological protocols should be applied in the forensic sciences. The data produced will be complementary to the basic biological studies used to identify the deceased. By analysing the deceased in their taphonomic environment and by trying to reconstruct the sequence of events, significant clues might be provided about the perpetrator and the *modus operandi*. In archaeothanatology it is only by performing a joint analysis of all available taphonomic observations that an effective interpretation of burial patterning can be provided.

Acknowledgements

The archaeological data for this contribution were collected as part of 'archéologie préventive' (Inrap) and partly funded by 'Maison des Sciences de l'Homme d'Aquitaine' (Projet Région Aquitaine – France) and by a grant from the French National Research Agency as part of a programme of investments for the future (ANR-10-LABX-52). A special thanks goes to Frances Holden and Christopher Knüsel for reviewing this article.

References

Blaizot, F. (2008) Réflexions sur la typologie des tombes à inhumation: restitution des dispositifs et implications chrono-culturelles. *Archéologie Médiévale*, **38**: 1–30.

Blaizot, F. (2014) From the skeleton to the funerary architecture: a logic of the plausible. *International Journal of the Science of Man*, **52**: 263–284.

Castex, D. (2009) From a burial ground to the discovery of an epidemical crisis. Biological identity and genotype. In: Holmgren, A. and Borg, G. (eds), *Handbook of Disease Outbreaks: Prevention, detection and control*. Nova Science Publishers: New York, pp. 23–48.

Castex, D., Kacki, S., Reveillas, H., Souquet-Leroy, I., Sachau-Carcel, G. *et al.* (2014) Revealing archaeological features linked to mortality increases. *International Journal of the Science of Man*, **52**: 299–318.

Duday, H. (2006) Archaeothanatology or the archaeology of death. In: Gowland, R. and Knüsel, C. (eds), *Social Archaeology of Funerary Remains*. Oxbow Books: Oxford, pp. 30–56.

Duday, H. (2009) *The Archaeology of the Dead. Lectures in archaeothanatology*. Oxbow Books: Oxford.

Duday, H., Le Mort, F. and Tillier, A.-M. (2014) Archaeology, application to the study of primary single burials. *Anthropologie: International Journal of Human Diversity and Evolution*, **52**: 235–246.

Souquet-Leroy, I., Réveillas, H. and Castex, D. (2015) The impact of epidemics on funerary practices in Modern France (16th–18th centuries). In: Tarlow, S. (ed.), Death and Burial in Post-medieval Europe. De Gruyter: Berlin. pp. 61–87.

Part III

Anti-, Peri- and Post-Mortem Modifications to the Body

20

Forensic Toxicology of Decomposed Human Remains

Richard Lloyd and Julie Evans

20.1 Introduction

As long ago as 1865, Dr Edward Pritchard, an English physician, was convicted of murder, on the basis of antimony detected in a number of internal organs of his wife, Mary, as well as in those of his wife's mother, one Mrs Taylor. Both bodies were exhumed when suspicion arose concerning the circumstances of their deaths following the revelation that Pritchard may have taken a mistress shortly before their demise (Trestrail 2007). Nowadays, although many laboratories focus on police casework involving non-fatal cases including drink-driving prosecutions and drug abuse screening, some toxicologists carry out medico-legal casework in order to assist a pathologist to determine the extent to which drugs – whether directly or indirectly – may have played a part in an otherwise unexpected or suspicious death. Although forming a small part of their work, forensic toxicologists may additionally undertake investigations into suspected homicidal cases, working on samples from exhumed, burnt or otherwise degraded bodies (Anderson and Torrance 2010). Compared to clinical work, however, many of the laboratory methods employed in the analysis of post-mortem samples are both complex and time-consuming, requiring a significant investment in both equipment and staff. Table 20.1, which gives examples of two recently reported methods for the analysis of hair and bone, clearly illustrates the degree of analytical complexity.

Until relatively recently, the determination of post-mortem drug levels was regarded by many as being analogous to the examination of concentrations observed in the living. On an assumed basis that once death occurred, drug concentrations in the body at the moment of death remained thereafter constant (largely as a result of the cessation of metabolic processes), it had been the case that, for many years, the amount of any drug detected in post-mortem samples would be compared directly to documented therapeutic and toxic levels in the living, and an opinion would be offered based on this simple reference.

It is now widely recognised, however, that the accurate interpretation of post-mortem toxicology carries with it significant challenges that are not encountered *in vivo* (Flanagan and Connally 2005; Leikin and Watson 2003). Successful interpretation requires a consideration of pharmacokinetic (the absorption, distribution, metabolism and excretion rates of drugs within an individual) as well as pharmacodynamic (the effects that a drug has on the body) data, including drug half-lives, distribution volume, plasma-protein binding and pKa values (Karch 2008a). Although beyond the scope of this chapter, recent work has acknowledged the significance of these pre-mortem factors on the accuracy of post-mortem toxicology, including knowledge of the quantity and route of the drug administered and whether there was any degree of established tolerance to the drug in question (Karch 2008b). An additional problem is the amount of time that may have elapsed between

Taphonomy of Human Remains: Forensic Analysis of the Dead and the Depositional Environment, First Edition.
Edited by Eline M.J. Schotsmans, Nicholas Márquez-Grant and Shari L. Forbes.

Table 20.1 Methods for preparing hair and bone for analysis by Gas Chromatography-Mass Spectrometry (GC-MS).

	Hair (Cordero and Paterson 2007)	Bone (Cornthwaite and Watterson 2014)
Cleaning	Shampoo and water, then dichloromethane (5 ml), isopropanol (5 ml), then dried with acetone (2 ml)	Phosphate buffer (0.1 M, pH 6.0), then methanol and acetone. Dried for 48 h then ground using grinding mill for 2 min then pulverised using ball mill for 1 min
Drug extraction	Hydrochloric acid (0.1 M, 2 ml), heated at 50°C for 16 h	Glacial acetic acid (100 µl) and acetonitrile:methanol (1:1,3 ml), then storage at −20°C for 12 h. Centrifuged at 1100 × *g* for 10 mins and supernatant evaporated to 1 ml under air at 70°C
Buffering	Phosphate buffer (0.1 M, 2 ml, pH 7.0) and potassium hydroxide (1 M, 200 µl)	Diluted to 4 ml with phosphate buffer (0.1 M, pH 6.0) and glacial acetic acid (100 µl).
Purification and derivatisation	Solid-phase extraction (SPE) cartridge conditioned with methanol (2 ml), then deionised water (2 ml), followed by phosphate buffer (0.1 M, 2 ml, pH 7.0). Acidic and neutral drugs then eluted with chloroform:isopropanol (80:20,2 ml), then basic drugs eluted with chloroform:isopropanol:ammonium hydroxide (80:17:3,2 ml). N-methyl-bis-triflouroacetamide (MBTFA) (15 µl), then dried down under nitrogen at 80°C until 1 ml remaining, transferred to microvials and evaporated to dryness under nitrogen at 80°C. Then N-methyl-N (trimethylsilyl) trifluoroacetamide (MSTFA) and 1% trimethylchlorosilane (TCMS) (30 µl) added and heated to 80°C for 1 hr. Further MBTFA (10 µl) then added and heated for further 30 min at 80°C	Solid-phase extraction plates conditioned with methanol (3 ml), phosphate buffer (3 ml) and distilled water (3 ml). Samples added then wells washed with phosphate buffer (0.1 M, pH 6.0, 3 ml) and acetic acid (0.1 M, 3 ml) then dried under vacuum for 5 mins at 400 mm Hg. After drying, wells rinsed with 3 ml methanol, then dried under vacuum for 10 mins at 400 mm Hg. Elution with ethyl acetate:isopropanol:ammonium hydroxide (80:17:3,4 ml), then evaporated to dryness under air at 70°C, then reconstituted in 100 µl ethyl acetate.
Analysis	1 µl injected into GC-MS	2 µl injected into GC-MS

administration of the drug and death, the so-called dose-death interval, which determines the extent to which a drug might be expected to have been absorbed and distributed (Lafrenière and Watterson 2009, 2010; Watterson and Desrosiers 2011). Other work has highlighted the role that age (Byard 2013; Drummer 2013), gender, body weight and disease may play in the responsiveness of an individual to a given dose of a given drug (Rowland and Tozer 2011).

If these variables are not problematic enough, individually let alone collectively, then one of the greatest interpretative challenges in post-mortem toxicology is the phenomenon whereby anatomical site variability of blood-tissue-drug ratios can be observed between different parts of the body, in a not yet wholly understood process known as post-mortem redistribution (Mußhoff *et al.* 2004; Tominaga *et al.* 2013).

Thus, although there is a very large body of clinical toxicology data relating to drug concentrations in the living, toxicologists are counselled in the pitfalls of attempting to make direct correlations with post-mortem findings (Jones 2011). The Holy Grail of post-mortem forensic toxicology is to be able to determine the amount of drug injected, swallowed, insufflated – or otherwise consumed – during life, from the evidence that can be gleaned after death. For the reasons already considered, as well as others to be discussed later in the chapter, attempts at back-extrapolation are fraught with danger. Progress has, however, been made in the case of a number of drugs (Ferner 2008), although arguably much of this work has only served to underline further the problems inherent in such attempts (Milroy and Forrest 2000; Wennig 2000b).

This is not to say, however, that post-mortem toxicological analysis can never provide definitive results. Although in the case of quantitative questions – relating to definitions of the quantity, or concentration of a drug – the results may be presented with significant reservations, in the case of qualitative assessments – determining, simply, whether or not a drug is present – entirely convincing results are frequently obtainable and have contributed to successful criminal prosecutions. In January 2000, the conviction of Dr Harold Shipman, a UK medical practitioner, was secured, in part, on the basis of morphine (as an important metabolite of diamorphine) being detected in a number of his victims. Although it is believed he killed somewhere between 220 and 240 of his patients over the course of his medical career, his conviction was for the murder of 15 patients, by the administration of lethal doses of diamorphine, demonstrated by toxicological analysis of skeletal muscle obtained from a number of bodies exhumed between 38 and 852 days following death (Pounder 2003).

20.2 Toxicological Matrices

Unlike recently deceased bodies where, in most instances, blood will be the tissue, or matrix, of choice for analysis, it is often the case with taphonomic work that blood is not available and other matrices must be tested. The remainder of this chapter, therefore, considers those other tissues that are used in forensic casework, examining the advantages and disadvantages of each, before presenting an actual case study, demonstrating the practical and legal application of toxicological analysis.

20.2.1 Soft Tissues and Fluids

Whereas blood and other fluids will often be lost in a burial environment within a short space of time, muscle is not only comparatively abundant, but is relatively slow to decompose, and a number of drugs have been detected over significant periods of time in this matrix (Christensen *et al.* 1985; Langford *et al.* 1998). One of the first morphine cases reported in the literature identified the drug after 5 months of burial (Worm *et al.* 1983); the 9 exhumations carried out as part of the Shipman investigation, mentioned above, were successfully analysed for morphine and other drugs between 38 and 852 days following death. Other drugs and poisons have been identified in various tissues years after burial including diazepam and furosemide (both 7.5 years) and parathion (17 years) (Grellner and Glenewinkel 1997; Käferstein *et al.* 1994; Sierra-Callejas and Pribilla 1978), while phenobarbital was identified in a body discovered in a hut, naturally mummified, 10 years after the individual was last seen alive (Giusiani *et al.* 2012). An advantage of muscle, furthermore, is that it does not contain certain enzymes found in other parts of the body that are responsible for the breakdown of drugs that contain an ester functional group in their chemical structure, including the cholinesterase inhibitors neostigmine and rivastigmine (Satoh *et al.* 2002). Although toxicologists have a limited amount of reference material from which to form opinions on post-mortem cases, the data available for drugs in skeletal muscle is perhaps better than that available for many other matrices (Rees 2011).

Toxicological analysis is also undertaken from time to time on other soft tissues or fluids (Drummer and Gerostamoulos 2002), including the liver (Mußhoff and Madea 2001), fat and lung tissue (Drummer 2004), and a limited amount of research has been carried out on brain (Kalasinsky *et al.* 2001), pleural effusions (Sims *et al.* 1999), vitreous humour (Scott and Oliver 2001), and even cerebrospinal fluid (Jenkins and Lavins 1998), synovial fluid (DeKing *et al.* 2014) and fly larvae (De Carvalho 2010), though the amount of data available renders many of these matrices unusable for all but the most simple qualitative assessments.

Although muscle and other tissues can be used for toxicological analysis, a number of drugs are unstable in the post-mortem environment (Robertson and Drummer 1995). Although these differences may in part be attributed to post-mortem redistribution, organic decomposition of the body also plays a part. While some drugs are known to remain chemically stable, others, such as nitro-benzodiazepines (a group of hypnotics containing many well-known drugs of abuse including diazepam and flunitrazepam, better known as the date-rape drug rohypnol) are commonly metabolised by bacteria that flourish in the typical post-mortem environment (Ferner 2008; Watterson and Donohue 2011).

Rates of decomposition are, however, variable, depending on factors such as ambient temperature and humidity (Skopp 2004). As a guiding principle, the more advanced the degree of putrefaction, the greater the analytical and diagnostic challenges facing the toxicologist, although qualitative data for a wide range of drugs has been published (Arnold *et al.* 1984). The question of drug recovery within biological environments has been examined by a number of authors (Butzbach 2010; Peters 2007), and a careful consideration of these findings is often useful when attempting to interpret the analysis of degraded tissues (Kennedy 2010).

An additional and important problem in post-mortem analysis, most especially in the case of mass graves, is contamination from items in close proximity to the body, including other corpses. Hence, control samples should always be taken from the environment in which the body is found or exhumed (Carter and Tibbett 2008). Commonly, several samples of soil will be taken from around the body, and in the case of conventional burials, samples of the coffin and its fittings, as well as any objects that might have been placed within the grave before burial are collected, in order to preclude the possibility of erroneous results (Dettmeyer *et al.* 2014).

20.2.2 Hair

Hair is a material that has an extensive literature and holds a mainstream place in forensic toxicology, largely because of the fact that it grows at a uniform rate and can, therefore, be regarded as a 'timeline' of drug use. It was first used in the 1960s as a marker of occupational exposure to heavy metals (Kintz 2008). By the late 1970s, however, improved methods of detection enabled the analysis of organic molecules, and the publication of the first report identifying morphine in the hair of heroin abusers (Baumgartner *et al.* 1979). Nowadays, hair is sampled regularly in pre-natal as well as pre-employment screening as well as in sport-related doping control tests and, in some countries, for driving licence regulatory purposes (Barbosa *et al.* 2013). Additionally, although traditionally used to demonstrate only chronic drug abuse, hair is now customarily taken in cases of drug-facilitated crime (DFC), particularly when a significant window of time has passed between the alleged offence and its reporting (Scott 2009). Such is the degree of confidence in hair as a reliable matrix that, since 2004, in the UK, it has been routinely analysed for selected HM Coroner cases in suspicious deaths (Lee *et al.* 2009).

When considering toxicology in decomposed remains, the great advantage of hair over other tissue types is its resistance to degradation. The opium habits of the poet John Keats, were detected in his hair nearly 170 years after his death (Baumgartner *et al.* 1989) and, remarkably, benzoylecgonine – the principal metabolite of cocaine – has been detected in the hair shafts of Chilean and Peruvian mummified corpses dating to 2000 BC (Cartmell *et al.* 1991); cocaine and alcohol have also been detected in the scalp hair of Inca child sacrifice victims (Wilson *et al.* 2013). One of the more interesting cases reported in the literature is that of a badly decomposed body discovered in a forest with so little soft tissue remaining that visual identification was impossible (Kintz 2004). Toxicological analysis undertaken on the hair revealed amounts of chlorpromazine, fluoxetine, carbamazepine and lorazepam (medications used most commonly as, respectively, anti-psychotic, anti-depressant, anti-epileptic and anxiolytics) that corresponded to the medication regime of a psychiatric patient who had been missing from a local hospital for some weeks. Identification was confirmed by DNA testing.

A very significant advantage that hair has over matrices such as blood, urine and muscle is that in many cases it can be used to distinguish between single exposure and chronic abuse. The reason for this is two-fold. First, the mechanism by which drugs are incorporated into hair – primarily into the growing shaft via the vascular hair follicle – has been fairly well understood for some time (Henderson 1993). Second, and of crucial importance in DFC work where it is essential to be able to construct extremely accurate timelines, the rate of growth of hair is generally uniform between individuals and is well-documented. Thus, it is known that hair grows at a rate of between 0.22 and 0.52 mm/day (Saitoh *et al.* 1969), and so by undertaking a multi-sectional analysis of hair, it is possible to construct a retrospective history of drug use extending commonly over a period of months or, in cases where especially long scalp hair is obtainable, for several years (Wada and Nakashima 2006). Using such a method, it has been possible for some time to reconstruct in detail the drug histories of exhumed bodies, even in cases of advanced decomposition (Tsatsakis *et al.* 2001), as is clearly demonstrated in the case study accompanying this chapter. Another advantage of hair compared to nails and bone is that, for a number of drugs, there appears to be a good correlation between known drug use and analytical findings (Mußhoff *et al.* 2006; Pepin and Gaillard 1997; Scheidweiler *et al.* 2005).

Like almost every other analytical technique used in the investigation of forensic casework, however, hair testing is not entirely problem free, and its results are not always unequivocal (Kintz 2014; Mußhoff and Madea 2007; Wennig 2000a). As well as having the potential to be altered by cosmetic processes, including dying, bleaching and permanent waving (Jurado *et al.* 1997), it has been clearly demonstrated that hair has a significant capacity to adsorb smoke, vapours and other contaminants from the external environment, as well as being porous to the extent that it can absorb sweat or other liquids, such that its weight can be increased by up to 18% (Kintz 2008). This final point alone clearly has important implications for toxicology undertaken on exhumation cases where, commonly, bodies buried in coffins are frequently found submerged in significant quantities of putrefactive liquid. In mass grave situations, therefore, the risk of obtaining false-positives from cross-contamination may be high (Kintz 2012), and although the detection of drugs in hair, where contamination is not possible, would constitute definitive evidence of exposure, the need to take soil samples from around the body itself will be of critical importance to the veracity of the results presented. Careful sample preparation is extremely important (Cooper *et al.* 2012). Recent work has also suggested that submersion in putrefactive fluids or submersion in water may cause decomposition of the hair root, with implications for toxicology intending to establish drug use close to the time of death (Wilson 2008; Koch *et al.* 2013). Additionally, it has been demonstrated that black hair incorporates greater quantities of drugs than does blond hair, and thus the possibility of racial bias might need to be taken into consideration (Henderson *et al.* 1998).

20.2.3 Nails

Like other analytical matrices, nails can prove to be extremely useful in certain specific cases. In clinical medicine, problems with hepatic metabolism can be predicted by analysing a particular enzyme found in the nails (Nishiyori *et al.* 2002); in cases where information regarding a patient's previous renal function is unknown, the determination of creatinine levels in the nail plate can be used, importantly, to distinguish chronic from acute renal failure (Tosti *et al.* 2002); additionally, nails are regarded as excellent evidential sources of drug exposure *in utero* (Skopp and Pötsch 1997).

In post-mortem work, too, although hair is frequently the preferred matrix, nail analysis has long been known to have particular strengths. A case report published in 2004 demonstrated the benefits of nail analysis in determining arsenic poisoning, resulting in a criminal conviction that might not have been obtained by other means (Daniel *et al.* 2004). In this case, an investigation was carried out into the unexplained death of a travelling salesman. He had previously been hospitalised on several occasions over a six-month period, suffering from generalised weakness and increasing weight loss. After his death, a dermatopathologist noticed unusual transverse lines on the finger nails which, on analysis, revealed significant levels of arsenic. This finding, along with an examination of the salesman's lifestyle, triggered the recollection of a similar case, whereby another salesman suffering almost identical symptoms died of unexplained causes. His body was exhumed and his nails were also found to demonstrate a periodic ingestion of arsenic. Taking account of a daily fingernail growth rate of around 0.1 to 0.15 mm, and plotting the frequency of the so-called Mees' lines on the nails of both victims with their appointments diaries it was, remarkably, possible to narrow the window of likely arsenic ingestion to the lunch counter of a particular department store where both men happened to eat when in one particular town. A waitress in the store was duly arrested and charged with murder.

This case highlights the usefulness of the nail as a matrix for the detection of certain poisons. One of the earliest post-mortem cases reported in the literature was that of a successful analysis being made following exhumation some seven months following burial (Pirl *et al.* 1983). A number of drugs have been qualitatively identified in nails though, compared to other matrices used in difficult cases, research in this area has been somewhat more limited. After the early work identifying arsenic in post-mortem cases, a number of laboratories looked at the detection of drugs of forensic interest in the nails of the living. The earliest study, published in 1984, demonstrated the capability of GC-MS to detect amphetamine and methamphetamine in the finger- and toenails of users (Suzuki *et al.* 1984). Work on amphetamine detection was continued with a comparative paper in 1989, examining detection of the drug in hair, sweat and saliva, as well as nails, finding that the drug could be detected in nails for 45 days following ingestion, compared to 18 days in hair and only 2 days in saliva (Suzuki *et al.* 1989). Little else appeared in the literature until 1998, when a significant study identified cocaine in 82.3% of post-mortem subjects, where only 27.7% had been positively identified using the conventional matrices of blood and urine (Garside *et al.* 1998). The following year, a study was published reporting the successful identification of cocaine and its metabolites, as well as a number of opiates in 46 post-mortem cases (Engelhart *et al.* 1998), and the same author continued this work, publishing a study in 2002 that claimed to discern consistently greater concentrations of cocaine metabolites and opiates in fingernails than in toenails (Engelhart and Jenkins 2002). More recently, a Chinese study has reported the successful detection of several opiates, including the primary heroin metabolite, 6-MAM, in fingernails although, again, the method used fresh, rather than taphonomic samples (Shen *et al.* 2014).

Despite these successes, a number of problems appear to hinder the extent to which nails can be usefully analysed. Perhaps the main difficulty is that there is still no firm understanding of the mechanism by which drugs are incorporated into nails, due to an incomplete understanding of how the nail plate itself grows and how the proximity of the vascular supply with sweat glands and sebaceous glands interacts to allow the incorporation of drugs into the keratin of the nails (Garside 2008). It is unclear, furthermore, whether it is possible that incorporation can take place via external contamination and, additionally, there are known instances where nails in post-mortem cases have shown no trace of drugs, while simultaneous blood and urine toxicology screens have tested positive, suggesting that nails may not provide evidence of peri-mortem drug use (Engelhart *et al.* 1998; Garside *et al.* 1998). Nails also appear to incorporate drugs at lower concentrations than hair, and the correlation with time of intake appears less well defined (Palmeri *et al.* 2000). Related to this problem is a seemingly considerable variability of pharmacokinetic measurements obtained from different subjects, even of the same sex and race (Ropero-Miller *et al.* 2000). Ropero-Miller, in the same paper, also makes the point that the method by which the nails are prepared for analysis – the way in which the drugs are extracted from the keratin – may also affect the results.

One of the greatest advantages of nail in exhumation cases is that it is extremely resistant to decomposition and will survive far beyond the period in which soft tissue or even hair in putrefied environments can be recovered (Suzuki *et al.* 1989). In the absence of hair it also has the very considerable advantage that, because of its rate of growth, like hair it can potentially be used to determine a drug ingestion timeline for perhaps up to 12 months in the case of the particularly slow growing great toenail (Fleckman 1985). Another significant advantage in exhumation work is that there is a much greater stability of drugs within the nail matrix, whereas the analysis of body fluids or tissues in such cases has been known to yield false negatives due to the breakdown of the target analytes (Palmeri *et al.* 2000).

20.2.4 Bone and Bone Marrow

The analysis of bone marrow aspirate is used as the preferred diagnostic tool in a number of clinical settings including haematology and oncology (Provan *et al.* 2009), though its application in post-mortem work is less well developed when compared to many other methods (Tattoli *et al.* 2014; Watterson 2006). It has been used successfully for estimating the post-mortem interval (Findlay 1976), for genetic typing (van Doorn *et al.* 2011) and, given its frequent implication in cases of unexpected death, there has been a long-standing interest in alcohol (ethanol) identification in marrow (Cartisier *et al.* 2011). Bone itself has been a source of research attention in recent years and has been found to be a useful repository of drugs that might not otherwise be detectable in the fluids or soft tissues of a decomposing body (McIntyre *et al.* 2000). Collectively, however, bone and bone marrow remain one of the least researched areas in post-mortem toxicology (McGrath and Jenkins 2009).

It might be expected that marrow could be a useful analyte, given that the cavity in which it is found is encased as a layer of hard and relatively impervious compact bone, as well as an outer 'skin', the periosteum, and is thus protected from both external contamination and internal deterioration (Roll *et al.* 2009). Given the resistance of finger and toe nails to decomposition and the excellent stability of drugs within them, bone collagen might equally be expected to be a useful target of analysis, given that it can survive burial for hundreds or even thousands of years. Although both tissues have received increasing attention in recent years, one of the problems associated with the use of bone and bone marrow remains the wide-ranging methods of both extraction and analysis reported in the literature. While the femur is regarded by many as the preferred source of marrow, success has also been achieved via aspiration from the vertebrae (Maeda *et al.* 2006), as well as by using marrow squeezed from the ends of cut ribs (Schloegl *et al.* 2006). Analysts have also reported the successful identification of morphine and codeine in the teeth of burnt, putrefied and skeletal remains (Cattaneo *et al.* 2003) and, more recently, have been able to identify and quantify opiates extracted from the clavicles of recently deceased forensic cases (Vardakou *et al.* 2014).

As well as a lack of consistency in sampling methodology, a significant problem is that, contrary to the situation with nails, the uptake of drugs into bone may be more easily reversible than initially suspected (Jenkins 2007). Results in closely controlled, experimental conditions have often been inconsistent. In one study, the corpse of a domestic pig – being anatomically and physiologically the closest animal analogue to a human body – was allowed to decompose and skeletonise for 2 years, following which 13 of its bones were analysed for the antidepressant medications with which it had been dosed before death (Desrosiers *et al.* 2012). Comparative analysis of the bones revealed differences of 33- to 166-fold, depending on the drug, although there were consistently closer ratios observed between the parent drug and its metabolite, in each case, varying from 1- to 8-fold. Indeed, in a series of controlled experiments undertaken by the same laboratory using pigs and rats, significant variability between the site of recovery was observed with a range of drugs (Watterson and Cornthwaite 2013). Given that it is a richly vascularised tissue, recent work has sought to correlate drug levels between bone marrow and blood, though the results have been disappointing (Cartisier *et al.* 2011; Wiebe and Watterson 2014). Finally, what must also be borne in mind is that no matter how well conceived and conducted experimental work might be, the extent to which results obtained from pig and rat models can be confidently extrapolated to actual human, forensic cases is a matter that requires careful consideration (Watterson *et al.* 2010).

This is not to say, however, that bone and bone marrow forensic analysis is without purpose. There is no doubt that both matrices can already be regarded as useful for the qualitative identification of a number of substances. Table 20.2 lists the drugs that have been detected, as listed in publications since 2008, as a supplement to the table published in Drummer (2008) (see also McGrath and Jenkins 2009). Although the precise mechanisms by which drugs enter and leave bones and bone marrow – and the ways in which these processes interact both before and after death – will require further investigation if they are to have greater forensic value, a new means of separating drugs from bone tissue, using microwave assisted extraction, has recently reported a significant improvement on the more common methods employed (Cornthwaite and Watterson 2014). Other work, using relatively recently deceased skeletonised rats, has reported discernible and useful analytical differences following acute and chronic drug exposure (Watterson *et al.* 2012).

Table 20.2 Examples of selected drugs of abuse detected in bone and bone marrow reported in the literature since 2008.

Drug class detected (Reference)	Conditions	Notes
Opioids (Watterson and Donohue 2011)	Experimental – skeletal rat tibiae, vertebrae and pelvis Bone and bone marrow (BM)	Successful extraction of meperidine using Microwave Assisted Extraction
Opioids (Lafrenière and Wattson 2010)	Experimental – skeletal rat femora and tibiae Bone and BM	Use of enzyme-linked immunosorbent assay (ELISA) for identification of fentanyl
Benzodiazepines (Delabarde *et al.* 2013)	Human skeletal forensic case. Bone, BM and adipocere	Positive for diazepam and nordiazepam using UPLC/MS-MS
Amphetamines, opiates and benzodiazepines (Tominaga *et al.* 2013)	Fresh human autopsy cases. Thoracic vertebrae, BM	Many drugs identified at time of death using GC-MS
Opiates (Vardakou *et al.* 2014)	Fresh human autopsy cases, BM from clavicle	Identification of morphine, codeine and 6-MAM by GC/MS
Opioids (Wiebe and Watterson 2014)	Experimental – skeletal rat bones, various	Identification of tramadol and *O*-desmethyltramadol using GC-MS
Benzodiazepines (Watterson *et al.* 2010)	Experimental – skeletal pig bones and BM, various	Identification of diazepam and nordiazepam using GC-MS
Benzodiazepines (Watterson and Botman 2009)	Experimental – rat BM	Identification of diazepam using ELISA

20.3 Case Study

The first part of this chapter has considered, from a theoretical perspective, the methods by which toxicological analysis can be undertaken on either decomposing or decomposed remains, examining the inherent strengths and weaknesses of each tissue type. What now follows is a case study based in part of the prosecution evidence presented in an actual (anonymous) criminal case heard in the UK Crown Court. From a toxicological perspective, the case was both lengthy and complex, beginning with the routine analysis of tissues from a recently-deceased nursing home resident, progressing to the examination of muscle and hair obtained from the exhumed bodies of other residents. Of particular interest in this case is the way in which hair was used decisively to prove that the drug charts of the deceased residents were an inaccurate record of their actual drug ingestion.

20.3.1 Background

This case involved the investigation of a number of residents in a care home. Concerns had been raised by members of staff about the care of residents and the behaviour of the manager. When a 97-year-old female resident died unexpectedly, a police investigation was instigated. The inquiry took two years to complete and culminated in a criminal conviction and custodial sentence.

20.3.2 Initial Case

Analysis of routine toxicology samples (blood, stomach contents and tissue from around the suspected injection sites) from the body of the 97-year-old resident that sparked the enquiry identified very high concentrations of tramadol that would offer a potential explanation for her death. Tramadol was an important finding, since the drug had never been prescribed to the deceased. Additionally, pethidine was detected, and although the concentration was not excessive, it was another drug that had not been prescribed. Fentanyl and midazolam were both detected, though in quantities consistent with their prescription. The deceased had, however, been prescribed diamorphine on the night leading up to her death which, according to her drugs chart, had been administered. Once in the body, diamorphine is quickly metabolised into other compounds, including morphine, which would ordinarily be detected in significant quantities after death. Blood analysis, however, revealed much lower concentrations of morphine than expected. There were, therefore, three significant inconsistencies with the toxicology in this case: the presence of two drugs that had not been prescribed, and a much lower than expected concentration of another. A summary of the toxicology findings in the initial case is provided below, in Table 20.3.

The higher concentration of tramadol in the blood from the arm over that in the leg may be explained by post-mortem redistribution. However, a needle puncture mark was observed below the right collar bone, suggesting that the drug may have been injected, thus explaining the elevation, if death had occurred before dispersal from the site of injection had taken place.

Table 20.3 Summary of toxicology (blood) results, initial case.

BLOOD (right arm)	BLOOD (left arm)	BLOOD (right leg)
Free Morphine – 3 µg/L	Tramadol – 33 mg/L	Tramadol – 18 mg/L
Total Morphine – 4 µg/L	Midazolam – 94 µg/L	Fentanyl – 2.6 µg/L
Fentanyl – 2.7 µg/L		Pethidine – 22 µg/L

Table 20.4 Summary of toxicology results (plucked hair), initial case.

Drugs	Segment 0–3 cm	Segment 3–6 cm	Segment 6–9 cm
Opiates	Not detected	Not detected	Not detected
Fentanyl	4.9 pg/mg	2.5 pg/mg	1.8 pg/mg
Midazolam	65 pg/mg	6 pg/mg	6 pg/mg
Tramadol	605 pg/mg	40 pg/mg	43 pg/mg

In view of the almost total absence of morphine, against a background of prescribed diamorphine, testing was undertaken on the hair of the deceased in an attempt to examine historic administration. The results are presented in Table 20.4.

The high concentration of tramadol in the first segment of hair could be entirely due to the presence of the roots and thus reflect the administration close to the time of death. The concentrations further down the shaft are relatively low and may be due to incorporation from sweat at around the time of death, although previous administration cannot be excluded. The findings with respect to the fentanyl and midazolam correlated with the deceased's prescribing history. Importantly, however, no opiates (including morphine) were detected in the hair, a finding completely at odds with the deceased's drug chart.

The primary suspect was the manager of the home, who initially denied any wrong doing. Police interviews with other residents of the home, however, suggested that they had been given medications that were not prescribed, and that medications prescribed had not been administered. Testing of hair from the living residents making these allegations (which are not reported here) supported their claims.

The police inquiry then turned to other residents who had died in suspicious circumstances, but where post-mortem examinations had not been conducted, and it was decided to exhume the bodies of three former residents.

20.3.2.1 Exhumation 1

This 89-year-old former resident was exhumed around 10 months after burial and samples, including hair, blood, thigh muscle and cavity fluid were taken for analysis. No drugs were detected in the hair sample or the cavity fluid. In view of these findings, no testing was performed on the blood samples (which were small) or the thigh muscles.

Of concern, however, was the absence of cyclizine, midazolam and morphine, drugs that were reportedly being administered via a syringe driver in the last hours of the deceased's life. Although the stability of cyclizine during putrefaction has not been studied, and midazolam can be lost post-mortem, morphine is known to be relatively stable, and thus some evidence of its use would be expected to be found in the cavity fluid, even after 10 months.

Overall, no evidence was found to support the view that drugs were a factor in the death, and there was no evidence that drugs that were not prescribed to the deceased had been administered in the months preceding death. There was, however, some evidence to suggest that drugs that were prescribed to the deceased (morphine, cyclizine, midazolam and oxycodone) may not have been administered.

20.3.2.2 Exhumation 2

The body of the third suspected victim was exhumed around 11 months after death, with samples of cut head hair, cavity fluid, stomach contents, nails and thigh muscle being taken for analysis. No blood could be recovered from the body.

Analysis of the cavity fluid detected midazolam (1 μg/L), diazepam (1.3 μg/L) and nordiazepam (0.4 μg/L), with no other drugs being identified. Midazolam (<2 mg in total) and clomipramine (<5 mg in total) were detected in the stomach contents. All of these were prescribed to the deceased.

The hair was analysed for a wide range of pharmaceutical drugs, the results of which are presented in Table 20.5.

While there was no evidence to support the view that the administration of drugs was a direct factor in the death, the condition of the body limited the usefulness of the analysis. Importantly, however, neither oxycodone nor cyclizine were detected in the cavity fluid, drugs which should have been present, as they were being administered via a syringe driver in the hours preceding death. Although the effect of decomposition can offer an explanation for their absence, the presence of midazolam (which is known to be unstable) would tend to suggest that decomposition of drugs was not complete and thus the findings cast doubt on oxycodone and cyclizine being administered as prescribed. What was of greater significance, however, was that the hair, although indicating diazepam usage, did not provide expected evidence of the large doses that had been prescribed to the deceased for many months preceding death.

20.3.2.3 Exhumation 3

The body of the fourth suspected victim was exhumed around 18 months after death. Samples of cavity fluid, thigh muscle and pubic hair were obtained and tested. Midazolam, morphine and fentanyl were detected in the cavity fluid with no other drugs being identified during the testing. Quantitative analysis of the thigh muscle tissues are summarised in Table 20.6.

Although the concentration of morphine detected was high, particularly in the left leg, the condition of the body and the large amount of fluid that was within the coffin prevented any firm conclusion being made in respect of whether the death was as a result of drug administration. The drug charts for the day of the death were unfortunately missing, although the deceased was prescribed diamorphine and thus the possibility that the morphine findings were from correctly administered doses could not be excluded. Midazolam findings were consistent with reported administration. Importantly, however, there was evidence that fentanyl had been administered, although there was no record of it having been prescribed.

Table 20.5 Summary of toxicology results (cut hair), Exhumation 2.

DRUGS	SEGMENT 0–3 CM	SEGMENT 3–6 CM	SEGMENT 6–9 CM	SEGMENT 9–12 CM
Midazolam	82 pg/mg	71 pg/mg	70 pg/mg	120 pg/mg
Temazepam	7 pg/mg	8 pg/mg	4 pg/mg	8 pg/mg
Nordiazepam	34 pg/mg	26 pg/mg	18 pg/mg	31 pg/mg
Diazepam	58 pg/mg	69 pg/mg	50 pg/mg	73 pg/mg

Table 20.6 Quantitative analysis on thigh muscle of Exhumation 3.

Drug	Left Thigh Muscle	Right Thigh Muscle
Morphine (free)	344 μg/g	70 μg/g
Midazolam	244 μg/g	302 μg/g
Fentanyl	53 μg/g	49 μg/g

Table 20.7 Quantitative analysis on pubic hair of Exhumation 3.

DRUGS	FIRST SEGMENT	SECOND SEGMENT	THIRD SEGMENT	FOURTH SEGMENT
Midazolam	88 pg/mg	84 pg/mg	60 pg/mg	41 pg/mg
Morphine	0.6 ng/mg	0.4 ng/mg	0.4 ng/mg	0.4 ng/mg
Fentanyl	4 pg/mg	4 pg/mg	4 pg/mg	4 pg/mg

Table 20.8 Summary of findings in the hair of the suspect compared to admissions.

Drug	Prescribed to Suspect	Admitted Use
Codeine	No	No (Yes[a)])
Morphine	No	No (Yes[a)])
Diazepam	No	No (Yes[a)])
Midazolam	No	No (Yes[a)])
Tramadol	No	No (Yes[a)])
Pethidine	Yes[b)]	No (Yes[a)])
Fentanyl	No	No (Yes[c)])
Oxycodone	No	No (Yes[a)])
Lorazepam	No	No (Yes[a)])

a) *Initially denied but admitted shortly before the trial*
b) *Prescribed but would not account for the findings in the hair as discontinued before the time period expected to be covered by the hair*
c) *Initially denied but admitted during the trial*

Segmental analysis of the pubic hair was then undertaken (Table 20.7). Despite having been prescribed both morphine and diamorphine in the six months before death, toxicology findings did not support the drug administration record, with very little evidence of administration being found.

20.3.3 Summary

Toxicology found evidence that drugs which were not prescribed to residents had been administered, while drugs that were prescribed (notably opiates and opioids) were in many cases not detected, suggesting strongly that they had not been administered. A similar pattern was identified in the hair of some of the current residents living at the home.

Analysis of hair from the manager of the home demonstrated a long standing history of the use of opiate and opioid use (morphine, pethidine, codeine, tramadol, fentanyl and oxycodone), as well as benzodiazepines (midazolam, lorazepam and diazepam) (Table 20.8), and she was duly charged.

Shortly before the trial, perhaps in light of the overwhelming evidence, the suspect admitted to taking drugs prescribed to residents for her personal use, though denied substituting drugs. She also admitted fabricating circumstances in order to gain additional drugs, again for her own use. On the basis of toxicology evidence, it was accepted by the defence that the suspect began to self-medicate with tramadol and that she later used diamorphine, diazepam, oxycodone, pethidine, midazolam and lorazepam prescribed to other residents. She admitted that she had used the diamorphine prescribed to the 97-year-old on the night of her death, thus accounting for the lack of appreciable morphine in the deceased. She pleaded guilty to the unlawful possession of drugs, and to falsifying records, and was convicted of the manslaughter of the 97-year-old female whose death sparked the inquiry.

If this case study demonstrates the practical application of drug analysis, what it also does is highlight the way in which the toxicological examination of taphonomic remains can be extremely useful. From a forensic perspective, importantly, what this case also underlines is the fact that the toxicological evidence obtained from degraded remains can be accepted as admissible evidence in a court of law.

20.4 Conclusion and Future Research

To summarise Karch (2007), post-mortem toxicology is a challenging area of forensic science and the interpretation of the results brings with it a unique set of very often significant challenges. A thorough understanding and reasoned consideration of a variable range of biological parameters – including the individual pharmacokinetic and pharmacodynamics aspects discussed in the introduction to this chapter – is necessary if the most accurate interpretation is to be provided. Additionally, detailed information about the circumstances and manner of death when known can, in many cases assist (Gruszecki *et al.* 2007). Knowledge of the drug habits of an individual can be of considerable help when assessing the likelihood of a detected concentration being primarily responsible for the death or it being simply an incidental finding (Karch 2001). Because of the range of samples the toxicologist might be expected to examine, and the condition in which those samples might be found, it is important to tailor analyses as closely as possible to the sample being presented, bearing in mind the question being asked. Only with a full knowledge of all available evidence will the toxicologist be able to provide the most reliable interpretation.

As for the future, there is the need for more comparative work between different post-mortem tissues, of the sort reported by Cingolani *et al.* in 2004, as research in this area may not only determine more precisely the benefits of respective tissues as toxicological matrices in their own rights, but may also serve further to elucidate the precise mechanisms by which drugs are incorporated and stored. This could be important, particularly for nails, where current methods are less well developed than those for hair. Bones and bone marrow, too, are comparatively under-represented in both the literature and in forensic practice, yet both show promise, bone marrow especially, as it a vascular medium, and is protectively sheltered within the long bones.

Although we are able to calculate drug concentrations from many different types of samples, the ability to calculate ante-mortem drug dosage by back-extrapolating from post-mortem findings remains elusive to forensic toxicologists (Karch 2013). The ever-increasing capability of analytical technology in conjunction with the development of new techniques and ever-improving pharmacokinetic modelling methods, however, have led to much improved and more accurate reporting in recent years. With further advances, and sustained research, this position can only improve.

References

Anderson, R.A. and Torrance, H.J. (2010) Forensic toxicology. In: White, P. (ed.), *Crime Scene to Court*. RSC Publishing: Cambridge, pp. 390–437.

Arnold, D., Naeve, W. and Arnold, W. (1984) Toxikologische Befunderhebungen an Fäulnisleichen. *Zeitschrift für Rechtsmedizin*, **93**: 151–164.

Barbosa, J., Faria, .J, Carvalho, F., Pedro, M., Queirós, O. *et al.* (2013) Hair as an alternative matrix in bioanalysis. *Bioanalysis*, **5**: 895–914.

Baumgartner, A.M., Jones, P.F., Baumgartner, W.A. and Blank, C.T. (1979) Radioimmunoassay of hair for determination of opiate-abuse histories. *Journal of Nuclear Medicine*, **20**: 748–752.

Baumgartner, W.A., Hill, V.A. and Blahd, W.H. (1989) Hair analysis for drugs of abuse. *Journal of Forensic Sciences*, **34**: 1433–1453.

Butzbach, D.M. (2010) The influence of putrefaction and sample storage on post-mortem toxicology results. *Forensic Science Medicine and Pathology*, **6**: 35–45.

Byard, R.W. (2013) Post-mortem toxicology in the elderly. *Forensic Science Medicine and Pathology*, **9**: 254–255.

Carter, D.O. and Tibbett, M. (2008) Cadaver decomposition and soil: processes. In: Tibbet, M. and Carter, D.O. (eds), *Soil Analysis in Forensic Taphonomy: Chemical and biological effects of buried human remains*. CRC Press: Boca Raton, pp. 29–51.

Cartisier, N., Bévalot, F., Fanton, L., Gaillard, Y. and Guitton, J. (2011) State-of-the-art of bone marrow analysis in forensic toxicology: a review. *International Journal of Legal Medicine*, **125**: 181–198.

Cartmell, L.W., Aufderhide, A. and Weems, C. (1991) Cocaine metabolites in pre-Columbian mummy hair. *The Journal of the Oklahoma State Medical Association*, **84**: 11–12.

Cattaneo, C., Gigli, F., Lodi, F. and Grandi, M. (2003) The detection of morphine and codeine in human teeth: an aid in the identification and study of human skeletal remains. *Journal of Forensic Odonto-Stomatology*, **21**: 1–5.

Christensen, H., Steentoft, A. and Worm, K. (1985) Muscle as an autopsy material for evaluation of fatal cases of drug overdose. *Journal of the Forensic Science Society*, **25**: 191–206.

Cingolani, M., Scavella, S., Mencarelli, R., Mirtella, D., Froldi, R. and Rodriguez, D. (2004) Simultaneous detection and quantitation of morphine, 6-acetylmorphine, and cocaine in toenails: comparison with hair analysis. *Journal of Analytical Toxicology*, **28**: 128–131.

Cooper, G.A.A., Kronstrand, R. and Kintz, P. (2012) Society of Hair Testing guidelines for drug testing in hair. *Forensic Science International*, **218**: 20–24.

Cordero, R. and Paterson, S. (2007) Simultaneous quantification of opiates, amphetamines, cocaine and metabolites and diazepam and metabolite in a single hair sample using GC-MS. *Journal of Chromatography B*, **850**: 423–431.

Cornthwaite, H.M. and Watterson, J.H. (2014) Microwave assisted extraction of ketamine and its metabolites from skeletal tissues. *Analytical Methods*, **6**: 1142–1148.

Daniel, C.R., Piraccini, B. and Tosti, A. (2004) The nail and hair in forensic science. *Journal of the American Academy of Dermatology*, **50**: 258–261.

De Carvalho, L.M.L. (2010) Toxicology and forensic entomology. In: Amendt, J., Campobasso, C.P, Goff, M.L. and Grassberger, M. (eds), *Current Concepts in Forensic Entomology*. Springer: London and New York, pp. 163–178.

DeKing, J., Hargrove, V.M. and Molina, D.K. (2014) Synovial fluid: an alternative toxicologic specimen? *The American Journal of Forensic Medicine and Pathology*, **35**, 154–156.

Delabarde, T., Keyser, C., Tracqui, A., Charabidze, D. and Ludes, B. (2013) The potential of forensic analysis on human bones found in riverine environment. *Forensic Science International*, **228**: e1–e5.

Desrosiers, N.A., Watterson, J.H., Dean, D. and Wyman, J.F. (2012) Detection of amitriptyline, citalopram and metabolites in porcine bones following extended outdoor exposure. *Journal of Forensic Sciences*, **57**: 544–549.

Dettmeyer, R.B., Verhoff, M.A. and Schütz, H.F. (2014) *Forensic Medicine: Fundamentals and perspectives*. Springer: Heidelberg.

Drummer, O.H (2004) Postmortem toxicology of drugs of abuse. *Forensic Science International*, **142**: 101–113.

Drummer, O.H. (2008) Drugs in bone and bone marrow. In: Jenkins, A.J. (ed.), *Drug Testing in Alternate Biological Specimens*. Humana Press: New Jersey, pp. 131–137.

Drummer, O.H. (2013) Post-mortem toxicology in the elderly. *Forensic Science Medicine and Pathology*, **9**: 258–259.

Drummer, O.H. and Gerostamoulos, J. (2002) Postmortem drug analysis: analytical and toxicological aspects. *Therapeutic Drug Monitoring*, **24**: 199–209.

Engelhart, D.A. and Jenkins, A.J. (2002) Detection of cocaine analytes and opiates in nails from postmortem cases. *Journal of Analytical Toxicology*, **26**: 489–492.

Engelhart, D.A., Lavins, E.S. and Sutheimer, C.A. (1998) Detection of drugs of abuse in nails. *Journal of Analytical Toxicology*, **22**: 314–318.

Ferner, R.E. (2008) Post-mortem clinical pharmacology. *British Journal of Clinical Pharmacology*, **66**: 430–443.

Findlay, A.B. (1976) Bone marrow changes in the post-mortem interval. *Journal of the Forensic Science Society*, **16**: 213–218.

Flanagan, R.J. and Connally, G. (2005) Interpretation of analytical toxicology results in life and at post mortem. *Toxicological Reviews*, **24**: 5–62.

Fleckman, P. (1985) Anatomy and physiology of the nail. *Clinics in Dermatology*, **3**: 373–381.

Garside, D., Ropero-Miller, J.D., Goldberger, B.A., Hamilton, W.F. and Maples, W.R. (1998) Identification of cocaine analytes in fingernail and toenail specimens. *Journal of Forensic Science*, **43**: 974–979.

Garside, D. (2008) Drugs-of-abuse in nails. In: Jenkins, A.J. (ed.), *Drug Testing in Alternate Biological Specimens*. Humana Press: New Jersey, pp. 43–65.

Giusiani, M., Chericoni, S. and Domenici, R. (2012) Identification and quantification of phenobarbital in a mummified body 10 years after death. *Journal of Forensic Sciences*, **57**: 1384–1387.

Grellner, W. and Glenewinkel, F. (1997) Exhumations: synopsis of morphological findings in relation to post-mortem interval. Survey on a 20-year period and review of the literature. *Forensic Science International*, **90**: 139–159.

Gruszecki, A.C., Booth, J. and Davis, G.G. (2007) The predictive value of history and scene investigation for toxicology results in a medical examiner population. *The American Journal of Forensic Medicine and Pathology*, **28**: 103–106.

Henderson, G.L. (1993) Mechanism of drug incorporation into hair. *Forensic Science International*, **63**: 19–29.

Henderson, G.L., Harkey, M.R. and Zhou, C. (1998) Incorporation of isotopically labelled cocaine into human hair: race as a factor. *Journal of Analytical Toxicology*, **22**: 156–165.

Jenkins, A.J. (2007) Pharmacokinetics: basic concepts and models. In: Karch, S.B. (ed.), *Pharmacokinetics and Pharmacodynamics of Abused Drugs*. CRC Press: Boca Raton, pp. 1–14.

Jenkins, A.J. and Lavins, E.S. (1998) 6-Acetylmorphine detection in postmortem cerebrospinal fluid. *Journal of Analytical Toxicology*, **22**: 173–175.

Jones, G. (2011) Postmortem toxicology. In: Moffat, A.C., Osselton, M.D., Widdop, B. and Watts, J. (eds), *Clarke's Analysis of Drugs and Poisons*. Pharmaceutical Press: London, pp. 176–189.

Jurado, C., Kintz, P., Menéndez, M. and Repetto, M. (1997) Influence of the cosmetic treatment of hair on drug testing. *International Journal of Legal Medicine*, **110**: 159–163.

Käferstein, H., Madea, .B, Sticht, G. and Sachs, H. (1994) Toxicological findings after several years of burial. *Acta Medicinae Legalis*, **44**: 439–442.

Kalasinsky, K.S., Dixon, M.M., Schmunk, G.A. and Kish, S.J. (2001) Blood, brain and hair GHB concentrations following fatal ingestion. *Journal of Forensic Sciences*, **46**: 728–730.

Karch, S.B. (2001) Alternate strategies for post-mortem drug testing. *Journal of Analytical Toxicology*, **25**: 393–395.

Karch, S.B. (2007) When the simple becomes complex – problems in post-mortem toxicology. *Journal of Toxicology. Clinical Toxicology*, **45**: 335.

Karch, S.B. (2008a) *Pharmacokinetics and Pharmocodynamics of Abused Drugs*. CRC Press: Boca Raton.

Karch, S.B. (2008b) *Post-mortem Toxicology of Abused Drugs*. CRC Press: Boca Raton.
Karch, S.B. (2013) Post-mortem toxicology in the elderly. *Forensic Science Medicine and Pathology*, **9**: 256–257.
Kennedy, M.C. (2010) Post-mortem drug concentrations. *Internal Medicine Journal*, **40**: 183–187.
Kintz, P. (2004) Value of hair analysis in post-mortem toxicology. *Forensic Science International*, **142**: 127–134.
Kintz, P. (2008) Drug testing in hair. In: Jenkins, A.J. (ed.), *Drug Testing in Alternate Biological Specimens*. Humana Press: New Jersey, pp. 67–81.
Kintz, P. (2012) Segmental hair analysis can demonstrate external contamination in post-mortem cases. *Forensic Science International*, **215**: 73–76.
Kintz, P. (2014) *Toxicological Aspects of Drug-Facilitated Crimes*. Academic Press: Waltham and San Diego.
Koch, S.L., Michaud, A.L. and Mikell, C.E. (2013) Taphonomy of hair – a study of postmortem root banding. *Journal of Forensic Sciences*, **58**: S52–S59.
Lafrenière, N.M. and Watterson, J.H. (2009) Detection of acute fentanyl exposure in fresh and decomposed skeletal tissues. *Forensic Science International*, **185**: 100–106.
Lafrenière, N.M. and Watterson, J.H. (2010). Detection of acute fentanyl exposure in fresh and decomposed skeletal tissues. Part II: The effect of dose-death interval. *Forensic Science International*, **194**: 60–66.
Langford, A.M., Taylor, K.K. and Pounder, D.J. (1998) Drug concentrations in selected skeletal muscles. *Journal of Forensic Sciences*. **43**: 22–27.
Lee, S., Cordero, R. and Paterson, S. (2009) Distribution of 6-monoacetylmorphine and morphine in head and pubic hair from heroin-related deaths. *Forensic Science International*, **183**: 7–77.
Leikin, J.B. and Watson, W.A. (2003) Post-mortem toxicology: what the dead can and cannot tell us. *Journal of Toxicology: Clinical Toxicology*, **41**: 47–56.
Maeda, H., Zhu, B.-L., Ishikawa, T., Oritani, S., Michiue, T. *et al.* (2006) Evaluation of post-mortem ethanol concentrations in pericardial fluid and bone marrow aspirate. *Forensic Science International*, **161**: 141–143.
McGrath, K.K. and Jenkins, A.J. (2009) Detection of drugs of forensic importance in postmortem bone. *American Journal of Forensic Medicine and Pathology*, **30**: 40–44.
McGrath, K.K. and Jenkins, A.J. (2009) Detection of drugs of importance in post-mortem bone. *The American Journal of Forensic Medicine and Pathology*, **30**: 40–44.
McIntyre, I.M., King, C.V., Boratto, M. and Drummer, O.H. (2000) Post-mortem drug analyses in bone and bone marrow. *Therapeutic Drug Monitoring*, **22**: 79–83.
Milroy, C.M. and Forrest, A.R.W. (2000) Methadone deaths: a toxicological analysis. *Journal of Clinical Pathology*, **53**: 277–281.
Muβhoff, F. and Madea, B. (2001) Fatality due to ingestion of tramadol alone. *Forensic Science International*, **116**: 197–199.
Muβhoff, F., Padosch, S., Steinborn, S. and Madea, B. (2004) Fatal blood and tissue concentrations of more than 200 drugs. *Forensic Science International*, **142**: 161–210.
Muβhoff, F., Driever, F., Lachenmeier, K., Lachenmeier, D.W., Banger, M. and Madea, B. (2006) Results of hair analyses for drugs of abuse and comparison with self-reports and urine tests. *Forensic Science International*, **156**: 118–123.
Muβhoff, F, and Madea, B. (2007) Analytical pitfalls in hair testing. *Analytical and Bioanalytical Chemistry*, **338**: 1475–1494.
Nishiyori, A., Sakata, R. and Fukuda, K. (2002) Single-strand conformation polymorphism analysis for alcohol dehydrogenase 2 (ADH2) genotyping using nail clippings. *Clinical Chemistry*, **48**: 563–564.

Palmeri, A., Pichini, S., Pacifici, R., Zuccaro, P. and Lopez, A. (2000) Drugs in nails: physiology, pharmacokinetics and forensic toxicology. *Clinical Pharmacokinetics*, **38**: 95–110.

Pepin, G. and Gaillard, Y. (1997) Concordance between self-reported drug use and findings in hair about cocaine and heroin. *Forensic Science International*, **84**: 37–41.

Peters, F.T. (2007) Stability of analytes in biosamples – an important issue in clinical and forensic toxicology? *Analytical and Bioanalytical Chemistry*, **388**: 1505–1519.

Pirl, J.N., Townsend, G.F., Valaitis, A.K., Grohlich, D. and Spikes, J.J. (1983) Death by arsenic: a comparative evaluation of exhumed body tissues in the presence of external contamination. *Journal of Analytical Toxicology*, **7**: 216–219.

Pounder, D.J. (2003) The case of Dr Shipman. *The American Journal of Forensic Medicine and Pathology*, **24**: 219–226.

Provan, D., Singer, C.R.J., Baglin, T. and Dokal, I. (2009) *Oxford Handbook of Clinical Haematology*. Oxford University Press: Oxford.

Rees, K.A. (2011) *The Distribution of Opiates, Cocaine and their Metabolites in Skeletal Muscle Tissue and Vitreous Humour as an Aid to Post-Mortem Toxicological Interpretation*. Unpublished PhD thesis, Bournemouth University: Bournemouth.

Robertson, M.D. and Drummer, O.H. (1995) Post-mortem drug metabolism by bacteria. *Journal of Forensic Science*, **40**: 382–386.

Roll, P., Beham, A. and Beham-Schmid, C. (2009) Post-mortem histological investigations of bone marrow in forensic medicine: an important issue for both the forensic and clinical pathologist. *Forensic Science International*, **186**: e17–e20.

Ropero-Miller, J.D., Goldberger, B.A., Cone, E.J. and Joseph, R.E. (2000) The disposition of cocaine and opiate analytes in hair and fingernails of humans following cocaine and codeine administration. *Journal of Analytical Toxicology*, **24**: 496–508.

Rowland, M. and Tozer, T.N. (2011) *Clinical Pharmacokinetics and Pharmacodynamics: Concepts and Applications*. Lippincott Williams & Wilkins: Baltimore.

Saitoh, M., Uzaka, M., Sakamoto, M. and Kobori, T. (1969) Rate of hair growth. In: Montagna, W. (ed.), *Advances in Biology of Skin: Hair growth*. Appleton-Century-Crofts: Oxford, pp. 183–194.

Satoh, T., Taylor, P., Bosron, W.F., Sanghani, S.P., Hosokawa, M. and La Du, B.N. (2002) Current progress on esterases: from molecular structure to function. *Drug Metabolism and Disposition*, **30**: 488–493.

Scheidweiler, K.B., Cone, E.J., Moolchan, E.T. and Huestis, M.A. (2005) Dose-related distribution of codeine, cocaine, and metabolites into human hair following controlled oral codeine and subcutaneous cocaine administration. *The Journal of Pharmacology and Experimental Therapeutics*, **313**: 909–915.

Schloegl, H., Rost, T., Schmidt, W., Wurst, F.M. and Weinmann, W. (2006) Distribution of ethyl glucuronide in rib bone marrow, other tissues and body liquids as proof of alcohol consumption before death. *Forensic Science International*, **156**: 213–218.

Scott, K.S. (2009) The use of hair as a toxicological tool in DFC casework. *Science and Justice*, **49**: 250–253.

Scott, K.S. and Oliver, J.S. (2001) The use of vitreous humour as an alternative to whole blood for the analysis of benzodiazepines. *Journal of Forensic Sciences*, **46**: 694–697.

Shen, M., Chen, H. and Xiang, P. (2014) Determination of opiates in human fingernail – comparison to hair. *Journal of Chromatography B*, **967**: 84–89.

Sierra-Callejas, J.L. and Pribilla, O. (1978) Exhumierung bei Verdacht auf Vergiftung – Retikulumzellsarkom. *Zeitschrift für Rechtsmedizin*, **81**: 335–340.

Sims, D.N., Lokan, R.J., James, R.A., Felgate, P.D., Felgate, H.E. *et al.* (1999) Putrefactive pleural effusions as an alternative sample for drug quantification. *The American Journal of Forensic Medicine and Pathology*, **20**: 343–346.

Skopp, G. (2004) Preanalytic aspects in post-mortem toxicology. *Forensic Science International*, **142**: 75–100.

Skopp. G. and Pötsch, L. (1997) A case report on drug screening of nail clippings to detect prenatal drug exposure. *Therapeutic Drug Monitoring*, **19**: 386–389.

Suzuki, O., Hattori, H. and Asano, M. (1984) Nails as useful materials for detection of methamphetamine or amphetamine abuse. *Forensic Science International*, **24**: 9–16.

Suzuki, S., Inoue, T., Hori, H. and Inayama, S. (1989) Analysis of methamphetamine in hair, nail, sweat, and saliva by mass fragmentography. *Journal of Analytical Toxicology*, **13**: 176–178.

Tattoli, L., Tsokos, M., Sautter, J., Anagnostopoulos, J., Maselli, E., Ingravallo, G. *et al.* (2014) Postmortem bone marrow analysis in forensic science: Study of 73 cases and review of the literature. *Forensic Science International*, **234**: 72–78.

Tominaga, M., Michiue, T., Ishikawa, T., Kawamoto, O., Oritani, S. *et al.* (2013) Postmortem analysis of drugs in pericardial fluid and bone marrow aspirate. *Journal of Analytical Toxicology*, **37**: 423–429.

Tosti, A., Baran, R. and Dawber, R.P.R. (2002) The nail in systemic disease and drug-induced changes. In: Baran, R., Dawber, R.P.R., de Berker, D.A., Haneke, E. and Tosti, A. (eds), *Baran and Dawber's Diseases of the Nails and their Management*. Blackwell Science Ltd: Oxford, pp. 223–329.

Trestrail III, J.H. (2007) *Criminal Poisoning*. Humana Press: New Jersey.

Tsatsakis, A.M., Tzatzarakis, M.N., Psaroulis, D., Levkidis, C. and Michalodimitrakis, M. (2001) Evaluation of the addiction history of a dead woman after exhumation and sectional hair testing. *The American Journal of Forensic Medicine and Pathology*, **22**: 73–77.

van Doorn, N.L., Wilson, A.S., Willerslev, E. and Gilbert, M.T.P. (2011) Bone marrow and bone as a source for postmortem RNA. *Journal of Forensic Sciences*, **56**: 720–725.

Vardakou, I., Athanaselis, S., Pistos, C., Papadodima. S., Spiliopoulou, C. and Moraitis, K. (2014) The clavicle as an alternative matrix in forensic toxicological analysis. *Journal of Forensic and Legal Medicine*, **22**: 7–9.

Wada, M. and Nakashima, K. (2006) Hair analysis: an excellent tool for confirmation of drug abuse. *Analytical and Bioanalytical Chemistry*, **385**: 413–415.

Watterson, J. (2006) Challenges in forensic toxicology of skeletonized human remains. *Analyst*, **131**: 961–965.

Watterson, J.H. and Botman, J.E. (2009) Detection of acute diazepam exposure in bone and bone marrow: influence of tissue type and the dose-death interval on sensitivity of detection by ELISA with liquid chromatography tandem mass spectrometry confirmation. *Journal of Forensic Sciences*, **54**: 708–714.

Watterson, J.H. and Cornthwaite, H.M. (2013) Discrimination between patterns of drug exposure by toxicological analysis of decomposed skeletal tissues. *Part II: amitriptyline and citalopram. Journal of Analytical Toxicology*, **37**: 565–572.

Watterson, J.H. and Desrosiers, N.D. (2011) Examination of the effect of dose-death interval on detection of meperidine exposure in decomposed skeletal tissues using microwave-assisted extraction. *Forensic Science International*, **207**: 40–45.

Watterson, J.H. and Donohue, J.P. (2011) Relative distribution of ketamine and norketamine in skeletal tissues following various periods of decomposition. *Journal of Analytical Toxicology*, **35**, 452–458.

Watterson, J.H., Desrosiers, N.A., Betit, C.C., Dean, D. and Wyman, J.F. (2010) Relative distribution of drugs in decomposed skeletal tissue. *Journal of Analytical Toxicology*, **34**: 510–515.

Watterson, J.H., Donohue, J.P. and Betit, C.C. (2012) Comparison of relative distribution of ketamine and norketamine in decomposed skeletal tissues following single and repeated exposures. *Journal of Analytical Toxicology*, **36**: 429–433.

Wennig, R. (2000a) Potential problems with the interpretation of hair analysis results. *Forensic Science International*, **107**: 5–12.

Wennig, R. (2000b) Threshold values in toxicology – useful or not? *Forensic Science International*, **113**: 323–330.

Wiebe, T.R. and Watterson, J.H. (2014) Analysis of tramadol and *O*-desmethyltramadol in decomposed skeletal tissues following acute and repeated tramadol exposure by gas chromatography and mass spectrometry. *Forensic Science International*, **242**: 261–265.

Wilson, A.S. (2008) The decomposition of hair in the buried body environment. In: Tibbet, M. and Carter, D.O. (eds), *Soil Analysis in Forensic Taphonomy: Chemical and biological effects of buried human remains*. CRC Press: Boca Raton, pp. 123–151.

Wilson, A.S., Brown, E.L., Villa, C., Lynnerup, N., Healey, A. *et al.* (2013). Archaeological, radiological, and biological evidence offer insight into Inca child sacrifice. *Proceedings of the National Academy of Sciences of the United States of America*, **110**: 13322–13327.

Worm, K., Steentoft, A. and Christensen, H. (1983) Experiences with exhumed material illustrated by a single case of morphine intoxication. *Journal of the Forensic Science Society*, **23**: 209–212.

21

Thermal Alteration to the Body

Tim J.U. Thompson, David Gonçalves, Kirsty Squires and Priscilla Ulguim

21.1 Introduction

There are few taphonomic processes that have as great and significant an effect on the body as burning. This highly transformative process can result in a broad range of changes to the soft and hard tissues, which in turn make recovery in the field and subsequent analysis extremely challenging. Within the archaeological and forensic contexts, it is not surprising that many view burned bone as being the most difficult of conditions to study – and as such, there are few researchers in the forensic or archaeological arenas who are working routinely with this material.

Specific terms used in relation to burned remains are discussed in more detail by Thompson (2009; 2015), but the key point is that while many terms are used interchangeably, they do have specific meanings. Thus 'burned remains' refers to remains that have been exposed to fire, 'cremated remains' refer to bodies that have been burned as part of a funerary process, and 'calcined remains' refer to those that have undergone alterations including calcination (thus suggesting an intense burning environment). These subtle differences in terms have important implications when describing the broader context of burning.

This chapter will explore the myriad ways in which heating and burning alters the human body, how these alterations influence our ability to successfully analyse the remains, and possible future directions for research and practice.

21.2 Soft Tissue Changes

Heating and burning have a dramatic effect on the whole body, but the soft tissues are particularly susceptible to damage. The source of the heat can have a great influence on the speed and extent of this damage. For example, a modern crematorium can reach temperatures of over 1,000°C with optimised air flow, whereas a fire in a garden may only reach 500°C and be more susceptible to local environmental weather. As the most external and superficial of the soft tissues, the skin will be affected first by fire. The exposure of the skin to heat causes the tissue to dehydrate, which results in shrinkage and splitting. This is problematic in the forensic context since this splitting may mimic non-heat related trauma, or may worsen peri-mortem damage. Splitting of the skin then speeds up the damage to the more internal structures. Hair and nails will also be damaged by the fire and melting (or 'clubbing') of these structures can occur. Following destruction of the skin, the muscles are exposed to the heat. As with the skin, the muscles experience shrinkage and contraction due to dehydration and ultimately will be physically destroyed by the heating.

Taphonomy of Human Remains: Forensic Analysis of the Dead and the Depositional Environment, First Edition.
Edited by Eline M.J. Schotsmans, Nicholas Márquez-Grant and Shari L. Forbes.

Before this point, the contraction of the muscles will result in the well-documented 'pugilistic attitude' position whereby the upper and lower limbs flex at the joints, presenting the body in a fighter's position (Symes *et al.* 2008). Historically this was used to determine that the individual was alive and struggling at the time of the fire, but has since been proven to be a result of dehydration and contraction of the muscles. The internal viscera will become directly exposed to the heat and fire once the skin and muscles have been destroyed. The heat will cause these organs to contract and they will also shrink in size. Note as well that heat will affect the body as a result of the fire, but also because of the heated air and gases that the victim will breathe into the body if still alive, thus damaging the respiratory system directly. Presence of this form of damage has been used to determine whether the victim was alive or dead during the fire event. When heating of the brain occurs, it is possible for bloodstains to be left on the internal surfaces of the cranial bones. This is referred to as a heat haematoma and can be misinterpreted as being the result of violence. Blood is also affected by heat. First, the proximity of the fire can cause the physical destruction of the blood cells. Second, the composition of the blood can be altered by the toxins breathed in by the victim. The classic example is with the build-up of carbon monoxide.

Note that the damage to the soft tissue will not occur uniformly across the body, but is rather determined by proximity to the heat source. Forensically this is useful since it allows for the fire scene to be reconstructed and body position to be determined relative to the fire through an analysis of thermal damage across the body (DeHaan 2008; Symes *et al.* 2008). Differences in proximity to the heat source are evident through the gradient of expression of heat-induced features, such as colour change and those discussed below.

While it is thought that the destruction to the soft tissues is relatively straightforward, heat-induced changes to the hard tissues are complicated and multifactorial. Nonetheless, a fuller understanding of these changes does allow one to comment confidently on the context of death or deposition.

21.3 Hard Tissue Changes

The changes to the hard tissues arguably have a greater impact on our ability to determine the identity of the deceased and the manner and context of death. Bone and teeth undergo four stages of transformation (Mayne Correira, 1997; Thompson 2004):

1) *Dehydration* occurs when the water is lost from the bone
2) *Decomposition* occurs when the organic material in the bone is lost
3) *Inversion* follows and marks the beginning of the changes in the inorganic component of the bone
4) *Fusion*, the final phase, occurs when the inorganic crystals start to coalesce and reorder

There is some debate as to the exact point at which these four stages will occur, and they are likely to alter as a result of a number of variables including temperature, duration of burning, oxygen supply, presence of clothing, etc. The *Fusion* stage has a considerable effect on our methods of osteoprofiling (constructing a biological identity) from the remains and this can occur in an average house fire setting (Thompson 2004).

In addition to these four general stages of transformation, there are a number of more specific heat-induced changes that occur in bone and can be linked strongly with the transformations detailed above. However, the two most significant of these phases are the second (*Decomposition*) and the fourth (*Fusion*). The loss of the organic material and the restructuring of the inorganic phase have been shown to be the precursor for the heat-induced changes that are routinely recorded on burned bone (Thompson 2005). These two changes have thus been labelled as *primary-level* heat-induced changes. All other heat-induced changes, such as changes to colour and the propagation of fractures are termed *secondary-level* changes, as they are the result of the *primary-level* changes (Thompson 2005, 2009).

While it may seem that these changes are so extensive that they preclude any deep understanding of a given set of burned human remains, this is not the case. The majority of information available to an anthropologist from unburned remains is also available from burned remains, but this requires greater effort and interpretation because of these overlapping changes.

21.3.1 Colour Change

Heat-induced colour change in bone and teeth is a macroscopic, secondary-level change resulting from chemical and physical alterations within the bone structure that occur progressively during heating (Thompson 2004). Colour data from forensic contexts enables the reconstruction of details of the combustion process through assessment of burn intensity and variability. As a highly visible indicator of heating, with regular stages, colour change has formed part of burned bone analysis since early studies (Baby 1954). Subsequent experimental research has provided a link between such colour change and primary-level changes in the bone structure (Bonucci and Graziani 1975; Shipman *et al.* 1984). However, interpretation is challenged by variables including other taphonomic processes, and the assessment of the variation of colour across surfaces (Mayne Correia 1997). Therefore, this approach requires a systematic and objective recording system, and is best employed in combination with other analytical methods (Devlin and Herrmann 2008; Sandholzer 2014; Shipman *et al.* 1984; Walker *et al.* 2008).

As bone is heated, increasing intensity and duration cause changes in the organic and inorganic phases of the bone structure and chemistry resulting in colour alterations from pale yellow through orange shades to brown, black, grey and then white (Bonucci and Graziani 1975; Devlin and Herrmann 2008; Ellingham *et al.* 2015; McCutcheon 1992; McKinley 2000; Munro *et al.* 2007; Nicholson 1993; Shipman *et al.* 1984; Thurman and Wilmore 1980; Ubelaker 1978) (Table 21.1). Similar changes have been recorded in tooth structures (Beach *et al.* 2008; Kharkanis *et al.* 2009; Sandholzer 2014; Sandholzer *et al.* 2014; Schmidt 2008). This colour change is mainly associated with the decomposition phase as organic content is reduced, while extended burning at higher temperatures usually results in white calcined bones indicating removal of organic matter and possible inversion and fusion in accordance with linked primary-level changes in bone (Ellingham *et al.* 2015; Thompson 2004). Equivalent colours may be attained through different temperature and duration combinations, meaning that colour is more useful for assessing intensity rather than specific temperatures (Duday 2009; Sandholzer 2014; Shipman *et al.* 1984). Such research has been successfully applied in anthropological and archaeological contexts, for example, Harvig *et al.* (2013) in part used colour to determine that bones in an Iron Age house were probably not heated within a pyre structure due to their interpretation of burn intensity. Other studies have used burn variation across articular surfaces to assess whether bones were burnt when articulated or disarticulated (Wolf 2011). Furthermore, colour evidence comprises an important indicator for the survival of organics for stable isotope and DNA analysis (Harbeck *et al.* 2011; Schwark *et al.* 2011; Walker *et al.* 2008).

Variables influencing colour change include exposure, duration, local environment, oxygen availability and fuel type and quantity. Fuel and oxygen availability imply differing combustion levels, heat release and flux rates (DeHaan 2002, 2008; Walker and Miller 2005; Walker *et al.* 2008). Meanwhile, exposure may be influenced by body position and condition, including the amount of soft tissue, blood and haemoglobin, marrow, fat and moisture which can protect bones and teeth and cause physical and chemical reactions during combustion (Binford 1963; DeHaan and Nurbakhsh 2001; Eckert *et al.* 1988; Schmidt 2008; Symes *et al.* 2008; Walker *et al.* 2008). In addition, colour may be altered

Table 21.1 Colour mapping of experimental colour data on burned bone with increasing temperature and primary level phase. Decomposition encompasses the change from yellow/brown to calcined white. 1: Dehydration, 2: Decomposition, 3: Inversion, 4: Fusion. YE: Yellow, BR: Brown, BL: Black, GR: Grey, WH: White.

	Shipman *et al.* 1984	Nicholson 1993	Munro *et al.* 2007	Walker *et al.* 2008	Phase (Thompson 2004)			
°C	Defleshed Animal Bone/Teeth	Defleshed Animal Bone	Defleshed Animal Bone	Fresh Defleshed Human Bone (Femur)	1	2	3	4
100					■			
150					■			
200	YE	BR	YE/BR	BR	■			
250	YE	BR			■			
300		BL	BR	BL	■	■		
350	BR				■	■		
400		GR	BL	BR/GR	■	■		
450	BR				■	■		
500		GR		BR/GR	■	■	■	
550	BL				■	■	■	
600		GR	GR/YE	GR	■	■	■	
650	WH					■	■	
700	WH	WH	WH/GR	GR		■	■	■
750	WH					■	■	■
800	WH	WH	WH	WH/GR		■	■	■
850	WH						■	■
900		WH	WH	WH			■	■
950	WH						■	■
1000				WH			■	■
1050							■	■
1100				WH			■	■

by other materials in the combustion environment, for example burning in proximity to metals may produce greens, yellows, pinks and reds (Dunlop 1978).

Bones may also be burnt or heated in natural or man-made fires prior to or following deposition; this could include cooking (Roberts *et al.* 2002; Subías 2002) or alteration of buried bone (Bennett 1999; Stiner *et al.* 1995). Bennett (1999) showed that subsurface colour change occurs in a similar fashion to surface burning, but that bone surface colour appears more uniform, most likely due to a more consistent exposure through the insulation, dispersal of the heat through the ground, and consistency of the burial medium.

Other activities can result in non-heat related bone colour change. In a recent archaeological study, microscopic analysis of black-coloured bones indicated that the colour resulted from treatment with bitumen, rather than heat-induced change, and this was interpreted as part of a funerary practice involving dismembering prior to burial (Argáez *et al.* 2011). Colour change similar to burning could apply if other substances are applied, for example ochre (hydrated iron oxide). In burial contexts, bone colour can also be altered by soil staining, pH level and the presence of trace elements (Oakley 1954; Shahack-Gross *et al.* 1997; Svenson and Wendel 1965). Finally, conservation may impact colour, including the application of consolidants such as paraloid or cyanoacrylate to prevent fragmentation of fragile elements. The liquid solution can cause darkening and reflective surface sheen or gloss, and if bones are insufficiently cleaned, any organic or inorganic materials on the bone surface will be fixed in place (Ulguim 2015).

The complexity and variation in bone surface colour change led Mayne Correia (1997) to question the value of any single bone colour in interpreting fire dynamics. However, colour data can be of value when detailed information on patterning across surfaces is collected. The transition of colours across elements represents a 'process signature' (Symes *et al.* 2008), which can be used to reconstruct past events. In order to assess this complexity a robust, repeatable and objective method is required. Shipman *et al.* (1984) employed a standardised method for assessing bone colour, using manual comparison with the Munsell Soil Colour Chart, which has become a standard assessment method (Kharkanis *et al.*, 2009; McCutcheon 1992; Munro *et al.* 2007). Shipman *et al.* (1984) did note the limitations in human colour perception and objectivity, and although the Munsell system allows more systematic recording of colour, it is a system designed for soil colour analysis, and can only provide a subjective assessment which is influenced by material state and light conditions. Additionally, the non-continuous nature of the data does not allow for easy comparison (Wolf 2011). Researchers are now investigating the use of different colour models such as RGB (Red-Green-Blue) and CIE *L*a*B* (a model defined by CIE, the Commission Internationale de l'Eclairage, with values for L*: lightness, a*: red-green values, b*: yellow-blue values which locates colour on a three-dimensional axis), together with digitised recording methods such as flat-bed scanners, digital photography and spectrophotometers to reduce subjectivity and permit fine-grained and statistical analysis of colour change and surface variation (Devlin and Herrmann 2008; Ulguim 2015; Walker *et al.* 2008) (Table 21.2).

Devlin and Herrmann (2008) recorded colour in cremated human remains at the Walker-Noe archaeological site using CIE L* a* B*, with spectrophotometers to collect accurate colour data which could be analysed statistically. When combined with accurate fragment location and identification in a GIS system, this accounted for variation across surfaces (Devlin and Herrmann 2008). Cranial fragments exhibited the whitest colouring with elevated yellow levels, indicating increased intensity, while appendicular bone provided lower white levels. They also noted the effect of soil staining occurring in the depositional environment. Ulguim (2015) applied RGB analysis to cremated remains, in this case a computer program captured RGB colours from a minimum of three points on bone surfaces to provide more objective information about burn patterning. Walker *et al.* (2008) used a different approach, creating average RGB analysis for the scanned bone surfaces. Cluster analysis of burnt

Table 21.2 Some advantages and disadvantages of commonly used colour systems.

Colour Recording System	Advantages	Disadvantages	Application to Burnt Bones and Teeth
Munsell	• Systematic and Standardised	• Subjective • Cannot easily account for surface colour variation • Developed for soil colour analysis • Colour coding difficult for statistical manipulation	Shipman *et al.* 1984
RGB	• Systematic and Standardised • Objective • Quantifiable and easily comparable	• Requires post-processing digital photograph calibration and analysis or expensive equipment	Walker *et al.* 2008; Ulguim 2015
CIE L* a* B*	• Systematic and Standardised • Objective • Quantifiable, and easily comparable	• Requires expensive equipment	Devlin and Herrmann 2008; Sandholzer 2014

tooth surface colour has also been used to further support the premise that colour change is linked to exposure and duration of heating (Sandholzer 2014).

In cases where equipment is lacking, photography may be used as a proxy with data capture via computer, though lighting conditions must be controlled and consistent, and the use of colour palettes for post-processing calibration is essential. Colour change alone cannot provide a full reconstruction of the combustion of burned remains, but it can provide a wealth of data which may be used in conjunction with microscopic analytical techniques such as histomorphology, X-Ray Diffraction and Fourier Transform Infrared Spectroscopy among others. In summary, the use of quantifiable, digitised techniques for such analysis of burnt hard tissues holds further promise for the interpretation of burn conditions and variation.

21.3.2 Changes in Mass

As has been noted, heat is a very destructive agent leading in some cases to the pyrolysis of soft tissues, shrinkage or amputation of the extremities (Bohnert *et al.* 2001). Therefore, full body mass of a cadaver is not at all a useful individualisation feature in forensic cases. On the other hand, the mass of fully skeletonised burned remains may not always be completely devoid of value for bioanthropological assessments. Mass loss occurs due to the removal of water and organics during a burning event (Hiller *et al.* 2003; Thompson 2004). Natural post-mortem decomposition – which also involves dehydration and organic decay (Collins *et al.* 2002; Karr and Outram 2012) – may mimic this, so mass loss is not an exclusive heat-induced change. In cases where the identification of heated bone and teeth is uncertain, mass may help confirm that the remains are indeed burned. Since burning exposure often differentially affects a body (Bohnert *et al.* 1998), this may result in unnatural antimere differences, thus suggesting that a heat-related event occurred (Figure 21.1). Regrettably, complete preservation of both antimeres is not often found when dealing with burned skeletal remains, so this approach certainly has its limitations.

It has been demonstrated that skeletal mass loss varies greatly. It may reach between 30 and 60% (Enzo *et al.* 2007; Grupe and Hummel 1991; Hiller *et al.* 2003; Munro *et al.* 2007; Person 1996), depending on factors such as temperature and pre-burning condition of the skeletal remains (e.g.

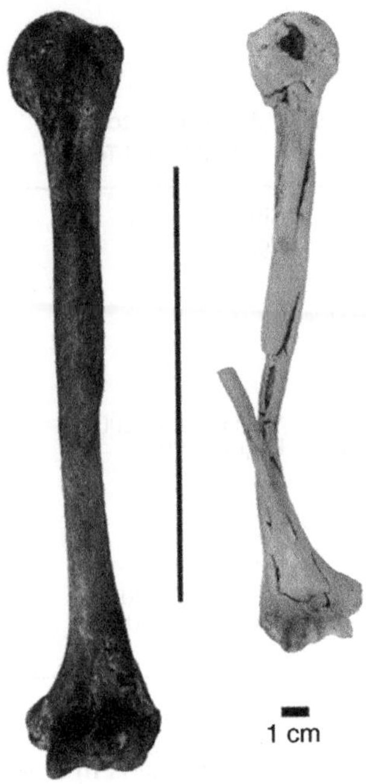

Figure 21.1 Left unburned humerus and right calcined humerus from individual 50 of the XXI Century Identified Collection of the University of Coimbra, subjected to controlled burning. The burned antimere presents substantial shrinkage and mass loss of 35.8%.

fresh vs. dry bones). Nonetheless, under specific circumstances, skeletal mass may still provide important insights (Gonçalves *et al.* 2015). The major advantage of the skeletal mass approach over other bioanthropological approaches – based on diagnostic features – is that it is not considerably affected by heat-induced fragmentation. Therefore, it can be used in addition to, or as an alternative to, more conventional and reliable methods which usually are more affected by fragmentation.

Studies based on modern crematoria can be used to devise reference data which then allows for skeletal mass to be used as a means of assessing the completeness of the remains or the minimum number of individuals from archaeological and forensic contexts (Gonçalves *et al.* 2015). Several of these references are available today (Bass and Jantz 2004; Chirachariyavej *et al.* 2006; Gonçalves *et al.* 2013a; Malinowski and Porawski 1969; May 2011; McKinley 1993; Van Deest *et al.* 2011; Warren and Maples 1997). In brief, very small masses are suggestive of incomplete remains, while very large masses are indicative of assemblages containing more than one individual (Duday *et al.* 2000; Gonçalves *et al.* 2015). Another potential use proposed for skeletal mass refers to sex estimation, since it is clearly sexually dimorphic (e.g. Malinowski and Porawski 1969; Van Deest *et al.* 2011). However, the application of this approach to sex estimation requires that burned skeletal remains are assuredly complete, belong to only one individual and are uniformly calcined, something that is often not the case in both forensic and archaeological contexts. Another potential of skeletal mass refers to the detection of preferential selection of specific anatomical parts for subsequent burial. Intentional behaviour can be detected by looking at general trends on the recovery of skeletal elements from the pyre and several methods have been proposed (Duday *et al.* 2000; Gonçalves *et al.* 2015; Lenorzer 2006; Richier 2005).

Although useful in some cases, skeletal mass analyses clearly have their own limitations. For instance, references refer only to calcined modern adult individuals (often quite aged) that were cremated in gas-fuelled retorts, so comparison with assemblages presenting other characteristics, such as non-calcined or non-adult remains, is problematic. Also, regional differences in skeletal mass have often been reported previously, so the selection of references is not straightforward, especially when dealing with archaeological populations (e.g. Bass and Jantz 2004; Gonçalves *et al.* 2013a). In addition, the mass of burned skeletal remains may be inflated by non-human aggregated materials and may be scattered or commingled, thus complicating or even precluding any comparative analysis (Kennedy 1996; Warren 2008).

It should also be noted that the dehydration and loss of the organic component which impacts on mass also results in the propagation of fractures. Traditionally, it has been argued that the presence of the soft tissues impacts the nature of the heat-induced fracture pattern. Thus fleshed bones exhibited U-shaped fractures running up the long-axis of the bone, while dry bone displayed rectangular grid-like fracture patters (Thompson 2009). More recent work has questioned the absoluteness of this principle, and argued that it is the presence of collagen within the bone, rather than the outer soft tissues *per se*, that may be more significant (Gonçalves *et al.* 2011; Thompson 2015). While the presence of fractures (and the resulting fragmentation) can impede the creation of a biological profile, it does not prevent it. Further work has demonstrated that it is entirely possible to differentiate heat-induced fracturing from that caused by peri-mortem violence (Fairgrieve 2008).

21.3.3 Dimensional Changes

Over the years, dimensional change has been one of the most researched heat-induced changes. That is probably because it is a major nuisance to bioanthropology, almost certainly being the most problematic heat-induced obstacle to the application of metric methods (such as those used for age and sex estimation). Although this phenomenon is not as troublesome when dealing with pre-calcined remains (Bradtmiller and Buikstra 1984; Gonçalves 2012; Thompson 2005), its impact on calcined bones and teeth cannot be overlooked.

Dimensional changes, both in the form of shrinkage and expansion, are due to several processes. They are partly caused by dehydration and the removal of the organic component of bones and teeth, but major changes occur only during the fusion stage of heat-induced skeletal transformation when pores previously filled by water and organic material are refilled as a result of the coalescence of the inorganic phase (Thompson 2005). Therefore, all these processes are expected to lead to shrinkage but, somewhat surprisingly and yet inexplicably, bone expansion has also been documented (Gonçalves 2012; Thompson 2005). This further complicates the application of metric methods, which are often used for the assessment of the biological profile. In summary, dimensional bone changes have been documented to vary between a 3.9% expansion and a 37.7% shrinkage (Bradtmiller and Buikstra 1984; Gonçalves 2012; Grupe and Herrmann 1983; Herrmann 1976; Holland 1989; Shipman *et al.* 1984; Strzalko and Piontek 1974; Thompson 2005). To date, the expansion events have been documented only in diaphyseal and epiphyseal dimensions of long bones and in tarsal bones (Gonçalves 2012; Thompson 2005). Sandholzer *et al.* (2013) observed that shrinkage ranged between 4.8% in teeth burned at 400°C and 32.5% in teeth burned at 800°C. Expansion has not yet been recorded for the dentition. Although the organic composition of teeth and bone is somewhat distinct, apparently this does not lead to considerable differences in heat-induced dimensional changes.

The potential of dimensional changes to aid in the identification of burned bone is quite narrow. It requires the presence of both antimeres to allow for a size comparison. If unnatural and significant bilateral asymmetry is present, this suggests that the skeletal remains were subjected to a burning event (Figure 21.1). However, it must be noted that other taphonomic agents can mimic heat-induced shrinkage. This is the case of post-depositional bone that gradually loses water and organic components (Piepenbrink 1986; Lynnerup 2010). In addition, trauma healed in a shortened position, due to overlapping of fractured ends, leads to unusual bilateral asymmetry. Also, pathological conditions such as *chondrodysplasia punctata* (Waldron 2009) or Ollier disease (Silve and Jüppner 2006) potentially result in the asymmetric shortening of bones.

Although the impact of dimensional changes on the applicability of metric methods is undeniable, their usefulness is not completely eradicated by heat exposure. In forensic contexts, bodies often display differential burning exposures and parts of the skeleton may not be severely affected by heat due to soft tissue insulation, thus making it possible to use conventional metric references on the skeletal elements. In cases where complete skeletalisation occurred and heat exposure clearly altered the size of bones and teeth – like those involving remains from archaeological contexts – other metric approaches must be used. For instance, a few comparative references have been compiled for sex estimation based on selected calcined remains that were heavily affected by shrinkage (Gonçalves *et al.* 2013b; Van Vark *et al.* 1996; Wahl 1996). Other procedures are based on the enlargement of the estimation intervals. For example, the interval for the age at death estimation of foetal burned remains must take into account heat-induced dimensional changes. Adapting the recommendations from Fairgrieve (2008), the bounds of that interval should be formed by:

1) the result of bone measuring taking the maximum heat-induced expansion into consideration (bone measurement*0.039 + bone measurement)
2) the result of bone measuring taking the maximum heat-induced shrinkage into consideration (bone measurement*0.377 + bone measurement)

21.3.4 Histological Changes

An essential aspect of analysing burned skeletal remains is an assessment of their macroscopic appearance. However, the study of histological changes that occur to heat-modified bone is equally as valuable. This form of analysis can provide useful information about burning conditions and their effect on skeletal material. Forbes (1941) was one of the first to recognise the value of conducting histomorphological (or thin-section) analysis on human burned bone. However, it was not until Herrmann (1977) conducted histomorphological analyses on archaeological material that this technique received the recognition that it deserved. Since then, the histological character of burned archaeological and modern bone has been examined as a means of understanding the microscopic changes that occur in bone as a result of burning processes (Bradtmiller and Buikstra 1984; Cattaneo *et al.* 1999; Fernández Castillo *et al.* 2013a, 2013b; Hanson and Cain 2007; Squires *et al.* 2011).

Histological changes of heat-modified skeletal remains are assessed by cutting thin-sections of bone and are subsequently examined under a microscope using plain polarised light and cross polarised light (Figures 21.2 and 21.3). There are many factors that can influence the histological changes to burned bone, such as the type of skeletal element, position of the body, temperature and duration of a fire. The microstructure of burned bone from archaeological and forensic contexts can be compared

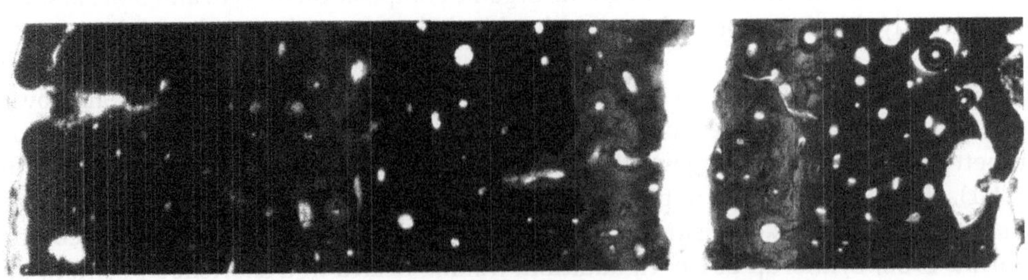

Figure 21.2 Histological detail of a cremated femur fragment from burial EL76NN (FN 549) from the Elsham (North Lincolnshire) cemetery seen under plane polarised light (Source: Reprinted with permission of North Lincolnshire Museum).

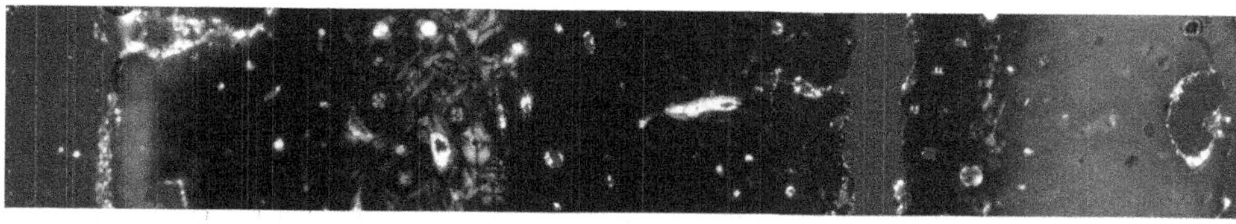

Figure 21.3 Histological detail of a cremated femur fragment from burial EL76NN (FN 549) from the Elsham (North Lincolnshire) cemetery seen under cross polarised light (Source : Reprinted with permission of North Lincolnshire Museum).

to experimental specimens, where temperature and conditions of burning are known, as a means of obtaining detailed information about burning environment (Squires 2015). It is widely recognised that increased temperatures and longer burning times result in bone with decreased organic content and increased fusion of inorganic bone mineral (hydroxyapatite), particularly when heated in excess of 700°C (Herrmann, 1977) – and although evident histologically, this technique is rarely employed by osteoarchaeologists and forensic anthropologists.

Shipman *et al.* (1984) noted that an examination of the histological changes to heat-modified bone is more accurate than relying on bone colour alone, although in most instances the colour of bone and its histological character correspond extremely well (Squires 2011). For example, white calcined bones with no microstructure and complete fusion of hydroxyapatite crystals indicates high intensity burning. However, there are instances where discrepancies occur. A good example of this was identified during the analysis of cremated human remains from the early Anglo-Saxon cemetery of Elsham (North Lincolnshire). Six out of 16 (38%) samples showed varying degrees of disagreement between the macroscopic appearance and the histological changes of cremated bone (Squires 2011). These observations all indicate that reducing conditions played a key role in the macroscopic appearance of bone fragments, whereas an examination of histological changes provided an insight into burning intensity. Therefore, when assessing burned skeletal remains, temperature, duration and oxidising conditions of a fire are of equal importance when considering the histological appearance of burned bone.

Unfortunately, the time-consuming nature of preparing thin-section samples often discourages the study of histological changes of burned bone (McKinley 1994). Sections of bone need to be extremely thin to identify key histological features through a microscope. Furthermore, heating bone results in dehydration and the loss of organic components, making bone more brittle and fragile. Consequently, cutting thin-sections is challenging, as samples frequently crumble during the initial stages of sample preparation. Therefore, the cortical bone of long bones should be employed when studying histological changes, owing to the more durable nature of these skeletal elements.

21.3.5 Crystalline and Elemental Changes

In addition to the visible changes that burning causes to bone, the microscopic structure will also be affected. Recent methodological advances (e.g. Thompson *et al.* 2011, 2013) have allowed researchers to study these changes and use them to discuss contexts of burning. Fundamentally, bone is a crystalline structure in the form of hydroxyapatite [$Ca_{10}(PO_4)_6(OH)_2$]. Since this structure has a large-surface area, it makes it very reactive. Researchers have long been aware of this feature, and understanding this allows one to comment on diagenetic change or stable isotopic variation. Crucially this structural change is predictable, although the duration of this change can vary. In living individuals, bone has a disordered structure comprised of small crystals with large strain. When bone is burned, this structure transforms into one with larger, better ordered crystals with a smaller strain between them. Note that this transformation is not a linear process, but rather occurs slowly at lower intensity burning and then increases as the intensity of burning increases. Crystalline changes will ultimately plateau at around 1,000°C.

Since this crystalline transformation is universal to all burning events, some bioarchaeologists attempted to correlate the degree of change with temperature of burning. Although there appears to be a solid correlation, the influence of uncontrolled and unknown variables on the nature of the burning event (i.e. oxygen availability, the presence of soft tissues, the use of accelerants, etc.) causes problems with the interpretation of results. Further complicating the widespread analysis and use of this correlation is the fact that different scientists use different methods or statistical techniques to examine this crystal change. One approach is to use X-ray Diffraction (XRD). This method allows one to examine the organisation of the crystal structure and has been used very successfully on burned bone (e.g. Enzo *et al.* 2007; Etok *et al.* 2007; Figueiredo *et al.* 2010; Rogers *et al.* 2010). Interestingly, some scientists have proposed that it is sensitive enough to speciate bone when burned (Beckett *et al.* 2011; Rogers *et al.* 2010; although also see Figueiredo *et al.* 2010 and Piga *et al.* 2013 for a counter argument). An alternative to the use of XRD is spectroscopy. Both Fourier transform infrared (FTIR) and Raman spectroscopy have been used to study burned bone, although the former is considerably more popular. Unlike XRD, spectroscopic methods examine the compounds that comprise the burned bone – which are a reflection of the crystal structure itself. In order to assess the degree of crystalline change using XRD or spectroscopy, it is necessary to use a statistical measure. One of the most discussed is the Crystallinity Index (CI), which is used with the FTIR spectrometer in particular. The traditional CI is defined as $CI = \{A_{565} + A_{605}\}/A_{595,}$ where A_x is the absorbance at given wavelength x. A baseline correction is usually applied between 750 and 450 cm^{-1} (Shemesh 1990; Thompson *et al.* 2011). Note that Thompson *et al.* (2013) recently suggested more appropriate calculations for assessing the degree of burning, while other scientists have used different equations to determine the same.

In the field, differences in heat-induced changes to crystallinity have been used in a variety of ways, such as to differentiate funerary practices, identify habitation sites and comment on pyre intensity (e.g. Butler and Dawson 2013; Piga *et al.* 2008; Schiegl *et al.* 2003; Squires *et al.* 2011). Generally these techniques seem to be most powerful when combined with other methods of analysis.

Burning has also been shown to alter the elemental composition of bone, and as with crystallinity changes described above, this is the result of the large highly-reactive surface area of bone microstructure. Despite some interest in the area (e.g. Grupe and Hummel 1991; Harbeck *et al.* 2011; Hummel *et al.* 1988), this remains the least well studied aspect of heat-induced change in bone – possibly because of the nature of the equipment and expertise required. Heat-induced changes in calcium, phosphorus, strontium, barium and lead have all been recorded, while changes in copper, zinc and magnesium seem to be independent of temperature (Grupe and Hummel 1991). Note that proportional changes in elements can also be the result of elemental uptake, but also the reduction in the organic phase (Grupe and Hummel 1991; Herrmann and Grupe 1988). Concentrations of elements have been used to determine whether bone has been burned or not, and in forensic contexts to state whether material presented to families from crematoria was actually bone (Brooks *et al.* 2006; Sillen and Hoering 1993). More recent work has focused on the impact of heating and burning on the results of radiocarbon and stable isotope analysis. With the former it has been shown that accurate dating is possible and that inter-laboratory accuracy is maintained with cremated bone (Olsen *et al.* 2007, 2013).

21.4 Conclusion and Future Research

Future work will need to address the problem of scattering and commingling in burned human skeletal remains, possibly following the work of Gonzalez-Rodriguez and Fowler (2013), who were able to discriminate the remains of several individuals using X-ray fluorescence and chemometric tools. Currently, bioarchaeologists and forensic anthropologists are quite powerless in doing this with cremated remains, therefore impacting on our methods of analysis (i.e. by limiting the range of our mass-related inferences). Another concern is related to method applicability. Current metric methods have large limitations. One reason for this is our inability to exactly assess the effect of heat-induced changes in a case-by-case basis. As a result, the selection of analytical methods can at times be ambiguous. Future research will necessarily have to address this question and eventually figure out a way of improving this important aspect of bioanthropological assessment of burned human skeletal remains. One means of addressing this is to combine methods, and refine the mapping between burn duration, intensity and the *primary-* and *secondary-level* heat-induced changes. This will enable more detailed investigation into the relative variation of bone change, which could indicate body position, tissue protection, combustion environment and exposure.

Overall the contribution of anthropologists, bioarchaeologists and forensic scientists to the study of burned and cremated human remains is increasing. Furthermore, the interpretations of these funerary and forensic contexts can be made with more confidence. This will continue as workers explore a greater range of burning contexts and practices.

References

Argáez, C., Batta, E., Mansilla, J., Pijoan, C. and Bosch, P. (2011) The origin of black pigmentation in a sample of Mexican prehispanic human bones. *Journal of Archaeological Science*, **38**: 2979–2988.

Baby, R. (1954) Hopewell cremation practices. *Papers in Archaeology, The Ohio Historical Society*, **1**: 1–7.

Bass, W.M. and Jantz, R.L. (2004) Cremation weights in East Tennessee. *Journal of Forensic Sciences*, **49**: 901–904.

Beach, J.J., Passalacqua, N.V. and Chapman, E.N. (2008) Heat-related changes in tooth color: temperature versus duration of exposure. In: Schmidt, C.W. and Symes, S.A. (eds), *The Analysis of Burned Human Remains*. Academic Press: London, pp. 137–144.

Beckett, S., Rogers, K.D. and Clement, J.G. (2011) Inter-species variation in bone mineral behaviour upon hearing. *Journal of Forensic Sciences*, **56**: 571–579.

Bennett, B.L. (1999) Thermal alteration of buried bone. *Journal of Archaeological Science*, **26**: 1–8.

Binford, L.R. (1963) An analysis of cremations from three Michigan sites. *Wisconsin Archaeologist*, **44**: 98–110.

Bohnert, M., Rost, T. and Pollak, S. (1998) The degree of destruction of human bodies in relation to the duration of the fire. *Forensic Science International*, **95**: 11–21.

Bohnert, M., Schmidt, U., Perdekamp, M.G. and Pollak, S. (2001) Extent of burn lesions: an analysis of 68 burned cadavers. *Archiv für Kriminologie*, **207**: 104–113.

Bonucci, E. and Graziani, G. (1975) Comparative thermogravimetric, X-ray diffraction and electron microscope investigations of burnt bones from recent, ancient, and prehistoric age. *Atti Memorie dell'Accademia Nazionale dei Lincei Scienze, Fisiche, Matematiche Naturali, Ser. 8 Sec. 2A*, **59**: 517–534.

Bradtmiller, B. and Buikstra, J.E. (1984) Effects of burning on human bone microstructure: a preliminary study. *Journal of Forensic Sciences*, **29**: 535–540.

Brooks, T.R., Bodkin, T.E., Potts, G.E. and Smullen, S.A. (2006) Elemental analysis of human cremains using ICP-OES to classify legitimate and contaminated cremains. *Journal of Forensic Sciences*, **51**: 967–973.

Butler, D.H. and Dawson, P.C. (2013) Accessing hunter-gatherer site structures using Fourier transform infrared spectroscopy: applications at a Taltheilei settlement in the Canadian Sub-Arctic. *Journal of Archaeological Science*, **40**: 731–1742.

Cattaneo, C., DiMartino, S., Scali, S., Craig, O.E., Grandi, M. and Sokol, R.J. (1999) Determining the human origin of fragments of burnt bone: a comparative study of histological, immunological and DNA techniques. *Forensic Science International*, **102**: 181–191.

Chirachariyavej, T., Amnueypol, C., Sanggarnjanavanich, S. and Tiensuwan, M. (2006) The relationship between bone and ash weight to age, body weight and body length of Thai adults after cremation. *Journal of the Medical Association of Thailand*, **89**: 1940–1945.

Collins, M.J., Nielsen-Marsh, C.M., Hiller, J., Smith, C.I., Roberts, J.P. *et al.* (2002) The survival of organic matter in bone: a review. *Archaeometry*, **44**: 383–394.

DeHaan, J.D. (2002) *Kirk's Fire Investigation*. Brady Publishing: New York.

DeHaan, J.D. (2008) Fire and bodies. In: Schmidt, C.W. and Symes, S.A. (eds), *The Analysis of Burned Human Remains*. Academic Press: London, pp. 1–16.

DeHaan, J.D. and Nurbakhsh, S. (2001) Sustained combustion of an animal carcass and its implications for the consumption of human bodies in fires. *Journal of Forensic Science*, **46**: 1076–1081.

Devlin, J.B. and Herrmann, N.P. (2008) Bone color as an interpretive tool of the depositional history of human cremains. In: Schmidt, C.W. and Symes, S.A. (eds), *The Analysis of Burned Human Remains*. Academic Press: London, pp. 109–128.

Duday, H. (2009) *The Archaeology of the dead: Lectures in archaeothanatology*. Oxbow Books: Oxford

Duday, H., Depierre, G. and Janin, T. (2000) Validation des paramètres de quantification, protocoles et stratégies dans l'étude anthropologique des sépultures secondaires à incinération. L'exemple des nécropoles protohistoriques du midi de la France. In : Dedet, B., Gruat, P., Marchand, G., Py, M. and Schwaller, M. (eds), *Archéologie de la mort, archéologie de la tombe au premier Âge du Fer*. AFEAF: Lattes, pp. 7–29.

Dunlop, J.M. (1978) Traffic light discolouration in cremated bones. *Medicine, Science and The Law*, **18**: 163–173.

Eckert, W.G., James, S. and Katchis, S. (1988) Investigation of cremations and severely burned bodies. *American Journal of Forensic Medicine and Pathology*, **9**: 188–200.

Ellingham, S.T.D., Thompson, T.J.U., Islam, M. and Taylor, G. (2015) Estimating temperature exposure of burnt bone – A methodological review. *Science and Justice*, **55**: 181–188.

Enzo, S., Bazzoni, M., Mazzarello, V., Piga, G., Bandiera, P. and Melis, P. (2007) A study by thermal treatment and X-ray powder diffraction on burnt fragmented bones from tombs II, IV and IX belonging to the hypogeic necropolis of 'Sa Figu' near Ittiri, Sassari (Sardinia, Italy). *Journal of Archaeological Science*, **34**: 1731–1737.

Etok, S.E., Valsami-Jones, E., Wess, T.J., Hiller, J.C., Maxwell, C.A. *et al.* (2007) Structural and chemical changes of thermally treated bone apatite. *Journal of Material Science*, **42**: 9807–9816.

Fairgrieve S (2008) *Forensic Cremation: Recovery and analysis.* CRC Press: Boca Raton.

Fernández Castillo, R., Ubelaker, D.H., Acosta, J.A.L. and de la Fuente, G.A.C. (2013a) Effects of temperature on bone tissue. Histological study of the changes in the bone matrix. *Forensic Science International*, **226**: 33–37.

Fernández Castillo, R., Ubelaker, D.H., Acosta, J.A.L., de la Rosa, R.J.E. and Garcia, I.G. (2013b) Effect of temperature on bone tissue: histological changes. *Journal of Forensic Sciences*, **58**: 578–582.

Figueiredo, M., Fernando, A., Martins, G., Freitas, J., Judas, F. and Figueiredo, H. (2010) Effect of the calcination temperature on the composition and microstructure of hydroxyapatite derived from human and animal bone. *Ceramics International*, **36**: 2383–2393.

Forbes, G. (1941) The effects of heat on the histological structure of bone. *Police Journal*, **14**: 50–60.

Gonçalves, D. (2012) *Cremains: The value of quantitative analysis for the bioanthropological research of burned human skeletal remains.* Unpublished PhD thesis. University of Coimbra: Coimbra.
Gonçalves, D., Campanacho, V., Thompson, T.J.U., Cunha, E. and Mataloto, R. (2015) The weight of the matter: examining the potential of skeletal weight for the bioarchaeological analysis of cremation at the Iron Age necropolis of Tera (Portugal). In: Thompson, T.J.U. (ed.), *The Archaeology of Cremation: Burned human remains in funerary studies.* Oxbow Books: Oxford, pp. 63–96.
Gonçalves, D., Thompson, T.J.U. and Cunha, E. (2011) Implications of heat-induced changes in bone on the interpretation of funerary behaviour and practice. *Journal of Archaeological Science*, **38**: 1308–1313.
Gonçalves, D., Cunha, E. and Thompson, T.J.U. (2013a) Weight references for burned human skeletal remains from Portuguese samples. *Journal of Forensic Sciences*, **58**: 1134–1140.
Gonçalves, D., Thompson, T.J.U. and Cunha, E. (2013b) Osteometric sex determination of burned human skeletal remains. *Journal of Forensic and Legal Medicine*, **20**: 906–911.
Gonzalez-Rodriguez, J. and Fowler, G. (2013) A study on the discrimination of human skeletons using X-ray fluorescence and chemometric tools in chemical anthropology. *Forensic Science International*, **231**: 407.e401–406.
Grupe, G. and Herrmann, B. (1983) Über das schrumpfungsverhalten experimentell verbrannter spongiöser knochen am beispiel des caput femoris. *Zeitschrift für Morphologie und Anthropologie*, **74**: 121–127.
Grupe, G. and Hummel, S. (1991) Trace element studies on experimentally cremated bone. I. Alteration of the chemical composition at high temperatures. *Journal of Archaeological Science*, **18**: 177–186.
Hanson, M. and Cain, C.R. (2007) Examining histology to identify burned bone. *Journal of Archaeological Science*, **34**: 1902–1913.
Harbeck, M., Schleuder, R., Schneider, J., Wiechmann, I., Schmahl, W.W. and Grupe, G. (2011) Research potential and limitations of trace analyses of cremated remains. *Forensic Science International*, **204**: 191–200.
Harvig, L., Kveiborg, J. and Lynnerup, N. (2013) Death in flames. human remains from a domestic house fire from Early Iron Age, Denmark. *International Journal of Osteoarchaeology*, **25**: 701–710.
Herrmann, B. (1976) Experimentelle und theoretische beiträge zur leichenbrand unter schung. *Homo*, **27**: 114–118.
Herrmann, B. (1977) On histological investigations of cremated human remains. *Journal of Human Evolution*, **6**: 101–103.
Herrmann, B. and Grupe, G. (1988) Trace element content in prehistoric cremated human remains. In: Grupe, G. and Herrmann, B. (eds), *Trace Elements in Environmental History.* Proceedings of the Symposium held 24–26 June 1987 at Göttingen. Springer-Verlag: Berlin, pp. 91–101.
Hiller, J.C., Thompson, T.J.U., Evison, M.P., Chamberlain, A.T. and Wess, T.J. (2003) Bone mineral change during experimental heating: an X-ray scattering investigation. *Biomaterials*, **24**: 5091–5097.
Holland, T.D. (1989) Use of the cranial base on the identification of fire victims. *Journal of Forensic Sciences*, **34**: 458–460.
Hummel, S., Schutkowski, H. and Herrmann, B. (1988) Advances in cremation research. *Actes des 3èmes Journées Anthropologiques*, **24**: 177–194.
Karr, L.P. and Outram, A.K. (2012) Bone degradation and environment: understanding, assessing and conducting archaeological experiments using modern animal bones. *International Journal of Osteoarchaeology*, **25**: 201–212.
Kennedy, K.A.R. (1996) The wrong urn: commingling of cremains in mortuary practices. *Journal of Forensic Sciences*, **41**: 689–692.
Kharkanis, S., Ball, J. and Franklin, D. (2009) macroscopic and microscopic changes in incinerated deciduous teeth. *Journal of Forensic Odontostomatology*, **27**: 9–19.

Lenorzer, S. (2006) *Pratiques funéraires du Bronze final IIIb au premier âge du Fer en Languedoc occidental et Midi-Pyrénées: Approche archéo-anthropologique des nécropoles à incinération.* Unpublished PhD thesis. University of Bordeaux: Bordeaux.

Lynnerup, N. (2010) Medical imaging of mummies and bog bodies, a mini-review. *Gerontology*, **56**: 441–448.

Malinowski, A. and Porawski, R. (1969) Identifikations Möglichkeiten menschlicher Brandknochen mit besonder Berücksichtigung ihres Gewichts. *Zacchia*, **5**: 1–19.

May, S.E. (2011) The effects of body mass on cremation weight. *Journal of Forensic Sciences*, **56**: 3–9.

Mayne Correira, P. (1997) Fire modification of bone: a review of the literature. In: Haglund, W.D. and Sorg, M.H. (eds), *Forensic Taphonomy: The postmortem fate of human remains.* CRC Press: Boca Raton, pp. 275–293.

McCutcheon, P.T. (1992) Burned archaeological bone. In: Stein, J.K. (ed.), *Deciphering a Shell Midden.* Academic Press: London, pp. 347–370.

McKinley, J.I. (1993) Bone fragment size and weights of bone from British cremations and the implications for the interpretation of archaeological cremations. *International Journal of Osteoarchaeology*, **3**: 283–287.

McKinley, J.I. (1994) The Anglo-Saxon Cemetery at Spong Hill, North Elmham. *Part VIII:* The cremations. East Anglian Archaeology Report 69, Norfolk Museums Service: Dereham.

McKinley, J.I. (2000) The analysis of cremated bone. In: Cox, M. and Mays, S. (eds), *Human Osteology: In archaeology and forensic science.* Cambridge University Press: Cambridge, pp. 403–421.

Munro, L.E., Longstaffe, F.J. and White, C.D. (2007) Burning and boiling of modern deer bone: effects on crystallinity and oxygen isotope composition of bioapatite phosphate. *Palaeogeography, Palaeoclimatology, Palaeoecology*, **249**: 90–102.

Nicholson, R.A. (1993) A morphological investigation of burnt animal bone and an evaluation of its utility in archaeology. *Journal of Archaeological Science*, **20**: 411–428.

Oakley, K. (1954) Evidence of fire in South African cave deposits. *Nature*, **174**: 261–262.

Olsen, J., Heinemeier, J., Bennike, P., Krause, C., Hornstrup, K.M. and Thrane, H. (2007) Characterisation and blind testing of radiocarbon dating of cremated bone. *Journal of Archaeological Science*, **35**: 791–800.

Olsen, J., Heinemeier, J., Hornstrup, K.M., Bennike, P. and Thrane, H. (2013) 'Old wood' effect in radiocarbon dating of prehistoric cremated bones? *Journal of Archaeological Science*, **40**: 30–34.

Person, A., Bocherens, H., Mariotti, A. and Renard, M. (1996) Diagenetic evolution and experimental heating of bone phosphate. *Palaeogeography, Palaeoclimatology, Palaeoecology*, **126**: 135–149.

Piepenbrink, H. (1986) Two examples of biogenous dead bone decomposition and their consequences for taphonomic interpretation. *Journal of Archaeological Science*, **13**: 417–430.

Piga, G., Guirguis, M., Bartoloni, P., Malgosa, A. and Enzo, S. (2008) A funerary rite study of the Phoenician-Punic necropolis of Mount Sirai (Sardinia, Italy). *International Journal of Osteoarchaeology*, **18**: 1–14.

Piga, G., Solinas, G., Thompson, T.J.U., Brunetti, A., Malgosa, A. and Enzo, S. (2013) Is X-ray diffraction able to distinguish between animal and human bones? *Journal of Archaeological Science*, **40**: 778–778.

Richier, A. (2005) Sépultures primaires à incineration: nouvelles données et nouvelles problématiques. In: *Mordant, C.* and Depierre, G. (eds), *Les pratiques funéraires à l'âge du bronze en France.* Comité des Travaux Historiques et Scientifiques: Paris, pp. 199–210.

Rogers, K.D., Beckett, S., Kuhn, S., Chamberlain, A. and Clement, J. (2010) Contrasting the crystallinity indicators of heated and diagenetically altered bone mineral. *Palaeogeography, Palaeoclimatology, Palaeoecology*, **296**: 125–129.

Roberts, S.J., Smith, C.I., Millard, A.R. and Collins, M.J. (2002) The taphonomy of cooked bone: characterizing boiling and its physico-chemical effects. *Archaeometry*, **44**: 485–494.

Sandholzer, M.A., Walmsley, A.D., Lumley, P.J. and Landini, G. (2013) Radiologic evaluation of heat-induced shrinkage and shape preservation of human teeth using micro-CT. *Journal of Forensic Radiology and Imaging*, **1**: 107–111.

Sandholzer, M.A. (2014) *Heat-induced Alterations of Dental Tissues.* Unpublished PhD Thesis. University of Birmingham: Birmingham.

Sandholzer, M.A., Baron, K., Heimel, P. and Metscher, B.D. (2014) Volume analysis of heat-induced cracks in human molars: A preliminary study. *Journal of Forensic Dental Science*, **6**: 139–44.

Schiegl, S., Goldberg, P., Pfretzschner, H.-U. and Conard, N.J. (2003) Paleolithic burnt bone horizons from the Swabian Jura: distinguishing between *in situ* fireplaces and dumping areas. *Geoarchaeology: An International Journal*, **18**: 541–565.

Schmidt, C.W. (2008) The recovery and study of burned human teeth. In: Schmidt, C.W. and Symes, S.A. (eds), *The Analysis of Burned Human Remain.* Academic Press: London, pp. 55–74.

Schwark, T., Heinrich, A., Preusse-Prange, A. and Von Wurmb-Schwark, N. (2011) Reliable genetic identification of burnt human remains. *Forensic Science International: Genetics*, **5**: 393–399.

Shahack-Gross, R., Bar-Yosef, O. and Weiner, S. (1997) Black-colored bones in Hayorim Cave, Israel: differentiating between burning and oxide staining. *Journal of Archaeological Science*, **24**: 439–446.

Shemesh, A. (1990) Crystallinity and diagenesis of sedimentary apatites. *Geochimica et Cosmochimica Acta*, **54**: 2433–2438.

Shipman, P., Foster, G. and Schoeninger, M. (1984) Burnt bones and teeth: an experimental study of colour, morphology, crystal structure and shrinkage. *Journal of Archaeological Science*, **11**: 307–325.

Sillen, A. and Hoering, T. (1993) Chemical characterization of burnt bones from Swartkrans. In: Brain, C.K. (ed.), *Swartkrans: a cave's chronicle of early man.* Transvaal Museum Monograph 8: Pretoria, pp. 243–249

Silve, C. and Jüppner, H. (2006) Ollier disease. *Orphanet Journal of Rare Diseases*, **1**: 37.

Squires, K.E. (2011) *An Osteological Analysis and Social Investigation of the Cremation Rite at the Cemeteries of Elsham and Cleatham, North Lincolnshire.* Unpublished PhD thesis. University of Sheffield: Sheffield.

Squires, K.E. (2015) The use of microscopic techniques in cremation studies: A new approach to understanding the social identity of cremation practicing groups from early Anglo-Saxon England. In: Thompson, T.J.U. (ed.), *The Archaeology of Cremation: Burned human remains in funerary studies.* Oxbow Books: Oxford.

Squires, K.E., Thompson, T.J.U., Islam, M. and Chamberlain, A. (2011) The application of histomorphometry and Fourier Transform Infrared Spectroscopy to the analysis of early Anglo-Saxon burned bone. *Journal of Archaeological Science*, **38**: 2399–2409.

Stiner, M.C., Kuhn, S.L., Weiner, S. and Bar-Yosef, O. (1995) Differential burning, recrystallization and fragmentation of archaeological bone. *Journal of Archaeological Science*, **22**: 223–237.

Strzalko, J. and Piontek, J. (1974) Wpływ spalania w warunkach zbliżonych do kremacji pradziejowych na morfologię kości. *Przegląd Antropologiczny*, **40**: 315–326.

Subías, S.M. (2002) Cooking in Zooarchaeology: Is this issue still raw? In: Miracle, P. and Milner, N. (eds), *Consuming Passions and Patterns of Consumption.* McDonald Institute of Archaeological Research: Cambridge, pp. 7–15.

Svensson, A. and Wendel, O. (1965) *The Techniques of Crime Scene Investigation*. New York: Elsevier.

Symes, S.A., Rainwater, C., Chapman, E., Gipson, D.R. and Piper, A. (2008) Patterned thermal destruction of human remains in a forensic setting. In: Schmidt, C.W. and Symes, S.A. (eds), *The Analysis of Burned Human Remains*. Academic Press: London, pp. 15–54.

Thompson, T.J.U. (2004) Recent advances in the study of burned bone and their implications for forensic anthropology. *Forensic Science International*, **146**: S203–S205.

Thompson, T.J.U. (2005) Heat-induced dimensional changes in bone and their consequences for forensic anthropology. *Journal of Forensic Sciences*, **50**: 185–193.
Thompson, T.J.U. (2009) Burned human remains. In: Blau, S. and Ubelaker, D. (eds), *Handbook of Forensic Anthropology and Archaeology*. Left Coast Press: Walnut Creek, pp. 295–303.
Thompson, T.J.U., Islam, M. and Bonniere, M. (2013) A new statistical approach for determining the crystallinity of heat-altered bone mineral from FTIR spectra. *Journal of Archaeological Science*, **40**: 416–422.
Thompson, T.J.U., Islam, M., Piduru, K. and Marcel, A. (2011) An investigation into the internal and external variables acting on Crystallinity Index using Fourier Transform Infrared Spectroscopy on unaltered and burned bone. *Palaeogeography, Palaeoclimatology, Palaeoecology*, **299**: 168–174.
Thompson, T.J.U. (2015) The Archaeology of Cremation: Burned human remains in funerary studies. *Studies in Funerary Archaeology Series*, Oxbow Press: Oxford.
Thurman, M. and Wilmore, L. (1980) A replicative cremation experiment. *North American Archaeologist*, **2**: 275–283.
Ubelaker, D. (1978) *Human Skeletal Remains: Excavation, analysis, interpretation*. Aldine: Chicago, IL.
Ulguim, P.F. (2015) Analysing cremated human remains from the southern Brazilian highlands: Interpreting archaeological evidence of funerary practice at mound and enclosure complexes in the Pelotas River Valley. In: Thompson, T.J.U. (ed.), *The Archaeology of Cremation: Burned human remains in funerary studies.* Oxbow Press: Oxford.
Van Deest, T.L., Murhad, T.A. and Bartelink, E.J .(2011) A re-examination of cremains weight: sex and age variation in a Northern Californian sample. *Journal of Forensic Sciences*, **56**: 344–349.
Van Vark, G.N. (1974) The investigation of human cremated skeletal material by multivariate statistical methods I. *Methodology. Ossa*, **1**: 63–95.
Van Vark, G.N., Amesz-Voorhoeve, W. and Cuijpers, A. (1996) Sex-diagnosis of human cremated skeletal material by means of mathematical-statistical and data-analytical methods. *Homo*, **47**: 305–338.
Wahl, J.K. (1996) Erfahrungen zur metrishen Geschlechtsdiagnose bei Leichenbränden. *Homo*, **47**: 339–359.
Waldron, T. (2009) *Palaeopathology*. Cambridge University Press: Cambridge
Walker, P.L. and Miller, K.W.P. (2005) Time, temperature, and oxygen availability: an experimental study of the effects of environmental conditions on the color and organic content of cremated bone. *American Journal of Physical Anthropology*, **40**: 222.
Walker, P.L., Miller, K.W.P. and Richman, R. (2008) Time, temperature, and oxygen availability: an experimental study of the effects of environmental conditions on the color and organic content of cremated bone. In: Schmidt, C.W. and Symes, S.A. (eds), *The Analysis of Burned Human Remains*. Academic Press: London, pp. 129–135.
Warren, M.W. (2008) Detection of commingling in cremated human remains. In: Adams, B.J. and Byrd, J.E. (eds), *Recovery, Analysis, and Identification of Commingled Human Remains*. Humana Press: Totowa, pp. 185–197.
Warren, M.W. and Maples, W.R. (1997) The anthropometry of contemporary commercial cremation. *Journal of Forensic Sciences*, **42**: 417–423.
Wolf, A. (2011) *Determining whether Spectrophotometer CIE L*a*b* Color Analysis is an Effective Alternative to Munsell Soil Color Charts for the Study Of Burnt Bones: Insights from analysis of Babedh-Dhra EB II-III Burnt Bone.* Unpublished Honours Thesis. Oberlin College: Oberlin.

22

Concealing the Crime: the Effects of Chemicals on Human Tissues

Eline M. J. Schotsmans and Wim Van de Voorde

22.1 Introduction

What is the best way to make a dead body disappear? This question is familiar to many forensic scientists. The internet and non-scientific literature provide a solution that triggers one's imagination: dissolving in acid. It is based on misconceptions and inspired by films and crime series such as 'Le Trio Infernal' (Girod 1974) or 'Breaking Bad' (Gilligan 2008–2013).

Perpetrators often try to conceal their crime by destroying evidence, hiding the corpse and hampering identification. Body disposal hinders (early) detection of the homicide, potentially destroys evidence and makes identification more difficult. Several methods and locations are used for this purpose. Most common are concealing the body or body parts in a cellar or attic, disposal in nature, burial, submerging in water or burning. Less common ways are encasing it in concrete, freezing it or (trying to) dissolve it in corrosives. The body disposal location and method of disposal depends on the motive, the offender's capabilities and experience, the crime site, the available means of transport, the victim–offender relationship, the offender's criminal sophistication level, the degree of planning, and the offender's knowledge of the body disposal site (Napier and Baker 2002).

A post-delictuous act that aims to facilitate transport or hide indications of homicide by hampering identification and concealing evidence, is called defensive mutilation[1] in forensic medicine. Attempts to hide the identity of a victim and prevent positive identification include dismemberment, decapitation, removal of fingers or teeth, disfigurement of the face, burning and dissolving the body in acid or alkaline substances (Aggrawal 2010; Rajs *et al.* 1998; Seidel and Fulginiti 2014). In cases of body disposal, the search and forensic investigation are challenging, dealing with decomposition, taphonomy, incomplete (dispersed) body (parts), difficult terrain, multiple crime scenes (crime site, transportation vehicle, deposition site), increased time lapse, loss of evidence, etc. In the case of a (presumably) dissolved body, the *corpus delicti* is missing, which makes the investigation even more difficult. Moreover, in forensic practice, experience with dissolved human remains is lacking, and knowledge is mostly anecdotal and not scientifically documented.

This chapter will focus on the effects of corrosive substances on human tissues and not by oral ingestion. Chemical injuries to the human gastrointestinal tract by ingested substances are described

1 Other subsets of mutilations are: aggressive mutilation, carried out as a result of a state of outrage that persists after the death of the victim; offensive mutilation resulting from the need to kill and carry out sexual urges, or by the need to inflict pain, injury or death while carrying out sexual urges; and necromantic mutilation, involving the severing or disfigurement of the face and genitalia of the victim, usually including the removal of body parts as trophies, symbols or for fetish reasons (Aggrawal 2010; Rajs *et al.* 1998; Seidel and Fulginiti 2014).

Taphonomy of Human Remains: Forensic Analysis of the Dead and the Depositional Environment, First Edition.
Edited by Eline M.J. Schotsmans, Nicholas Márquez-Grant and Shari L. Forbes.

in several case studies and forensic medicine and toxicology books (e.g. Byard 2015; Derelanko and Auletta 2014; Matshes *et al.* 2008; Vij 2009).

This contribution will provide definitions and case examples, followed by an overview of the existing experimental research. Finally, a serial killer case from Belgium is provided, which shows the importance of experimental research in a criminal investigation.

Because forensic cases of bodies exposed to caustic substances are infrequently reported in the forensic literature, and sometimes only briefly mentioned, not all reported cases are described in great detail.

22.2 Corrosive Substances: Definitions and History

According to the Material Safety Data Sheets (MSDS), a corrosive is a chemical that causes visible destruction of, or irreversible alterations in, living tissue by chemical action at the site of contact (www.msdsonline.com). The word 'corrosive' was first used in English in the 14th century and is derived from the Latin word 'corrodere' meaning to gnaw away (Chambers and Chambers 2008).

There are two types of corrosive materials: acids and alkalis. The acidity or alkalinity of a substance is specified by pH, a logarithmic measure of hydrogen ion concentrations expressed on a scale from 1 to 14. Solutions with a pH of less than 7 are acidic, solutions with a pH greater than 7 are alkaline or basic, while pH 7 is considered to be neutral (Burke 2013). The strength of an acid or a base is defined as the degree of ionisation of the acid or base in water. Substances with a pH of less than 2 are called strong acids and those with a pH greater than 12 are considered to be strong bases (Fire 2009).

The terminology of corrosive substances is not always consistently used or clearly defined. Technically, the correct terminology for an acid is 'corrosive' and for a base is 'caustic'. However, those words are often used as synonyms (Burke 2013). Moreover, the general public tend to use the term 'acid' inaccurately for all corrosives. MSDS and the US Department of Transportation (DOT) do not differentiate between the words corrosive and caustic. Following this, in this chapter the words corrosive and caustic are also used as synonyms.

Although chemistry as a science was only established after the 16th century, when the idea arose that changes of individual substances under the influence of heat, solvents or reagents could be considered as a subject of special study, chemistry has been preceded by many centuries of human activity and dates back to prehistoric times (Leicester 1956). Ancient authors such as Herodotus or Pliny the Elder described products, which have the nature of being acidic or basic. However, at that time they were not given these terms (Bailey 1932; Koller *et al.* 2005). In some texts, the effects of chemicals on dead bodies are mentioned. For example, in the 1st century AD, Pliny the Elder describes lime in his book 'Natural History'. Pliny explains the lime cycle and how to form hydrated lime from quicklime (called 'Calcis' or 'Calx'). Furthermore, he mentions applications of limestone, gypsum, plaster, chalk, slaked lime and quicklime with their use in medicine, agriculture, as building materials or cleaning products (Bailey 1932). Interestingly, in chapter XVII, Pliny describes the corrosive properties of lime and the effect of lime on dead bodies and grave goods:

> It is known that bodies of the dead, which are buried in coffins of this material, consume away within forty days, with the sole exception of the teeth. We know further that mirrors, body-scrapers, clothes and shoes, buried with the dead become petrified. … If fastened to the bodies, even of living men, it consumes the flesh (Bailey 1932).

Clearly, the misconception that lime accelerates decay started many years ago.

Once scientifically discovered and industrially manufactured, acids and bases were rapidly adapted into the areas of warfare and criminal attacks. In the 19th, 20th and 21st centuries, there are many examples of the application of these products in domestic or industrial accidents, as well as in personal attacks and warfare (Fire 2009; Josset and Hall 2014; Magnuson *et al.* 2012). Well known are the socially, politically or religiously motivated acid attacks in countries such as Bangladesh (Anwary 2003; Kumar Das *et al.* 2015; Mannan *et al.* 2004), Cambodia (Waldron *et al.* 2014), Colombia (Guerrero 2013), India (Kachan *et al.* 2015), Jamaica (Branday *et al.* 1996), Hong Kong (Young *et al.* 2002), Uganda (Asaria *et al.* 2004) and many other countries. The intention of this acid violence that is often pre-meditated, is to maim, disfigure, torture or kill (Mannan *et al.* 2007; Milton *et al.* 2010). Different to the acid attacks are criminal offences with corrosives in order to facilitate disappearance of the victim. Those offences are related to homicide and classified as defensive mutilation. They differ from chemical assault and from domestic and industrial chemical burns because it is driven by different motivations.

22.3 The Effect of Corrosive Substances on Human Tissues: Case Examples

The chemical substances that are most often used in forensic practice are described in this section. They are based on case examples, mostly derived from the media. Clearly, the number of forensic cases that mention the use of chemicals to conceal a crime is higher than the available scientific and experimental literature, described in the next section.

22.3.1 Acids

Acids are materials that release hydrogen ions (H^+) when placed in water. They present a long list of hazards in the literature on hazardous materials. They can be corrosive, explosive, water reactive, toxic, combustible, etc. There are inorganic and organic acids. Organic acids are combustible, while the inorganic acids will not burn. Inorganic acids are stronger than the organic acids at the same concentration. Furthermore, inorganic acids are more chemically reactive than organic acids (Fire 2009).

Inorganic acids can generally be identified by hydrogen at the beginning of the formula, because few other compounds begin with hydrogen (Burke 2013). A well-known inorganic acid is **sulphuric acid (H_2SO_4)**. It is one of the strongest acids known and, depending on the concentration, used in industry as a corrosive agent as well as a source of sulphates. Its corrosiveness destroys tissue, and vapours released from it are strong irritants. Moreover, it greatly damages many metals (Fire 2009). One of the most infamous historical cases of defensive mutilation with the application of sulphuric acid is the case of the Romanovs. After the execution of the Russian Tsar Nicholas II and his family in 1918, it was said that their bodies were buried and covered with acid. In 1991, the remains of Tsar Nicholas's family were exhumed and appeared to be skeletonised. The dental remains, skeletal remains and soil samples suggested exposure to a corrosive agent. Later, the offenders revealed that sulphuric acid was used to cover the identity of the Romanovs. The acid had not destroyed the DNA of bone and teeth, therefore identification was successful (Abramov *et al.* 2015; Aufderheide 2003; Jackson 2002; Maples and Browning 1994; Slater 2007).

Another case also dates back to the beginning of the 20th century. In April 1934, Georges Sarrejani, alias 'Sarret', was executed by guillotine in Aix-en-Provence (France). Together with his two mistresses, he killed several people for insurance money, and amongst those he dissolved two victims in sulphuric acid (Larue 2009). His murders inspired filmmaker Francis Girod, who produced a Franco-Italian-German film 'Le Trio Infernal' in 1974.

Similar methods to eliminate bodies of victims were used by the English serial killer John George Haigh in the 1940s, known as 'the acid bath murderer'. He dissolved his victims in concentrated sulphuric acid and was hanged in 1949 (Lowe 2015; Oates 2014).

Sulphuric acid, in order to 'melt away', is one of the methods applied by the Italian mafia. Grillo and Cascino (2011) describe how tanks full of acid, torture instruments and human remains were found at the property of criminals from the Sicilian mafia 'Casa Nostra'.

Other reported strong inorganic acids are halogen acids such as **hydrochloric acid (HCl)** and **hydrofluoric acid (HF).** Hydrochloric acid is found naturally in the stomach to aid the digestion and has many industrial uses as a chemical agent in the production of plastics (Fire 2009). Hydrofluoric acid is used widely in the chemical industries, electronics manufacturing, glass etching, melting and cleaning, but also in domestic settings such as household rust removers and compressed air dusters (Xingang *et al.* 2014). Death has been reported from body surface burns of only small areas (Anderson and Anderson 1988; Bertolini 1992).

Amongst the forensic cases, there are two examples from the USA and France. In 2013, a 27-year-old man from Washington stood accused of strangling his girlfriend and trying to cover up the crime by placing her body in a plastic tub filled with acid. The police found episodes of the US television series 'Breaking Bad' on the perpetrator's DVD player and a room mate confirmed that this was his favourite show. In Breaking Bad (Gilligan 2008–2013), the main character disposed of several corpses by soaking them in vats of hydrofluoric acid (Moaba 2013).

In Toulouse (France), a murder plot inspired by the same TV series took place. Three French men between 19 and 23 years murdered a 23-year-old student over a drugs debt. The perpetrators purchased a plastic trunk to place the body in and covered it with hydrochloric acid. They went back to the victim's flat several times to inspect the state of the body. Sources suggested that air fresheners were used to mask the smell of disintegrating flesh. After 10 days, the body was discovered by the victim's mother, and found to be in an advanced stage of decomposition (Sims 2015).

In forensic practice, it is not always clear which acid has been used. A case from the UK describes a woman who stabbed her 3-year-old daughter to death before covering her with a corrosive with the intention to 'dissolve her away'. The pathologists, who carried out the post-mortem examination, were unable to identify what corrosive substance was applied to the child's body, but a pH indicator test (litmus paper test) indicated that it was an acid rather than an alkaline. The mother was declared unfit for trial (BBC 2010).

22.3.2 Alkalis

Some alkalis are as powerful corrosives as many acids. Alkalis, also known as bases or caustics, are defined as compounds that contain the hydroxide ion (OH^-). They are ionic compounds and therefore inorganic compounds, known as the chemical opposites of inorganic acids. The chemical reaction that demonstrates this is the 'neutralisation reaction', in which an acid and a base react to form a salt and water (Fire 2009). One such powerful base is **sodium hydroxide (NaOH)**, also known as caustic soda, lye or white caustic, easily extracted from household drain cleaner.

Ubelaker and Sperber (1988) describe a case study from 1979, when a 19-year-old female went missing in Nebraska (USA). She remained missing for 8.5 years until her remains were found in an unused cistern. Dental examination revealed an unusual appearance, inconsistent with a body lying undisturbed for nine years. The labial surfaces of the maxillary anterior dentition had a chalky white colour, similar in appearance to that seen in decalcified enamel. The cranium and mandible also showed perforation and corrosion. Two years later, the perpetrator was brought to trial for murder. His testimony suggested that, after killing the girl, he had made an attempt to disfigure the cadaver beyond recognition, by pouring lye or 'some other highly caustic substance' over the face. The use of a corrosive alkaline substance was confirmed by measuring the pH of the floor of the cistern, which was much more alkaline than reference samples of sludge-like materials (Ubelaker and Sperber 1988).

Another case is that of Mexican drug dealer Santiago Meza Lopez, who was arrested in 2009, after long being on the Federal Bureau of Investigation's (FBI) most wanted list. Lopez's nickname was 'El Pozolero', the soupmaker, and he was accused of having killed and dissolved more than 300 bodies in caustic soda (Sanchez 2013).

A more recent example dates back to 2015, when a 21-year-old man pleaded guilty to murdering a Glasgow student during a night out. After killing the girl, he went to a local shop to buy 6 litres of sodium hydroxide in an attempt to destroy her body. It is not clear in which state the victim's body was in when detected (*HMA v Alexander Benjamin Pacteau* 2015).

Another alkaline substance, mentioned in a high number of case studies, is lime. Lime is a generic term for **quicklime (CaO)** (also called unslaked lime or burnt lime), **hydrated lime ($Ca(OH)_2$)** (variously known as slaked lime) and other lime derivatives such as hydraulic lime, which contains impurities such as silica and alumina. The reasons behind the use of lime are diverse, ranging from aiming to preserve the body, prophylactic reasons and to accelerate decay (e.g. Schotsmans *et al.* 2015; 2017). In the following case descriptions, lime was used with the intention to accelerate decay. Unfortunately, it is not always clear whether quicklime or hydrated lime was applied.

The earliest records of a homicide victim covered with lime go back to 1931. The Chicago police discovered a woman packed in quicklime (Laudermilk 1932). This statement led to the first study of lime on decay, detailed in the next section.

In 1942, workmen discovered skeletonised remains beneath a stone slab in the cellar of a Baptist chapel in southeast London. Slaked lime had been spread over the body. Police found out that the remains matched a lady who went missing 15 months before. She appeared to be killed by her husband who consequently was found guilty and hanged (Jackson and Jackson 2008).

Jones (1987) analysed a burial of a woman discovered in 1980 in Oklahoma (USA). The victim had been covered with hydrated lime and buried for an unknown period. It was assumed that the perpetrator had the intention to accelerate decomposition but the opposite effect occurred. Upon exhumation, forensic scientists noticed little decomposition and maggot activity was minimal.

In 1981, in a shallow grave in Tennessee (USA), W. Bass recovered the body of a man who disappeared a year earlier. Lime was dumped over his body. Bits of dry tissue remained on some of the bones, but most of the remains were skeletonised after one year of burial (Bass and Jefferson 2003).

Manhein (1996) describes a body, buried for 4.5 years, sealed in heavy plastic and secured with tape. Upon excavation, extensive 'adipocere' was present, with pink colouring visible in some muscle tissue and an intense odour of putrefaction (Chapters 1 and 2). The body was well preserved. After 5 years of burial, positive identification was made using fingerprints from the disarticulated fingers. Analysis of the contents of the bag suggested that lime had been placed with the remains (Manhein 1996). In this case, it is not clear if the adipocere or lime were chemically analysed. Experiments by Forbes *et al.* (2005) show that a burial environment containing lime significantly inhibits adipocere formation.

Hochrein et al. (1999) compiled information on forensic cases involving buried bodies gathered from newspaper articles in the USA. One case involved a federal drug informant who was buried in a prepared grave. Lime was used with the intent of accelerating decomposition. Instead, it helped to preserve the remains for two years. Another case involved a two-year burial with large amounts of lime laid out on the bottom of the grave and poured out on top of the victim. The lime had hardened into a concrete-like consistency and acted as a preservative and drying agent. Hochrein (2002) also reported a victim disposed of in a sinkhole and covered with layers of hay, trash and lime. Investigators wanted to know if the lime was poured into the sinkhole prior to the deposition of the body, which would suggest planning and preparation for the homicide. Examination demonstrated that the lime had washed down and seeped beneath the victim. It did not constitute a pre-deposited layer on which the remains were placed.

Ivan Stambolic, a former Serbian president, was abducted and killed in 2000 by Slobodan Milosevic's Special Operations Unit. Three years later his body was found in a shallow, lime-covered grave in Belgrade (Serbia) (Declercq 2003; Green 2003).

In Belgium, a woman was convicted of the murder of her husband in 2002. She gave her husband sleeping pills and tried to bury him alive in the garden, covered with lime because she 'read on the internet that it would expedite putrefaction' (De Buck 2004).

In 2008, a 27-year-old girl was abducted and strangled in Aalten in The Netherlands. The perpetrator buried her in his garden and covered her with 25 kg of lime that he had bought in a nearby shop (Rechtbank Zutphen 2010).

In another Dutch case from 1994, a man was convicted of killing 11 young women. Some of them had been buried in quicklime (Lambrix 1996).

Another example of forensic lime cases was documented in Costa Rica. Congram (2008) described the search for a clandestine burial in 2004. A person had been murdered, placed in a shallow grave and covered with lime and cement. After 2.5 years of burial, skeletonised human remains were discovered with liquefying soft tissue found at the base of the grave.

In 2011, the French police dug up the bodies of a mother, her 4 children and their 2 dogs in a garden in Nantes. They appeared to have been shot by the father, wrapped in hessian sacks, and buried with quicklime (Chrisafis 2011).

As mentioned earlier, the Italian mafia follow macabre rituals after executing their victims. D'Errico *et al.* (2011) describe a case of two men killed and completely covered with lime by members of the mafias in Southern Italy. When the pathologists arrived at the scene around 48 hours post-mortem, the caustic effects of the quicklime represented full thickness burns on the face and reddish areas on the trunk of the victims.

Another forensic case with lime is briefly described by Komar *et al.* (2012). The authors found a homicide victim buried in a remote area. The perpetrator had applied a layer of lime to the grave before depositing the victim face down. As such, full facial features were captured in the lime as a 'death-mask'. The authors tried to capture the impression with a 3D laser scanner but failed. Attempts to stabilise the lime cast were also unsuccessful because of the fragility of the cast.

Other highly alkaline substances, with lime as the major constituent, are cement and concrete. Body disposal in concrete and/or cement is meant to hide evidence rather than hamper identification. Cement is a common binder within building materials and widely used throughout the world and through history. Cement consists of a mixture of lime and clay, which have been fired together with other additives such as gypsum. Nowadays, Portland cement is the most common type of cement, developed in Britain in the 19th century AD. Portland cement contains varying percentages of lime, silicon dioxide and alkali oxides. When sand and gravel are added to cement, concrete is formed. Concrete is widely used to create foundations, walls and architectural structures (Sherman and Larkin 2005). Case studies on concealing in concrete are described in this volume in Chapters 33 and 34. Other cases are detailed by Toms *et al.* (2008) and Preuss *et al.* (2006). All these reports show that setting corpses in concrete slows decay, does not prevent smell and complicates the estimation of the post-mortem interval (PMI).

In some cases, it can be observed if the concrete was hand mixed or machine mixed. Furthermore, collaboration with concrete companies might be helpful for PMI estimation. Morel (2005) described how police detectives asked a concrete company to help with the investigation of a murdered body found in concrete in Las Vegas. The concrete company applied three of its laboratory techniques to define specific qualities of the concrete that would be indicative of age: the depth the concrete was carbonated, the relative porosity of the paste and the degree of cement hydration. As a result, the police had a more precise timeline to investigate a smaller group of missing person reports, and was subsequently able to identify the victim.

22.4 Research on Corrosive Agents and Decomposition

The case studies above show that perpetrators often use easily obtainable products when they aim to 'dissolve' their victims. This includes household corrosive chemicals and building materials. Similar observations are made regarding acid attacks and chemical assault. A study by Mannan *et al.* (2007) showed that from the 1960s onwards the most common chemical for assault was sodium hydroxide, obtained from household drain cleaner. Not surprising, lye is listed as an agent of assault in the USA. In developing countries, sulphuric acid is the main agent for assault, because it is easily obtainable from car batteries (Mannan *et al.* 2007).

There is a gap in the literature regarding the effects of chemical agents on different tissues of the human body. The few existing studies are presented below. Because the tissues and the concentrations of the substances differ in each study, the results are presented by individual study, rather than by substance. Table 22.1 gives an overview of the corrosive agents that are most often reported in forensic cases (see section 22.3) with reference to experimental research.

22.4.1 Experimental Research

Hartnett *et al.* (2011) investigated the effects of household chemicals on human tissues in order to solve a forensic case. Five different human tissues (bone, tooth, hair, fingernails and skin/muscle/fat) were immersed into six different corrosive agents. These agents consisted of hydrochloric acid, sulphuric acid, sodium hydroxide (lye), sodium hypochlorite (bleach, NaClO), organic septic cleaner (consisting of bacteria and enzymes) and Coca Cola®, which has an unknown concentration of phosphoric acid (H_3PO_4). Tap water was used as a control. The results of this study demonstrated that hydrochloric acid was the most destructive. It consumed most tissue within 24 hours. Sulphuric acid was the second-most destructive agent, but not as fast as hydrochloric acid. Bleach, lye and cola had no structural effects on the hard tissues of the body, but altered the appearance and integrity of the

Table 22.1 Corrosive agents that are most often reported in forensic practice with references to experimental research.

	Corrosive agent	Chemical formula	Experimental research
Acids	Sulphuric acid	H_2SO_4	Grillo & Cascino 2011; Hartnett *et al.* 2011; Cope & Dupras 2009; Mazza *et al.* 2005
	Hydrochloric acid	HCl	Hartnett *et al.* 2011; Cope & Dupras 2009; Mazza *et al.* 2005
	Hydrofluoric acid	HF	
Alkalis	Sodium hydroxide	NaOH	Christensen & Myers 2011; Hartnett *et al.* 2011; Cope & Dupras 2009
	Quicklime	CaO	Schotsmans *et al.* 2012, 2014a, 2014b; Laudermilk 1932
	Hydrated lime	$Ca(OH)_2$	Schotsmans *et al.* 2012, 2014a, 2014b; Thew 2000

hair, nails and soft tissue. Organic septic cleaner and tap water had no effect on any of the tested human tissues.

Mazza *et al.* (2005) studied the effects of four different acids on human dentition. In 37% solution of hydrochloric acid, the teeth were completely dissolved after 14 h of immersion, while after 90 h in 96% sulphuric acid, the destruction of the samples was still incomplete. In 65% nitric acid (HNO_3), the teeth underwent complete dissolution after 12 h. In aqua regia (chloroazotic acid) (hydrochloric/nitric acid 3:1), it took 17 h.

A similar result was obtained by Cope and Dupras (2009), who examined the effects of four household chemical products on human teeth in a 24 h period of exposure. Hydrochloric acid was the most detrimental chemical. Sulphuric acid enacted minimal alterations to the teeth apart from some etching and discolouration. Phosphoric acid resulted in variable changes of the organic and inorganic compounds of the teeth and sodium hydroxide resulted in little to no change.

Grillo and Cascino (2011) conducted two experiments with sulphuric acid. In the first experiment, a pork knuckle was left in pure sulphuric acid. After 30 minutes, the piece of pork had a brown appearance. After two days, the muscle structures were loose and after six days the bone began to erode, but remained complete. The second experiment consisted of a pork knuckle in sulphuric acid, activated with water. This reaction was much more violent, resulting in the bone being completely dissolved after two days.

An experiment with a different aim was published by Christensen and Myers (2011), who looked into the effects of aquatic environments of varying pH on bovine bones. Solutions of different pH levels were prepared with tap water in combination with nitric acid (representing pH 1 and pH 4) and sodium hydroxide (representing pH 10 and 14). The neutral (pH 7) and moderately basic (pH 10) solutions had little effect on the bone, while all other solutions affected the bone to some degree. Extreme pH levels significantly affected the integrity and physical appearance of the bone, completely dissolving it in the case of pH 1 and degrading it considerably in the case of pH 14. A similar result was obtained by Baglieri (2015) who observed the macroscopic damage of five American household chemicals: Acidic Toilet Bowl Cleaner®, Lime-Away®, Septic Tank Cleaner®, Heavy Duty Stripper and Cleaner® and Pequa Drain Cleaner® on pig ribs. The results showed that the alkaline product Pequa Drain Cleaner® (pH 11–12) was the most destructive, reducing the ribs to fragments due to its main agent potassium hydroxide (KOH). The other household chemicals had minor macroscopic effects.

Regarding research of lime on decomposition, the earliest experiments date back to 1932. Experiments with quicklime on a dead owl and pieces of beef were conducted over 4 weeks. Despite the short time frame of the experiments and the rather small subjects, Laudermilk was the first researcher who proved that lime neither destroys bodies nor accelerates decay (Laudermilk 1932). Seventy years later, the effects of quicklime and hydrated lime on entire pig carcasses were studied by Thew (2000) and Schotsmans *et al.* (2012, 2014a,b)The results showed that lime retards the rate of decomposition if present in a burial environment, but does not stop it. Since lime is only applied to the outside of a body, putrefactive decay continues from the inside by microorganisms derived from the body itself. Bacterial populations on the exterior of the carcass are reduced by lime, but not eliminated. The end result is skeletonisation.

22.4.2 Issues Regarding Experiments with Chemicals

The sections above show that, while there are many forensic cases of chemicals used to facilitate disappearance, the experimental scientific research is minimal. It is not straightforward to simply describe the effects of particular chemicals on human remains because of several reasons. First, not all tissues in a human body consist of the same material, with some tissues being more resistant than others. Corrosive substances act differently on soft tissue, bone, teeth, hair and nails.

Other variables are the quantity and concentration of the substance and the fact that the chemical is only applied to the outside of a body. While contact with alkaline and acid substances can cause several types of skin reactions from mild irritation to full thickness burns, it is a misconception that corrosives accelerate decay and destroy bodies. If the depositional environment becomes too alkaline or too acid, bacteria will not flourish, and the bacterial breakdown of organic matter will be slowed down or even stopped. To illustrate this, lime is often used as a disinfectant during mass disasters or mass burials (De Ville de Goyet 2004). Acetic acid has been commonly used in medicine for the disinfection of wounds and prophylaxis of the plague (Ryssel *et al.* 2009). Moreover, the use of chemicals will not only stop bacteria, it will also affect the attractiveness of the cadaver to insects or other microorganisms. Mann *et al.* (1990) describe a case from the Anthropological Research Facility (ARF) at Tennessee. A badly damaged hand was removed from a decaying body at the ARF for fingerprinting. The police laboratory placed the hand in a jar of formalin. When the hand was put back with the body, the maggots would not feed on it, even after months of exposure outdoors. Based on this, Mann *et al.* (1990) advised to consider chemical exposure if a body part of a decomposing body shows no signs of destruction.

Another difficulty in the study of chemicals on decay is the use of body parts and tissue sections during experiments, instead of complete bodies. It is hard to extrapolate results of experiments with cubes of tissue to whole carcasses with complete viscera. Whole bodies have their internal organs with the entire bacterial community still present, and a different surface area to volume ratio than cubes of tissue. When a corrosive agent is applied to the outside of a carcass, the remains will continue to deteriorate from the inside outwards by microorganisms derived from the body itself. Hydrochloric acid might consume a portion of a human body as seen in Hartnett *et al.* (2011). The French case example from Toulouse, described above (Sims 2015), shows that destroying an entire human body did not work that easily with the same product. Similarly, experiments with sections of pig tissue covered by quicklime and hydrated lime indicated that lime easily desiccates a small cube of tissue (Laudermilk 1932; Schotsmans *et al.* 2012), while whole pig carcasses covered with lime did not desiccate (Schotsmans *et al.* 2014a,b; Thew 2000).

A final issue regarding experiments with chemicals is the hazard for the researchers (and the perpetrator) themselves. Experiments with chemicals on entire carcasses require the greatest care for the executor. Careful selection and use of adequate personal protective equipment (PPE) should protect the individual from hazards effecting the respiratory system, skin, eyes, face, hands, feet, head and body. PPE should be used in conjunction with other protective methods such as exposure control procedures. Moreover, careful consideration should be given to the choice of the right container in which the experiment will take place and the effect the chemical can have on the container (e.g. steel bath tub, plastic barrel, etc.).

22.5 Case Study: The Pandy Case

22.5.1 Introduction

In 2002, a Belgian court convicted Andras Pandy, a Hungarian priest, and his daughter Agnes for the murder of at least six of their relatives between 1986 and 1990. Pandy had an incestuous relationship with three of his daughters. Family members were eliminated as soon as the incestuous secret was about to be revealed to the outside world. For many years, Pandy misguided police investigators with clear explanations about the disappearance of his family members. He pretended that they had moved abroad and he created false postcards and letters, allegedly written by the disappeared family members, to show that he was still in touch with them.

In 1992, two years after the last disappearance, Agnes attempted to report her father to the police for sexual abuse and the disappearance of several family members. Police investigation remained limited and Agnes's statement was put aside. However, during the aftermath of another infamous Belgian serial killer case and paedophile scandal 'the Dutroux affairs' (1996), police and law authorities decided to re-open (c)old cases and look for errors and oversights.

In 1997, Agnes was interrogated and confessed to participating in the murders of her disappeared mother and siblings by assisting her father. She explained that the victims were lead to the basement of their house and then shot or killed with a sledgehammer. Next, the corpses were sawn into pieces and put in a barrel with Cleanest® (currently known as Destop®), a product used to unblock drains. After a few days the liquid was poured down the drain and the harder (osseous) remnants were dumped in the bin of a nearby abattoir.

Despite the accusations of his daughter, Pandy denied any involvement in the disappearance of their relatives, nor in having incestuous relationships with his daughters. Thorough searches in his houses revealed a few unidentifiable human dental and osseous fragments under the concrete floor in the basement and empty plastic containers of Cleanest®.

With the accused denying every involvement and in the absence of solid evidence, the investigation reached a dead end. Moreover, there was no forensic literature to support the case and preliminary tests of the product to unblock drains on non-human mammal tissue were disappointing. Therefore, the investigating judge requested that a team of scientists carry out an experiment with the product and human remains following the detailed descriptions by Agnes.

22.5.2 Experimental Set-up

The experiment was carried out in 1998 at the faculty of medicine from the University of Leuven (Belgium). The University of Leuven maintains high ethical standards in research involving human tissues. To be consistent with the well-developed rules and conditions of the ethical committee, only body parts of a person who donated his/her body to the university could be used for this experiment. The remaining human remains were carefully buried afterwards. The experiment was justified by being the only possible way in searching for the truth. It was carried out by a multidisciplinary team, consisting of a forensic pathologist, toxicologists, geneticists, forensic odontologist and anthropologist, in collaboration with the Belgian Disaster Victim Identification team of the Belgian Federal Police.

According to Agnes, Cleanest® was used to dissolve parts of dismembered bodies, including the head, by immerging them in a barrel for 5 to 8 days at room temperature. She stated that the product was not renewed and no fresh product was added.

Preliminary tests with animal tissue did not give the expected results. After in-depth research, it was revealed that Cleanest® was taken over by another manufacturer in 1994, which changed the original formula. The original formula of the product, as used by Pandy between 1986 and 1990, was not commercially available anymore and had to be re-created by the forensic toxicologists of the team. It consisted of sulphuric acid, a salt (sodium dichromate $Na_2Cr_2O_7$) and the emulsifier Eumulgin®[2].

The experiment was set up in three phases. First, the lungs, heart, stomach, spleen, one kidney, head (including 5 teeth), hands and feet were put in a perforated basket. The teeth consisted of the lower canines (33 and 43), lower premolars (34 and 44) and one lower molar (47)[3]. The basket was submerged in a 100 litre PVC (polyvinyl chloride) barrel filled with 50 litres of the original formula of Cleanest®. Five hours later, in the second phase, a lower leg was added to the basket. After 25 hours, the second lower leg was also put into the barrel.

2 The authors decided not to publish the exact concentrations because of ethical reasons.

3 Dental numbering based on the International Standards Organisation Designation System (ISO-3950 notation).

The whole process took place in a laboratory with a fume cupboard. Everything was filmed and photographed. The temperature of the substance was systematically measured and its appearance regularly described. The content was automatically stirred and inspected at regular time intervals by lifting the basket with the remains. The changes to the human tissue were photographed and described from a morphological, anthropological and odontological point-of-view. Bone tissue was sampled several times during the process to investigate for the survival of DNA.

22.5.3 Results

The product led to an initial exothermic chemical reaction during the first 24 hours, reaching a maximum temperature of 79°C after 5 hours. The temperature normalised to room temperature after 36–48 hours (Figure 22.1). The rise of temperature was accompanied with foam production and irritant vapours.

Within one hour of immersion, the human body parts were severely damaged, leading to unrecognisable facial features, loss of soft tissue and partial skeletonisation (Figure 22.2). After five hours, the organs, hands and feet were completely dissolved (i.e. absent) and the head was reduced to the thickest parts of the cranium with unrecognisable jelly brain fragments (Figure 22.2). One tooth (34) was removed for further inspection.

After five days, the initial violet coloured fluid was turned into dark, syrupy oil. Filtering the fluid revealed fragments of the cranium, consisting of a part of the occipital bone (50 × 80 mm) with a few porous grey osseous fragments of the occipital and temporal bone (pars petrosa) (Figure 22.2). Only three of the four remaining teeth were recovered (33, 44 and 47). Tooth 43, the lower canine, disappeared totally (Figure 22.3). The lower leg, which was put into the basket 5 hours after the onset of the experiment, did not have any soft tissue left and showed erosion at the bone surface. The second lower leg, added during the third phase, 25 hours after the start of the experiment, was still covered with soft tissue but showed damage to the skin. The tibia and fibula were intact without any damage.

Forensic odontological examination of the remaining teeth showed erosion of the dental enamel, with partially dissolved dentine of the roots of the teeth (Figure 22.3). However, radiographically the pulp chamber and root canals were still discernable, indicating that the teeth could potentially be used for identification.

Forensic genetic DNA analysis of the bone samples could not reveal one single DNA profile, from one hour of submersion onwards.

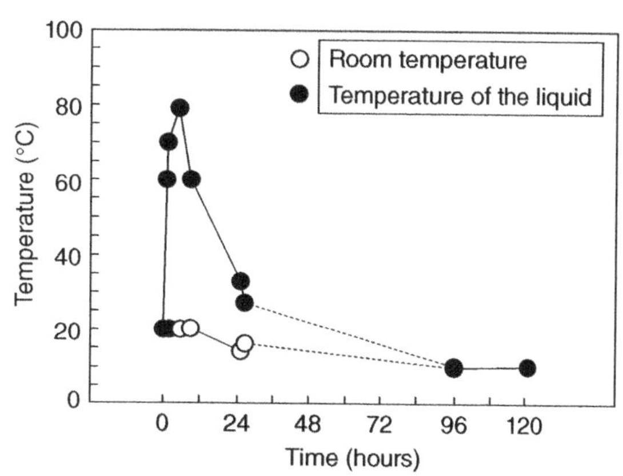

Figure 22.1 Room temperature and temperature of the fluid, indicating an exothermic reaction during the initial 24 hours of the experiment, reaching a maximum temperature of 79°C after 5 hours (source: J. Tytgat, image courtesy: Rep EX/98-44).

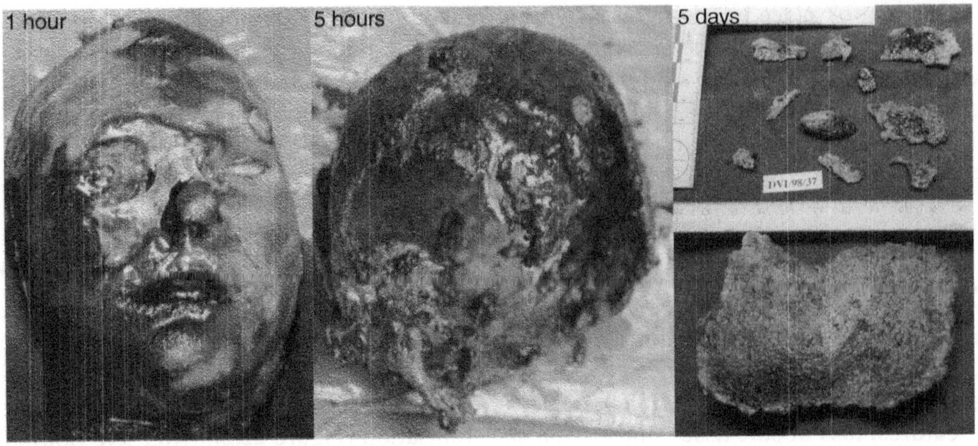

Figure 22.2 One hour after the onset of the experiment, the head showed unrecognisable facial features. After five hours, the head was reduced to the thickest parts of the cranium. After five days, only a part of the occipital bone and a few porous grey osseous fragments of the occipital and temporal bones remained (photos: J. Stragier, image courtesy: Rep EX/98-44).

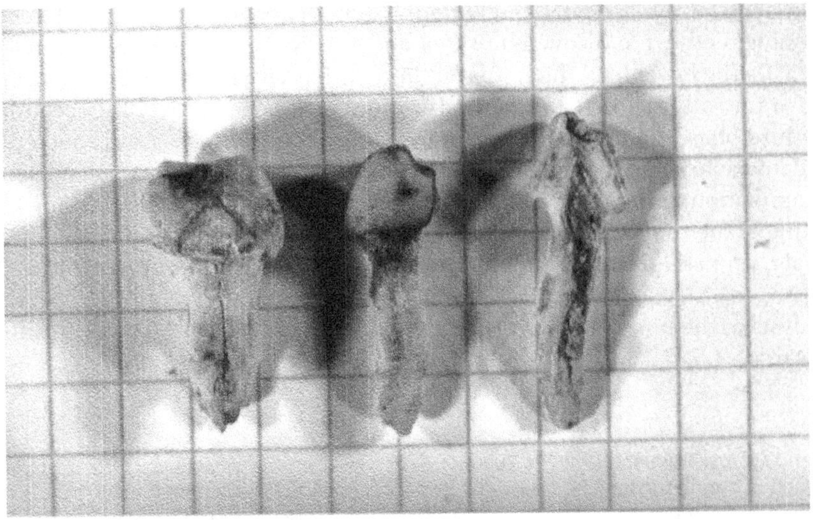

Figure 22.3 Image of the three recovered teeth (47, 44 and 33), five days after the experiment. The teeth show erosion of the enamel with partially dissolved dentine of the roots. Radiographically, the pulp chamber and root canals were still discernable, indicating that the teeth could potentially be used for identification. 1 square is 5 mm (photo: E. De Valck, image courtesy: Rep EX/98-44).

22.5.4 Conclusions of the Experiment

At the time, the available product, Cleanest®, was capable of dissolving human body parts in a very short time. Within a few hours, the remains were reduced to a syrupy oily substance with undefinable fragments, a few eroded porous bones and eroded teeth. The experiment showed that the initial exothermic reaction played an important role in the dissolving process. The lower legs, that were added 5 and 25 hours after the onset of the experiment, were not dissolved, less degraded and still recognisable.

During a criminal investigation, one of the main concerns is the identification of the victim. Clearly, this product hampered identification. Within one hour, DNA appeared to be completely destroyed. Only forensic odontology, using radiographic examination of teeth remnants and, depending on the remaining bone fragments, anthropological examination of the bony fragments, could potentially be useful for victim identification.

Andras Pandy was sentenced to life imprisonment in 2002 and died in prison in 2013 at the age of 86. He kept denying all charges until his death. His daughter Agnes received a 21-year sentence for being an accomplice in the murders. Her lawyers raised mitigating factors. Agnes acted under the tyrannical pressure of her father who raped her regularly and forced her into the killings of her mother and siblings. Further investigation speculated that Pandy and Agnes may have committed several additional murders of non-relatives, but has not been proven to date.

22.6 Conclusion

The case examples in this chapter demonstrate that a perpetrator's intent towards further concealment of evidence and hampering identification might be reflected in introduced chemicals. They include easily attainable substances such as sulphuric acid, hydrochloric acid, hydrofluoric acid or sodium hydroxide, and building materials such as lime or concrete.

Dissolving bodies with chemicals is a relatively rare phenomenon, not often encountered in forensic literature and practice (because they are not detected?). In this chapter, the number of forensic cases that describe the use of chemicals is higher than the available scientific literature and experimental research on the effects of corrosives on decay. Unfortunately the experiments usually follow the crime, when harm is already done.

One should be careful when mixing science with anecdotal information. A substance that burns the skin will not necessarily destroy a whole body. Some tissues are more resistant than other tissues. The quantity and concentration of the product, and the fact that the chemical is only applied to the outside of a body, also plays a role. More quantitative and qualitative data on the effects of different common corrosive agents on complete human bodies are necessary.

The Pandy serial killer case is a good example of investigation that was initially stopped because of a lack of evidence. Andras Pandy and his daughter Agnes successfully made body parts disappear. If the judge had not asked for the experiments, Pandy would not have been caught and Agnes would never have been believed. In Belgium, the media and several leading authorities in the medical and ethical field condemned the experiment. However, the results showed that the experiment had proven to be essential for sustaining justice. It might even have prevented more murders. The other side of the coin is that the Pandy case might inspire other perpetrators to do the same, just like the aforementioned films and crime series. Fortunately products used to clear drains are not as strong nowadays, because of ecological regulations, and the original product Cleanest® does not exist anymore. At least, the revealed forensic cases and existing scientific research show that it is not easy to dissolve a body completely in chemicals.

Acknowledgements

The authors would like to thank all the people who were involved in the Pandy experiment, in particular the crime investigators, the members of the Belgian Victim Identification Team, B. Bulthé, J.-J. Cassiman, P. Daenens, R. Decorte, E. De Valck, J. De Winne, J. Tytgat and M. Vandenbruaene.

References

Abramov, A., Veselovskaya, E., Dolgov, A., Engovatova, A.V., Mednikova, M.B. *et al.* (2015) Forensic archaeology in the Russian Federation. In: Groen, W.J.M., Marquez-Grant, N. and Janaway, R.C. (eds), *Forensic Archaeology*. Wiley-Blackwell: Chichester, UK, pp. 139–148.

Aggrawal, A. (2010) *Necrophilia, Forensic and Medico-Legal Aspects*. Boca Raton: CRC Press.

Anderson, W.J. and Anderson, J.R. (1988) Hydrofluoric acid burns of the hand: mechanism of injury and treatment. *Journal of Hand Surgery*, **13**: 52–57.

Anwary, A. (2003) Acid violence and medical care in Bangladesh. Women's activism as carework. *Gender and Society*, **17**: 305–313.

Asaria, J., Kobusingye, O.C., Khingi, B.A., Balikuddembe, R., Gomez, M. and Beveridge, M. (2004) Acid burns from personal assault in Uganda. *Burns*, **30**: 78–81.

Aufderheide, A.C. (2003) *The Scientific Study of Mummies*. Cambridge University Press: Cambridge.

Baglieri, G. (2015) The effects of household corrosive chemicals on pig bone and human tissue. *Journal of Undergraduate Anthropology*, **5**: 35–50.

Bailey, K.C. (1932) *The Elder Pliny's Chapters on Chemical Subjects*, Part II: Arnold and Co: London.

Bass, W.M. and Jefferson, J. (2003) *Death's Acre*. Putman: New York.

BBC (2010) *Birmingham acid douse woman unlawfully killed daughter*, www.bbc.com/news/uk-england-birmingham-11642178 (Accessed 28 December 2015).

Bertolini, J.C. (1992) Hydrofluoric acid: a review of toxicity. *Journal of Emergency Medicine*, **10**: 163–168.

Branday, J., Arscott, G.D.L., Smoot, E.C., Williams, G.D. and Fletcher, P.R. (1996) Chemical burns as assault injuries in Jamaica. *Burns*, **22**: 154–155.

Burke, R. (2013) *Hazardous Materials Chemistry for Emergency Responders*. CRC Press: Boca Raton.

Byard, R.W. (2015) Caustic ingestion – A forensic overview. *Journal of Forensic Sciences*, **60**: 812–815.

Chambers, W. and Chambers, R. (2008) *Chambers 21st Century Dictionary*. Harrap Publishers: Edinburgh.

Chrisafis, A. (2011) *Mother and four children found buried in French garden, The Guardian*, www.theguardian.com/world/2011/apr/22/nantes-family-murder (Accessed 20 November 2015).

Christensen, A.M. and Myers, S.W. (2011) Macroscopic observations of the effects of varying fresh water pH on bone. *Journal of Forensic Sciences*, **56**: 475–479.

Congram, D.R. (2008) A clandestine burial in Costa Rica: prospection and excavation. *Journal of Forensic Sciences*, **53**: 793–796.

Cope, D.J. and Dupras, T.L. (2009) The effects of household corrosive chemicals on human dentition. *Journal of Forensic Sciences*, **54**: 1238–1246.

D'Errico, S., Turillazzi, E., Pomara, C., Fiore, C., Monchiotti, F. and Fineschi, V. (2011) A novel macabre ritual of the Italian mafia. *American Jounal of Forensic Medicine and Pathology*, **32**: 44–46.

De Buck, W. (2004) *Nu dood ik hem zelf*. Het Nieuwsblad. Mediargus: Brussels.

De Ville de Goyet, C. (2004) Epidemics caused by dead bodies: a disaster myth that does not want to die. *Pan American Journal of Public Health*, **15**: 297–299.

Declercq, I. (2003) *Stambolic gevonden*. Knack. Mediargus: Brussels.

Derelanko, M.J. and Auletta, C.S. (2014) *Handbook of Toxicology*. CRC Press: Boca Raton.

Fire, F.L. (2009) *The Common Sense Approach to Hazardous Materials*. PennWell: Tulsa.

Forbes, S.L., Stuart, B.H. and Dent, B.B. (2005) The effect of the burial environment on adipocere formation. *Forensic Science International*, **154**: 24–34.

Gilligan, V. (2008–2013) *Breaking Bad*, 5 seasons, 62 episodes.

Green, P.S. (2003) A Serbian mystery unravels with a crackdown on gangsters, *The New York Times*, www.nytimes.com/2003/04/09/world/a-serbian-mystery-unravels-with-a-crackdown-on-gangsters.html (Accessed 20 December 2015).

Grillo, M. and Cascino, F.M. (2011) Method of concealment of corpses in mafia related homicides: melting in strong acids. *Proceedings of the American Academy of Forensic Sciences*, **17**: 254.
Girod, F. (1974) *Le trio infernal*, comédie noire, 107 min.
Guerrero, L. (2013) Burns due to acid assaults in Bogota. *Burns*, **39**: 1018–1023.
Hartnett, K.M., Fulginiti, L.C. and Di Modica, F. (2011) The effects of corrosive substances on human bone, teeth, hair, nails and soft tissue. *Journal of Forensic Sciences*, **56**: 954–959.
HMA v Alexander Benjamin Pacteau 2015, www.scotland-judiciary.org.uk/ (Accessed 20 December 2015).
Hochrein, M.J., Gabra, J. and Nawrocki, S.P. (1999) The buried body cases content analyses project: patterns in buried body investigations. *Proceedings of the 51st Annual Meeting of the American Academy of Forensic Sciences*, Orlando.
Hochrein, M.J. (2002) An autopsy of the grave: recognizing, collecting and preserving forensic geotaphonomic evidence. In: Haglund, W.D. and Sorg, M.H. (eds), *Advances in Forensic Taphonomy*. CRC Press: Boca Raton, pp. 45–69.
Jackson, A.R.W. and Jackson, J.M. (2008) *Forensic Science*. Pearson Education Limited: Essex.
Jackson, S. (2002) *No Stone Unturned. The story of Necrosearch International*. Kensington Publishing Corporation: New York.
Jones, A.M. (1987) An unusual atypical gunshot wound. *American Journal of Forensic Medicine and Pathology*, **8**: 338–341.
Josset, P. and Hall, A.H. (2014) History of chemical burns and scope of the problem. In: Maiback, H.I. and Hall, A.H. (eds), *Chemical Skin Injury. Mechanisms, prevention, decontamination, treatment*. Springer: London, pp. 1–19.
Kachan, T., Ram, P., Tandon, A. and Krishan, K. (2015) Acid violence in India – A modern day sombre reality? *Burns*, **41**: 1372–1373.
Koller, J., Baumer, U., Kaup, Y. and Weser, U. (2005) Herodotus' and Pliny's embalming materials identified on ancient Egyptian mummies. *Archaeometry*, **47**: 609–628.
Komar, D.A., Davy-Jow, S. and Decker, S.J. (2012) The use of a 3-D laser scanner to document ephemeral evidence at crime scenes and post-mortem examination. *Journal of Forensic Sciences*, **57**: 188–191.
Kumar Das, K., Olga, L., Peck, M., Morselli, P.G. and Salek, A.J.M. (2015) Management of acid burns: experience from Bangladesh. *Burns*, **41**: 484–492.
Lambrix, Y. (1996) Oud-gevangene onthult seriemoorden in tv-uitzending. *Het Belang van Limburg*. Hasselt: Mediargus: Hasselt.
Larue, S. (2009) *Les nouvelles affaires criminelles de France*. De Borée: Paris.
Laudermilk, J.D. (1932) Concerning quicklime burial. *The American Journal of Police Science*, **59**: 59–63.
Leicester, H.M. (1956) *The Historical Background of Chemistry*. John Wiley & Sons: New York.
Lowe, G. (2015) *The Acid Bath Murders. The trials and liquidations of John George Haigh*. The History Press: London.
Magnuson, M.L. Satzger, R.D., Alcaraz, A., Brewer, J., Fetterolf, D. *et al.* (2012) Guidelines for the identification of unknown samples for laboratories performing forensic analyses for chemical terrorism. *Journal of Forensic Sciences*, **57**: 636–642.
Material Safety Data Sheets, www.msdsonline.com (Accessed 20 November 2015).
Manhein, M.H. (1996) Decomposition rates of deliberate burials: a case study of preservation. In: Haglund, W.D. and Sorg, M.H. (eds), *Forensic Taphonomy: The postmortem fate of human remains*. CRC Press: Boca Raton, pp. 469–482.
Mann, R.W., Bass, W.M. and Meadows, L. (1990) Time since death and decomposition of the human body: variables and observations in case and experimental field studies. *Journal of Forensic Sciences*, **35**: 103–111.

Mannan, A., Ghani, S., Clarke, A. and Butler, P.E.M. (2007) Cases of chemical assault worldwide: a literature overview. *Burns*, **33**: 149–154.

Mannan, A., Ghani, S., Sen, S.L., Clarke, A. and Butler, P.E.M. (2004) The problem of acid violence in Bangladesh. *The Journal of Surgery*, **2**: 39–43.

Maples, W.R. and Browning, M. (1994) *Dead Men Do Tell Tales*. Broadway Books: New York.

Matshes, E.W., Taylor, K.A. and Rao, V.J. (2008) Sulfuric acid injury. *American Journal of Forensic Medicine and Pathology*, **29**: 340–345.

Mazza, A., Merlati, G., Savio, C., Fassina, G., Menghini, P. and Danesino, P. (2005) Observations on dental structures when placed in contact with acids: experimental studies to aid identification processes. *Journal of Forensic Sciences*, **50**: 406–410.

Milton, R., Mathieu, L., Hall, A.H. and Maibach, H.I. (2010) Chemical assault and skin/eye burns: two representative cases, report from the Acid Survivors Foundation, and literature review. *Burns*, **36**: 924–932.

Moaba, A. (2013) Breaking bad murder Jason Hart accused of using acid technique, The Huffington Post, www.huffingtonpost.com/2013/06/27/breaking-bad-murder_n_3511285.html (Accessed 2 December 2015).

Morel, K. (2005) A concrete body of evidence. *The American Edge*, **9**: 1–3.

Napier, M.R. and Baker, K.P. (2002) Criminal personality profiling. In: James, S.H. and Nordby, J.J. (eds), *Forensic Science: An introduction to scientific and investigative techniques*. CRC Press: Boca Raton, pp. 531–550.

Oates, J. (2014) *John George Haigh, the Acid-bath Murderer. A portrait of a serial killer and his victims.* Pen and Sword Books: Barnsley.

Preuss, J., Strehler, M., Dressler, J., Risse, M., Anders, S. and Madea, B. (2006) Dumping after homicide using setting in concrete and/or sealing with bricks – Six case reports. *Forensic Science International*, **159**: 55–60.

Rajs, J., Lundstrom, M., Broberg, M., Lidberg, L. and Lindquist, O. (1998) Criminal mutilation of the human body in Sweden – A thirty year medico-legal and forensic psychiatric study. *Journal of Forensic Sciences*, **43**: 563–580.

Rechtbank, Zutphen (2010) *Rechterlijke uitspraak Joanne Noordink*. Jure Béta: Zutphen.

Ryssel, H., Kloeters, O., Germann, G., Schäfer, Th., Wiedermann, G. and Oehlbauer, M. (2009) The antimicrobial effect of acetic acid – An alternative to common local antiseptics? *Burns*, **35**: 695–700.

Sanchez, L. (2013) El pozolero, legado de muerte. El Universtal, http://archivo.eluniversal.com.mx/notas/915149.html (Accessed 28 December 2015).

Schotsmans, E.M.J., Denton, J., Dekeirsschieter, J., Ivaneanu, T. *et al.* (2012) Effects of hydrated lime and quicklime on the decay of buried human remains using pig cadavers as human body analogues. *Forensic Science International*, **217**: 50–59.

Schotsmans, E.M.J., Denton, J., Fletcher, J.N., Janaway, R.C. and Wilson, A.S. (2014a) Short-term effects of hydrated lime and quicklime on the decay of human remains using pig cadavers as human body analogues: laboratory experiments. *Forensic Science International*, **238**: 142.e1–142e.10.

Schotsmans, E.M.J., Fletcher, J.N., Denton, J., Janaway, R.C. and Wilson, A.S. (2014b) Long-term effects of hydrated lime and quicklime on the decay of human remains using pig cadavers as human body analogues: field experiments. *Forensic Science International*, **238**: 141.e1–141.e13.

Schotsmans, E.M.J., Van de Vijver, K., Wilson, A.S. and Castex, D. (2015) Interpreting lime burials. A discussion in light of lime burials at St Rombout's cemetery in Mechelen, Belgium (10th–18th centuries). *Journal of Archaeological Science Reports*, **3**: 464–479.

Schotsmans, E.M..J, García-Rubio, A., Edwards, H.G.M., Munshi, T., Wilson, A.S. and Rios, L. (2017). Analysing and interpreting lime burials from the Spanish Civil War (1936–1939): a case study from La Carcavilla cemetery. *Journal of Forensic Sciences*.

Seidel, A.C. and Fulginiti, L.C. (2014) The first cut is the deepest: looking for patterns in cases of human dismemberment. In: Martin, D.L. and Anderson, C.P. (eds), *Bioarchaeological and Forensic Perspectives on Violence*. Cambridge University Press: Cambridge, pp. 63–82.

Sherman, S.C. and Larkin, K. (2005) Cement burns. *The Journal of Emergency Medicine*, **29**: 97–99.

Sims, A. (2015) French students dissolve body in acid after killing girl in breaking bad murder plot, *The Independent*, www.independent.co.uk/news/world/europe/french-students-dissolve-body-in-acid-after-killing-girl-in-breaking-bad-murder-plot-10447943.html (Accessed 20 December 2015).

Slater, W. (2007) *The Many Deaths of Tsar Nicholas II: Relics, remains and the Romanovs*. Routledge: Abington.

Thew, H.A. (2000) *Effects of Lime on the Decomposition Rate of Buried Remains*, MSc thesis, University of Indianapolis.

Toms, C., Rogers, C.B. and Sathyavagiswaran, L. (2008) Investigation of homicides interred in concrete – the Los Angeles experience. *Journal of Forensic Sciences*, **53**: 203–207.

Ubelaker, D.H. and Sperber, N.D. (1988) Alterations in human bones and teeth as a result of restricted sun exposure and contact with corrosive agents. *Journal of Forensic Sciences*, **33**: 540–548.

Vij, K. (2009) *Textbook of Forensic Medicine and Toxicology. Principles and practice*. Noida: Elsevier.

Waldron, N.R., Kennifer, D., Bourgois, E., Vanna, K., Noor, S. and Gollogly, J. (2014) Acid violence in Cambodia: the human, medical and surgical implications. *Burns*, **40**: 1799–1804.

Xingang, W., Yuanhai, Z., Liangfang, N., Chuangang, Y., Chunjiang, Y. *et al*. (2014) A review of treatment strategies for hydrofluoric acid burns: current status and future prospects. *Burns*, **40**: 1447–1457.

Young, R.C., Ho, W.S., Ying, S.Y. and Burd, A. (2002) Chemical assaults in Hong Kong: a 10-year overview. *Burns*, **28**: 651–653.

23

Distinguishing between Peri- and Post-Mortem Trauma on Bone

Cristina Cattaneo and Annalisa Cappella

23.1 Introduction

In trauma analysis, the correct timing of a skeletal injury with respect to death is of paramount importance. For every single lesion it is always necessary to evaluate whether it occurred prior to (ante-mortem), around the time of (peri-mortem), or after death (post-mortem) (Sauer 1998). This is required for all types of traumatic lesions, whether they stem from blunt force injury, sharp force or gunshot/ballistic (or high velocity) wounds, and can be extremely challenging (Passalacqua and Rainwater 2015; Symes *et al.* 2014). A detailed analysis is thus indispensable whenever bone traumatic injuries are found, in order to distinguish them from taphonomic or voluntary post-mortem alterations (Symes *et al.* 1998). This means that it is important to evaluate the location, morphology and significant characteristics of all injuries, and to interpret the nature of trauma and the possible weapons involved (Hart 2005). The resulting pattern of trauma will contribute to the interpretation of both cause of death and events around death in the medico-legal setting (Sauer 1998).

This chapter will describe the present-day approaches in interpreting peri- and post-mortem trauma, and illustrate their limitations and pitfalls. Furthermore, it will provide alternative approaches and future recommendations for this particular kind of research.

23.2 Peri- and Post-Mortem Trauma

Distinguishing between a post-mortem and peri-mortem lesion on skeletal remains is one of the most challenging yet crucial issues in forensic anthropology, because it might determine the difference between a homicide and a natural death.

The term 'peri-mortem trauma' means, etymologically, around, and therefore before or after death, and clearly implies the impossibility of defining the lesion as ante- or post-mortem. The term is more frequently used in forensic anthropology than in forensic pathology, because the latter discipline has the advantage of dealing with soft tissue which, if well preserved, makes differentiating between ante-mortem and post-mortem easier. In ante-mortem trauma, when skin is still present, blood will actively be pumped into the soft tissues from and around the broken arteries, giving a classical microscopic image of red blood cells packed into the soft tissue where they should not be. In addition, several other cells including biochemical markers of inflammation are released, indicating a vital reaction, which causes for example, the typical macroscopic reddening around the wound. A post-mortem lesion does not produce this effect on surrounding tissues. Forensic anthropology

Taphonomy of Human Remains: Forensic Analysis of the Dead and the Depositional Environment, First Edition.
Edited by Eline M.J. Schotsmans, Nicholas Márquez-Grant and Shari L. Forbes.

and archaeology, usually deal with bone, which in most of these cases is deprived of soft tissue (or decomposed if present) and therefore presents a different scenario: blood travels in Haversian canals and within hydroxyapatite cases; therefore, even when fresh, these canals do not allow for active blood extravasation into the tissue. Therefore, one has to look for signs of active bleeding at the margins of the fracture, in soft tissue residues in and around bone, or for the survival of biochemical markers of inflammation. On dry bone this may be extremely difficult due to the scarce survival of all these elements after putrefaction.

On a dry bone, anthropologists can only verify if the fracture is or looks 'fresh' or not. A peri-mortem fracture can be compared to the fracture produced when a fresh green branch breaks – it has 'bent', which reflects the turgidity and elasticity of the young branch; a post-mortem fracture reflects the pattern left in a dry old branch: clear cut and neat. Nevertheless, the fact that the fracture looks fresh and thus can be classified as peri-mortem does not mean that it was related to the period around death. A peri-mortem fracture could be related to the ante-mortem period (days or even weeks before death) when signs of healing cannot yet be perceived (macroscopically), or to the post-mortem period (months or years after death) when decomposition has not yet caused the loss of all elastic features (collagen, elastin, other organic components of the bone tissue which give the bone elasticity).

The term 'post-mortem damage' (taphonomic alteration) refers to bone lesions occurring after 'green' or elastic properties have gone and can often be related to taphonomic factors, such as carnivore activity, surface erosions, sun bleaching, weathering, etc., but also to accidental events produced by human activity, transportation and fortuitous trauma. The definition is easier in theory than in practice, for example, chewing marks of carnivores on fresh tissue are usually erroneously called by default, post-mortem, because one assumes that animal scavenging occurs after death. However, sometimes they may be peri-mortem since chewing frequently occurs on bone, which is still full of organic components.

To define peri- and post-mortem, anthropologists usually adopt parameters based solely on macro-morphologic appearance (Galloway 1999; Moraitis and Spiliopoulou 2006; Moraitis *et al.* 2009; Symes *et al.* 2014; Ubelaker 1991, 1996; Ubelaker and Adams 1995; Wieberg and Wescott 2008), but the most significant influence on fracture morphology depends on the moisture content of the bone, which sometimes has nothing to do with the chronology of the fracture (Dirkmaat 2008, 2012; Evans 1957; Jonsens 1985; Moraitis and Spiliopoulou 2006; Symes *et al.* 2014' Ubelaker 1996; Wieberg and Wescott 2008). A 'green fracture', typical of fresh bone tissue, has characteristics that differ greatly from those exhibited by a so-called 'dry fracture', typically formed on dried bone. Fracture characteristics are closely related to the moisture content and the quantity of collagen matrix (which gives flexibility to the bone tissue). This means that at or around the time of death, the bone tissue is characterised by the same features observable also in living bone tissue (with the same properties of strength, elasticity and flexibility). Once bone tissue begins to lose its original components, such as the collagen matrix and content of water or humidity (because of decomposition), its own properties will change radically and invariably. At this point bone tissue becomes gradually 'dry', and therefore less flexible and resistant to subsequent stress (Harkess *et al.* 1996; Johnson 1985).

However, there may be a phase in which the properties of bone tissue will present characteristics intermediate between 'green' and 'dry', thus causing intermediate responses that will be more difficult to interpret. Hence it is impossible to specify an exact time at which the bone properties will be clearly of the peri or post type. In conclusion, what is determinant for changes in tissue properties is not only the passing of time since death, but also all cumulative effects resulting from the process of decomposition, taphonomic events and environmental factors that arise over time in specific environments (Calce and Rogers 2007; Moraitis *et al.* 2009; Sauer 1998; Ubelaker 1996; Wieberg and Wescott 2008).

Therefore, the contribution that osteology and anthropology can give is often limited by the few indicators, which are classically described to be 'diagnostic', between peri- and post-mortem trauma. Those indicators can be misleading and tricky and, by definition, cannot clearly define trauma as precisely before or after death. All this may lead to an inaccurate interpretation of trauma (Dirkmaat 2008, 2012; Symes *et al.* 2012, 2014). Even more confusing is the use of the terms ante-, peri- and post-mortem trauma by forensic pathologists. In forensic medicine, the term post-mortem refers literally to the period after death, ante-mortem refers to the period before death and peri-mortem refers to 'at or near the time of death'. In contrast, as explained above, for anthropologists, peri-mortem refers to a longer period when the bone is still green. It would be useful to find criteria, which can make the world of anthropology closer to that of the pathology of soft tissues.

It is important to figure out how to correctly deal with trauma analysis on skeletal remains when it is fundamental to distinguish between peri- and post-mortem lesions (Galloway 1999). The diagnosis of peri-mortem versus post-mortem needs to be based on reliable criteria for achieving such a result – criteria which at times are requested to go beyond reasonable doubt. For this reason, it is necessary to consider all limitations and unsolved questions around this important issue, in order to clarify the current state of knowledge and to develop or improve the approaches, which are still inadequate, not only to distinguish between peri-mortem and post-mortem but to turn peri-mortem into a clear ante-mortem or post-mortem fracture (Dirkmaat 2008; Sauer 1998; Symes *et al.* 2014; Ubelaker and Adams 1995, 1996).

23.2.1 Macroscopic Criteria Used by Forensic Anthropology: Morphological Fractures Characteristics

The characteristics of a fracture depend entirely on the type of bone response to injury, as mentioned above. This is based on bone proprieties that are subjected to changes due to the decomposition process, passing of time and also different environmental factors, to which the skeletal remains could be exposed (Calce and Rogers 2007).

Peri-mortem lesions, which occur when the bone tissue is still fresh, and able to absorb stress due to its high moisture content and original presence of tissue components, are almost the same as in living tissue. The high moisture content and richness in the bone matrix components determine high elasticity and plasticity, which ensure better tolerance, even in cases of great stress and strain before failure and fracture. This is very typical of living bone tissue, bone tissue around the time of death or in the very early stages of the decomposition process, unless some particular taphonomic factors intervene (Calce and Rogers 2007; Ubelaker and Adams 1995).

As soon as the organic matrix begins to degrade after death and the moisture content starts to decrease, the consequence will be the decrease in elasticity of the bone tissue. In this sense, the response will follow models of fracture and deformation completely different to those produced in fresh bone. Dry bone is characterised by little moisture content and organic matrix that causes more rigidity and brittleness as well as the loss of the typical viscoelastic properties of the original tissue (Johnson 1985; Symes *et al.* 2014). In the presence of these new properties, a fracture can be produced as a result of much less stress and will be characterised by a set of fractures different from those given by a fracture occurring in a fresh bone.

Several authors have claimed that it is possible to distinguish fairly easily between peri- and post-mortem fractures on the basis of specific macro-morphological characteristics of the fracture, which are in their opinion closely correlated with bone quality and properties (Galloway *et al.* 1999; Moraitis *et al.* 2009; Ubelaker 1991). They state that the proper assessment of trauma appears totally dependent on the characteristics of the fracture, such as fracture morphology, outline of fracture, angle and tactile roughness of the fracture margins (Moraitis and Spiliopoulou 2006;

Moraitis *et al.* 2009; Ubelaker 1997; Ubelaker and Adams 1995; Wheatley 2008; Wieberg and Wescott 2008), and last but not least, the colour of the margins fractured (Karr and Outram 2012a, 2012b; La Croix 2013). Few studies have focused on the problem of validity and reliability of such common criteria when they are applied to human skeletal remains on a large scale. This verification has been limited by the lack of human remains where different kinds of fractures (peri- and post-) are known and certain. In addition, not much is known about potential modification of original lesions with relation to time or as a consequence of environmental factors.

Conventional literature states that in general, the peri-mortem nature of an injury is sometimes indicated by the breaking pattern, which is more complex than that of a dry bone; concentric, circular and spiral fractures are usually typical of green fractures (fractures occurring in living or defleshed bone) (Figure 23.1). Patterns for dry bone (Ubelaker and Adams 1995) fractures include production of several small fragments, brittle flaking or shattering, and surface cracking (Maples 1986). Ubelaker and Adams (1995), as well as the common experience of the authors, have however demonstrated that unfortunately many types of fractures, both attributed to the ante- and post-mortem type, can occur regardless of how dry or elastic the bone is.

In addition, other features of peri-mortem fractures are bone tear, breakaway notches and plastic deformation, with the adhering of small fracture fragments adjacent to the fracture site or impact (Moraitis *et al.* 2009).

The fracture angle and colour are other additional features considered by Wieberg and Wescott (2008) as the main characteristics in the determination of post-mortem trauma: dry bone usually shows irregular to jagged fracture edges, which are often lighter in colour than the darkened adjacent bone (Ubelaker and Adams 1995). On dry bone, the fractures also exhibit breakage almost at a right-angle to their long axes with almost flat ends (seen in the perpendicular, parallel or diagonal breakage, as shown in Figure 23.2.

On the contrary, smooth, often bevelled, sharp fracture edges with sporadic sharp projections are associated with peri-mortem trauma and so are smooth fracture surface and obtuse or acute fracture angles (Figure 23.3). In this latter case, these morphological aspects indicate that the injury was inflicted when the bone still had elastic properties (Moraitis *et al.* 2009).

According to many authors (Bonnichsen 1979; Morlan 1984; Quatrehomme and Alunni 2013; Ubelaker and Adams 1995; Ubelaker 1997; Villa and Mahieu 1991; Wieberg and Wescott 2008), green fractures are characterised by smooth fracture edges usually of the same colour as the rest of the adjacent bone; thus colour staining can be present due to decomposition fluids, blood, soil, dirty water,

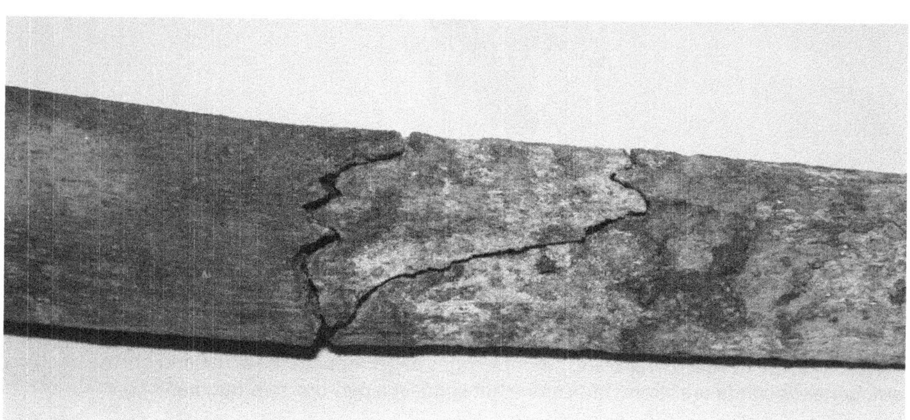

Figure 23.1 Example of a green fracture (peri-mortem breakage) with a complex fracture pattern.

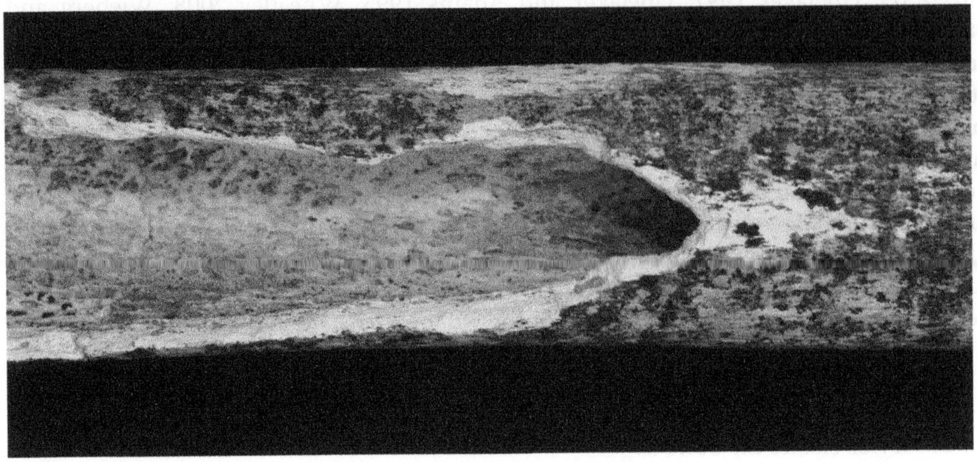

Figure 23.2 Post-mortem breakage to a dry human femur. The fracture is characteristic of dry bone fractures: the fracture edges are irregular and jagged and lighter in colour than the darker adjacent tissue.

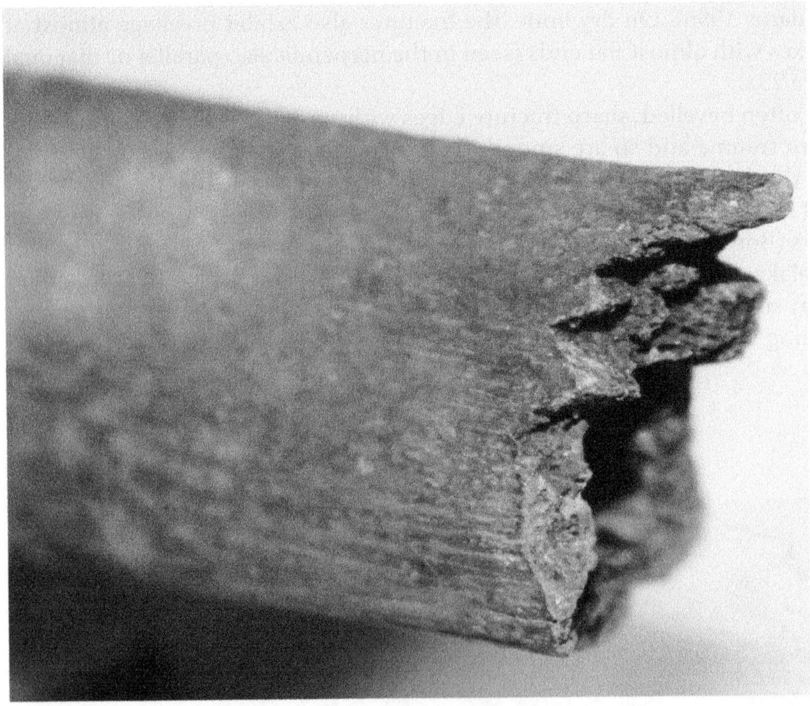

Figure 23.3 Human tibia fracture: the bevelled, sharp and smooth edges together with the acute and obtuse fracture angles as well as the homogeneous colour are strong indicators that suggest a peri-mortem trauma.

Table 23.1 Morphological comparison between fresh and dry bone features according to the literature (Johnson 1985; Wieberg and Wescott 2008)

Fracture Features	Fresh Bone Characteristics	Dry Bone Characteristics
Outline	Radial pattern circling diaphysis	Perpendicular/horizontal fracture surface
Colour surface	Homogeneous colour with external bone	Heterogeneous colour with external bone
Surface	Smooth	Rough
Fracture angle	Obtuse and acute angles	Right angles
Other	Loading point present	Loading point absent
Other	Fracture front never crosscut epiphyseal ends	Fracture front can crosscut epiphyseal ends

leaf stains and organic matter. In this sense, if the colour is homogenous for both fracture margins and the external bone layer, the fractures could be considered to be peri-mortem, since both have been exposed for the same time to staining materials. On the contrary, the difference in colour of post-mortem trauma is connected to the fact that the fracture occurred a long time after death and so the fracture surface has a different colour (usually lighter) than the adjacent external layer because it was exposed at a later time. The coloration of fracture edges should be used with caution given its very variable nature, which depends on the depositional environment. This caution was also suggested by several authors (Morlan 1984; Moraitis *et al.* 2009; Symes *et al.* 2014; Wieberg and Wescott 2008), who reported an equalisation of colour between fracture margins and external cortical bone, over time.

To explain the differences between peri- and post-mortem trauma in bone, a brief summary is presented in Table 23.1.

Despite the numerous publications on the subject, the criteria for distinguishing between peri- and post-mortem lesions are based on observations of fractures involving long bones or bone elements, characterised by cortical tissue. On the contrary, when considering spongy tissue or bones where the cortical component is not present as a main constituent (Figure 23.4), one should take into account that behaviour of bone fractures may be very different; this specific phenomenon has not yet been investigated.

Furthermore, different contexts can modify the bone tissue properties differently and, as a result, produce diversified responses to the same post-mortem stress, perhaps not easily interpretable. A typical example is burial within a closed environment, such as inhumation in a coffin, where wet conditions and putrefaction fluids derived from decomposition could be retained and thus creating a moist environment, so that the original bone keeps its pseudo-elastic properties for longer. As such, wet environments may produce changes that may mimic peri-mortem bone damage (Calce and Rogers 2007; Moraitis *et al.* 2009; Morlan 1984; Wieberg and Wescott 2008).

Clearly, not only is it macroscopically difficult to verify whether a dry bone fracture was produced in life or not, it is also difficult in specific scenarios to distinguish between peri- versus post-mortem fractures.

23.2.2 Microscopic Analysis as a Potential Support in the Diagnosis of Peri- versus Post-Mortem Trauma

Most studies focus on macroscopic morphological fracture characteristics to differentiate bones, which have been fractured in a fresh state or from those broken in a dry or mineralised state. Very few

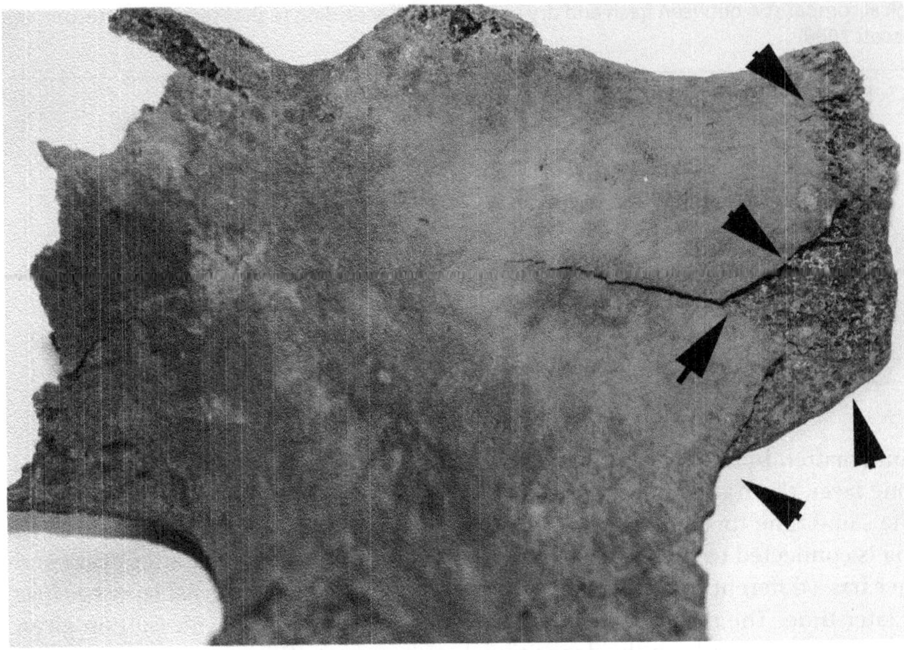

Figure 23.4 A known peri-mortem fracture of the ilium: the morphological appearance of a similar fracture is to all effects more difficult to assess and requires much more caution since it does not respond totally to the parameters suggested for long bones.

scientists examine the microscopic properties of bone fractures in an attempt to describe microscopic pattern differences existing between wet/elastic and dry bones (Hanaue *et al.* 2007; Pechnìkova *et al.* 2011) or other changes linked to taphonomy (Shipman 1981). Pechnìkova *et al.* (2012) studied over 900 osteons (fresh and dry) in which they verified if the fracture line respects the Haversian system structure in fresh bone and passes around it (as opposed to through it). The rationale behind this was that in fresh bone, fractures would follow the lines of least resistance, whereas in dry bone a fracture would randomly cut through a less differentiated structure (Figure 23.5). The results of this study revealed no statistically significant differences in the pattern of osteon fracturing between fresh and dry bone, confirming that osteon fracture pattern cannot help in the diagnosis of peri- versus post-mortem bone fractures. However, this analysis did seem to be useful for distinguishing between high-energy blast and low-energy blunt force trauma on fresh bone (Pechnìkova *et al.* 2012).

When in doubt concerning the peri-mortem nature of a fracture, it may be worth looking for an answer through extrinsic elements, that is, indicators that have nothing to do with bone but may reveal that a tool has been applied on the surface of that specific bone. The fact that tool marks or residues may be found near a fracture can help prove the criminal nature of that lesion. For such cases, scanning electron microscopy with energy dispersive X-ray spectroscopy (SEM-EDX) can be extremely useful to search for metal particles, which can give important evidence in trauma analysis and whose presence has been proven to persist for long-time near bone lesions (Amadasi *et al.* 2012; Berryman *et al.* 2010; Gibelli *et al.* 2012; Pechnìkova *et al.* 2012; Taborelli *et al.* 2012; Vermeij *et al.* 2012). The presence of gunshot, sharp force and blunt force tool residues, could function as markers of 'peri-mortality' if found in a bone lesion of skeletal remains. Additionally, metal residues not only give important evidence with respect to the timing of a fracture/lesion, but they might also provide important information regarding type of trauma and potential tools that might have

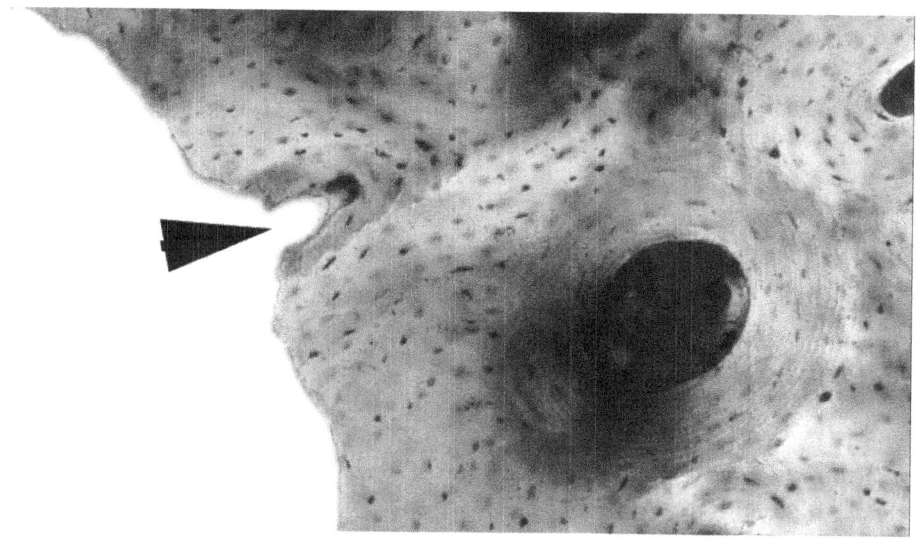

Figure 23.5 A thin undecalcified bone section showing a post-mortem fracture of a tibia. The fracture line, as indicated by the black arrow, passes through a Haversian system. In some other cases, the fracture line respects the Harversian structures and passes around them, showing no significant differences to what happens in fresh bone tissue.

produced the lesion (Figure 23.6) (Amadasi *et al.* 2014; Gibelli *et al.* 2012; Pechnìkova *et al.* 2012). As always, contamination from the environment needs to be taken into consideration and should be excluded before drawing conclusions (Gibelli *et al.* 2012). Of course, residues can be related also to post-mortem criminal activity such as dismemberment; however, the pattern and distribution of the cut or the saw marks is indicative of this kind of action. In conclusion, microscopic analysis of metal particles (light microscopy and SEM) could add important information to the morphological examination. However, caution is required in forensic contexts concerning contamination. It is also important to acknowledge that this approach is not biological proof of the ante-mortem nature of a fracture but only of the application of a tool on the bone.

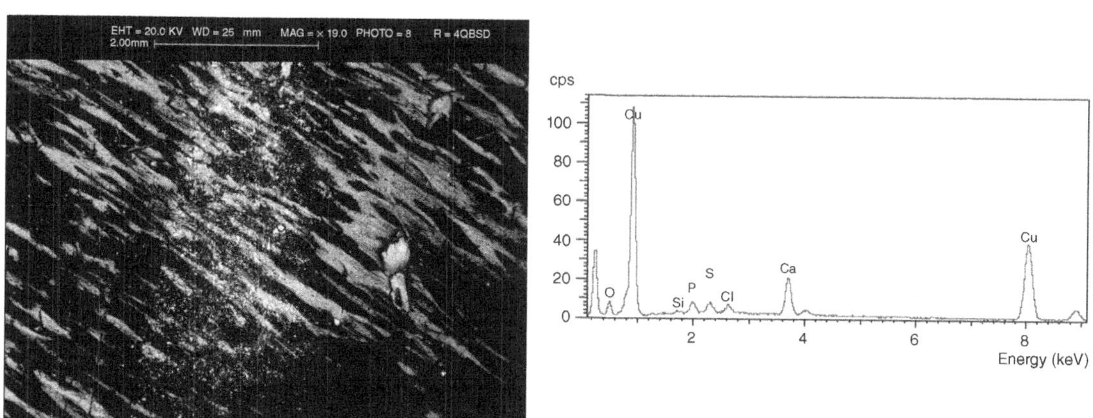

Figure 23.6 Left: A backscattered electron image of some copper (Cu) particles detected on a bone hit with a copper bar (Cu inside). Right: The X-ray spectrum of the particles detected on the same sample.

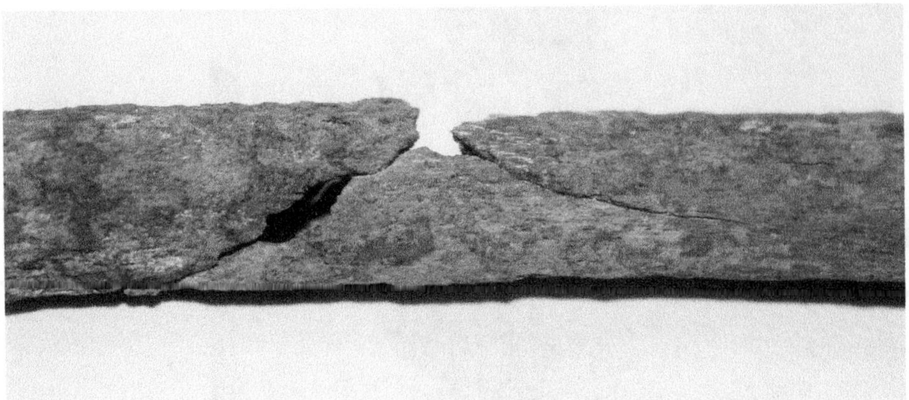

Figure 23.7 An example of a fracture for which the assessment is difficult due to the presence of diverse characteristics, some distinctive of fresh bone fractures, some typical of dry bone.

23.2.3 Problems Concerning Trauma Interpretation: Successful Outcomes and Limits of Current Methods

Within forensic science, it is crucial not to assess a fracture wrongly. If peri-mortem lesions are not diagnosed correctly, the resulting lack of evidence of peri-mortem trauma will hinder the detection of lethal events and vital trauma. Despite many publications, which report results on the differentiation between peri- and post-mortem trauma based on macro-morphological parameters, for example differences in colour, angle, morphology of fracture margins and in fracture outline, there is little research that observes the real reliability and effectiveness of these criteria. As mentioned previously, this is due particularly to the lack of research on known peri- and post-mortem osteological material on which one can conduct similar assessments. Two studies (Cappella *et al.* 2014a,b) on a known skeletal collection (the Milano skeletal collection) have focused on the evaluation of correct or incorrect interpretation of known peri- and post-mortem trauma in bones, based on the standard criteria used, as described in the previous paragraphs. The studies aimed at detecting limits, repeatability and problems in interpreting trauma potentially related to cause and manner of death. The availability of skeletal remains with known peri- and post-mortem trauma, as well as the known causes of death, allowed the authors to conduct a study concerning the role of taphonomy in altering or transforming peri-mortem lesions correlated with death. Clearly, the interference of environmental taphonomic factors may contribute to pre-existing lesions by altering them or create new skeletal damage and fractures, an aspect that makes it harder for anthropologists to correctly assess trauma (Figure 23.7).

The first study (Cappella *et al.* 2014a) focused on macro-morphologic trauma analysis and was performed on several skeletons for which the cause of violent death was known and from which autopsy reports with a description of the bone lesions were available. Upon excavation, more damage to the skeletonised remains had been performed, therefore the skeletons presented known peri- and post-mortem trauma. Observations were carried out in order to verify if and how the diverse types of trauma survive after 15 years of inhumation (and 20 years after death) (Figure 23.8). In this study, the comparison between autopsy findings (fractures on fresh bones) and the anthropological findings on skeletonised remains 20 years later showed important results concerning the persistence of some specific lesions, which can lead to a correct interpretation of trauma. This work also highlights the role of taphonomy in complicating the interpretation of trauma by hiding important peri-mortem

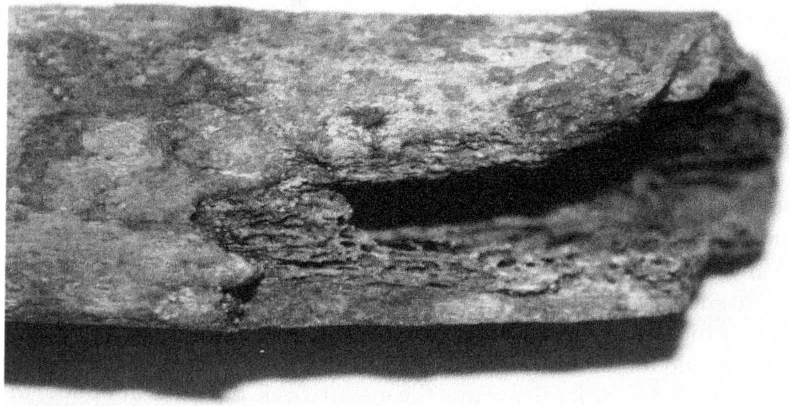

Figure 23.8 An example of the appearance of a fracture observed at autopsy (after 20 years of inhumation). The fracture still shows characteristics of peri-mortem trauma. However, some features are transformed by the taphonomic effects, which render evaluation more difficult especially when spongy bones have to be considered.

features and adding a consistent number of new post-mortem alteration/fractures, which often alter pre-existing peri-mortem lesions, particularly regarding blunt force trauma.

The study revealed that gunshot and sharp force lesions do not change considerably and remain highly specific, even though similar lesions caused by taphonomic events can be found and may result in being easily misinterpreted at anthropological analysis. On the other hand, blunt force trauma was clearly more altered by taphonomy. An additional study by Capella *et al.* (2014b) investigated the latter in more detail and concentrated on blunt force trauma, one of the most challenging lesions whose assessment appeared to be extremely difficult in the previous study. The aim was to verify the validity and reliability of the macro-morphologic parameter on a consistent number of fractures (over 200) of known origin from skeletons selected from the Milano skeletal collection. This research was carried out with the intent of highlighting the limits of these common criteria, which proved to be unsatisfactory and difficult to apply to cancellous/spongy bone. The results showed that the application of the criteria described in the previous paragraphs, applied to over 200 fractures of known origin by two experienced anthropologists, was a partial failure. It illustrated a high number of errors (inter- and as well as intra-observer errors) as well as incorrect interpretations on the type of trauma (peri- or post-mortem), in particular, but not only, on spongy bone.

Both studies highlight the difficulty and problems that lie behind 'fracture timing', especially for fractures that occur on spongy bone which displays a thin cortical surface; the structural differences between long bones and flat or short bones (such as pelvic bone, vertebrae, ribs, etc.) may play a crucial role in exhibiting specific morphological features in the case of injury as well as with taphonomical effects. Considering that the distinction between peri- and post-mortem fractures is based solely on macro-morphologic parameters and that these last ones have been mainly established on the characteristics observed in cortical tissue of long bone, it appears evident that we need to developed new models and parameters for assessing peri- and post-mortem trauma.

23.3 Alternative Solutions for Distinguishing Between Peri- and Post-Mortem Trauma on Bone

Clearly, there is a need to focus on further fundamental parameters and markers, until the interpretation of skeletal lesions becomes clear. Since the parameters commonly used in anthropology are essentially based on morphological characteristics and of dubious utility in some circumstances, it is clear that there is a need for different criteria such as biological markers, to distinguish between ante- or post-mortem trauma. Therefore anthropology has to adopt certain methods of pathology. This can only be achieved through the search for traces of vitality from the fracture, for example haemorrhaging and markers of inflammation. The use of such additional indicators is fundamental (Cattaneo *et al.* 2010; Clark 1996; Kondo and Ishida 2010; Kondo *et al.* 2002; Madea *et al.* 2010; Oehmichen 2004; Singer and Clark 1999). Cattaneo *et al.* (2010) have shown that microscopic residues of soft tissue do remain in bone, which may indicate the presence of an inflammatory reaction and therefore that the fracture was vital (e.g. fibrin and red blood cell clots). In their pilot study, the fracture margins of macerated bone (fresh bone treated in order to assume the macroscopic aspect of dry bone) of individuals who died from a trauma at known times (ranging from 10 min to 60 days) were observed microscopically. Although soft tissue was no longer visible on the bone, signs of inflammation and bone repair could clearly still be seen with histochemical and immunohistochemical techniques. Further research needs to be performed, in parallel with novel proteomic techniques, in order to investigate the potential of biochemical markers. However, the search for biomarkers indicating a vital reaction in decomposed and osseous material is an ambitious goal. Very little is known about the taphonomy of microscopic blood cells and bone elements. For example, how often can the presence of well-defined red blood cells in tissue be reliably detected? In other words, can blood or bone cells, if not well preserved, be mistaken for something else or vice versa? How long do these elements survive microscopically? Clearly, microscopic taphonomy and taphonomy of biological markers and cells are disciplines that are in the initial stages: the bases have still to be set.

23.3.1 Blood as a *Biomarker* of Vitality in Peri-Mortem Skeletal Lesions and the Survival of Red Blood Cells in Bone

The use of biomarkers might be a possible aid in the diagnosis of the timing of lesions, and as a subject is closely related to the estimation of survival time for ante-mortem lesions. The detection of specific biomarkers such as the blood components and the inflammatory mediators/proteins with advanced techniques could give information concerning vital reaction in a lesion, first and foremost in terms of timing of survival: haemorrhage, blood extravasation and infiltration, haematoma formation and haemostatic clots are all signs which could help to distinguish a vital and therefore ante-mortem lesion from a post-mortem one, especially with reference to the concept of vitality. Although many studies have clarified the haemorrhage phases, the coagulation cascade and the healing process from a physiological and timing point of view (Clark 1996; Hernandez-Cueto *et al.* 2000; Kondo and Ishida 2010; Kondo *et al.* 2002; Madea *et al.* 2010; Raekallio 1976; Singer and Clark 1999), these elements have never been explored and verified in bone lesions of decomposed corpses and skeletal remains.

A study by Cappella *et al.* (2015a) was performed on the decomposition of red blood cells (erythrocytes) in decomposing human cadaver blood. Isolated cells of the blood were monitored at different times of decomposition using SEM in order to discover and identify all possible morphological changes acquired by erythrocytes during decomposition. To facilitate their correct identification, it was important to avoid possible mistakes that could derive from the presence of similar contaminants from the natural environment, in particular botanical structures. In the literature, it is often assumed that the detection of erythrocyte-like cells on skeletal remains (even ancient) demonstrates

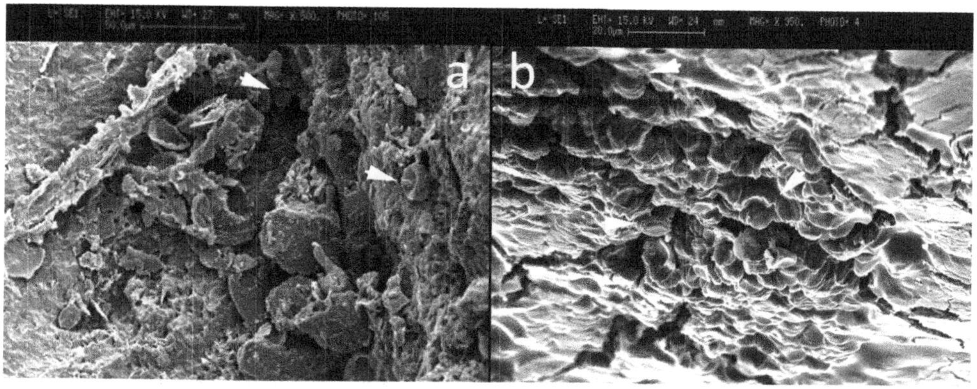

Figure 23.9 (a) SEM analysis of erythrocyte-like structures (arrows) in a fracture margin of skeletal remains; the interpretation of these structures becomes very difficult and botanic/mycological contamination needs to be considered. (b) Erythrocytes visible by SEM in an archaeological bone artificially dipped in human fresh blood.

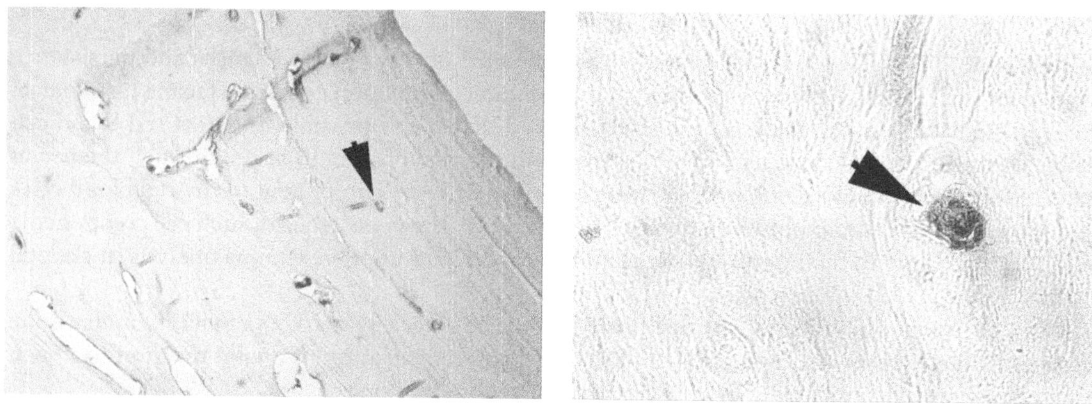

(a) (b)

Figure 23.10 Immunohistochemical analysis, which uses antibody anti-Human Glicophorin A in detecting residues from erythrocytes even when these are highly degraded (after 2 months of decomposition in air): the Glicophorin A protein persists longer in decomposing bone tissue. The brownish coloration (as indicated by the black arrows) suggests the persistence of such residues (confirming their own origin), which are useful indicators of blood.

the presence of erythrocytes (Charlier *et al.* 2008; Maat 1991; Melki *et al.* 2011; Setzer *et al.* 2013). It is not often taken into consideration that the origin may be different from blood (Charlier *et al.* 2008; Melki *et al.* 2011; Schweitzer *et al.* 2007; Setzer *et al.* 2013). It is very easy to confuse erythrocytes with botanical elements, such as spores and pollens derived from contamination (Figure 23.9).

Cappella *et al.* (2015b) showed that although there are diagnostic features useful in identifying red blood cells from botanical structures, some spores are very similar to decaying red blood cells. In addition, further interesting questions emerged, for example – what happens to red blood cells in decomposing bone tissue and how can they be visualised through light microscopy? Do red blood cells remain present in skeletal remains? And finally, if erythrocytes are no longer recognisable by morphology because of their deterioration, could they still be detected by using more sensitive techniques like immunohistochemistry?

In another study, changes of blood components, namely erythrocytes, within decomposing cortical and trabecular bone were monitored with light microscopy during decomposition (Figure 23.10)

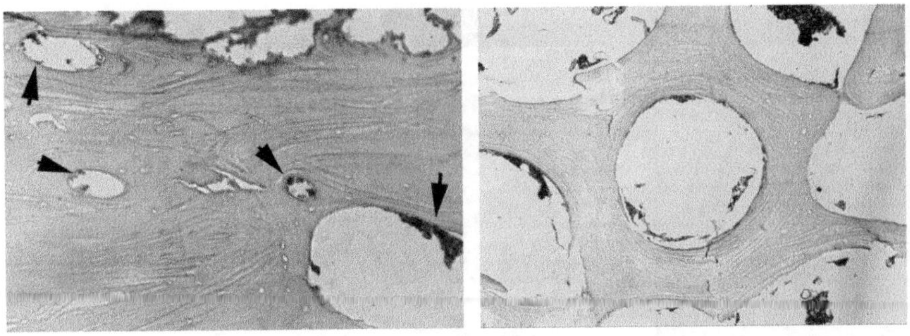

(a) (b)

Figure 23.11 In cemetery skeletal remains (inhumed for 15 years) it is still possible to identify blood residues thanks to the sensitive immunohistochemical techniques. This technique demonstrates the presence of erithrocytic residues in some Haversian canals and in bone marrow spaces. If degraded erythrocytes are no longer detectable morphologically, they can still be identified by such techniques, as can the presence of haematomas or blood clots or similar biomarkers, which could still be traceable after so many years in fracture margins.

(Capella *et al.* 2015b). The aim of this study was a detailed observation of changes and persistence of red blood cell components over time and in different decomposition conditions using histological and immunohistochemical analysis. The study showed that it was possible to detect red blood cell residues, even in skeletal remains with a post-mortem interval of over 15 years, through the use of sensitive techniques such as looking for Glycophorin A (GLYA, a component of the red blood cell's membrane) through immunohistochemistry (Figure 23.11). The persistence of such cell components could play a key role in the interpretation of trauma and could improve trauma analysis in skeletal remains (Figure 23.12).

Clearly, the above studies show the need for methods of detecting markers of vitality in dry bone fractures. To date, based on experience of real cases, a demonstration of a vital reaction has been obtained on decomposed skin by the authors but not yet on dry bone.

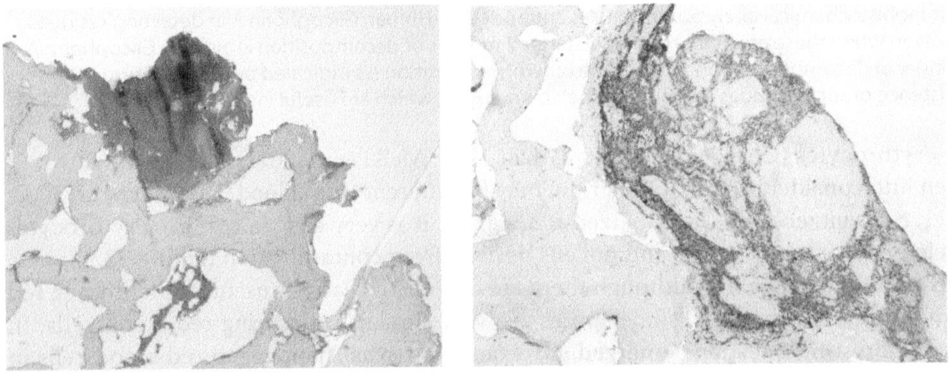

(a) (b)

Figure 23.12 In (a) a clot composed of blood materials (erythrocytes and platelets) was visible in the thin bone section obtained from a fracture margin of a vital skull fracture (40X magnification). The survival time of the individual (3 hours) was sufficient for the appearance of signs of vitality, e.g. the clot. In (b) a higher magnification (200X) of the same clot stained by anti-Glycophorin A antibody, which made it possible to prove the haematic nature of such material.

23.4 Conclusion

The timing of a bone lesion with respect to death requires a high degree of certainty. The current status of anthropological knowledge applying macroscopic methods does not allow for such precision. Detecting biomarkers as specific indicators of vitality and survival to an injury, could enable us to solve the common problems encountered in the interpretation of ante-, peri- and post-mortem injuries due to the absence of perceptible bone signs at a macroscopical, microscopical and radiographical level (Cattaneo *et al.* 2010). In order to do this, it is fundamental to study how cellular and biochemical markers react to time and taphonomy. The presence of inflammation markers, and therefore the presence and persistence of soft tissue and biomolecular elements, must become the future of forensic anthropology. Only in-depth knowledge of blood component taphonomy and of taphonomic models related to the decomposing bone tissue at different stages, will lead the correct way of interpreting trauma in bones.

References

Amadasi, A., Brandone, A., Rizzi, A., Mazzarelli, D. and Cattaneo, C. (2012) The survival of metallic residues from gunshot wounds in cremated bone: a SEM-EDX study. *International Journal of Legal Medicine*, **126**: 525–531.

Amadasi, A., Gibelli, D., Mazzarelli, D., Porta, D., Gaudio, D. *et al.* (2014) Assets and pitfalls of chemical and microscopic analysis on gunshot residues in skeletonized bodies: a report of five cases. *International Journal of Legal Medicine*, **129**: 819–824.

Berryman, H.E., Kutyla, A.K. and Russell, D.J. (2010) Detection of gunshot primer residues on bone in an experimental setting-an unexpected finding. *Journal of Forensic Science*, **55**: 488–491.

Bonnichsen, R. (1979) Pleistocene bone technology in the Beringian Refugium. *Archaeological Survey of Canada*, **89**: 1–280.

Calce, S.E. and Rogers, T.L. (2007) Taphonomic changes to blunt force trauma: a preliminary study. *Journal of Forensic Science*, **52**: 519–527.

Cappella, A., Amadasi, A., Castoldi, E., Mazzarelli, D., Gaudio, D. and Cattaneo, C. (2014a) The difficult task of assessing perimortem and post-mortem fractures on the skeleton: a blind test on 210 fractures of known origin. *Journal of Forensic Science*, **59**: 1598–1601.

Cappella, A., Castoldi, E., Sforza, C. and Cattaneo, C. (2014b) An osteological revisitation of autopsies: comparing anthropological findings in exhumed skeletons to their respective autopsy reports in seven cases. *Forensic Science International*, **244**: 315.e1–10.

Cappella, A., Stefanelli, S., Caccianiga, M., Rizzi, A., Bertoglio, B., Sforza, C. and Cattaneo, C. (2015a) Blood or spores? A cautionary note on interpreting cellular debris on human skeletal remains. *International Journal of Legal Medicine*, **129**: 919–926.

Cappella, A., Bertoglio, B., Castoldi, E., Maderna, E., Di Giancamillo, A., *et al.* (2015b) The taphonomy of blood components in decomposing bone and its relevance to physical anthropology. *American Journal of Physical Anthropology.* **158**: 636–645.

Cattaneo, C., Andreola, S., Marinelli, E., Poppa, P., Porta, D. and Grandi, M. (2010) The detection of microscopic markers of hemorrhaging and wound age on dry bone. *The American Journal of Forensic Medicine & Pathology*, **31**: 22–26.

Charlier, P., Georges, P., Bouchet, F., Huynn-Charlier, I., Carlier, R. *et al.* (2008) The microscopic (optical and SEM) examination of putrefaction fluid deposits (PFD). Potential interest in forensic anthropology. *Virchows Archive*, **453**: 377–386.

Clark, R.A.F. (1996) *The Molecular and Cellular Biology of Wound Repair*. Plenum Press: New York.

Dirkmaat, D.C., Cabo, L.L., Ousley, S.D. and Symes, S.A. (2008) New perspectives in forensic anthropology. *American Journal of Physical Anthropology*, **51**: 33–52.
Dirkmaat, D.C. (2012) *A Companion to Forensic Anthropology*. Wiley-Blackwell: Chichester, UK.
Evans, F.G. (1957) Stress and Strain in Bones. *Charles C.* Thomas: Springfield.
Galloway, A., Symes, S.A., Haglund, W.D. and France, D.L. (1999) The role of forensic anthropology in trauma analysis. In: Galloway, A. (ed.), *Broken Bones: Anthropological analysis of blunt force trauma*. Charles C. Thomas: Springfield, pp. 5–31.
Galloway, A. (1999) The biomechanics of fracture production. In: Galloway, A. (ed.), *Broken Bones: Anthropological analysis of blunt force trauma*. Charles C. Thomas: Springfield, pp. 35–62.
Gibelli, D., Mazzarelli, D., Porta, D., Rizzi, A. and Cattaneo, C. (2012) Detection of metal residues on bone using SEM-EDS-Part II: Sharp force injury. *Forensic Science International*, **223**: 91–96.
Hanaue, K., Katakura, A., Kasahara, K., Kamiyama, I., Takaki, T. *et al.* (2007) Course of fracture line in sagittal splitting of human mandible. *The Bulletin of Tokyo Dental College*, **48**: 163–170.
Harkess, J.W., Ramsey, W.C. and Harkess, J.W. (1996) Principles of fractures and dislocations. In: Rockwood, C.A. Jr., and Green, D.P. (eds), *Fractures in Adults*. Lippincott Company: Philadelphia, p. 48.
Hart, G.O. (2005) Fracture pattern interpretation in the skull: differentiating blunt force from ballistics trauma using concentric fractures. *Journal of Forensic Science*, **50**: 1276–1281.
Hernandez-Cueto, C., Girela, E. and Sweet, D. (2000) *Advances in the Diagnosis on Wound Vitality: A review*. Lippincott Williams & Wilkins: Philadelphia, pp. 21–31.
Johnson, E. (1985) Current developments in bone technology. *Advance Archaeological Method & Theory*, **8**: 157–235.
Karr, L.P. and Outram, A.K. (2012a) Bone degradation and environment: understanding, assessing and conducting archeological experiments using modern animal bones. *International Journal of Osteoarchaeology*, **25**: 201–212.
Karr, L.P. and Outram, A.K. (2012b) Tracking changes in bone fracture morphology over time environment, taphonomy and the archaeological record. *Journal of Archaeological Science*, **39**: 555–559.
Kondo, T., Ohshima, T., Mori, R., Guan, D.W. and Ohsima, K. (2002) Immunohistochemical detection of chemokines in human skin wounds and its application to wound age determination. *International Journal of Legal Medicine*, **116**: 87–91.
Kondo, T. and Ishida, Y (2010) Molecular pathology of wound healing. *Forensic Science International*, **203**: 93–98.
La Croix, M.N. (2013) *A Study of the Impact on Weathering upon The Minimal Force Required to Fracture Bone*. Unpublished MSc Thesis. Boston University: Boston.
Maat, G.J.R. (1991) Ultrastructure of normal and pathological fossilized red blood cells compared with pseudopathological biological structures. *International Journal of Osteoarchaeology*, **3**: 209–214.
Madea, B., Saukko, P., Oliva, A. and Musshoff, F. (2010) Molecular pathology in forensic medicine. Introduction. *Forensic Science International*, **203**: 3–14.
Maples, W. (1986) Trauma analysis by the forensic anthropologist. In: Reichs, K.J. (ed.), *Forensic Osteology: Advances in the identification of human remains*. Charles C. Thomas: Springfield, pp. 218–228.
Melki, J.A.D., Martin, C.C.S. and Zerbini, T. (2011) Scanning electron microscopy as an auxiliary method in the study of exhumed bones. *Forensic Science International*, **206**: e67–e70.
Moraitis, K. and Spiliopoulou, C. (2006) Review: identification and differential diagnosis of perimortem blunt force trauma in tubular long bones. *Forensic Science, Medicine & Pathology*, **2**: 221–229.
Moraitis, K., Eliopoulos, C. and Spiliopoulou, C. (2009) Fracture characteristics of perimortem trauma in skeletal material. *The Internet Journal of Biological Anthropology*, **3**: http://ispub.com/IJBA/3/2/11380 (Accessed 15 September 2015).

Morlan, R.E. (1984) Toward the definition of criteria for the recognition of artificial bone alterations. *Quaternary Research*, **22**: 160–171.

Oehmichen, M. (2004) Vitality and time course of wounds. *Forensic Science International*, **144**: 2–3.

Pechnìkova, M., Porta, D. and Cattaneo, C. (2011) Distinguishing between perimortem and postmortem fractures: are osteons of any help? *International Journal of Legal Medicine*, **125**: 591–595.

Pechnìkova, M., Porta, D., Mazzarelli, D., Rizzi, A., Drozdova, E. *et al.* (2012) Detection of metal residues on bone using SEM-EDS. Part I: Blunt force injury. *Forensic Science International*, **223**: 87–90.

Passalacqua, N.V. and Rainwater, C.W. (2015) *Skeletal Trauma Analysis: Case studies in context.* Wiley-Blackwell, John Wiley & Sons: Chichester, UK.

Quatrehomme, G. and Alunni, V. (2013) Bone trauma. In: Siegel, J. and Saukko, P. (eds), *Encyclopedia of Forensic Science.* Elsevier Science & Technology: Amsterdam, pp. 89–96.

Raekallio, J. (1976) Timing of wounds in forensic medicine. *The Japanese Journal of Legal Medicine*, **30**: 125–136.

Sauer, N.J. (1998) The timing of injuries and manner of death: distinguishing among antemortem, perimortem and postmortem trauma. In: Reichs, K.J. (ed.), *Forensic Osteology: Advances in the identification of human remains.* Charles C. Thomas: Springfield, pp. 321–332.

Schweitzer, M.H., Wittmeyer, J.L. and Horner, J.R. (2007) Soft tissue and cellular preservation in vertebrate skeletal elements from the Cretaceous to the present. *Proceedings of the Royal Society B*, **274**: 183–197.

Setzer, T.J., Sundell, I.B., Dibbley, S.K. and Les, C. (2013) Technical note: a histological technique for detecting the cryptic preservation of erythrocytes and soft tissue in ancient human skeletonized remains. *American Journal of Physical Anthropology*, **152**: 566–568.

Shipman, P. (1981) Applications of scanning electron microscopy to taphonomic problems. *Annals of the New York Academy of Sciences*, **276**: 357–385.

Singer, A.J. and Clark, R.A. (1999) Cutaneous wound healing. *New England Journal of Medicine*, **347**: 738–746.

Symes, S.A., Berryman, H.E. and Smith, O.C. (1998) Saw marks in bone: introduction and examination of residual kerf contours. In: Reichs, K.J. (ed.), *Forensic Osteology: Advances in the identification of human remains.* Charles C. Thomas Publisher LTD: Springfield, pp. 389–409.

Symes, S.A., L'Abbe, É.N., Chapman, E.N., Wolff, I. and Dirkmaat, D.C. (2012) Interpreting traumatic injury to bone in medicolegal investigations. In: Dirkmaat, D.C. (ed.), *A Companion to Forensic Anthropology.* Wiley-Blackwell: Chichester, UK, pp. 340–389.

Symes, S.A., L'abbé, E.N., Stull, K.E., Lacroix, M. and Pokines, J.T. (2014) Taphonomy and the timing of bone fractures in trauma analysis. In: Pokines, J.T. and Symes, S.A. (eds), *Manual of Forensic Taphonomy.* CRC Press: Boca Raton, pp. 341–365.

Taborelli, A., Gibelli, D., Rizzi, A., Andreola, S, Brandone, A. and Cattaneo, C. (2012) Gunshot residues on dry bone after decomposition: a pilot study. *Journal of Forensic Science*, **57**: 1281–1284.

Ubelaker, D,H, (1991) Perimortem and postmortem modification of human bone. Lessons from forensic anthropology. *Anthropologie (Brno)*, **29**: 171–174.

Ubelaker, D.H. and Adams, B.J. (1995) Differentiation of perimortem and postmortem trauma using taphonomic indicators. *Journal of Forensic Science*, **40**: 509–512.

Ubelaker, D.H. (1997) Taphonomic applications in forensic anthropology. In: Haglund, W.D. and Sorg, M.H. (eds), *Forensic Taphonomy: The postmortem fate of human remains.* CRC Press: Boca Raton, pp. 77–90.

Vermeij, E.J., Zoon, P.D., Chang, S.B., Keereweer, I., Pieterman, R. and Gerretsen, R.R (2012) Analysis of microtraces in invasive traumas using SEM/EDS. *Forensic Science International*, **214**: 96–104.

Villa, P. and Mahieu, E. (1991) Breakage patterns of human long bones. *Journal Human Evolution*, **21**: 27–48.

Wheatley, B. (2008) Perimortem or postmortem bone fractures? An experimental study of fracture patterns in deer femora. *Journal of Forensic Science*, **53**: 69–72.
Wieberg, D.A.M. and Wescott, D.J. (2008) Estimating the timing of long bone fractures: correlation between the postmortem interval, bone moisture con- tent, and blunt force trauma characteristics. *Journal of Forensic Science*, **53**: 1028–1034.

24

Collection Care and Management of Human Remains

Rebecca C. Redfern and Jelena J. Bekvalac

24.1 Introduction

Taphonomy is a process that continues after the recovery of human remains. Many archaeologists regard the deposition of material within an archive or a curating institution as the end of the post-excavation journey. The holding of collections by institutions is often viewed as a process, which has minimal risk; one, which compared to the 'real world', is safe and secure. However, museological and taphonomic research has shown that this is not the case. Taphonomy is a constant action and institutions often have unique environments, with their own risks and processes. This chapter focuses on aspects of collection care and management of human remains that can have significant impacts on (forensic) anthropological research. It is concerned with the origin of collections, documentation issues, collection care strategies and conservation actions, and how these can impact on the human remains held for research.

24.2 Collection Origin and Deposition

Institutions across the world are responsible for the curation of many hundreds of thousands of human remains. The research potential and value of these remains, beyond the evidence for the individual, is dictated by their origin and mode of deposition. These two factors are explored below, focusing on the origin of many British collections and international case studies.

In Britain, the development of commercial archaeology in the early 1990s and the introduction of planning legislation (Schofield *et al.* 2011) has meant that for many archives, the majority of their holdings have been professionally excavated and are supported by a comprehensive site archive, providing that which Stodder (2008) has described as the 'critical link' between excavation and analysis. Simply put, there is documentation to record what has happened to the human remains and their associated artefacts, from their burial location to box in the archive. Within many countries in Europe, archaeological material is typically held by local or nationally funded government institutions, and organised at town/city and regional level. These institutions range from local history centres, museums or huge warehouses. Their staff maintains and curates all of the artefacts, finds, paper and digital records about the site and any specialist reports generated by or related to that excavation, such as carbon 14 dating information. These resources are accessible to researchers but also to the general public, under the governance of a member of staff.

Commercial archaeology differs significantly from research-led excavations, to the extent that it is often referred to as developer-led archaeology. In this context, only the council planners, site owners

Taphonomy of Human Remains: Forensic Analysis of the Dead and the Depositional Environment, First Edition.
Edited by Eline M.J. Schotsmans, Nicholas Márquez-Grant and Shari L. Forbes.

and developers dictate where excavations will take place, and in Britain this is increasingly tied to the re-development of Victorian-built areas of cities and major infrastructure projects (e.g. highways). Although this has created an urban bias in sample origin, projects such as Crossrail and Eurotunnel have enabled excavations in areas, which have never been excavated or have only been subject to small-scale investigations. For example, Charterhouse in London (Sutton's hospital at Charterhouse) was founded in the medieval period, but its building and grounds had never been subject to large-scale excavations until recently, when excavations preceding Crossrail construction work uncovered part of a 14th-century Black Death cemetery (Crossrail 2013).

A smaller number of archaeological collections may be deposited with a local or regional archive, subsequent to excavations undertaken by community projects or local archaeological groups, individual finders (Portable Antiquities Scheme 2014) and in London, from specific projects aimed at examining the history of the River Thames and foreshore (Thames Discovery Programme 2014). These should have sufficient documentation to allow an assemblage history to be accurately recorded; there are also cases where holdings are transferred to another institution or sold, and such actions are governed by professional standards (Museums Association 2008).

From a forensic perspective, some of the most interesting holdings in Britain are skeletal collections, which are of known age-at-death and sex and are typically post-medieval in date (16th to 19th centuries AD). Research based on early modern human remains can improve age-at-death and sex estimation methods (Cardoso *et al.* 2014). The majority of these excavations are in response to urban renewal projects (Adams *et al.* 2006; English Heritage 2011; McKinley 2008), and these samples are providing a wealth of new research opportunities, because in many cases there is very good preservation of organic remains and coffin furniture (Wilson *et al.* 2013). In turn, this has developed research into the social aspects of death and funerary rites in these periods (Tarlow 1998, 2011). This information has been found to be very useful when establishing whether single burials in non-normative locations, such as in boundary ditches or estuary islands, are early modern or in fact more recent in date. In many cases, following analysis, post-medieval samples are re-buried according to the conditions set out in the burial licence (Ministry of Justice 2015), according to the Burial Act 1857 and Disused Burial Grounds (Amendment) Act 1981. However, the data are deposited and available for future research (Boston *et al.* 2009; Miles *et al.* 2008; Wilson *et al.* 2013). Nevertheless, the frequently negative impact of differences in excavation techniques and recording methods cannot be forgotten, such as some pathologies not being photographed or only a limited suite of measurements being recorded. Nonetheless, licences issued by the Ministry of Justice frequently allow for many known individuals to be kept for research (Cowie *et al.* 2008; Henderson *et al.* 2013).

The majority of excavated individuals are anonymous, because the overwhelming majority of excavations have taken place either at cemeteries where the funerary rites did not involve a method of commemoration that has survived to the present day, or else in time periods where coffin plates were not used in funerary practices, or were very expensive (Mahoney-Swales *et al.* 2011; Tarlow 2011). Nevertheless, contextual information supplied through excavation has meant that in a few cases, the identity of some individuals has been established through the use of burial records and cemetery plans. Typically though, where present and legible, coffin plates are used to assign identity. The rise in popularity of family history has also enabled the lives of a few individuals to be established in more detail. For example, Mrs Milborough Maxwell was excavated from Chelsea Old Church in 2000 and is curated by the Museum of London (MoL). Subsequently, she was included in a stable isotope mobility study and found to be non-local, probably from the Caribbean (Trickett 2006). Mrs Maxwell was included in the 'Skeletons. London's buried bones' collaborative exhibition curated by the Wellcome Trust and MoL (2008). After the exhibition, a descendent of Mrs Maxwell contacted the Museum to visit her remains again, and provided a wealth of information about her life, including documentation showing that she had spent most of her life in Jamaica.

The burial environment of crypts permits the excellent preservation of coffins and coffin furniture (Cox 2001; Association of Diocesan and Cathedral Archaeologists 2010), and individuals from these internments are more likely to be identified compared to their lower-status counterparts, because of the greater use of coffin plates by this status group and burial records kept by each church. To date, only two 18th- and 19th-century crypt populations are curated in Britain, both from London: the population from St Bride's Church, revealed after the church was bombed in the Second World War (MoL curates them *in situ*); and the population excavated from Christ Church, Spitalfields, curated by the Natural History Museum (NHM) under a faculty licence (Cox 1996, 1997). In both populations, a large proportion of the individuals have been identified by their coffin plates, and extensive work has been undertaken to establish their life histories using wills, death certificates (est. 1837) and parish records.

A number of British, European and North American natural history and medical museums curate collections of known and anonymous individuals, who died within the last 300 years. These were assembled through the donation or acquisition of bodies/skeletons to the individual museums, either from medical sources or by the excavation of more recent burial grounds, such as the Portuguese 'Old Lisbon Collection' (1805–1975) (Cardoso 2006) and the sample held by the Universitat Autònoma de Barcelona in Spain (Rissech and Steadman 2011). Some museums held or continue to hold remains, whose acquisition is contested, particularly the remains of indigenous peoples, institutionalised, socio-economically and politically disenfranchised individuals (Bauer-Clapp and Pérez 2014; Fforde *et al.* 2002; Turner 2005) (see also: de la Cova 2012). Changes in museum practice have meant that in many cases, these individuals have been repatriated and/or reburied (Clegg *et al.* 2013). The ethics of whether these individuals should be retained, because their study is argued to be invaluable, is an issue that should not be shied away from by those wishing to study their remains. For example, in 18th-century England, Charles Byrne – the Irish Giant – did his utmost to prevent his body being anatomised by John Hunter, but Hunter was successful and included Byrne's skeleton and casts of his body parts in his anatomical collection, which was later acquired by the Royal College of Surgeons (London); Byrne's continued curation and display is contested (Doyal and Muinzer 2011; Muinzer 2013).

24.3 Collection Management

24.3.1 Documentation

Documentation is essential in order to curate and research a collection. It is central to museum life and also a professional standard, 'documentation should include a full identification and description of each item, its associations, provenance, condition, treatment and present location' (International Council of Museums 2006). Documentation strategies vary considerably, reflecting not only the different sizes of various institutions, but also their staff capacity and resources, particularly when it comes to human remains (Giesen *et al.* 2013). No documentation system will be error-free and with the development of separate curatorial and collection manager roles, often the provenance and history of an object is not investigated, because greater emphasis is placed on research, and its physical care and documentation in the present, rather than what happened to it in the past (Mulkerin 2013). Standards of record keeping are also impacted by the greater reliance of data inputting by volunteers and web-based crowd-sourcing projects, particularly as curatorial and documentation officer roles are being cut due to budget constraints. With all of these issues affecting documentation, it is often necessary to return to the original documentation, which recorded the material's accession to the museum, but also to investigate the donor or collector, and to verify all information pertaining to the remains (Clegg 2009; Mulkerin 2013).

Returning human remains to their place of origin, repatriation, is a highly complex and emotive endeavour, and has fundamentally changed museum practice and professional attitudes both in North America, Britain and Australasia (amongst others, Cassman *et al.*, 2007; Fforde *et al.* 2002; Clegg *et al.* 2013; Giesen 2013; Kakaliouras 2012; Tayles 2009; Turner 2005; Walker 2008). This legal process first began in the USA in 1990 with the implementation of the Native American Grave Protection and Repatriation Act (1990, Amended) (NAGPRA), which created a legislative framework to enable institutions and federally recognised First Nation communities to work together to repatriate human remains and cultural objects; this Act has been amended over time to better serve its relevant parties. Until this Act came into law, supported in the UK by the Department of Culture, Media and Sports' (2005) Guidelines for the Care of Human Remains in Museums, institutions were in many cases unable to repatriate holdings because of the legislative Acts governing their institution. Furthermore, the return of human remains to indigenous communities was not a process that had been considered to be part of Western museum practice. Nevertheless, this process facilitated the opportunity for institutions to verify their holdings, and to confirm if documentation was correct. Such tasks have highlighted the perils of repatriating human remains without involving a physical anthropologist, because of inconsistencies in both the documentation and human remains (Clegg and Bonney 2010). Ousley (2001) provides an example from the Smithsonian Institution (Washington, DC). In 1870, an incomplete cranium was collected by a US Army doctor and donated to the Army Medical Museum. The remains were transferred to the Smithsonian Institution in 1898, and the original documentation stated that this entry was the skull of a Kiowa Indian, killed while trying to steal a horse. Re-examination of the remains found that they were an adolescent who had suffered massive blunt force trauma to their head and face. The ancestry was established as being white. In reality, this Native American may well have been a European child who had been rescued or captured by the Kiowa people and brought up as a member of their community (Ousley 2001). This case shows the importance of verifying and questioning extant records but also having a holistic approach to identity, particularly during this period of American history (Knudson and Stojanowski 2009; Ousley 2001).

The need to rigorously investigate all extant documentation, because of potential errors generated by transcription and the transfer of holdings, is exemplified by a case published by the NHM (Clegg 2009). Work on a repatriation claim for Aboriginal Australians from Tasmania, identified one individual who had very clear discrepancies in their documentation. The remains in question had originally been part of the Royal Army Medical Corps collection in the early 19th century. They were then transferred to Oxford University where a catalogue had been written in 1880, before the collection was finally accessioned to the NHM some years later. The NHM database and index card stated that the skull was of an adult Aboriginal male from Tasmania, but noted that it had been listed in the original 1880 catalogue as being European. Anthropological analysis of the remains demonstrated that the skull was from a robust white adult female. Two months of research in numerous institutions showed that the error had arisen at Oxford University, where the documentation was changed despite the original catalogue entry, showing that the skull derived from a white female convict who had been transported to Australia for manslaughter. As she had died under sentence in 1854, the law allowed her remains to be anatomised. It was very common in the 1800s for military medical personnel stationed outside of the UK to donate the remains of indigenous people and prisoners to medical schools and natural history institutions in their home countries (Clegg 2009; Fforde 2004; Fforde *et al.* 2002).

Documentation also provides detailed information about the injuries observed on human remains. Bauer-Clapp and Pérez (2014) published their re-examination of Yaqui remains from Sonora (Mexico). In 1902, a group of Yaqui were killed by Mexican Troops at Sierra de Mazatán, and their bodies left in the open. These Yaqui had undertaken a rescue-raid on a series of haciendas to retrieve members of their community, who had been forced to work on these estates by the Mexican authorities

(Bauer-Clapp and Pérez 2014). Three months after the event, the remains of 12 individuals were collected by Hrdlička and deposited at the American Museum of Natural History in New York. Hrdlička had written in his journal about the site and state of bodies. In addition, he took photographs and notes, which stated that he did not retrieve all of the skulls, because they were so 'shattered' (Bauer-Clapp and Pérez 2014). These notes and historical information about the weapons used by Yaqui people and the Mexican Army allowed the anthropologists to understand more fully the trauma observed on these remains, for example, that blunt force injuries had been caused by a blow to the head with the butt of a Mauser rifle – standard issue to the Mexican troops at this time. Their examination also permitted them to distinguish between the retrieval of body trophies by the Mexican Army (Chacon and Dye 2008) and cut marks made by Hrdlička when he was removing the crania. The results of their study established scientifically that it had been a massacre rather than a battle, thereby providing new and important insights into this period of Yaqui history during this process of repatriation (Bauer-Clapp and Pérez 2014).

Morphometric and ancestry studies rely heavily on museum collections, as shown by the examples from the Smithsonian and NHM. Nevertheless, there may be crucial discrepancies between a person's biological identity, origin and the documentary information, particularly as information is transcribed over time. This has important repercussions for both repatriation work and the use of historic data sets in contemporary research. For example, repatriation work by NHM for the Torres Strait people (Australia) has found that many individuals, classified on their accession information as being from this locale, are not actually Indigenous Islanders (Bonney and Clegg 2011). Examination of the Howells Craniometric 'Test' data set made available online by Auerbach (2014) shows many discrepancies between the documentation information and Howell's comments, especially with regard to age, sex and ancestry/geographical origin. Therefore, practitioners must consider the reliability and applicability of these data.

24.3.2 Collection Care

In contemporary museum practice, the physical curation of the holdings is usually the responsibility of several different specialists: the curator of the collections, conservators and collection care practitioners. These professionals work together to ensure that the integrity and completeness of the collections are rigorously maintained to a high standard of care. In Britain today, these standards are set nationally and judged by an accreditation standard (Arts Council for England 2011). Furthermore, a huge amount of information is made available online by the various professional bodies representing these groups in the UK and elsewhere (Collections Trust 2014). The standards are also addressed in guidance documents specific to human remains in Britain (Department for Culture Media and Sport 2005; English Heritage and The Church of England 2005). However, because of the huge variability in expertise, funding and resources between curating institutions (e.g. Smith *et al.* 2012), inadequate collection care may have a detrimental effect on holdings (Heritage Preservation and the Institute of Museum and Library Services 2004). Moreover, not all countries have official standards of care, which leads to considerable variation in collection management across the world.

The storage facility chosen to curate human remains is the most significant determining factor for their long-term integrity, and covers every aspect from the building to the bag in which the remains are placed. There are numerous recollections in the literature about storing unprotected human remains outside or in completely inappropriate rooms (Cassman and Odegaard 2007). First, the physical environment of the store plays a crucial role. Factors such as humidity, fluctuating temperatures, exposure to daylight, pests and water ingress have well-documented impacts on the integrity of bone and teeth, and over a short space of time, can dramatically alter the observation of features (e.g. anatomical landmarks or pathology), particularly when remains become mouldy (Cassman and

Odegaard 2007; Janaway *et al.* 2001) The recommended standards for the curation of skeletonised non-indigenous human remains states that they should be stored in a secure room, which has a dry, cool and stable environment (55% ± 5% relative humidity in the UK), is not subject to water ingress, and whose environmental conditions are regularly monitored (British Association for Biological Anthropology and Osteoarchaeology Code of Practice 2010).

The packaging of remains also significantly impacts on their integrity, and if not carried out correctly will result in breakage, especially if the human remains are subject to frequent handling and movement – whether within a building or between institutions (Cassman and Odegaard 2007; Janaway *et al.* 2001) (Figure 24.1). For the purposes of long-term archiving, in order to ensure that the human remains are effectively managed, not only to maintain integrity but also to permit research, it is recommended by many British institutions and the British Association for Biological Anthropology and Osteoarchaeology (BABAO) (2010) that as a minimum standard, conservation-grade cardboard boxes should be used to store the human remains, with acid-free pads of tissue to act as supporting layers at the base and top of the container; bubble-wrap is not suitable for long-term use and newspaper is not appropriate even as a temporary measure (BABAO 2010), because of the gases used to make wrap and the inks used in printing.

The individual's remains should be bagged according to body area and side, using appropriately sized clear, 500 gauge plastic bags, which are perforated. The remains should be identified using at least two loose Tyvek© labels marked with permanent black ink, with the site name and unique

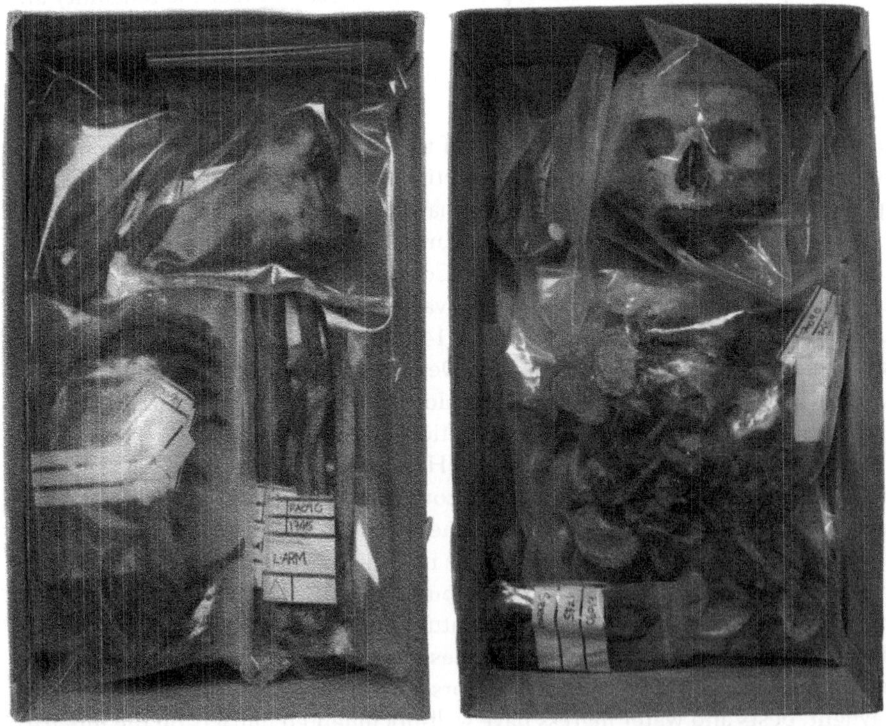

Figure 24.1 Image showing how human remains are packed at the Museum of London (Source: © *Museum of London*).

identifying number in each bag (BABAO 2010). The use of clear plastic bags means that the bones inside can be observed without having to remove them from the bag; the perforations allow for dispersion of any water or condensation that has developed because of water ingress; and the box is strong enough to avoid collapse and will remain rigid for many decades, allowing boxes to be securely stacked in the store.

The overwhelming majority of institutions do have protocols in place to manage risks for a variety of situations (i.e. loans managed by the institution's registrar) (Hillhouse 2012), and the best way to manage emergencies, such as salvage plans (e.g. Museum of London and Harwell Document Restoration Services 2013). These actions and workflows are usually documented by institutions to ensure that protocols conform to professional standards and recovery strategies are in place, such as 'buddy' institutions that assist with conservation, storage and inventories. Where applicable, such events (i.e. exhibitions) should be added to the object's documentation and labelling of salvage material in these cases is invaluable. For example, the medieval Raunds cemetery collection curated by Bradford University, UK, was damaged during an explosion in a nearby laboratory. Despite being stored appropriately, some of the remains were damaged by debris, and now have changes, which could mimic blunt and sharp force trauma (Pers. Comm. J. Buckberry).

The cumulative impact of collection care and conservation strategies on curated human remains can be significant, particularly in the absence of information about the products used. What must be recognised are the frequent competing needs of the conservator and anthropologist, particularly with the use of consolidants to ensure that the materials survive from excavation to deposition, and for display in exhibitions (Johnson 2001; Panagiaris 2001). Today, it is much more common for specialists to work together to find the best solution (McGowan and LaRoche 1996), However, in the past, this was not the case and often conservation strategies were implemented that have had significant knock-on effects, frequently compounded by a lack of documentation about the products used (Johnson 2001; Odegaard and Cassman 2001; Panagiaris 2001). These strategies can have lasting consequences for collections, particularly when budgets and resources do not allow these to be reversed – when possible!

This is demonstrated by the case of an Anglo-Saxon adult female burial that was excavated from the River Thames foreshore in 1990 (Redfern and Mant, unpublished). The site archive stated that the burial had been removed for micro-excavation off-site, because of the good preservation of organics; this had taken place 24 years before re-analysis. Preliminary observation of the skeleton identified over 50 points of peri-mortem breakage, which appeared at first-glance to be a peri-mortem bladed-weapon injury to the pelvis; all of the breaks had been messily repaired using an unknown adhesive (Figure 24.2). Fortunately, the re-analysis of the human remains coincided with the training of conservation students by the MoL Conservation Department. This opportunity provided the time and resources to enable the majority of adhesive to be removed, which took several weeks of work by two students. Each of the breaks was subsequently re-examined using a light microscope, which clearly showed morphological differences between breaks and thereby allowed peri-mortem trauma and post-mortem taphonomic damage to be differentiated (Loe 2008). A passing remark about this skeleton to a colleague revealed that they had been on site when the burial was lifted, and they explained that the inhumation had been 'chopped' in two using a spade so that it could be more easily removed by a crane, and lifted over the buildings facing the foreshore – this explained the marks on the pelvis. The osteologist, who examined the human remains, glued the skeleton back together to make it easier for recording.

Genomic studies are increasing year-on-year and provide unrivalled insights into past health, origin of diseases and the physical characteristics of past people (Anastasiou and Mitchell 2013; Bauer *et al.* 2013). Studies from the late 1980s onwards have investigated the impact of conservation treatments on such work (e.g. Barnes and Thomas 2006; Lee *et al.* 2010; Moore *et al.* 1989), but more recent

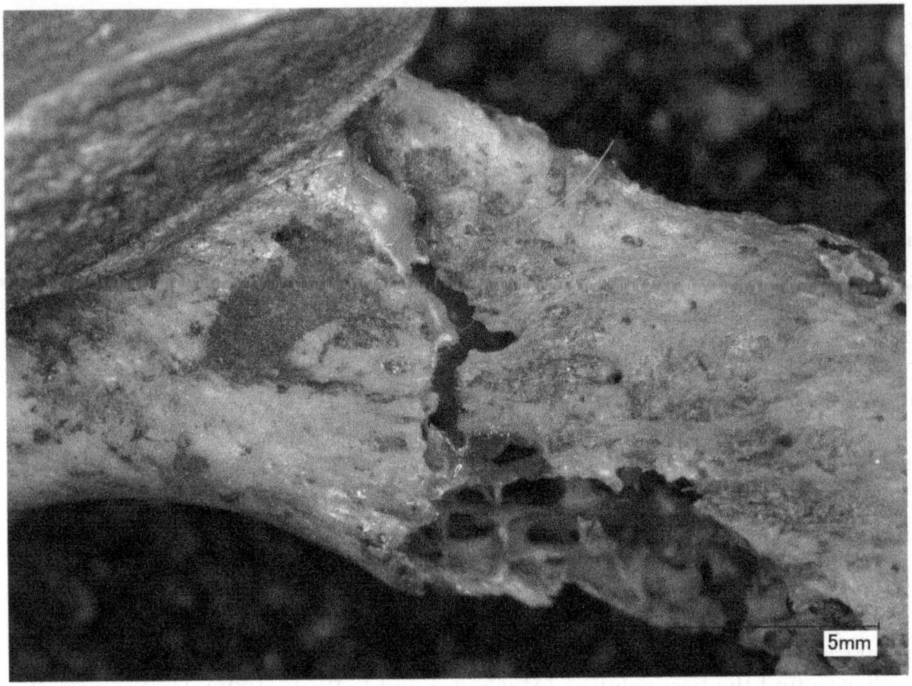

Figure 24.2 Example of a break repaired using an unknown adhesive in an adult Anglo-Saxon female skeleton. Close-up view shows the superior aspect of the right transverse process of the 2nd thoracic vertebra (Source: © *Museum of London*).

studies suggest that techniques are now sophisticated enough to successfully extract and analyse DNA from both treated and untreated bone and tissue (Gilbert *et al.* 2005; Paireder *et al.* 2013). There is also a greater awareness about the differential preservation of DNA within the human skeleton and dentition (Misner *et al.* 2009), and the imperative to develop minimally invasive or non-destructive extraction methods (Hofreiter 2012). Institutions have also experienced a change in the way they view their collections, with a greater awareness that they should be understood as biobanks (European Middle Eastern and African Society for Biopreservation and Biobanking), and therefore require new ways of being managed (Buś and Allen 2014). However, such developments also raise new ethical issues that have yet to be fully engaged by curating institutions: how does information given to a genetic databank by a researcher become linked to a museum record, and should people wanting to use it also seek the consent of the museum? The web-based dissemination of genomic data may also lead to people uncovering genetic relationships to known or anonymous individuals that are held in collections, and which has implications for current repatriation guidelines.

Another contentious issue is the sampling of human remains, especially when they concern remains from Indigenous Communities (Colwell-Chanthaphonh 2010; Harry 2009; Shelton and Marks 2001). It is an increasingly difficult aspect of collection care to manage, because techniques are developing incredibly rapidly, and the demand for samples appears to be insatiable. Institutions must also cope with the consequences of historical sampling, which greatly impact on research, from macroscopic to imaging studies (Figures 24.3 and 24.4). However, the demands of genomic research must be balanced against an institution's need to maintain collection integrity for the long term. For example, the use of incremental counts to establish the age of an individual is very accurate, particularly in infant material (Cartsen 2014; Naji *et al.* 2014). The analysis can only be done on a sectioned tooth,

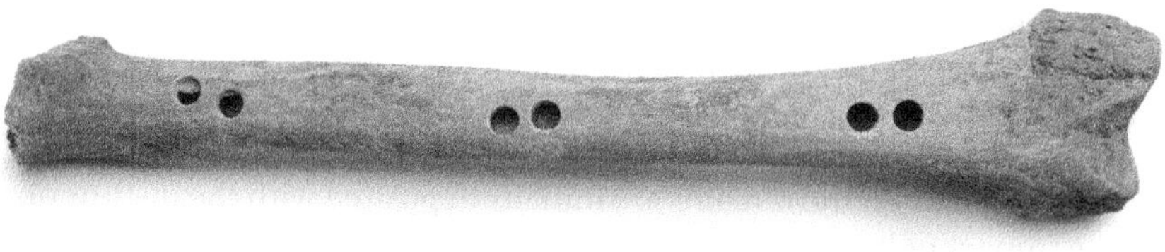

Figure 24.3 Example of multiple samples taken from a femur using a drill technique (Source: © *Museum of London*).

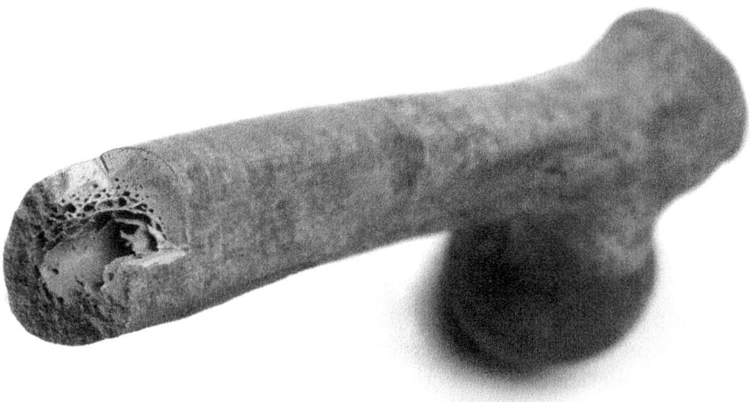

Figure 24.4 Example of a femur with saw marks caused by sampling (Source: © *Museum of London*).

an irreparable action, which has significant implications for macro- and microscopic studies of dental health and wear (Figure 24.5) and those wishing to undertake incremental and bulk stable isotope studies of diet and mobility. All of these studies have the potential to significantly contribute to (forensic) anthropological methods (Beaumont *et al.* 2013; Font *et al.* 2015a; 2015b; Pasveer *et al.* 1998; Prince *et al.* 2008). Therefore, the needs of the current project must be weighed against other known (and potential future) requests, and the need to maintain the integrity of the collection. These reasons have contributed to institutions across Europe and the Americas introducing policies, which are weighted towards protecting their collections. Anecdotally, we have perceived a shift in demand away from institutions with strict protocols, to smaller ones that lack the expertise and/or are not networked to get help and advice, or to collections outside of the UK, where stringent procedures are not in place. From our personal experience, the ways in which sampling has been undertaken at MoL has rapidly been transformed over the past decade, and this can be entirely explained by the presence of specialist curators.

The primary reason for continuing to hold human remains in institutions is the unique research contribution they can make to a range of scientific and clinical disciplines (Department for Culture Media and Sport 2005; Jones and Harris 1998). This statement is reiterated by many museum policies (The British Museum 2006; The Horniman Museum and Gardens 2013). However, making collections accessible for research increases their risk of damage. Condition reports for all holdings are standard practice within museums, and the majority of institutions have protocols in place to govern transport and other aspects of loan agreements: lighting, storage, display mounts and cases, etc. (Genoways and Ireland 2003). However, for human remains not on display, this may be unfeasible for practical reasons alone: if the holdings are very large, a lack of specialist training that would allow a curator to distinguish between older/more recent breaks and peri-mortem trauma, and funding to cover time and specialist staff to perform this duty. Therefore, many institutions attempt to manage this by comparing extant remains with original recording forms, archaeological context sheets or other documentation. As outlined above, these sources may be wholly inadequate and therefore condition reports should be undertaken when the remains are initially deposited with the institution. The only study to investigate the impact of handling on human remains from teaching and research is the survey by Caffell *et al.* (2001). Their study of two cemetery samples held by Bradford University in 1999, which had entered their collections in the 1980s, contains many significant and worrying findings. They discovered that there had been detrimental and/or significant damage to both collections, individuals had lost and/or gained bones and/or teeth, elements had been broken, pathological changes had been damaged, and there was a direct relationship between frequency of use and the amount of damage observed (Caffell *et al.* 2001). Our personal experience of managing collections at MoL and other institutions, including the crypt population from St Bride's, supports these findings. It is collections with named individuals, frequently used to generate methods, which have the most pressure put upon them.

24.4 Conclusion

Taphonomy is a process that does not stop at the doors of a curating institution. Often that institution can cause more damage to human remains than being in a crypt for several hundred years could achieve. As with all aspects of curatorial practice and collection care, a balance must be achieved between making collections available – the purpose of holding them – and maintaining their integrity for future generations. The past decade has seen the rapid development of techniques and methods, many designed and tested on such collections, but the destructive nature of many achievements means that an irrecoverable price has been paid for this success (Figures 24.3–24.5). Despite training and research, as a discipline it is often forgotten that these are the remains of people who will not return – their remains cannot be regenerated – and we should not shy away from such ethical issues.

This chapter has provided an overview of the key aspects of museum curation and collection care management. This is based on professional experience of the authors working in Britain, predominantly on archaeologically derived skeletons, but many of these issues are universal to museum practice and not limited to human remains. The importance of questioning and searching documentation and understanding the origin of collections are the key areas, which we perceive to have the greatest impact on forensic anthropological research, but they are rarely considered in the forensic literature.

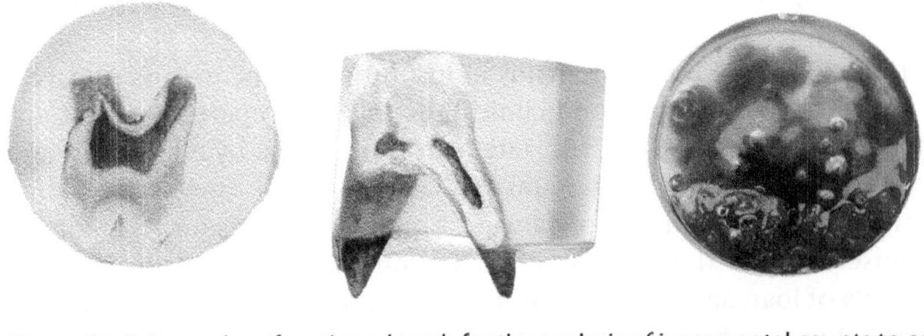

Figure 24.5 Examples of sectioned teeth for the analysis of incremental counts to establish the age of an individual. The one on the right 'exploded' whilst being mounted in resin (Source: © *Museum of London*).

Acknowledgements

The authors would like to thank the Conservation and Collection Care teams at the Museum of London, Dr Heather Bonney (NHM London), Dr Jo Buckberry (University of Bradford) and Dr Margaret Clegg (UCL).

References

Adams, J., Brickley, M., Buteux, S., Adams, T. and Cherrington, R. (2006) *St Martin's Uncovered: Investigations in the churchyard of St Martin's-in-the-Bull-Ring, Birmingham, 2001*. Oxbow Books: Oxford.

Anastasiou, E. and Mitchell, P.D. (2013) Palaeopathology and genes: investigating the genetics of infectious diseases in excavated human skeletal remains and mummies from past populations. *Historical Medical Genetics: Skeletal disorders*, **528**: 33–40.

Arts Council for England (2011) Accredition scheme for museums and galleries in the United Kingdom: accreditation standard. http://www.artscouncil.org.uk/media/uploads/pdf/accreditation_standard_english_web.pdf (Accessed 14 April 2015).

Association of Diocesan and Cathedral Archaeologists (2010) Archaeology and burial vaults. *A guidance note for churches. Association of Diocesan and Cathedral Archaeologists Guidance Note* **2**. http://www.archaeologyuk.org/adca/documents/ADCAGuidanceNote2.pdf (Accessed 14 April 2015).

Auerbach, B.M. (2014) Howells craniometric 'test' data set, vol. **2014**. http://web.utk.edu/~auerbach/HOWL.htm (Accessed 14 April 2015).

British Association for Biological Anthropology and Osteoarchaeology (2011) Code of Practice. http://www.babao.org.uk/index/cms-filesystem-action/code%20of%20practice.pdf (Accessed 14 July 2015).

Barnes, I. and Thomas, M.G. (2006) Evaluating bacterial pathogen DNA preservation in museum osteological collections. *Proceedings of the Royal Society*, **273**: 645–653.

Bauer-Clapp, H.J. and Pérez, V.R. (2014) Violence in life, violence in death, resiliency through repatriation: bioarchaeological analysis and heritage value of Yaqui skeletal remains from Sonora, Mexico. In: Martin, D.L. and Anderson, C.P. (eds), *Bioarchaeological and Forensic Perspectives on Violence: How violent death is interpreted from skeletal remains*. Cambridge University Press: Cambridge, pp. 171–191.

Bauer, C.M., Niederstätter, H., McGlynn, G., Stadler, H. and Parson, W. (2013) Comparison of morphological and molecular genetic sex-typing on mediaeval human skeletal remains. *Forensic Science International: Genetics*, **7**: 581–586.

Beaumont, J., Gledhill, A., Lee-Thorp, J. and Montgomery, J. (2013) Childhood diet: a closer examination of the evidence from dental tissues using stable isotope analysis of incremental human dentine. *Archaeometry*, **55**: 277–295.

Bonney, H. and Clegg, M. (2011) Heads as memorials and status symbols: the collection and use of skulls in the Torres Strait Islands. In: Bonogofsky, M. (ed.), *The Bioarchaeology of the Human Head: Decapitation, deformation and decoration*. University Press of Florida: Florida, pp. 51–66.

Boston, C., Boyle, A., Gill, J. and Witkin, A. (2009) 'In the vaults beneath'. Archaeological recording at St George's Church, Bloomsbury. *Oxford Archaeology Monograph No. 8*, Oxford Archaeology: Oxford.

British Association for Biological Anthropology and Osteoarchaeology Code of Practice (2010).

Buś, M.M. and Allen, M. (2014) Collecting and preserving biological samples from challenging environments for DNA analysis. *Biopreservation and Biobanking*, **12**: 17–22.

Caffell, A.C., Roberts, C.A., Janaway, R.C. and Wilson, A.S. (2001) Pressures on osteological collections: the importance of damage limitations. In: Williams, E. (ed.), *Human Remains. Conservation, retrieval and analysis*. Proceedings of a conference held in Williamsburg, 7–11 November 1999, British Archaeological Press S934, pp. 187–197.

Cardoso, H.F.V., Abrantes, J. and Humphrey, L.T. (2014) Age estimation of immature human skeletal remains from the diaphyseal length of the long bones in the postnatal period. *International Journal of Legal Medicine*, **128**: 809–824.

Cardoso, H.F.V. (2006) Brief communication: The collection of identified human skeletons housed at the Bocage Museum (National Museum of Natural History), Lisbon, Portugal. *American Journal of Physical Anthropology*, **129**: 173–176.

Cartsen, W. (2014) Echoes from birth – mutual benefits for physical and forensic anthropology for applying increment counts in enamel of deciduous teeth for aging. *Anthropologischer Anzeiger*, **71**: 87–103.

Cassman, V. and Odegaard, N. (2007) Storage and transport. In: *Cassman, V*., Odegaard, N. and Powell, J. (eds), *Human Remains. Guide for museums and academic insitutions*. Altamira Press: Oxford, pp. 103–128.

Cassman, V., Odegaard, N. and Powell, J. (eds) (2007) *Human Remains. Guide for museums and academic institutions*. Altamira Press: Oxford.

Chacon, R.J. and Dye, D.H. (2008) Introduction to human trophy taking. An ancient and widespread practice. In: Chacon, R.J. and Dye, D.H. (eds), *The Taking and Displaying of Human Body Parts as Trophies by Amerindians*. Springer: Berlin, pp. 5–31.

Clegg, M. (2009) The problem of provenance: inaccuracies, changes and misconceptions. In: Lewis, M. and Clegg, M. (eds), *Proceedings of the 9th Annual Conference of the British Association for Biological Anthropology and Osteoarchaeology*, British Archaeological Reports S1918, pp. 119–122.

Clegg, M. and Bonney, H. (2010) Setting the record straight: improving the quality of early museum records. *American Journal of Physical Anthropology*, **50**: 81.

Clegg, M., Redfern, R.C., Bekvalac, J. and Bonney, H. (eds) (2013) *Global Ancestors: Global perspectives on human remains and museum repatriation*. Oxbow Books: Oxford.

Collections Trust (2014) Risk management. http://www.collectionstrust.org.uk/risk-management/risk-management-homepage (Accessed 15 April 2015).

Colwell-Chanthaphonh, C. (2010) Remains unknown: repatriating culturally unaffiliated human remains. *Anthropology News*, **51**: 4–8.

Cowie, R., Bekvalac, J. and Kausmally, T. (2008) *Late 17th to 19th Century Burial and Earlier Occupation at All Saints, Chelsea Old Church, Royal Borough of Kensington and Chelsea*. MoLAS Archaeology Studies 18, Museum of London: London.

Cox, M. (1996) *Life and Death in Spitalfields, 1700 to 1850*. CBA Occasional Papers No. 21, Council for British Archaeology: York. http://archaeologydataservice.ac.uk/archives/view/cba_op/op21.cfm (Accessed 14 April 2015).

Cox, M. (1997) Crypt archaeology after Spitalfields: dealing with our recent dead. *Antiquity*, **71**: 8–10.

Cox, M. (2001) Crypt archaeology: an approach. *Institute of Field Archaeologists Technical Paper Number* 3. http://citeseerx.ist.psu.edu/viewdoc/download?doi=10.1.1.112.5229andrep=rep1andtype=pdf (Accessed 20 Sept 2015).

Crossrail (2013) Crisis and the black death. http://www.crossrail.co.uk/news/articles/new-research-shows-crossrails-charterhouse-skeletons-were-black-death-victims (Accessed 14 April 2015).

de la Cova, C. (2012) Patterns of trauma and violence in 19th-century-born African American and Euro-American females. *International Journal of Paleopathology*, **2**: 61–68.

Department for Culture Media and Sports' (2005) *Guidance for the Care of Human Remains in Museums*. DCMS: London.

Doyal, L. and Muinzer, T. (2011) Should the skeleton of 'the Irish giant' be buried at sea? *British Medical Journal*, **343**: d7597.

English Heritage (2011) The heritage of death. *Conservation Bulletin* **66**. https://historicengland.org.uk/images-books/publications/conservation-bulletin-66/ (Accessed 20 September 2015).

English Heritage and The Church of England (2005) *Guidance for Best Practice for the Treatment of Human Remains Excavated from Christian Burial Grounds in England*. English Heritage. https://content.historicengland.org.uk/images-books/publications/human-remains-excavated-from-christian-burial-grounds-in-england/16602humanremains1.pdf/ (Accessed 14 April 2015).

European Middle Eastern and African Society for Biopreservation and Biobanking. http://www.esbb.org/ (Accessed 14 April 2015).

Fforde, C. (2004) *Collecting the Dead. Archaeology and the Reburial Issue*. Gerald Duckworth and Co Ltd: London.

Fforde, C., Hubert, J. and Turnbull, P. (eds) (2002) The Dead and Their Possessions: Repatriation in priniciple, policy and practice. Routledge: London.

Font, L., Jonker, G., van Aalderen, P.A., Schiltmas, E.F. and Davies, G.R. (2015a) Provenancing of unidentified World War II casualities: application of strontium and oxygen isotope analysis in tooth enamel. *Science and Justice*, **55**: 10–17.

Font, L., van der Peijl, G., van Leuwen, C., van Wetten, I. and Davies, G.R. (2015b) Identification of the geographical place of origin of an unidentified individual by multi-isotope analysis. *Science and Justice*, **55**: 34–42.

Genoways, H.H. and Ireland, L.M. (2003) *Museum Administration: An introduction*. Altamira Press: Oxford.

Giesen, M. (ed.) (2013) *Curating Human Remains. Caring for the dead in the United Kingdom*. Boydell and Brewer: Woodbridge.

Giesen, M., McCarrison, K. and Park, V. (2013) Dead and forgotten? Some observations on human remains documentation in the UK. In: Giesen, M. (ed.), *Curating Human Remains: Caring for the dead in the United Kingdom*. Boydell and Brewer: Woodbridge, pp. 53–64.

Gilbert, M.T.P., Rudbeck, L., Willerslev, E., Hansen, A.J., Smith, C. *et al.* (2005). Biochemical and physical correlates of DNA contamination in archaeological human bones and teeth excavated at Matera, Italy. *Journal of Archaeological Science*, **32**: 785–793.

Harry, D. (2009) Indigenous peoples and gene disputes. *Chicago-Kent Law Review*, **84**: 147.

Henderson, M, Miles, A., Walker, D., with Wroe-Brown, R. and Connell, B. (2013) *'He being dead yet speaketh': Excavations at three post-medieval burial grounds in Tower Hamlets, East London, 2004–10*. Museum of London Monograph Series 64, Museum of London Archaeology: London.

Heritage Preservation and the Institute of Museum and Library Services (2004) The Heritage Health Index Report on the state of America's collections. https://www.heritagepreservation.org/HHI/full.html (Accessed April 2015).

Hillhouse, S. (2012) Assess and manage risk in collections care: a *Collections Care How To* Guide. http://www.collectionstrust.org.uk/news/share-museums-east-how-to-guide-to-assess-and-manage-risk-in-collections-care (Accessed 15 April 2015).

Hofreiter, M. (2012) Nondestructive DNA extraction from museum specimens. *Methods in Molecular Biology*, **840**: 93–100.

International Council of Museums (2006). *ICOM Code of Ethics for Museums*. http://icom.museum/fileadmin/user_upload/pdf/Codes/code_ethics2013_eng.pdf (Accessed 15 April 2015).

Janaway, R.C., Wilson, A.S., Caffell, A.C. and Roberts, C.A. (2001) Human skeletal collections: the responsibilities of project managers, physical anthropologists and conservators, and the need for standardized condition assessment. In: Williams, E. (ed.), *Human Remains. Conservation, retrieval and analysis*. Proceedings of a conference held in Williamsburg, 7–11 November 1999, British Archaeological Reports S934. pp.199–208.

Johnson, J. (2001) A long-term look at polymers used to preserve bone. In: Williams, E. (ed.), *Human Remains. Conservation, retrieval and analysis*. Proceedings of a conference held in Williamsburg, 7–11 November 1999, British Archaeological Reports S934, pp. 99–104.

Jones, D.G. and Harris, R.J. (1998) CA forum on anthropology in public: archaeological human remains: scientific, cultural, and ethical considerations. *Current Anthropology*, **39**: 253–264.

Kakaliouras, A.M. (2012). An anthropology of repatriation. Contemporary physical anthropology and Native American ontologies of practice. *Current Anthropology*, **53**: S210–221.

Knudson, K.J. and Stojanowski, C.M. (2009) *Bioarchaeology and Identity in the Americas*. University Press of Florida: Gainesville.

Lee, E.J., Luedtke, J.G., Allison, J.L., Arber, C.E., Merriwether, D.A. and Steadman, D.W. (2010) The effects of different maceration techniques on nuclear DNA amplification using human bone. *Journal of Forensic Sciences*, **55**: 1032–1038.

Loe, L. (2008) Peri-mortem trauma. In: Blau, S. and Ubelaker, D.H. (eds), *Handbook of Forensic Archaeology and Anthropology*. Left Coast Press: Walnut Creek, pp. 263–283.

Mahoney-Swales, D., O'Neill, R. and Willmott, H. (2011) The hidden material culture of death: coffins and grave goods in late 18th and early 19th-Century Sheffield. In: King, C. and Sayer, D. (eds), *The Archaeology of Post-Medieval Religion*. Boydell and Brewe: Woodbridge, pp. 215–232.

McGowan, G.S. and LaRoche, C.J. (1996) The ethical dilemma facing conservation: care and treatment of human skeletal remains and mortuary objects. *Journal of the American Institute for Conservation*, **35**: 109–121.

McKinley, J. (2008) The 18th Century Baptist Chapel and Burial Ground at West Butts Street, Poole. Wessex Archaeology: Salisbury.

Miles, A., Powers, N., Wroe-Brown, R. and Walker, D. (2008) *St Marylebone Church and Burial Ground in the 18th and 19th Centuries: Excavations at St Marylebone School, 1992 and 2004–6*. Museum of London Archaeology Monograph Series 46, Museum of London: London.

Ministry of Justice. (2015). Apply for an exhumation licence. https://www.gov.uk/apply-for-an-exhumation-licence (Accessed 14 April 2015).

Misner, L.M., Halvorson, A.C., Dreier, J.L., Ubelaker, D.H. and Foran, D.R. (2009) The correlation between skeletal weathering and DNA quality and quantity. *Journal of Forensic Sciences*, **54**: 822–828.

Moore, K.M., Murray, M.L. and Schoeninger, M.J. (1989) Dietary reconstruction from bones treated with preservatives. *Journal of Archaeological Science*, **16**: 437–446.

Muinzer, T.L. (2013) A grave situation: an examination of the legal issues raised by the life and death of Charles Byrne, the 'Irish Giant'. *International Journal of Cultural Property*, **20**: 23–48.

Mulkerin, M.S. (2013) Elephants never forget, but museums do. Investigating under-documented objects in museum collections. *Collection: A Journal for Museum and Archive Professionals*, **9**: 149–166.

Museum of London and Harwell Document Restoration Services (2013) *Salvage Pocket Guide*. London: Museum of London.

Museums Association (2008) *Code of Ethics for Museums*. London: Museums Association.

Naji, S., Colard, T., Blondiaux, J., Bertrand, B., d'Incau, E. and Bocquet-Appel, J.-P. (2014) Cementochronology, to cut or not to cut? *International Journal of Paleopathology*, doi:10.1016/j.ijpp.2014.05.003.

Odegaard, N. and Cassman, V. (2001) Treatment and invasive actions. In: Cassman, V., Odegaard, N. and Powell, J. (eds), *Human Remains. Guide for museums and academic institutions*. Altamira Press: Oxford, pp. 77–96.

Ousley, S.D. (2001) Lessons learned from the repatriation program at the National Museum of Natural History, Smithsonian Institution. *International Colloquim on the First Americans*, pp. 16–19.

Paireder, S., Werner, B., Bailer, J., Werther, W., Schmid, E. *et al.* (2013) Comparison of protocols for DNA extraction from long-term preserved formalin fixed tissues. *Analytical Biochemistry*, **439**: 152–160.

Panagiaris, G. (2001) The influence of conservation treatments on physical anthropology research. In: Williams, E. (ed.), *Human Remains. Conservation, retrieval and analysis.* Proceedings of a conference held in Williamsburg, 7–11 November 1999, BAR International S934, pp. 95–98.

Pasveer, J., Buck, A. and van Huystee, M. (1998) Victims of the Batavia mutiny: physical anthropological and forensic studies of the Beacon Island skeleton. *Bulletin of the Australian Institute for Maritime Archaeology*, **22**: 45–50.

Portable Antiquities Scheme (2014) https://finds.org.uk/ (Accessed 14 April 2015).

Prince, D.A., Kimmerle, E.H. and Konigsberg, L.W. (2008) A Bayesian approach to estimate skeletal age-at-death utilizing dental wear. *Journal of Forensic Sciences*, **53**: 588–593.

Redfern, R.C. and Mant, M. (unpublished) Analysis of a human skeleton from 67 Upper Thames Street, Bull Wharf Lane, EC4. Museum of London: London.

Rissech, C, and Steadman. D.W. (2011) The demographic, socio-economic and temporal contextualisation of the Universitat Autònoma de Barcelona collection of identified human skeletons (UAB collection). *International Journal of Osteoarchaeology*, **21**: 313–322.

Schofield, J., Carmen, J. and Belford, P. (2011) *Archaeological Practice in Great Britain. A heritage handbook*. Springer: London.

Shelton, B.L. and Marks, J. (2001) Genetic markers not a valid test of native identity. *Indigenous Peoples Council on Biocolonialism, Briefing Paper*. http://www.ipcb.org/publications/briefing_papers/files/identity.html (Accessed 14 April 2015).

Smith, M., Kneller, P., Elliott, D., Young, C., Manley, H. and Osselton, D. (2012) Multidisciplinary analysis of a mummified Egyptian cranium previously identified as a medieval execution victim. *Archaeological and Anthropological Sciences*, **4**: 75–89.

Stodder, A.L.W. (2008) Taphonomy and the nature of archaeological assemblages. In: Katzenberg, M.A. and Saunders, S.R. (eds), *Biological Anthropology of the Human Skeleton*. John Wiley & Sons: London, pp. 71–113.

Tarlow, S. (1998) Romancing the stones: the graveyard boom of the later 18th century. In: Cox, M. (ed.), *Grave Concerns: Death and burial in England 1700–1850*. Council for British Archaeology Monograph **113**. pp. 33–43.

Tarlow, S. (2011) *Ritual, Belief and the Dead in Early Modern Britain and Ireland*. Cambridge University Press: Cambridge.

Tayles, N. (2009) Repatriation – a view from a recieving end: New Zealand. In: Lewis, M.E. and Clegg, M. (eds), *Proceedings of the 9th Annual Conference of the British Association for Biological Anthropology and Osteoarchaeology*. British Archaeological Reports S1918, pp. 131–135.

Thames Discovery Programme (2014) http://www.thamesdiscovery.org/ (Accessed 14 April 2015).

The British Museum (2006) The British Museum policy on human remains. http://www.britishmuseum.org/PDF/HumanRemains.pdf (Accessed 14 April 2015).

The Horniman Museum and Gardens (2013) Collections development policy. http://www.horniman.ac.uk/media/_file/collections-development-policy.pdf (Accessed 14 April 2015).

Trickett, M. (2006) *A Tale of Two Cities: Diet, health and migration in post-medieval Coventry and Chelsea through biographical reconstruction, osteoarchaeology and isotope biogeochemistry*. Unpublished PhD Thesis. University of Durham: Durham.

Turner, T.R. (ed.) (2005) *Biological Anthropology and Ethics. From repatriation to genetic identity*. State University of New York Press: New York.

Walker, P.L. (2008) Bioarchaeological ethics: a historical perspective on the value of human remains. In: Katzenberg, M.A. and Saunders, S.R. (eds), *Biological Anthropology of the Human Skeleton*. Wiley Liss Inc: New York, pp. 3–39.

Wellcome Trust and Museum of London (2008) Skeletons: London's buried bones. http://wellcomecollection.org/exhibitions/skeletons (Accessed 12 July 2015).

Wilson, A.S., Powers, N., Montgomery, J., Buckberry, J., Beaumont, J.. *et al.* (2013) 'Men that are gone … come like shadows, so depart': research practice and sampling strategies for enhancing our understanding of post-medieval human remains. In: Dalglish, C. (ed.), *Archaeology, The Public and the Recent Past*. Boydell and Brewer: Woodbridge, pp. 145–162.

Part IV

Case Studies

25

The Use of Volatile Fatty Acid Biomarkers to Estimate the Post-Mortem Interval

Arpad A. Vass

25.1 Introduction

Determining the post-mortem interval (PMI) has always been challenging and remains one of the most difficult tasks facing the investigator, because both exogenous and endogenous factors differ for every death scene. The most constant variable associated with a death scene is typically the corpse itself. While the environment, manner of death and disposition of the corpse can change dramatically, all the victims, while alive, had physiological parameters spanning a relatively narrow life sustaining range. For this reason, the use of biomarkers has been among the more reliable methods for determining the PMI. Biomarkers can be grouped into two broad categories: organic markers usually obtained from soft tissue, used when the decedent is in the pre-skeletonisation phase of decomposition, and inorganic markers, which are typically utilised during the post-skeletonisation phase. This case study describes the use of one group of available organic biomarkers (volatile fatty acids – VFAs) as a means of determining the PMI.

VFAs are molecules with a carbon chain of six carbons or fewer. They can be formed from the microbial breakdown of food in the intestinal tract or derived from the breakdown of fat and muscle during the decomposition process. There are many VFAs, but only three have been shown to be important as PMI indicators in human decomposition based on their reproducibility, longevity in the environment and stability. These are: propionic acid (with 3 carbon atoms) CH_3CH_2COOH; butyric acid (with 4 carbon atoms) $CH_3(CH_2)_2COOH$; and valeric acid (with 5 carbon atoms) $CH_3(CH_2)_3COOH$. Some VFAs can be found as straight chains (e.g. n-valeric) and some as branched chains (e.g. iso-valeric) and are usually termed saturated fatty acids (alkanes), which means that they are composed entirely of single bonds. They are called VFAs because in an acid environment they form a gas, but in an alkaline environment they form a salt, which is not only stable but also water soluble. When human soft tissue decomposes in an aerobic environment, the process is typically alkaline due to proteolysis and the formed salts migrate with the leachate from the decedent and can be easily extracted from clothing, soil, bedding, etc.

25.2 Methods and Collection

In this particular death scene, the corpse of an adult male was found lying in a small clearing in a forested area in the Eastern region of the USA. Visual inspection of the corpse indicated that he was in Stage 3 (active decay) of decomposition. Some insect (maggot) activity was noted on the ground

Taphonomy of Human Remains: Forensic Analysis of the Dead and the Depositional Environment, First Edition.
Edited by Eline M.J. Schotsmans, Nicholas Márquez-Grant and Shari L. Forbes.

surrounding the corpse; however, little activity was apparent on the corpse itself. All indications suggested that the individual had decomposed where he was found and had not been moved. Animal scavenging was at a minimum.

Initially, the investigator must always evaluate which methods of determining the PMI are best suited for the particular set of circumstances that present themselves. These can include the collection of insect material, soil, tissue, air samples, clothing, bone, fingernails, microorganisms (fungi, microbes), etc. (Table 25.1). While these methods might vary depending on the death scene, the collection of temperature and humidity data remains mandatory. This collection includes the temperature and humidity at the time of discovery, data from the nearest National Weather Service station (NWS) for a period of time and collection from the death scene for a period of at least 3 days (usually 4–5). A comparison can then be made between the death scene and NWS data, in order to be able to correct for differences caused by elevation, sun exposure, shading, moisture, etc. The basic formula (1,285/temperature at the death scene in Celsius = days of weather to collect) can provide the investigator with some idea of the amount of weather data required that would be useful for these PMI determinations (Vass 2011). The value 1,285 (±110) is the accumulated degree day (ADD), where a VFA leaching from the body (fat and muscle) ceases. In simple terms, ADDs are an accumulation of average daily temperatures (in Celsius) over time. The cessation of leaching could be the result of a lack of remaining soft tissue, mummification, or if the body had been treated with chemicals that stop the decomposition process (either autolysis or putrefaction) at a cellular level. When using VFA analysis, it is important to determine whether the body is mummified, since this could prematurely stop the leaching of VFAs, even though soft tissue might remain. In such cases, the result of the VFA analysis would indicate a minimum time. If too much time has passed since mummified (before discovery), then no VFA chemicals would be detectable.

In this particular case, the temperature at the death scene at the time of discovery was 55°F (13°C), therefore 1,285/13 = 99 days, therefore 3 months of weather data were requested from the nearest NWS station (Table 25.2). This included temperature and humidity data. The 90 day average, after correcting for differences at the death scene (average of 3.2 °F cooler), was 65°F (18°C) and 73% humidity.

While several methods could have been applied to this particular case, only two (VFA analysis and entomology) were selected. VFA analysis was chosen primarily because significant amounts of soft tissue remained on the decedent and entomology was chosen, due to the large populations of insects

Table 25.1 Evaluating the best PMI method more than 48 hrs post-mortem (not all listed).

Primary Methods	Rationale for Use
Volatile fatty acids (VFAs)	Used when significant soft tissue remains on corpse
Inorganic indicators	Primarily used when mummified or mostly skeletonised
Microbes	16S RNA profiles/succession
Entomology	Best pre-skeletonisation
Tissue biomarkers	Early decomposition (<3 weeks)
Hair/fingernails	DNA degradation/(keratin markers – not temperature dependent)
Bone	Citrate analysis (requires rib bone in contact with soil) Primarily skeletonised remains.
Air samples – *odor mortis* (free and soil headspace)	Used if soft tissue present or absent, corpse moved and/or buried

Table 25.2 Results of VFA analysis from soil collected underneath the decedent.

VFA	Conc. (mmol)	Gram dry weight soil (7.52 g/10 g)	Dilution factor (20 ml water/ 10 g soil)	Final corrected VFA value	Ratio
n-butyric	1.88	0.752	×2	5.0	0.495
iso-butyric	1.83	0.752	×2	4.9	0.485
n-valeric	0.92	0.752	×2	2.4	0.238
iso-valeric	1.91	0.752	×2	5.1	0.505
propionic	3.79	0.752	×2	10.1	1

that were present at the time of discovery (although not actually on the decedent). Inorganic analysis and bone citrate are more useful techniques as the corpse approaches skeletonisation. Nails, tissue collection methods and microbial assessments are best used earlier in the decomposition cycle, as air sampling was not yet sufficiently developed as a valid technique at the time of this incident.

As observed in the photograph of the decedent (Figure 25.1), he was lying in contact with the ground and was not wearing any clothing. Any leachate from the decedent would saturate the ground directly beneath him. While clothing makes a valuable sorbent material, it is not always possible to obtain unstained material as a control, since all the clothing becomes saturated with decomposition fluids. In this case, soil samples for VFA analyses were collected from underneath the corpse and an appropriate control soil was collected approximately 10 m (~32 feet) from the decedent. The best location for collection of test material is under the thorax, but this is not always possible depending on the circumstances, for example, animal scavenging. In these cases, collection under any area with a large muscle mass (such as the thigh region) will suffice. Since the area was relatively flat (uphill

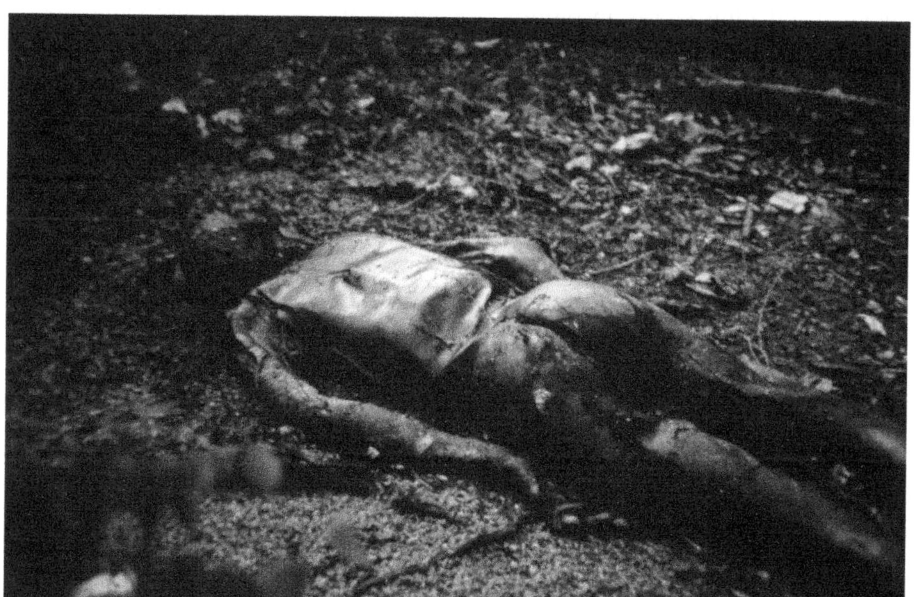

Figure 25.1 Image of the decedent. Estimated total body decomposition approximately 55–60%.

slopes being absent), collection of control soil at a greater distance from the corpse is required in order to avoid any possibility of cross-contamination, which may be the case if one were to collect soil uphill/upslope. Only a small amount of soil needs to be collected (~100 g) and this was placed in a clean metal evidence can. In cases where the body has been moved, severely scavenged, or simply is not present, the pH of the soil solution (Vass *et al.* 1992) should be tested prior to collection. Soil that has been exposed to decomposition products in an aerobic environment (above ground/surface) will, in many cases, have an elevated soil solution pH when compared to control soil solutions. If the pH of the collected soil solution is not alkaline (a solution is considered alkaline if the pH is greater than 7.0), then it is unlikely that VFAs can be detected with any reliability. Entomological evidence was also collected at the time of soil collection, packaged and sent to a qualified forensic entomologist for evaluation.

25.2.1 Volatile Fatty Acids

One of the advantages in using VFA analysis is the simplicity of the laboratory procedure. A simple water extract (2:1 water:soil – used if large amounts of soft tissue remain, or 1:1 – if minimal tissue remains), which can also be used for materials other than soil (clothing, fabrics, etc.), is all that is required (Vass *et al.* 1992). The procedure, designed to be used with common laboratory instrumentation such as a liquid chromatograph, gas chromatograph (GC) or the more sophisticated gas chromatograph-mass spectrometer (GC-MS) available in almost every crime laboratory (or university) in the world, is completely adequate for these analyses. In this case, a 2:1 (water:soil) extract was selected utilising 10 g of collected soil. After addition of the water, the sample was mixed and then centrifuged to separate the soil particles from the water. The VFAs, being water soluble, would then be concentrated in the water phase. The analysis yielded 0.92 mmol of n-valeric acid, 1.83 mmol of iso-butyric acid, 3.79 mmol of propionic acid, 1.91 mmol of iso-valeric and 1.88 mmol of n-butyric acid. These concentrations were then adjusted to accommodate any dilutions and the soil moisture (Table 25.2). Initial research in the early 1990s using VFAs (Vass *et al.* 1992) took into account the weight of the individual and adjusted the absolute VFA concentrations accordingly. Difficulty in obtaining correct weight information, especially if the decedent was unidentified, introduced uncertainty and was ultimately deemed unnecessary. Recent procedures (not only in VFA analysis, but also in inorganic analyses, tissue biomarkers, etc.) now rely more heavily on the ratios between the VFAs, or other markers, rather than absolute values. These are calculated and presented in Table 25.2. VFA concentrations in the control samples were below detectable levels, so no adjustment of these values was necessary.

VFA analyses, like many others, are effectively utilised by relating their abundance to ADDs. In the USA, temperature is usually recorded in Fahrenheit, so any temperature obtained from the NWS must first be converted to Celsius. In this case, the hourly weather data obtained from the NWS was first converted to daily averages (F) and recorded on a spreadsheet after correcting for temperature differences at the death scene as described earlier. These values were then converted to Celsius. At this point, ADD values were calculated by accumulating (in reverse order) the average daily temperature in Celsius. This was performed for the entire 90 days of collected NWS data (Table 25.3). The day the decedent was discovered is considered time zero and the average temperature on that day was calculated as 8.33°C. Therefore the ADD value for the day before discovery is 8.33. The average temperature for the day prior to the day of discovery was 9.44°C, therefore two days before discovery the ADD value is 8.33 + 9.44 or 17.77 (17.78 in Table 25.3 due to rounding issues). This is back calculated for the entire 90 days.

There are three places where the ratios between n-butyric, iso-butyric and iso-valeric acid are almost identical and are highlighted by circles in Figure 25.2. These equate to approximately 160–170

Table 25.3 Determination of ADD range for interpretation of VFA results.

Daily average (F)	Celsius	ADD	Days pre-discovery	
			~	
73	22.78	825.09		
69	20.56	804.54	60	
67	19.44	785.09		
71	21.67	763.42		
72	22.22	741.20		range of formula
75	23.89	717.31		based method
72	22.22	695.09	55	for determining
72	22.22	672.87		PMI (52–57 days)
73	22.78	650.09		
70	21.11	628.98		
65	18.33	610.65		
66	18.89	591.76	50	range based on
68	20.00	571.76		VFA analysis
65	18.33	553.42		(48–50 days)
62	16.67	536.76		
54	12.22	524.54		
57	13.89	510.65	45	
63	17.22	493.42		
62	16.67	476.76		
54	12.22	464.54		
58	14.44	450.09		
62	16.67	433.42	40	
57	13.89	419.54		
60	15.56	403.98		
			~	
51	10.56	114.44		
51	10.56	103.89	10	
53	11.67	92.22		
53	11.67	80.56		
52	11.11	69.44		
51	10.56	58.89		
49	9.44	49.44		
50	10.00	39.44		
52	11.11	28.33		
51	10.56	17.78		
49	9.44	8.33		
47	8.33	0.00	decedent found	
				Av. 90 day Temp = 65°F (18°C)
				Av. 90 day Humidity = 73%

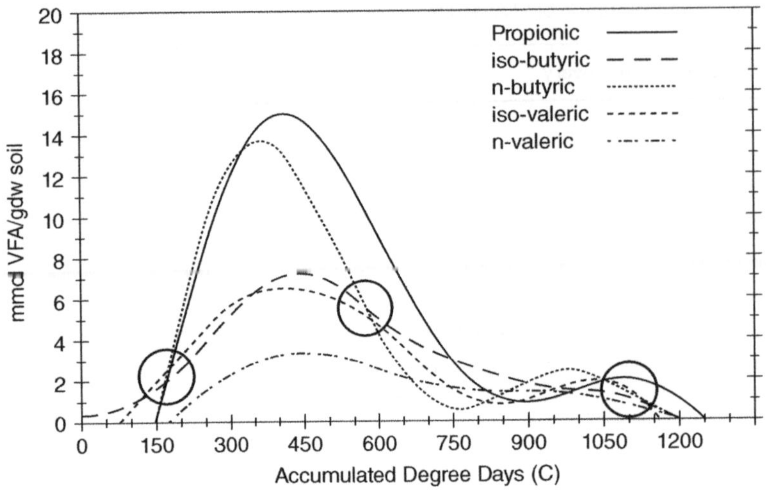

Figure 25.2 Possible ADD values when the decedent could have died based on VFA results (Source: Reprinted with permission of *Journal of Forensic Sciences* © 1992 ASTM International).

ADDs, 565–575 ADDs and 1,080–1,090 ADDs. After evaluating the proportion of propionic acid present (2 times greater) and the proportion of n-valeric acid (0.24), the only ADD range, which could apply, is the range of 565–575 ADDs. The ADD range of 160–170 would indicate early decomposition, which is clearly not the case, and as the 1050–1250 ADD range is approached, the corpse would be significantly more skeletonised than that observed, which also confirms that the 565–575 ADD range is the correct region to be evaluating. The closest ADD range in Table 25.3 encompassing the ADD range of 565–575 is 592–553 or 48–50 days prior to discovery and this would be the result of the VFA analysis. Interestingly, in this particular case, the corrected VFA value actually matches the *y*-axis value. This is because the weight correction factor of 1.000 in the original reference (weight range of 100–199 lbs (45–90 kg) would not have altered these values. This is not always the case, hence the value of switching to a ratio-based method and eliminating the weight estimation factor.

25.2.2 Formula-Based Method

The value of 1,285 (Figure 25.2) was an interesting discovery. The number was identified as the ADD value when VFAs could no longer be measured or detected in the leachate from a decomposition event. There is an error around this value of ±110 ADD, so the actual range would be 1,175–1,395 ADDs. This does not necessarily imply total skeletonisation – only that VFA liberation had ceased (e.g. mummification, etc.). This relatively constant value is therefore the basis for a formula-based method of determining the PMI (Vass 2011). This method has been developed to provide the investigator with a rapid estimate of the PMI while awaiting the results of the laboratory-based procedures. This can be a lengthy process, depending on the type of analysis or laboratory backlogs. In order to obtain this estimate, the investigator must determine the amount of total body decomposition, which has occurred. This does not necessarily need to be a single value, but can be a range of values. In this particular case, the abdominal cavity is beginning to collapse, which signifies approximately 50% decomposition. Both arms and both legs have begun to collapse, indicating slightly more advanced decomposition than 50%, so in this case a range of 55–60% was assigned to the decedent. Uncertainty by the investigator simply would increase the range to 45–70% or 40–75%, etc.

Using 1,285 as a basis, this value (signifying 100% decomposition based on VFA liberation) is multiplied by the decimal percentage of the estimated range of decomposition – in this case 55% and

60% resulting in 707–771 (ex. 1285 × 0.55 = 707). These values are ADDs and can be used without further mathematics, but it has been determined that of the four major taphonomic variables, which affect human decomposition (temperature, moisture, pH and the partial pressure of oxygen), temperature and moisture most significantly impact the decomposition process. Thus a more accurate result is obtained if these variables are also taken into account. Since the formula-based method is an equation with the numerator being decomposition and the denominator being environmental variables, the ADD values are then divided by temperature and humidity. When 707 ADDs is divided by the average temperature in Celsius (C) and humidity over the 90 days of corrected NWS data (18°C and 73% humidity), a result of 52 is obtained (707/(0.0103 × 18 × 73)) = 52 days and for 771/13.53 = 57 days (refer to reference for further explanation of the 0.0103 constant). The result is now in DAYS and no longer ADDs. When plotted on Table 25.3, there is remarkable agreement between the laboratory-based method of determining the PMI and the calculated formula-based method, which can be obtained at the death scene.

25.3 Conclusion

Investigative resolution of this case indicated that the decedent died 50 days prior to discovery. This was in agreement with VFA analysis of the soil and the results of the entomological study. Both of these techniques have a reported error range of approximately two days/month. The result of the formula based method (52–57) days, which was calculated only one day after discovery of the decedent, was accurate enough to allow for a rapid search of missing persons and an eventual identification of the decedent. Due to the ease of collection, extraction and analysis, VFAs have been used successfully in many forensic investigations worldwide.

References

Vass, A.A., Bass, W.M., Wolt, J.D., Foss, J.E. and Ammons, J.T. (1992) Time Since Death determinations of human cadavers using soil solution. *Journal of Forensic Sciences*, **37**: 1236–1253.

Vass, A.A. (2011) The elusive universal post-mortem interval formula. *Forensic Science International*, **204**: 34–40.

26

A Taphonomic Study Based on Observations of 196 Exhumations and 23 Clandestine Burials

Roosje de Leeuwe and W.J. Mike Groen

26.1 Introduction

This chapter summarises and compares the taphonomic observations on buried human remains, collected over a 9-year time period by forensic archaeologists from the Netherlands Forensic Institute (NFI).

There are two forensic archaeologists at the NFI, one employed in 2006 and a second in 2009. The main case work of the NFI forensic archaeologists consists of assisting the police during searches for missing and presumably buried persons, and also at crime scenes involving buried or scattered human remains and/or objects. The observations on hu man taphonomy presented in this chapter derive from three different types of victims:

1) individuals buried in a clandestine grave
2) unknown individuals buried in a cemetery grave
3) individuals who may have died a suspicious death and buried in a cemetery grave

In The Netherlands, a crime scene with a clandestine buried victim occurs on average three times a year, giving a total of 23 between 2006 and 2014. In addition, the forensic archaeologists also assist the police during exhumations performed at regular cemeteries. These exhumations either concern the identification of an unknown person (also known as *Nomen Nescio* or NN exhumations), or exhuming a corpse for a follow-up forensic investigation in cases of a suspicious death (regular exhumations).

26.2 Background on the Exhumations Carried out by the NFI

Before 2010, DNA sampling of an unidentified corpse for the missing person's database was not a standard procedure in The Netherlands. Unidentified individuals were buried as unknown persons in nameless graves. However, between 2010 and 2014, a total of 183 unidentified persons were exhumed at 44 different cemeteries, in order to extract their DNA. The physical remains were carefully dug up using archaeological techniques and forensic protocols to ensure that they were recovered complete and in a controlled environment. This also allowed the taphonomic observations to be recorded. The remains were then transported to a mobile autopsy tent, usually erected somewhere in the cemetery, where the forensic pathology department took samples for DNA analysis from a femur and a tooth and sometimes from other skeletal parts. After examination and sampling, the remains of the NN were buried in a separate place in the same cemetery or relocated to another cemetery for reburial.

Taphonomy of Human Remains: Forensic Analysis of the Dead and the Depositional Environment, First Edition.
Edited by Eline M.J. Schotsmans, Nicholas Márquez-Grant and Shari L. Forbes.

Of the exhumed individuals, 10 had an unknown burial date, leaving 173 individuals with known burial dates and thus the duration of their burial. Regular exhumations for follow-up investigation were less numerous: 23 in total.

The above-mentioned forensic excavations, NN exhumations and regular exhumations provided a good insight into decomposition stages and other taphonomic factors – encountered at clandestine burial sites and regular cemeteries, as different (taphonomic) observations were standardised and recorded during the NFI casework on specifically designed forms for this purpose. In this chapter, different variables (e.g. time, decomposition stage, body bags, soil type, burial depth, water context, coffins, trees and fauna) are assessed and discussed in relation to human decomposition processes below ground. Additionally, each variable is examined on its relevance to the taphonomic differences encountered between NN exhumations, regular exhumations and forensic excavations.

26.3 Variables

26.3.1 Decomposition Stage

Decomposition was scored on the NFI scale, based on Clark *et al.* (1997), who described decomposition in 10 stages, on a scale from 1 to 10, with 1 being a fresh corpse and 10 completely skeletonised. Nearly all corpses in forensic archaeological NFI cases are past the bloated stage (i.e. maximum swelling), which is stage 6 according to Clark *et al.* (1997). The next stage, stage 7, describes the visual onset of decomposition, when gases are released from the corpse, soft tissues putrefy and blood is totally destructed. In several NFI cases involving exhumations and excavations, the decomposition of the corpse was past the bloated stage, while externally the corpse still looked intact. This phenomenon is probably caused by slower or even arrested decomposition underground. The timescale for the decomposition of buried corpses is different from the one above ground. The scale of Clark *et al.* (1997) does not have an additional scale for this phenomenon, possibly because their scale was based on above-ground decomposition, where this stage takes place rapidly. The NFI scale used in this chapter is based on Clark *et al.* (1997) and modified for buried (B) corpses. The difference in stages 1 to 6 in Clark's scale are almost irrelevant for buried corpses in The Netherlands, because they are commonly encountered in an advanced decomposition stage. Therefore stages 1 to 6 in Clark's scale are combined in the NFI scale, for use during excavations and exhumations by a forensic archaeologist:

- Stage B-0: Fresh to bloated (Clark *et al.* (1997) stages 1 to 6)
- Stage B-1: Visually, the human remains look intact, but are past the bloated stage (no signs of bloat or decomposition, but possible smell of decomposition)
- Stage B-2: The human remains are in an advanced state of decomposition (Clark *et al.* (1997) stage 7)
- Stage B-3: The human remains are partly skeletonised (Clark *et al.* (1997) stage 8)
- Stage B-4: A skeleton with soft tissue parts, in particular ligaments (Clark *et al.* (1997) stage 9)
- Stage B-5: A skeleton without soft tissue parts (Clark *et al* (1997) stage 10)

As described above, the decomposition stages for all 219 human remains excavated or exhumed between 2006 and 2014 in The Netherlands are presented in Figure 26.1 and divided into regular exhumations, NN exhumations and forensic excavations.

In Figure 26.1, the linear line represents the mean for each specified case type. The forensic excavations display the steepest line (striped). This suggests a faster decomposition in clandestine burials. The results obtained from regular exhumations (solid line) seem to be similar to the results obtained from the forensic excavations. The NN exhumations (dotted line) produce the shallowest line, suggesting that the bodies of the NN individuals decompose slower on average. The differences in the

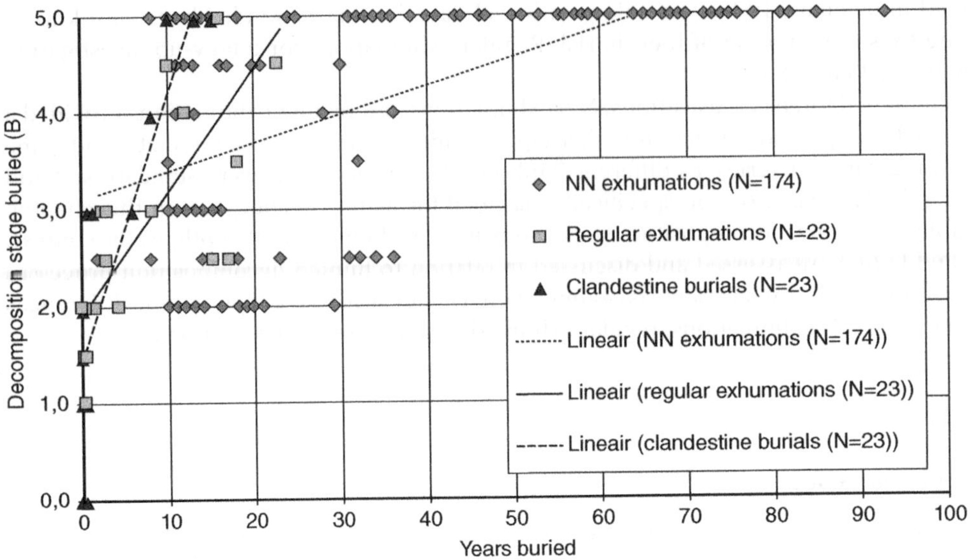

Figure 26.1 Decomposition stage of 219 human bodies, as observed during exhumations and forensic excavations. The *x*-axis correlates with the number of years that the bodies have been buried. The *y*-axis gives the observed decomposition stage.

decomposition rates are probably mainly related to the difference in the treatment of the corpse prior and during burial. For example, unknown individuals are often buried in plastic body bags, while a corpse in a clandestine grave can be buried naked or with a minimum of wrapping.

26.3.2 Duration of Burial

The most obvious taphonomic variable of a human burial is time. Given enough time, all human remains will skeletonise and eventually either disintegrate entirely leaving only a discoloration in the soil or fossilise into stone. Any other decomposition stages, for example, the presence of adipocere, are only temporary. Under favourable circumstances however, a human skeleton – even including (some) soft tissues – can stay intact for millennia. There is a significant difference in the NFI databases in relation to the forensic excavations and the exhumations. The individuals that were exhumed for identification (NN exhumations) purposes were buried between 2 and 93 years at the time of their exhumation. The oldest NN burial dated to 1920. In contrast, the burial period of individuals buried in clandestine graves rarely exceeded a few months to a couple of years, ranging between 5 days and 15 years. The range associated with regular exhumation for follow-up investigation is 1 month to 23 years.

26.3.3 Body Bags

One of the most influential factors in the decomposition process is the use of a body bag. The steepness of the lines in Figure 26.1 is strongly dependant on the use of plastic body bags. Dead interred at regular cemeteries will sometimes be buried in a body bag. Victims in clandestine graves might be wrapped in plastic, producing a similar effect to that of the use of a plastic body bag. Most other wrapping materials disintegrate and decay more easily, including modern eco-friendly biodegradable body bags. Plastic body bags were encountered in 80 of the 173 NN exhumations (45%) and in 11 of the 23 regular exhumations (48%). Table 26.1 shows the number of body bags used in cemetery burials per time period, for the total of 196 graves with a known burial date.

Table 26.1 Exhumed human bodies with and without body bag at regular cemeteries, per time period.

Burial period	N without body bag	N with body bag	Percentage with a body bag	Average decomposition stage
1920–1939	8	–	0%	5
1940–1959	59	–	0%	5
1960–1969	5	3	38%	5
1970–1979	3	11	79%	4.4
1980–1989	5	11	69%	4.1
1990–1999	7	44	86%	3.3
2000–2014	18	22	55%	3.1

Body bags were used for various reasons, most likely because the corpses were in a stage of decomposition and therefore easier to transport in a bag. Inside a body bag, decomposition slows down due to the closed environment causing a lack of oxygen. Table 26.1 shows a relatively low decomposition stage for corpses dating to the 1990s when plastic body bags were used more frequently in The Netherlands. The average decomposition stage for the 1990s is only marginally higher than the most recent ones dating to the 21st century.

The influence of a body bag on the decomposition stage also depends on the type of bag. In the 1960s, synthetic plastic bags (polymers) were used. The oldest synthetic purpose-designed body bag encountered during an exhumation that was still intact, dated to 1971. The plastic of these early body bags often hardened and was easily torn when pulled at. Usually the bodies inside these hardened plastic bags were skeletonised, or showed a few localised soft tissue parts with adipocere. In the 1980s and 1990s, Dutch body bags were made of a more durable plastic. To insure that the body would decompose, these bags were sometimes opened inside the coffin, just before the burial. The closed body bags usually slowed the decomposition process and resulted in a combination of bones, adipose and liquid substance of bodily fluids inside these bags. Since the early 21st century, most Dutch body bags are made of biodegradable plastics and also seem to be used less during burials.

The best-preserved corpses, that is in the earliest stage of decomposition (up to stage B-3), were the individuals buried in the 1990s, which was related to the strong body bags. It also made a difference whether a body bag was closed or open before the burial. Specifically, in closed body bags, the anaerobic conditions were ideal for adipocere formation. In closed body bags, the average decomposition stage was B-3.0 (at an average of 16 years buried). In open bags, the average decomposition stage was B-4.1 (at an average of 20 years buried). This would, generally speaking, translate to a decomposition rate of 5.4 years/B-stage for closed bags and 5.0 years/B-stage for open bags.

26.3.4 Soil Type

The Netherlands consists almost entirely of soft soils such as peat, clay or sand, or a combination of these. Also, being the proverbial Low Countries, Dutch ground water levels are relatively high. As of 1997, it is prohibited by law to bury people below groundwater level;[1] therefore many Dutch cemeteries are raised with sand. This sand is loose, porous and permeable to oxygen and water. Of the total of 196 exhumations, 137 (70%) were exhumed in sandy soils and 51 (26%) were exhumed in

1 'Besluit op de Lijkbezorging' (1997, paragraph 4, article 5).

Table 26.2 Decomposition rate per soil type, without a plastic wrapping.

	Sand	Clay	Peat	Tomb	Total
Forensic excavation	12	3	0	0	**15**
Regular exhumation	10	1	0	1	**12**
NN exhumation	14	3	0	3	**20**
Total	**36**	**7**	**0**	**4**	**47**
Average decomposition stage (B)	3.2	3.0			
Average number of years buried	9.8	13.7			
Decomposition rate (years/B-stage)	3.0	4.6			

clay. Forty-nine of the latter exhumations dated to the 1950s and only two dated post-1997. In four exhumations (2%) there was no soil, as these were tombs or 'basement' graves. Four exhumations (2%) took place on loess soil, a specific type of fine silt.

The taphonomic influence of the soil type can only be considered for burials without a body bag, as the plastic wrapping blocks the interaction with the soil. All human bodies buried before 1974 were completely skeletonised. This means that after, at the most, 36 years under ground in either clay or sandy soil, human remains in The Netherlands will be skeletonised if buried in regular cemeteries. In comparison, the oldest non-skeletonised human body buried in a closed body bag dated to 1974 (decomposition stage B-2.5). The oldest non-skeletonised human body buried – not wrapped in a plastic covering – dated to 1993. Only 20 NN exhumations – buried without a body bag – were associated with human bodies buried after 1974. In 12 regular exhumations and 15 clandestine burials also, no plastic wrapping was found (i.e. body bag or plastic covering). The total of excavated/exhumed bodies that were not wrapped in plastic is 47 (Table 26.2).

The average decomposition stage in sandy soils was more advanced than in clay soils. In The Netherlands, it takes on average 3 years in sandy soils for a corpse to degrade a stage. In clay soils this is over 4.5 years. Decomposition occurs faster in sandy soils, as most of these soil types are more permeable to oxygen and water than clay soils. Experience from the casework in The Netherlands shows that clay soil seals off buried corpses from the oxygen supply and produces a reasonably airtight environment. In several searches for missing persons where cadaver dogs were used, the clay soil notably prevented gases to seep through and possibly even absorb smells, causing the cadaver dogs to miss the buried victim (who were later found by other means). This observation should be taken into account when using cadaver dogs to locate missing persons that are presumably buried in a clay soil.

26.3.5 Burial Depth

The depth of a burial naturally influences the oxygen supply and the temperature. In theory, the deeper the burial the longer it takes to decompose, because with increasing depth, animals have less access to the remains, temperature decreases and oxygen supply diminishes (Rodriguez 1997). In Dutch cemeteries, the minimum burial depth (i.e. the thickness of the ground column above the lid of the coffin) required by Dutch law is 65 cm (2 feet). The maximum number of individuals that may be buried in a single grave (above each other) is 3, making the maximum burial depth 180 cm (6 feet). Unidentified persons are often buried in the top layer, 65 to 100 cm (2 to 3 feet) below the ground. Cemeteries do this on purpose, because there may be a need to exhume these individuals in the future. The observed influence of the burial depth in cemeteries is therefore seemingly negligible, if compared to other variables such as the presence of a body bag or the soil type.

Clandestine burials, as encountered in The Netherlands, have an average depth of ca. 33 cm below the ground level (to the upper side of the body) and an average depth of the grave-pit of 74 cm below ground level. The depth of a clandestine grave-pit is dependent on the soil type; it is easier to dig in sandy soils than it is in clay soils. The average grave depth of a clandestine grave in sandy soils was 79 cm (n = 17), whereas the average grave depth in clay soils was 52 cm (n = 4). Two graves were dug in peat (65 and 70 cm deep). The shallowest clandestine graves were encountered in clay soils, with a thin layer of clay only a few centimetres thick covering the corpse in two cases. The deepest clandestine graves were found in sandy soils, with two graves deeper than 170 cm. The depth of a sandy grave also seems to depend on the direct environment of the grave, as the presence of trees in the vicinity can prevent the digging of a deep grave, due to the roots being in the way. Twenty-two of the clandestine graves were dug by hand, mostly using some sort of shovel. One shallow grave was dug in sand without the use of any tools (bare hands).

26.3.6 Water Context

Of the 174 unknown persons exhumed for identification purposes, at least 85 were originally found in water. As for some of the NN cases, the circumstances of the discovery are unknown, and this number is probably even higher in reality (at least 50%). Water influences the decomposition process and the completeness of the body. In four NN exhumations, only one human torso was encountered during the exhumation, and in another just a lower leg.

Experience has shown that knowing in advance if the person to be exhumed is a water corpse is beneficial to the process of exhuming. This information helps, for example, to understand that the human remains about to be exhumed could be incomplete and therefore saves time looking extensively for the 'missing' body parts. The NFI database also shows that Dutch water corpses are commonly placed in a plastic body bag, as many of these corpses were discovered in an advanced stage of decomposition. Some exhumed remains were double or triple bagged.

A separate case file involved the exhumation of 29 victims of the 1953 North Sea flood disaster. Nearly all of these remains were complete corpses. This is very likely related to a fast recovery after the disaster, with a minimal amount of time in between death, floati ng and burial.

26.3.7 Coffins

All individuals associated with regular exhumations were buried in a coffin and only two of the unidentified individuals were buried without one. The quality of the material that was used to make the coffins, varied from solid oak to ply wood. Most of the unidentified individuals were buried in simple, cheap and available coffins, made out of, for example, 'oak veneer', which is bonded wood. These coffins often start to disintegrate after three years. As soon as a coffin begins to disintegrate the decomposition process accelerates. Sometimes the lid of the coffin was pushed in deliberately by the cemetery personnel – with the aid of an excavator – to enhance the decomposition process. Only one NN individual buried in a 'cheap' coffin had an intact coffin; the cheap coffins of other NN individuals were falling apart and had usually entirely disintegrated. Disintegration is common in coffins of three years and older, but has also been observed in even newer ones. On one occasion, an expensive lacquered wooden coffin was reused in an NN burial. Older, pre-1960 NN burials have been observed to have better-quality coffins, and oak was commonly used before the 1960s. A few exhumations contained welded zinc linings inside the wooden coffin, closing the access of oxygen. This is standard procedure in repatriations where coffins are transported across an international border. Sometimes a zinc lining was used inside coffins of NN individuals, when a crime was suspected. This had the advantage that the human body was much better preserved and protected against damage. Zinc, like other metals, has the property of preserving the organic material it is in contact with.[2] Within the forensic clandestine burials, no corpses were buried in a coffin or anything with a similar function.

26.3.8 Tree Roots

On several occasions, severe bone degradation was observed in human remains exhumed from graves with a tree in the vicinity. All skeletal elements exhumed under tree roots were observed to be very brittle. It is assumed that the roots of the trees absorbed the soft tissue and minerals from the remains, until the skeletal elements disintegrated. It is observed that, in general, trees have a very destructive influence on buried remains underneath them.

26.3.9 Fauna

The only frequently observed wildlife in coffins or body bags in The Netherlands are springtails (Collembola). Unfortunately, little is known about the influence of springtails on the decomposition of humans, except that they seem to feed on the organic remains. For Dutch exhumations, it is known that these hexapods can still be present in graves dating back decades and that they are able to find their way into seemingly inaccessible places.

Most of the Dutch clandestine burials lacked any fauna. This is possibly due to the maritime climate in The Netherlands, the high groundwater levels, soil conditions or other local factors. It often seems to be too cold for blowflies, although on some rare occasions, a few live fly maggots (Diptera) and unidentified worms were observed. Earthworms (Lumbricina) are nearly always present in a grave, but seem to be of little influence.

26.3.10 Other Variables

Other variables to take into account when assessing taphonomy of buried human remains are the age at death, whether or not a corpse has been autopsied and if the corpse was already in a stage of decomposition at the time of discovery, or at the time of burial. Furthermore, extreme habits (ranging from top sports to drug use or intense medication) also influence the decomposition rate. The latter aspects are often not known at the time of exhumation or excavation, specifically in unknown individuals. Experience has shown that it is desirable to have knowledge of all the above-mentioned variables before exhumation, in order to be able to predict what to expect or to find in a grave. A police report describing the find circumstances helps. If a human body has undergone an autopsy, decomposition will be in a more advanced state and, in some cases, loose body parts might be placed in the grave at a later stage. This occurs when the remains are buried, but some parts are still at the laboratory for further examination or identification purposes, such as the jaw, the head or the hands. One example is when the skull is used for a facial reconstruction.

26.4 Cemetery versus Clandestine Burials

What are the most significant differences in human taphonomy observed in graves exhumed at regular cemeteries versus graves excavated at clandestine locations? NFI data show that a wrapping, either of a body bag or other plastics, has the largest influence on the decomposition process, as observed in exhumations and excavations. Eight out of the 23 clandestine buried human bodies were wrapped in plastic. This is nearly 35%, a lower percentage than the use of body bags in regular cemetery burials

2 This is a well-documented observation in archaeology (e.g. Watson 1998, 2004).

(i.e. 46%). However, on a clandestine buried corpse, the plastic is usually not fully airtight. The corpse will therefore decompose faster than one buried in a closed plastic body bag. Oxygen supply rather than a difference in temperature and burial duration seem to be the other two important factors in all types of burials encountered by the NFI. The amount of oxygen supply not only depends on the wrapping, but also on the soil type and burial depth. Since clandestine buried corpses are shallower on average, this could result in faster decomposition.

26.5 Conclusion

Several taphonomic variables observed by the NFI forensic archaeologists in 196 exhumations and 23 excavations were discussed in this chapter. The statistics behind these variables confirm what is written in the literature (e.g. Grellner and Glenewinkel 1997; Manhein 1997; Mant 1987). Clearly, decomposition depends on factors such as time, oxygen supply, soil type, burial depth, etc. Additionally, this study has shown that decomposition stages for human bodies decomposing above ground have to be slightly altered to be of use for burials. Also, according to the NFI database, human bodies that are buried without a body bag (plastic coverings), in sandy soils, within the vicinity of a tree, or in a shallow grave, decompose faster. Finally, an important observation to keep in mind when using cadaver dogs, is that hardly any smell seems to seep through from clandestine burials in (Dutch) clay soil.

References

Clark, M.A., Worrell, M.B. and Pless, J.E. (1997) Postmortem changes in soft tissues. In: Haglund, W.D. and Sorg, M.H. (eds), *Forensic Taphonomy. The postmortem fate of human remains*. CRC Press: Boca Raton. pp. 151–164.

Grellner, W. and Glenewinkel, F. (1997) Exhumations: synopsis of morphological and toxicological findings in relation to the postmortem interval. Survey on a 20-year period and review of the literature. *Forensic Science International*, **90**: 139–159.

Manhein, M.H. (1997) Decomposition rates of deliberate burials: A case study of preservation. In: Haglund, W.D. and Sorg, M.H. (eds), *Forensic Taphonomy. The postmortem fate of human remains*. CRC Press: Boca Raton, pp. 469–481.

Mant, A.K. (1987) Knowledge acquired from post-War exhumations. In: Boddington, A., Garland, A.N. and Janaway, R.C. (eds), *Death, Decay and Reconstruction. Approaches to archaeology and forensic science*. Manchester University Press: Manchester, pp. 65–78.

Rodriguez, W.C. (1997) Decomposition of buried and submerged bodies. In: Haglund, W.D. and Sorg, M.H. (eds), *Forensic Taphonomy. The postmortem fate of human remains*. CRC Press: Boca Raton, pp. 459–467.

Watson, J. (1998) Organic artefacts and their preservation. In: Bayley, J. (ed.), *Science in Archaeology. An agenda for the future*. English Heritage: London, pp. 225–235.

Watson, J. (2004) *Organic Material Associated with Metalwork from the Anglo-Saxon Cemetery at Mount Pleasant, Kent*. Centre for Archaeology Report 8, English Heritage: London.

27

Case Studies on Taphonomic Variation between Cemetery Burials

Karl Harrison and Emily Cline

27.1 Introduction

This chapter aims to consider the nature of taphonomic variation in instances of buried human remains, and more specifically the manner in which patterns of decay and preservation might differ over short distances, such as within the bounds of a single cemetery or churchyard. Further to considering general observations on the understanding of the chief significant variables in burial taphonomy, this chapter will briefly sketch out two archaeological case studies that will assist in emphasising the main points followed by forensic case applications.

This first of these sketches details the excavation of burials in the 18th- and 19th-century cemetery attached to the Royal Hospital Haslar (UK), and considers the aggressive effect on human remains and associated funerary fittings of free water percolation through an acidic burial environment, and in addition the very localised instances of organic preservation that can result from metal ion inhibition, resulting in variances of preservational signatures between adjacent interments. The second sketch outlines the medieval vault burials of St Bees Man and St Bees Lady, in the south chancel of St Bees Priory (UK). In considering St Bees Man, the effect of human intervention in the form of efforts to embalm his soft tissues and the restriction of the immediate burial environment within a lead coffin, contrasts with the relatively unprotected skeletonised remains of St Bees Lady. The final sketch extends the consideration of taphonomic agents in burial environments by outlining how an improved understanding of the effect of these complex variables can be applied to contemporary forensic investigations. Such applications are briefly touched upon in an outline of a formal exhumation from a cemetery, and the recovery of remains from a clandestine grave filled with highly organic potting compost as a replacement for the natural clay fill.

It is noteworthy that the wellspring of so much contemporary research on the subject of burial taphonomy is derived from William Bass's erroneous estimation of the time since death of the body of Colonel William Shy, a Confederate Officer subject of an unauthorised exhumation in a Civil War Cemetery (Bass 1984). In this instance, Bass informed the police investigating that they were seeking to identify the body of a 24- to 28-year-old male who had been dead for a year. While the biological profile was correct, Colonel Shy has been dead for 113 years (Bass 1997).

27.2 Burial Taphonomy: Examples of Cemetery Burials

The cemetery is an environment that is increasingly becoming of interest to burial archaeologists. The secular or municipal cemetery has grown in popularity since the 18th century, and as a

Taphonomy of Human Remains: Forensic Analysis of the Dead and the Depositional Environment, First Edition.
Edited by Eline M.J. Schotsmans, Nicholas Márquez-Grant and Shari L. Forbes.

consequence will continue to develop as a locus for archaeological endeavour (Rugg 2000). While human remains in these locations frequently present as a relatively orderly array of single or multiple coffined inhumations with little or no intercutting or stratigraphic complexity, they can on occasion host unusual examples of deposition within monumental effigies (Stirland 1990), or apparently suspicious additions of seemingly hasty and clandestine burials to formal interments, such as the 16th-century double inhumation at the Lady Chapel of Mount Grace, Osmotherley, North Yorkshire, UK (Roberts *et al.* 1992).

The variables acting to degrade or preserve buried remains have perplexed forensic anthropologists and archaeologists for a generation. From the statement: 'At present there is little information pertaining to estimation of time since death of a buried body' (Rodriguez and Bass 1985), the interaction of taphonomic variables was subject to consideration in progressively greater detail; Waldron (1987) considered the action of bacteria, moulds and invertebrates to be the chief agents of decomposition, alongside dispersal by vertebrates and the chemical action of soil water and acids. Cox and Bell (1999) reflected on the variable survival of remains associated with a high profile UK serial killing, considering the spectrum of factors that might explain the partial nature of the recovered skeletal elements. They regarded these factors as being the nature of recovery, pre-depositional dispersal, abrasion, exfoliation, microstructural diagenesis, digestion, gnawing, insect damage, rootlet damage and soil depth, type and hydrology. Of particular relevance to the preservation of soft tissue is the formation of adipocere through the conversion of intrinsic body fats (Fieldler *et al.* 2009; Thali *et al.* 2011).

Recent research has not advanced a quantified understanding of the interaction of identified variables in a burial environment, but it has served to emphasise the point that dramatic instances of preservation or decay can result from a combination of environmental variables (depth of burial, climatic conditions, physical condition of the soil) and methods of burial or the nature or treatment of the remains (Lowe *et al.* 2013; Vass 2001).

27.2.1 The Royal Hospital Haslar

The Royal Hospital Haslar is located on the Gosport peninsula in Hampshire, UK, on land that was purchased by the Crown for the construction of a hospital in 1744. Early plans show the eventual hospital building located on a spit of fluvioaluvial sand and gravel surrounded by salt marshes and estuarine silts, and indicate the allotment of ca. 9 acres (ca. 3.6 hectares) for a burial ground adjacent to the hospital complex. This burial ground, known as the Paddock, was in use between 1753 and 1826, at which time burial in the hospital grounds was prohibited, the area reported as being '...thick with buried bodies and scattered tombstones...' (Lloyd and Coulter 1963).

In total, five seasons of excavation have been undertaken in the Paddock, with the aim of identifying distinctions in burial patterns inside and outside the formal boundaries of the cemetery; a series of exploratory machine trenches were cut across the area in 2005 by Oxford Archaeology to evaluate the position, condition and number of the underlying burials (Oxford Archaeology 2005). This was then followed by four seasons of excavation undertaken by Cranfield University (2007–2009 and 2013). The first three of these seasons concentrated on interments within the burial ground and the last on its boundary and the burials located beyond it (Shortland *et al.* 2008).

Within the Paddock, the burials appeared to have been single inhumations cut in arranged rows. Instances of multiple burials appear to be restricted to outside the formal cemetery (two triple burials were located in 2005, a double burial in 2009 and an interment of four individuals recorded in 2013) (Gilbert 2013). The Paddock interments generally featured a moderate to poor degree of skeletal preservation, with occasional preservation of pine coffin fragments (Hazell 2008) and coffin nails ubiquitous in the graves, indicating comprehensive coffining of remains prior to burial. The grave fills were generally unfavourable to organic survival, the Paddock being dominated by a mildly

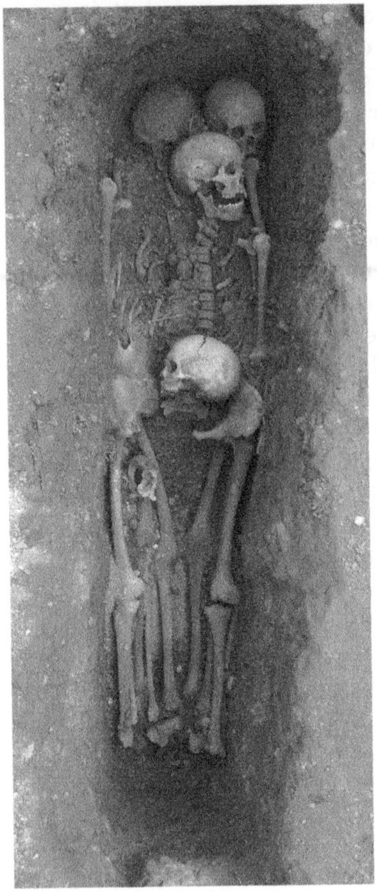

Figure 27.1 Working shot of interment with 4 individuals at Haslar Royal Hospital, 2013, illustrating distinction between dark silty grave fill and sand/gravel natural geology (image reprinted with permission of K. Harrison).

acidic sand and gravel geology that allowed the rapid percolation of rain water through the grave. Those graves that did retain the best-preserved remains tended to feature a darker stoneless silt as the immediate burial matrix, directly surrounding those skeletons (Figure 27.1). It was unclear whether this silt represented the inclusion of buried humic topsoil stripped from the modern surface of the Paddock by successive efforts of landscaping, or was formed as a consequence of the decomposition of coffins around the remains.

In his unpublished thesis, Martin (2011) examined in detail the characteristics of decomposition associated with burial Has2008/B102. The skeleton in question had been subject to an obvious craniotomy as part of an exercise in dissection or post-mortem examination. In addition to this, Martin suggested that an observed peri-mortem fracture to the right clavicle, the absent sternum and the pronounced degradation to the anterior rib ends might be consistent with a thoracotomy.

While the degree of organic survival across the site was generally poor, there was one particular instance of preservation by metal ion inhibition, whereby the biocidal action of copper items in graves was noted as being an agent of protection of organic material (Janaway 1983; Janaway and Scott 1989). In the Haslar Royal Hospital burial ground, two fragments of cloth thought to have formed part of a burial shroud and each ca. 20 m across were recovered fastened to a copper pin.

Given an opportunity to consider relative levels of decay and preservation over an extensive site, the dominating effect of aggressive conditions in this instance primarily mildly acidic soil conditions and a free-draining sand-gravel matrix that promoted water percolation through the graves, can be seen to provide generally predictable conditions of preservation. This general pattern seen across burials at the Royal Hospital Haslar has been shown to be subject to specific modifications which might represent subtle natural variations (i.e. an improved degree of skeletal preservation in the siltier grave fills), or striking alterations induced by human activity (i.e. either the post-mortem examination of a body affecting the ultimate presentation of excavated remains, or the inclusion of a copper shroud pin prompting the preservation of fragile fabrics).

27.2.2 St Bees Priory

One of the authors has recently completed a review of material associated with the remains of St Bees Man and St Bees Lady, which were discovered in 1981 during an excavation of St Bees Priory in St Bees, Cumbria, UK (Cline 2014). Architectural evidence suggested that a structure had stood on the site around 1290 AD and was abandoned prior to the dissolution of the Priory in 1539 (Todd 2013). The 1981 excavation season concentrated on an area south of the chancel, where 'the soils were mostly of boulder clay overlaying a bedrock of red-sandstone, with the common feature of a highly variable water table' (Chapman 1995). The foundations of a building were uncovered along with 12 associated burials, interpreted as being comprised of two distinct groups; an area associated with the burials of monks and another area destined to secular interments (O'Sullivan 1982). Two of these burials belonging to the latter secular group – St Bees Man and St Bees Lady – were located within a stone vault, which would have been aligned to the chancel aisle's midline. The fill of the vault was described as being a loose sandy brown loam with small sandstone rubble. On removal of this fill, the vault was found to contain a lead coffin and a skeleton (SK100), laid side-by-side.

The lead coffin was more accurately described as a 'lead wrap', as it was comprised of a sheet of lead that had been cut and placed around the body of St Bees Man (Knüsel *et al.* 2010). On initial recording, it was noted that a small perforation in the lead sheet was present at the foot of the coffin. On opening, it was found to contain a shrouded figure that was subject to a post-mortem examination by forensic pathologist Dr Edmund Tapp (Tapp and O'Sullivan 1982). The body of St Bees Man was found to be wrapped in two linen shrouds, both well-preserved and covered in a resinous substance as a form of embalming, at first thought to be beeswax (Todd 2013), but later identified as a pine resin (Knüsel *et al.* 2010). On removal of the shrouds, the body of St Bees Man was found to be so well preserved that Dr Tapp could examine all of the major organs. He noted that the body was intact with some damage associated with fungal colonisation of the right foot (Tapp and O'Sullivan 1982). The skin and tissues initially appeared to be pink, but rapidly turned yellow-brown on exposure to air. Head, beard and pubic hair all survived, and in addition a wreath of long human hair was arranged around the body's neck and shoulders. A high degree of preservation was noted in the hands, with fingernails present and fingerprints observed. The subcutaneous tissues featured blood that had a fresh appearance both within the vessels and in the thoracic cavity. In contrast with the preserved body of St Bees Man, the female skeleton SK100 was recovered lying supine next to the lead coffin with no survival of soft tissues, some fragmentation of her skeletal remains and a high concentration of lead percolating into the surrounding soil fill.

In the case of St Bees Man, Chapman (1995) states that 'decay ceased shortly after the formation of a layer of adipocere'; however, it is unclear how far the formation of adipocere had progressed – the only evidence of adipocere recorded at autopsy were crystalline nodules found within the serous cavity and other internal organs. It has been suggested that adipocere survives well in anaerobic conditions such as sealed lead coffins (Chamberlain and Pearson 2001). Where adipocere is present, it has been shown to be 'an important factor in retarding the ultimate decomposition process' (Mant 1987), but it has also been observed to form at a slower rate in coffined burials (Forbes *et al* 2005b). Preservation, decomposition and adipocere formation all depend upon the method of burial and the physical conditions of the burial environment; soil type and soil pH affect the formation of adipocere (Forbes *et al.* 2005a,c). A significant amount of research has been conducted into the formation of adipocere (Forbes *et al.* 2005a,b,c; Schoenen and Schoenen 2013; Ubelaker and Zarenko 2011), as well as the archaeological presentation of adipocere formation (Fiedler *et al.* 2009; Thali *et al.* 2011), but none mention its formation as crystals within soft tissues.

It is likely that preservation was initially induced by the formation of an anaerobic environment within the lead coffin, and the potential for heavy metals to inhibit enzyme activity (Carter and Tibbet 2008), but that prior to this, early efforts taken to preserve the soft tissue by wrapping and embalming would have been crucial. An embalming process including the application of preservative substances and the use of cloth strips to wrap the body was being utilised in the mid-1300s, but more typically involved the removal of the internal organs (Chamberlain and Pearson 2001). The striking preservation of the soft tissues was brought about by a combination of factors; the application of an embalming resin, sealing within a lead coffin and deposition within the stone vault, but while the chemical nature of the burial environment may have assisted in the preservation of St Bees Man, the skeleton of the woman beside him demonstrates the importance of a combination of preservative agents acting in concert. Moreover, the lead traces evident in the soil fill surrounding SK100 underline the chemical feedback at work in the burial vault. The proximity of these two burials, coupled with their marked difference in preservation, makes the case of St Bees an important case study, despite the age of much of the associated research.

27.2.3 Forensic Applications

It is a relatively easy task to consider what wide-ranging environmental variables might be responsible for generalised states of degradation across a broad sample of a cemetery population, as at the Royal Hospital Haslar. Likewise, a range of analytical techniques such as X-ray Diffraction (XRD), Fourier Transform Infrared Spectroscopy (FTIR) or the assessment of DNA preservation might be used to better grasp the interaction between a number of taphonomic agents acting to bring about dramatic instances of preservation within an otherwise undifferentiated cemetery, as with St Bees Man (Barta *et al.* 2014). Furthermore, it is clear that these investigations not only assist in shedding light on Bass's dilemma outlined at the start of this chapter; the complex problem of taphonomy in burial environments, but also that the review of material in the archaeological record can be at least as informative as formal experiment through the use of taphonomic facilities.

Beyond the production of standard tools, such as models for aiding the estimation of post-mortem interval, it is not always straightforward to see in which circumstances an improved understanding of burial taphonomy might aid forensic investigations. Consequently, two short examples are appended here.

27.2.3.1 Strategy for a Formal Exhumation

In 2006, one of the authors (KH) acted as a Crime Scene Manager in the formal exhumation of a coffined burial from a municipal cemetery in the English Midlands. The male decedent had died under suspicious circumstances two years previously and buried in the same year, and a re-investigation had highlighted a need to conduct a second post-mortem examination on his remains.

In planning for the excavation and successful recovery of the body, it was important to consider the likely condition of the remains. In speaking with the cemetery's sexton, it became clear how small alterations in landform and hydrology might affect the nature of individual grave environments. Over much of the cemetery the water table was low enough that it had no effect on the burials, but in the area of the exhumation, dug graves had a tendency to become water-logged. The grave diggers would counter this effect when mourners attended graveside committal services by retaining the leaves collected from the cemetery and filling the flooded grave bases with them to prevent splashing at the lowering of the coffin.

On exhumation, it became clear that the clay subsoil and waterlogged environment had acted to preserve the coffin and ensure the integrity of the body. In this instance, the surrounding coffin was of a solid timber construction. Had it been made from fibreboard or environmentally-friendly cardboard, then the wet burial matrix would have rapidly compromised its structure. At post-mortem, it became apparent that the male's organs, having been examined during the original post-mortem, had afterwards been placed in a plastic bag within the thoracic cavity and had consequently been subject to advanced decomposition, whereas the subdermal fat still associated with the body had undergone conversion and stabilisation as adipocere.

The coffin was opened at the mortuary prior to the post-mortem examination, where it was apparent that the evisceration during the first post-mortem two years previously and the embalming of the superficial tissues had succeeded in preserving the body such that a full and thorough re-examination could be undertaken.

27.2.3.2 An Unusually Adapted Burial in a Clandestine Burial

In 2010, one of the authors (KH) acted as a forensic archaeologist assisting a police force in the English Home Counties in the search for a clandestine burial of a male decedent in his eighties last seen alive in 2005. The search area was the back garden of a domestic property, the natural subsoil of which was a dense grey clay. The male's body was found in a ca. 1.2 m grave, wrapped loosely in a tarpaulin that failed to cover the peripheral elements such as the left hand, lower legs and top of the head. On excavating the grave, it was clear that the natural grey clay subsoil had been removed from the grave when it was excavated and replaced with an organic-rich potting compost apparently brought in for the purpose.

While the male's torso was protected by the tarpaulin and as a consequence much of the associated soft tissue had survived, primarily as a fragile layer of skin containing a soft, semi-liquid adipocere, the exposed parts in direct contact with the potting compost fill had skeletonised entirely. This pattern of focused decomposition could only be explained by three taphonomic variables; improved water percolation through the grave, oxygen-rich void spaces in the light grave fill, and the microbial action of the potting compost itself.

In both of these forensic examples, an understanding of the interaction of taphonomic agents, in part gained through consideration of examples offered in the archaeological record, has assisted in the reconstruction of crime scene formation processes, which in turn facilitate an optimal recovery of human remains and associated evidence, and the presentation of these observations in court. It seems unlikely that we will ever be afforded a comprehensive understanding of taphonomic variation in cemetery inhumations, but a combination of a mature and appropriate experimental programme and an improved consideration of case studies drawn from archaeology and forensic practice assist in sophisticating our view.

27.3 Conclusion

Much has been written about the taphonomic fate of human remains, and the impact of complex environmental factors in the assessment of preservation and decay. This chapter has sought to achieve two ends; first, it demonstrates the clear link between the archaeological and forensic records, and the importance, particularly for forensic anthropologists and archaeologists, of being able to understand and draw upon instances of taphonomic study derived from non-forensic contexts. Second, it emphasises the importance of case review as a means of not only supplementing, but also driving the agenda for taphonomic experimentation. The case studies and forensic applications presented here have little ostensibly in common, other than that each of them presents levels of complexity beyond competent experimental design, and as such offers valuable if perplexing insights into the nature of human decomposition.

References

Barta, J.L., Monroe, C., Crockford, S.J. and Kemp, B.M. (2014) Mitochondrial DNA preservation across 3,000-year-old northern fur seal ribs is not related to bone density: implications for forensic investigations. *Forensic Science International*, **239**: 11–18.

Bass, W. (1984) Time interval since death: A difficult decision. In: Rathbun, T.A. and Buikstra, J.E. (eds), *Human Identification: Case studies in forensic anthropology*. Charles C. Thomas: Springfield, pp. 136–147.

Bass, W. (1997) Outdoor decomposition rates in Tennessee. In: Haglund, W.D. and Sorg, M.H. (eds), *Forensic Taphonomy: The postmortem fate of human remains*. CRC Press: Boca Raton, pp.181–186.

Carter, D.O. and Tibbet, M. (2008) Cadaver decomposition and soil: processes. In: Carter, D.O. and Tibbett, M. (eds), *Soil Analysis in Forensic Taphonomy: Chemical and biological effects of buried human remains*. CRC Press: Boca Raton, pp. 29–51.

Chamberlain, A.T. and Pearson, M.P. (2001) *Earthly Remains: The history and science of preserved human bodies*. Oxford University Press: New York.

Chapman, S. (1995) *St Bees, Cumbria: A report on the human remains excavated from the south side of the Priory Church in 1981*. Unpublished MA dissertation, University of Leicester: Leicester.

Cline, E. (2014) *St Bees Man: A cold case review*. Unpublished MSc thesis, Cranfield University: Cranfield.

Cox, M. and Bell, L. (1999) Recovery of human skeletal elements from a recent UK murder inquiry: preservational signatures. *Journal of Forensic Sciences*, **44**: 945–950.

Fiedler, S., Buegger, F., Klaubert, B., Zipp, K., Dohrmann, R. *et al.* (2009) Adipocere withstands 1,600 years of fluctuating groundwater levels in soil. *Journal of Archaeological Science*, **36**: 1328–1333.

Forbes. S.L., Stuart, B.H. and Dent, B.B. (2005a) The effect of the burial environment on adipocere formation. *Forensic Science International*, **154**: 24–34.

Forbes, S.L., Stuart, B.H. and Dent, B.B. (2005b) The effect of the method of burial on adipocere formation. *Forensic Science International*, **154**: 44–52.

Forbes, S.L., Stuart, B.H. and Dent, B.B. (2005c) The effect of soil type on adipocere formation. *Forensic Science International*, **154**: 35–43.

Gilbert, C. (2013) *Excluded? Investigating graves outside the burial ground at Royal Hospital Haslar*. Unpublished MSc thesis, Cranfield University: Cranfield.

Hazell, Z. (2008) *Haslar, Gosport, Hampshire: Waterlogged wood remains from Royal Hospital Haslar*. Unpublished report of the Research Department Report Series. English Heritage.

Janaway, R.C. (1983) Textile fibre characteristics preserved by metal corrosion: the potential of SEM studies. *The Conservator*, 7: 48–52.

Janaway, R.C. and Scott, B.G. (1989) *Evidence Preserved in Corrosion Products: New fields in artifact studies*. United Kingdom Institute for Conservation: London.

Knüsel, C.J., Batt, C.M., Cook, G., Montgomery, J., Müldner, G. *et al.* (2010) The identity of the St Bees Lady, Cumbria: an osteobiographical approach. *Medieval Archaeology*, **5**: 271–311.

Lloyd, C. and Coulter, J.L. (1963) *Medicine and the Navy 1200–1900*. E. & S. Livingstone: Edinburgh.

Lowe, A.C., Beresford, D.V., Carter, D.O., Gaspari, F., O'Brien, R.C. *et al.* (2013) The effect of soil texture on the degradation of textiles associated with buried bodies. *Forensic Science International*, **231**: 331–339.

Mant, A.K. (1987) Knowledge acquired from post-War exhumations. In: Boddington, A., Garland, A.N. and Janaway, R.C. (eds), *Death, Decay and Reconstruction: Approaches to archaeology and forensic science*. Manchester University Press: Manchester, pp. 65–78.

Martin, N. (2011) *Death, Dissection and Deposition: The use of forensic archaeothanatology to examine eighteenth and nineteenth century burial practices at the Royal Hospital Haslar*. Unpublished MSc thesis, Cranfield University: Cranfield.

O'Sullivan, D. (1982) *St Bees Man: The discovery of a preserved medieval body in Cumbria*. Proceedings of the Palaeopathology Association, 4th European Meeting, Antwerp.

Oxford Archaeology (2005) *The Paddock. The Royal Naval Hospital Haslar, Gosport*, Archaeological Evaluation Report 2786, Oxford Archaeology: Oxford.

Roberts, C., Manchester, K. and Storey, A. (1992) Margaret Clitheroe: skeletal identification of an historical figure? *Forensic Science International*, **57**: 63–71.

Rodriguez, W.C. and Bass, W.M. (1985) Decomposition of buried bodies and methods that may aid in their location. *Journal of Forensic Sciences*, **30**: 836–852.

Rugg, J. (2000) Defining the place of burial: what makes a cemetery a cemetery? *Mortality*, **5**: 259–275.

Schoenen, D. and Schoenen, H. (2013) Adipocere formation – The result of insufficient microbial degradation. *Forensic Science International*, **226**: 301.e1–301.e6.

Shortland, A.J., Masters, P., Harrison, K., Williams, A. and Boston, C. (2008) Burials of eighteenth-century naval personnel: preliminary results from excavations at the Royal Hospital Haslar, Gosport (Hants). *Antiquity*, **82**: 317.

Stirland, A. (1990) The late Sir Thomas Reynes: a medieval identification. *Journal of the Forensic Science Society*, **30**: 39–43.

Tapp, E. and O'Sullivan, D. (1982) *St Bees Man: The autopsy*. Proceedings of the Palaeopathology Association, 4th European Meeting, Antwerp.

Thali, M.J., Lux, B., Lösch, S., Rösing, F.W., Hürlimann, J., Feer, P. *et al.* (2011) 'Brienzi' – The blue Vivianite man of Switzerland: time since death estimation of an adipocere body. *Forensic Science International*, **211**: 34–40.

Todd, J. (2013) The St Bees Man and the medieval way of death. Lecture, St Bees website, www.stbees.org.uk/history/stbeesman/stbees_man2_todd.html (Accessed 24 January 2016).

Ubelaker, D.H. and Zarenko, K.M. (2011) Adipocere: what is known after over two centuries of research. *Forensic Science International*, **208**: 167–172.

Vass, A.A. (2001) Beyond the grave-understanding human decomposition. *Microbiology Today*, **28**: 190–193.

Waldron, T. (1987) The relative survival of the human skeleton: implications for palaeopathology. In: Boddington, A., Garland, A.N. and Janaway, R.C. (eds), *Death, Decay and Reconstruction: Approaches to archaeology and forensic science*. Manchester University Press: Manchester, pp. 55–64.

28

Forensic Entomology Case Studies from Mexico

Leonardo R. Flores Pérez, Humberto Molina Chávez, Manuel Nava Hernández and Fray M. Pérez Villegas

28.1 Introduction

Cadaver degradation goes through a series of phenomena, which starts at the time of death and continues until all components of the corpse are returned to the ecosystem. As such, a decomposing body can be seen as a highly dynamic system in which decomposition is a continuous process, determined by different abiotic and biotic factors that have an impact on the transformation of the body as well as its conservation.

Forensic entomology is the study of insects and other arthropods for criminal investigation (Byrd and Castner 2010). This science has gained recognition since the first case report by a French physician, Louis F.E. Bergeret (1814–1893), in the second half of the 19th century, who estimated the post-mortem interval (PMI) of an individual based on the life cycle of insects. From the early stages after death, insects are attracted to a decomposing body. Their arrival depends on several factors and happens in a determined sequence, producing a succession of species (Carvalho *et al.* 2004). The entomologist knows that these patterns can provide useful information for the coroner, the ministry and the police, so that they can elucidate possible criminal cases (Goff *et al.* 2004). The correct estimation of PMI is useful for orienting and re-orienting an investigation, accepting or rejecting an alibi, or to shed light on peri-mortem and post-mortem activities. More details about the theoretical aspects of forensic entomology can be found in Chapter 13 of this volume.

Some insect species have a wide geographical distribution and can be found in most continents, while others are specific to the biogeographic area. The common species in Mexico have been reported (Flores 2009; Flores *et al.* 2008; Martínez *et al.* 2007; Molina *et al.* 2013; Nava *et al.* 2015; Valdés *et al.* 2008; Vázquez *et al.* 2007; Villamil *et al.* 2007). The present chapter deals with two case studies related to forensic entomological investigations in Mexico: Mexico City (D.F.) and the State of Hidalgo. They demonstrate how the analysis of insects assisted in the resolution of criminal cases from Mexico City's Attorney General Office. The case studies do not contain any details and are anonymous.

28.2 Case Study from Mexico City

The case study presented from Mexico City relates two death bodies discovered in 2009. In the spring, a father reported his two children missing. A report was filed with the authorities in charge of missing

Taphonomy of Human Remains: Forensic Analysis of the Dead and the Depositional Environment, First Edition.
Edited by Eline M.J. Schotsmans, Nicholas Márquez-Grant and Shari L. Forbes.

persons. The disappearance occurred in Mexico City, at a place known as Sierra de Guadalupe, at the centre of the Mexican Valley and is a Natural Protected Area (NPA). Sierra de Guadalupe is located to the north of Mexico City, on the border between Mexico City and Estado de Mexico. The soil, lithosol and haplic phaeozems, lies on top of eruptive rocks, in a dry and temperate climate (Cedillo *et al.* 2008). The weather conditions in Sierra de Guadalupe consist of cyclonic precipitation, usually from June to September, with the highest values reached during August and September (Salinas 1994). The geographical and weather data were taken into consideration during the analysis of this case.

By the end of spring 2009, Mexico City Police Department (*Policía Judicial del Distrito Federal*) received an anonymous call reporting that two human bodies were located in a deserted area, with concrete structures for electrical wiring and abundant herbaceous vegetation and bushes. This location was distinctive as it is an ecologically disturbed place that is illegally used as a dumping site on the outskirts of the city. Even though, both bodies were located at the same site, the context related to their deposition was different.

28.2.1 Body 01

This corpse corresponded to a 15- to 17-year-old female. It was covered in synthetic material bags and placed within a suitcase, which was torn on one side. The body was fully dressed but did not have footwear. The individual was placed in a genupectoral position (i.e. prone posture resting on the knees and upper part of the chest). The upper limbs were flexed, crossing the chest, and the flexed lower limbs were taped to the waist. The cadaver was in the liquefaction stage (colliquative phase). Dermal detachment in thorax, hands, feet and scalp was observed, as well as blisters, lingual protrusion and different stages of insect growth (Gisbert *et al.* 2004; Prieto *et al.* 2004). The pathologist established the cause of death as strangling by constriction of the upper airways.

28.2.2 Body 02

The remains of the second body corresponded to a 20-year-old male wrapped in black synthetic bags. The body was fully dressed and was wearing shoes. It was positioned on its side (lateral decubitus position) with tape around the upper and lower limbs. The body also presented the same characteristic signs as the first body, including liquefaction, blisters, dermal detachment at the thorax, hands, feet and scalp, lingual protrusion and different stages of insect growth (Gisbert *et al.* 2004; Prieto *et al.* 2004). The cause of death was strangling by constriction of upper airways, as in body 01.

28.2.3 Entomological Analysis of Body 01 and Body 02

The live entomological specimens were collected in fixative solution, following collection procedures based on Higley and Haskell (2001). They were immediately taken to the Laboratory of Forensic Entomology at Mexico City's Attorney General Office (Procuraduria General de Justicia de la Ciudad de México), which has an available insect facility, to confirm developmental stages and taxonomical identification.

The temperature data were obtained from a meteorological station near the site through the climatological portal of the National Autonomous University of Mexico (UNAM). The recorded average values were recorded at 22.5°C, the highest maximum temperature reached 30.7°C and the minimum temperature was 14.7°C.

For taxonomic identification, the width and length of the collected non-living species was measured as described by Day and Wallman (2006), followed by rinsing and montage for observation of immature stages, as described by Palacios and Mejía (2007). The species were identified using general and specific taxonomic references of dipterous species in larva and adult phases described by Florez and Wolff (2009), Sukontason *et al.* (2007) and Whitworth (2006). Recovered living organisms were taken to an appropriate facility in order to enable their development according to

Table 28.1 Identified species from two bodies at Mexico City.

Family	Species	Developmental Stage	Cadaver/Body n°
Muscidae	*Synthesiomyia nudiseta*	L-III Larvae with a range of 10.25 to 11.96 mm in length	01
		Coarctata type puparium with a 6.15 mm average length	
		Adults (imagos) with 1.4 mm average length	
Calliphoridae	*Lucilia sericata*	L-III Larvae with 12.98 to 14.47 mm length range	01
		Coarctata type pupas with 8.22 mm average length	
Muscidae	*Synthesiomyia nudiseta*	L-III Larvae with 12.25 to 13.21 mm length range	02
Fanniidae	*Fannia scalaris*	Coarctata type pupariums, 6.15 mm long	02
		Coarctata type pupas with a range of 4.6 to 5.19 mm in length	

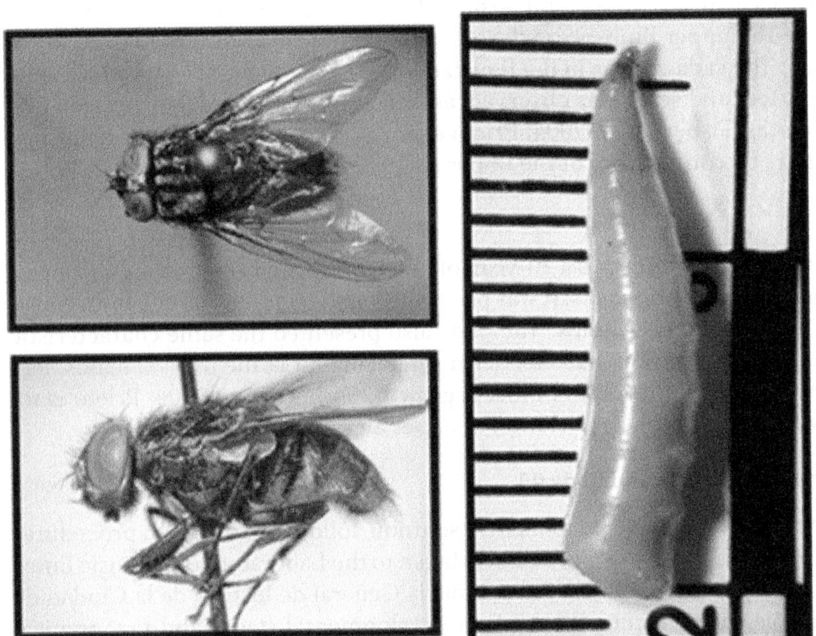

Figure 28.1 Adult and larva of *Synthesiomyia nudiseta*.

Byrd and Tomberlin (2010), aiming to monitor their development until the adult stage and proceed with the taxonomic identification of juvenile (immature) phases collected from the body. Based on the previous information, the species could be identified (Table 28.1).

The species *Synthesiomyia nudiseta* (Figure 28.1) was found on both bodies. This species is an urban diptera, which is synanthropic and associated with cadaveric decomposition of human remains. It has great forensic relevance as an indicator of minimum time since death, particularly for this case, as it is the longest living species of those associated with the remains. Organisms in different developmental stages were found, such as third instar vermiform larvae with a well-developed cephaloskeleton, a slightly longer dorsal view than ventral and four or five thick lobes on the prothoracic spiraculum. Caudal or posterior spiraculums displayed sinuous looking openings or slits. During the forensic investigation, the same characteristics were found in the empty puparia gathered from the site, the corpse, the clothing and objects. Furthermore, the presence of imagos (those in the last stage of growth during metamorphosis and prior to adult stage) and their following comparison to adults grown in the laboratory, enabled the observation of organisms in the adult stage, that displayed body colour ranging from black to light grey, antennae with filiform arista in the cephalic region and orange coloured flagellomere (same colour found in palps). On the dorsal region of the thorax, grey and black stripes were present, with two pairs of dorsocentral presutural silks and a prealar silk as well, and no villus in pleuras or hairs on anemiperon. In terms of developmental periods, the author's experience in Mexico reports an adult emergence period ranging from 19 to 22 days with a 20.4°C temperature on average, considering temperature variations ranging between 18 and 22°C. This enabled the estimation of the minimum PMI (mPMI) of 20 to 21 days for both corpses, prior to the date of discovery.

However, even though *S. nudiseta* was taken as the ruling species to estimate the PMI, an ecological succession in the body could be observed. Other identified organisms on body 01 included dipterous species, such as *Lucila sericata* and *Chrysomyia rufifacies*, as well as beetles belonging to Silphidae and Staphilinidae families.

The presence of the blowfly *L. sericata*, which was found in both immature (larvae and empty pupal cases) and adult stages, indicated the completion of a developmental cycle, from egg to adult, which is similar to the observations of *S. nudiseta*. However, the latter species display longer developmental periods than the first species (Higley and Haskell 2001; Molina *et al.* 2006). This was considered as a part of the ecological process of cadaver degradation, but not as a time of death indicator.

The second body also displayed the presence of *F. scalaris* (Figure 28.2). The first corpse was found inside a plastic bag placed within a suitcase at the same location and was therefore more sealed than corpse 02, which was found wrapped only in plastic bags.

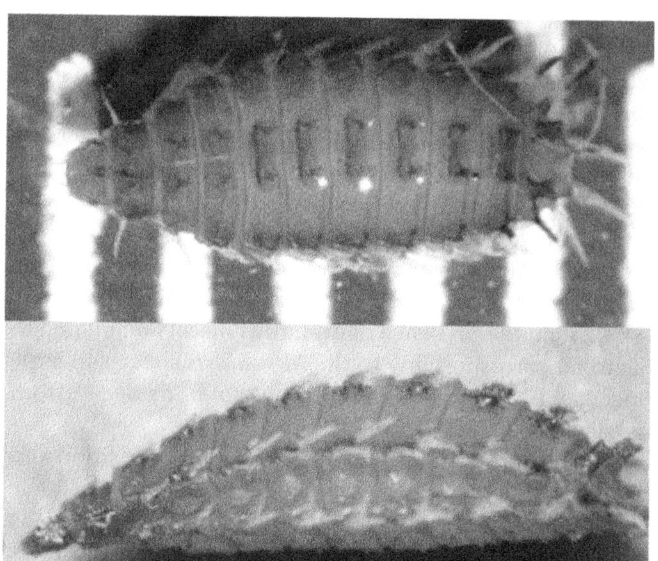

Figure 28.2 Larva of *Fannia scalaris*.

The identification of the victims was established, and based on entomological data it could be concluded that the bodies had been located in the Sierra de Guadalupe natural reserve, the location that corresponded to the hometown of the individual that had initially reported them as missing. In his statements, the father of the children mentioned that he could not have been present at the time these crimes had been committed. However, the time of death established for both cadavers, 20 to 21 days prior to discovery, pointed to the father as the possible perpetrator for the death of both his son and daughter.

Based on entomological data and additional other evidence, an apprehension order against the father was issued, and he was charged for murdering his children. The father finally confessed before the authorities that he had deprived his children of liberty and life due to marital and financial issues. He declared that he had tried to commit suicide, but had failed. Consequently, he transported the children to the illegal dump side and called the police to report them missing. He also confirmed that the time between the murder and the findings corresponded to the periods established by entomologic indicators.

28.3 Case Studies from Hidalgo State

This section presents three cases from the eastern state of Hidalgo, Mexico. Hidalgo is located in the Central Region of México. It has a semi-dry, temperate climate in the north and central part of this region, while the south of Hidalgo is temperate, sub-humid and humid. It is located between Sierra Madre Oriental and Mexico's highlands, with the presence of submontane, coniferous forests, pine-oak forests and xeric scrublands. There are different soils, from pelic vertisol to haplic phaeozem.

Body 1 corresponds to a male that was buried in the municipal pantheon at the centre of Hidalgo State. The corpse was exhumed 41 days after burial at the request of the police (Table 28.2). The cadaver presented an advanced stage of decomposition. Associated dipterous larvae were collected, which appeared to have morphological characteristics corresponding to Phoridae larvae. Their general morphology displayed a whitish muscidiform larva with a variable length of 5 to 6 mm, 12 metamere and small dorsal and lateral projections in the form of horns alongside the body. Sclerotic teeth were observed together with prothoracic spiracles in an oval shape and caudal spiracles on a protrusion in the shape of a plate with a cleft that forms lobes with straight openings, an individual characteristic of dipterous larvae from Phoridae, *Megaselia scalaris,* shown in Figure 28.3. It is a species frequently associated with buried cadavers in an advanced stage of decomposition, where bigger dipterous, such as Calliphoridae notably have difficulty accessing the body (Carvalho and Mello-Pantiu 2008; Rodríguez and Bass 1983).

Body 2 was excavated in the region known as Valle del Mezquital, in the Municipality of Actopan, where the climate is dry and xerophytic plants predominate. The remains were skeletonised and corresponded to a female individual who had received mortuary treatment before burial (Table 28.2). Forensic investigations related to the case established the presence of dipterous insects belonging to the Phoridae family, finding exuvias (exoskeletons) corresponding to the *M. scalaris* species in large quantities. This species of forensic importance can be found at different stages of body decay, from the initial stages to the ones observed in this case.

The third body was buried in a shallow grave. It displayed an advanced stage of decomposition and there was evidence of exposure to fire (Table 28.2). The discovery was made in a rural area at Valle del Mezquital, during the rainy season. The male corpse was buried supine with 60 to 70% of its body surface burned. The soil in which the body was buried was highly compacted and consisted of a layer of organic matter. The organisms found on the body were mainly collected from the head and torso regions and the surrounding soil layers, thus not only from the natural orifices of the body. The insects

Table 28.2 Bodies discovered at Hidalgo State.

Cadaver n°	Date of discovery	Deposit	State of decomposition	Inhumation period
1	Feb. 2011	Buried in wooden coffin, at pantheon	Advanced stage of decomposition	41 days
2	Oct. 2011	Buried	Skeletonised. No remaining soft tissue	60 months
3	Aug. 2011	Buried	Advance stage of decay with alterations due to direct exposure to fire	[a]13–15 days

a) estimated PMI.

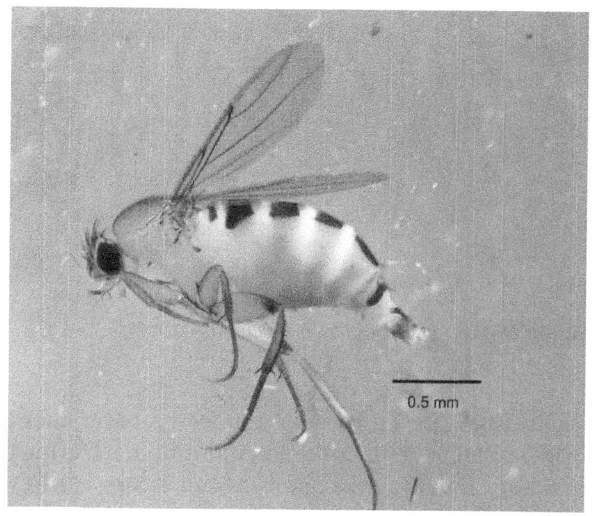

Figure 28.3 Adult of *Megaselia scalaris*.

appeared to belong to the Muscidae group, and more specifically to *Synthesiomyia nudiseta*. Pupae from the same family were also collected from the soil. Anderson (2010) highlighted that arthropod fauna colonising charred bodies could be correlated with the colonisation of unburned bodies. However, arthropod fauna might appear prematurely, probably due to skin slits and openings caused by burning. A PMI ranging from 13 to 15 days was estimated.

The above case studies show that the duration of the different stages of decomposition in buried corpses depends on different biotic and abiotic features, including soil compaction, depth of the burial site and inherent characteristics of the body, season, pH, oxygenation and polluting agents in the soil, types of vegetation, animals and other organisms (Gaudry 2010; Janaway *et al.* 2009; Pakosh and Rogers 2009; Simmons *et al.* 2010; Stokes *et al.* 2009). For forensic cases, these factors must be taken into consideration, as well as human intervention, whether caused by criminal or funerary reasons.

It is also important to highlight the importance of collecting all evidence, no matter how small it seems, since the presence of one single specimen – whether an exuvia, pupa or any other insect remain – can indicate that there were insects at the place of the findings, which might establish their relation to the cadaver.

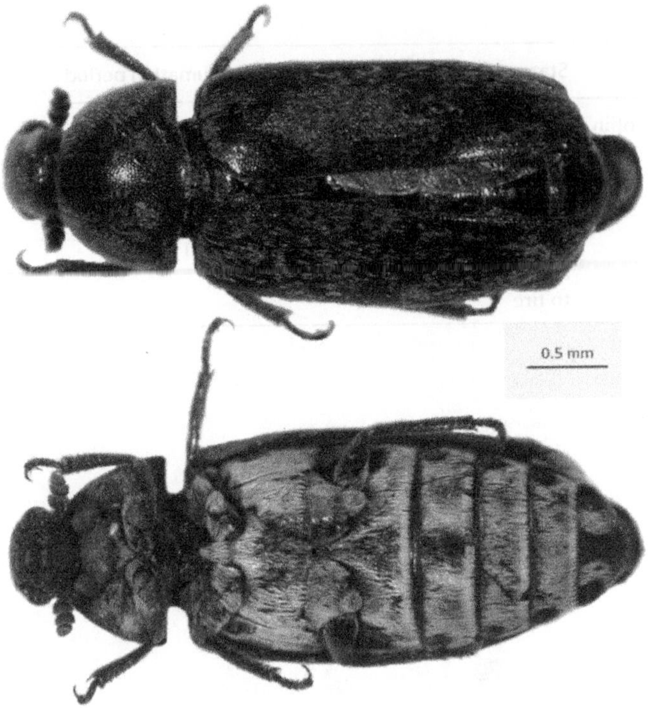

Figure 28.4 Adult of *Dermestes maculatus*.

Disturbing the corpse at the time of recovery has a great influence on the available entomological evidence found in the laboratory or morgue. During this procedure, organism collection must be carried out carefully. The organisms can escape easily, which makes their collection difficult, especially with the Staphylinidae, Silphidae and Histeridae beetle families. Therefore, it is important to undertake a thorough inspection of every piece of clothing the corpse was wearing, or the bag in which it was carried, as well as any area of the body where insects could be located, including the nasal cavities, such as in cadaver 03 where most Dermestidae (Figure 28.4) and Cleridae organisms were collected.

Wounds or lesions, as well as other post-mortem artefacts (e.g. produced by scavengers), are also features that affect the arrival and habitation of insects or sarcosaprophagous arthropods (Klippel and Synstelien 2007). Anderson (1997) notes that insects are attracted to exposed wounds in order to feed from them and lay eggs and, as a secondary measure, are drawn to the natural orifices of the body. In the same way that insects are drawn to the corpse, scavengers are also attracted by insects and can remove large portions of soft tissue (Anderson 2010). During the collection of organisms, we must consider not only the insects present on the body, but the evidence left by the first colonisers. When human remains are found, some of the insects leave an unmistakable trace of their presence, such as larvae exuvias, empty pupas and peritrophic membrane (Anderson 2010).

28.4 Conclusion

The study of a cadaveric ecosystem is a difficult task. Amongst the sarcosaprophagous entomofauna, insects are usually the first organisms to arrive at a dead body, colonising it in a predictable sequence determined by the stages of decomposition. Some insects are directly attracted by the body (necrophagous species), whereas other predatory species (necrophilous species) are attracted by insects that use the cadaver as a resource. There are many differences amongst sarcosaprophagous entomofauna, based on multiple variables such as location, weather, pre- and post-mortem lesions on the body, the presence of plants, animals, other organisms, etc. Sarcosaprophagous entomofauna are essential organisms for decomposition and the corpse's resource to complete its degradation cycle. Furthermore, everything usually happens as a well-defined process, even though the unexpected and its variants can multiply infinitely. Normally, there is a succession of organisms that fulfil their role as experimented performers; they meet certain periods of time, cover stages, respect 'hierarchies', have a timely entrance on stage, etc. This last feature is what enables us to use sarcosaprophagous insects as indicators with which to determine circumstances of forensic transcendence. If the succession of insects follows a pattern, the presentation of well-selected organisms can help establish the time since death occurred.

The data reported in this chapter show the sarcosaprophagous entomofauna present on dead bodies in Mexico and how the analysis of insects can assist with the resolution of criminal cases from Mexico. It can be useful for other cases related to clandestine burials, and the study of forensic entomology in general.

References

Anderson, G.S. (1997) The use of insects to determine time of decapitation: a case-study from British Columbia. *Journal of Forensic Sciences*, **42**: 947–950.

Anderson, G.S. (2010) Factors that influence insect succession in carrion. In: Byrd, J. and Castner, J. (eds), *Forensic Entomology: The utility of arthropods in legal investigations*. CRC Press: Boca Raton, pp. 201–250.

Byrd, J.H. and Castner, J.L. (2010) Insect of forensic importance. In: Byrd, J. and Castner, J. (eds), *Forensic Entomology: The utility of arthropods in legal investigations*. CRC Press: Boca Raton, pp. 39–126.

Byrd, J.H. and Tomberlin, J.K. (2010) Laboratory rearing of forensic insects. In: Byrd, J. and Castner, J. (eds), *Forensic Entomology: The utility of arthropods in legal investigations*. CRC Press: Boca Raton, pp. 177–200.

Carvalho, C.J.B. and de Mello-Pantiu, C.A. (2008) Key to the adults of the most common forensic species of Diptera in South America. *Revista Brasileira de Entomología*, **52**: 390–406.

Carvalho, L.M.L., Thyssen, P.J., Goff, M.L. and Linhares, A.X. (2004) Observations on the succession patterns of necrophagous insects on a pig carcass in an urban area of southeastern Brazil. *Aggrawal's Internet Journal of Forensic Medicine and Toxicology*, **5**: 33–39.

Cedillo, A.O.L., Rivas, S.M.A. and Rodríguez, C.F.N. (2008) Estudio de los suelos en la Sierra de Guadalupe. Sitio de estudio: Cañadas la mora 1 y la mora 2, determinación de granulometría, porosidad y permeabilidad. *Revista Sistemas Ambientales*, **2**: 1–11.

Day, D.M. and Wallman, J.F. (2006) Width as an alternative measurement to length for post-mortem interval estimations using *Calliphora augur* (Diptera: Calliphoridae) larvae. *Forensic Science International*, **159**: 158–167.

Flores, P.L., Sánchez, H., Ibáñez, S. and García, M.D. (2008). Insectos sarcosaprofagos asociados a la descomposición cadavérica de Sus scrofa en Texcoco, México. *Entomología Mexicana*, **7**: 768–774.

Flores, P.L. (2009) *Sucesión de entomofauna cadavérica utilizando como biomodelo cerdo blanco, Sus scrofa*. Tesis de Doctorado. Colegio de postgraduados. México.

Florez, E. and Wolff, M. (2009). Descripción y Clave de los Estadios Inmaduros de las Principales Especies de Calliphoridae (Diptera) de Importancia Forense en Colombia. *Neotropical Entomology*, **38**: 418–429.

Gaudry, E. (2010). The insects colonization of buried remains. In: Goff, M.L., Amendt, J., Campobasso, C.P. and Grassberger, M. (eds), *Current Concepts in Forensic Entomology*. Springer: Dordrecht, pp. 273–312.

Goff, M.L., García, M.D., Arnaldos, S.M. and Lozano, R.E. (2004). Entomología cadavérica: fundamentos y aplicación. Referencia a la entomología española. In: Gisbert, C.J.A. (ed.), *Medicina Legal y Toxicología*. Elsevier: Barcelona, pp. 253–262.

Gisbert, C.J.A., Villanueva, E. and Gisbert, M.S. (2004). Fenómenos cadavéricos. In: Gisbert, C.J.A. (ed.), *Medicina Legal y Toxicología*. Elsevier: Barcelona, pp. 191–213.

Higley, L.G. and Haskell, N.H. (2001). Insects: development and Forensic Entomology. In: Byrd, J. and Castner, J. (eds), *Forensic Entomology: The utility of arthropods in legal investigations*. CRC Press: Boca Raton, pp. 287–300.

Janaway, R.C., Wilson, A.S., Díaz, G.C. and Guillen, S. (2009) Taphonomic changes to the buried body in arid environments: an experimental case study in Peru. In: Ritz, K., Dawson, L. and Miller, D. (eds), *Criminal and Environmental Soil Forensics*. Springer: London, pp. 341–356.

Klippel, W.E. and Synstelien, J.A. (2007) Rodents as taphonomic agents: bone gnawing by brown rats and gray squirrels. *Journal of Forensic Sciences*, **52**: 765–773.

Martínez, R.H., Escoto, R.J. and Tafoya, F. (2007) Sucesión de insectos necrófagos en Sus scrofa, durante el periodo estacional de primavera en la ciudad de Aguascalientes. *Entomología Mexicana*, **6**: 880–884.

Molina, C.H.A., Luy, Q.J., Nava, H.M. and Galindo, M.N.E. (2006) Datos preliminares de dípteros relacionados con el proceso de descomposición cadavérica en la Cd. de México. *Entomología Mexicana*, **5**: 925–93.

Molina, C.H.A., Nava, H.M., Luy, Q.J., Miranda, G.B., Gutiérrez, R.S. and Galindo, M.N.E. (2013) Distribución de dípteros asociados con las fases de degradación cadavérica en humanos en el Distrito Federal. México. *Entomología Mexicana*, **12**: 1749–1755.

Nava, H.M., Avelino, R.J.C., Molina, C.H.A., Luy, Q.J. and Arana, M.F. (2015) Coleópteros asociados a la descomposición de materia orgánica animal en un área de la zona lacustre de Xochimilco, México. *Entomología Mexicana*, **2**: 498–504.

Pakosh, C.M. and Rogers, T.L. (2009) Soft tissue decomposition of submerged, dismembered pig limbs enclosed in plastic bags. *Journal of Forensic Sciences*, **54**: 1223–1228.

Palacios, J.G. and Mejía, B.E. (2007) *Tecnicas de colecta, montaje y preservación de microartropodos edaficios*. Las Prensas de Ciencia, UNAM México.

Prieto, J.L., Magaña, C. and Douglas, H.U. (2004). Interpretation of postmortem change in cadavers in Spain. *Journal of Forensic Science*, **49**: 918–923.

Rodriguez, W.C. and Bass, W.M. (1983) Insect activity and its relationship to decay rates of human cadavers in east Tennessee. *Journal of Forensic Sciences*, **28**: 423–432.

Salinas, M.A. (1994) *Geomorfología de la Sierra de Guadalupe y riesgos naturales*. Tesis. Geografía. Facultad. de Filosofía y Letras de la UNAM, México.

Simmons, T., Adlam, R.E. and Moffart, C. (2010). Debugging decomposition data – Comparative taphonomic studies and the influence of insects and carcass size on decomposition rate. *Journal of Forensic Sciences*, **55**: 8–13.

Stokes, K.L., Forbes, S.L., Benninger, L.A., Carter, D.O. and Tibbett, M. (2009) Decomposition studies using animal models in contrasting environments: evidence from temporal changes in soil chemistry and microbial activity. In; Ritz, K., Dawson, L. and Miller, D. (eds), *Criminal and Environmental Soil Forensics*. Springer: London, pp. 357–376.

Sukontason, K.L., Bunchu, N., Chaiwong, T., Kuntalue, B. and Sukontason, K. (2007). Fine structure of the eggshell of the blowfly, *Lucilia cuprina*. *Journal of Insect Sciences*, **7**: 9.

Valdés, P.M., Sánchez, F., Rodríguez, S. and Anderson, G. (2008). Artrópodos de importancia forense sobre carroña de cerdo en el semidesierto de Coahuila, México. *Entomología Mexicana*, **7**: 692–697.

Vázquez, S.R., Stephano, V.D., Marín, H.C., Rodríguez, C.A., Flores, M.J. and Díaz, T.P. (2007) Dípteros necrófagos del estado de Nuevo León, México. *Entomología Mexicana*, **6**: 885–888.

Villamil, R.E., Galindo, N. and Navarrete, J.L. (2007) Caracterización de la coleopterofauna asociada a cadáveres de *Mus musculus* L. en la reserva ecológica del pedregal. *Entomología Mexicana*, **6**: 885–888.

Whitworth, T. (2006) Keys to the genera and species of blow flies (Diptera: Calliphoridae) of America North of Mexico. *Proceedings of the Entomological Society of Washington*, **108**: 689–725.

29

Recovery of Skeletonised Human Remains and Textile Degradation: a Case Study

Rob C. Janaway and Nicholas Márquez-Grant

29.1 Introduction

Within an investigation, it is not only necessary to consider taphonomic aspects of the conditions of the body, but clothing and other textiles also provide a valuable source of information. An overview of clothing degradation in depositional environments is provided by Stuart and Ueland in this book (Chapter 9). In this chapter, the current procedure of the examination of an outdoor crime scene in the UK will be presented from the perspective of a forensic archaeologist and anthropologist, followed by a case study that highlights the analysis of certain taphonomic factors, including textile degradation.

29.2 Outdoor Recovery of Skeletonised Human Remains

The presence of skeletonised human remains in surface depositions outdoors can be found in a number of contexts. These may be in an area of woodland, in a rail embankment, in the wooded area near a motorway, on a mountain and so on. The remains might be encountered in a number of ways: an articulated skeleton; a body where the skeletal remains are scattered; only parts of a skeleton, which may still have some soft tissue attached; or the skeletal remains may have been affected by environmental factors modifying the body such as scavenging. The body might be clothed, or there may be no evidence of clothing, or in a sleeping bag, or perhaps wrapped in material that has disappeared with the passage of time. The body may have been there for weeks, perhaps months or even years; and the person may have died there, or in a criminal case, perhaps even killed in a different location and later transported and deposited in this outdoor area. The circumstances surrounding death may have been criminal or there may have been no criminal intent at all, for example, in a natural, accidental or suicidal death. Nevertheless, the location where the remains have been found will be regarded as a crime scene.

Taking a random example of human remains scattered in an area of woodland with evidence of textiles, food wrappers and bottles, the forensic strategy may include the following questions to be answered whilst investigating the crime scene. These questions may have been led by police work and then fed to the crime scene investigators. Some of the questions can be answered by forensic scientists such as anthropologists, archaeologists, entomologists, botanists, etc.:

- Are these human bones?
- Do the remains represent one person?

Taphonomy of Human Remains: Forensic Analysis of the Dead and the Depositional Environment, First Edition.
Edited by Eline M.J. Schotsmans, Nicholas Márquez-Grant and Shari L. Forbes.

- Who is this person?
- How long has the person been dead/been present there?
- When did this happen?
- How did the body arrive at this location?
- Has there been any third-party involvement or foul play?
- What is the manner and cause of death?
- Are all the remains present or are some of them missing and require further search?

Ultimately these questions can be placed under the umbrella of two main issues to address:

1) the identification of the victim
2) has any crime being committed and if so, can the perpetrators be brought to justice?

If there have been criminal activities involved, these questions might trigger certain lines of enquiry. How can forensic scientists tackle these questions and provide an opinion at the scene, prior to any analysis post-scene in the mortuary or laboratory?

The process for the examination of an outdoor scene from the perspective of forensic archaeology and anthropology includes:

1) Arrival at the scene and briefing with detectives and crime scene investigators/scientific support officers; in particular liaising with the Crime Scene Manager.[1] During the brief, the scientist (archaeologist, anthropologist) will be able to ask questions regarding when the remains were discovered and by whom. There might be information on who this person could be and background information on the last sighting of this person, criminal record or links, etc. This may be setting some bias however in the investigation, as to whether it is likely to be criminal activity or not (i.e. any absence of criminal links or records in the past). There is always a dynamic synergy between the scientists and the Crime Scene Manager.
2) Assessing the scene for visible material evidence or traces including a visual assessment (walkthrough) of the area, inner and outer cordons, ensuring access paths are clear, discussing what type of evidence may be required (e.g. are soil samples required before further trampling of the scene? Are soil samples going to provide any evidence? Should they be collected in case this turns out to be criminal? These questions may be better answered after the visual walkthrough). This visual assessment will allow the observation of the human body or human remains,[2] provide a preliminary assessment of whether they are scattered or not, whether semi-buried under soil and vegetation through the passage of time, whether there are branches covering the body intentionally, etc.
3) After a walkthrough, in conjunction with the Crime Scene Manager and any other forensic scientists or police officers (e.g. photographers, police search teams, and less so, exhibit officers) present, a forensic strategy will be formulated: how is the team going to approach the scene? Which steps will be taken regarding documentation, methods of recovery, what will be recovered first, what will be recovered last, whether the area will be searched after recovery, etc? This can be dynamic (e.g. if during recovery, entomological evidence is uncovered).
4) The scene and evidence are recorded (bones, plotting position of bones, position and orientation of body, other artefacts, etc.). Certain observations can be made to form a preliminary opinion about the scene. If there is an experienced anthropologist: age and sex of the deceased, position of the body whether abnormal (e.g. if hands are tied) or normal (e.g. lying on its back), whether

1 Some of these terms are those used mainly in the UK police system, although these roles may be similar in other countries. For more information about the UK system, see Janaway (2015).
2 We are here providing the perspective of forensic anthropology, where the surface remains are likely to be skeletonised, and at least potentially scattered.

the damage on the body is post-mortem due to the activity of scavengers, whether there is any evidence of foul play, an opinion on post-mortem interval.

5) Recovery of the material evidence and human remains, followed by possible post-scene recovery if required.

It is obvious that every step of this process is documented, alongside all the other information on scene arrival, people present, date and time, etc. At the end of the process an expert witness report has to be written by the forensic scientists. More details about the sequence of procedures to examine a crime scene are outlined by Gardner and Bevel (2009) and Gardner (2012).

29.3 Case Study

This case study involves the body of an elderly man that had been lying next to a tree by a rural roadside in northern England, UK, for 35 months. The scene was attended and processed by a forensic archaeologist/anthropologist, forensic botanist and Scenes of Crime Officers (SOCOs) from the police force in question. The case has been selected because it illustrates a number of taphonomic issues and site formation processes.

29.3.1 Scene Examination

The human body found at the scene was clothed and tied up with a mixture of polymer sheathed (insulated) industrial cable and cable ties, and enclosed in a number of black PVC refuse sacks. From information provided by the police and initial observations at the scene, it was assumed that these would have been transported to the location and rolled down a sloping bank at the side of a minor road, coming to rest against the trunk of a mature European ash tree (*Fraxinus excelsior*). When the remains were found by two men exercising their dogs, all the exposed parts of the body were fully skeletonised. The unclassified road adjacent to the scene runs in an east-west alignment. The verge to the north of the road slopes down steeply to the surrounding arable farmland, and is colonised by extensive vegetation, including mature trees. Further to the north of the ash tree was a wooden fence line that separates the verge from a field under arable cultivation. The combination of the slope and density of the vegetation meant that the body when dumped was visible from neither the road nor the fields.

Prior to disposal, the head had been wrapped in a plastic refuse sack secured around the neck. Examination revealed that roots had grown into the plastic refuse sack and a plastic cable tie had been tied around the neck. The body was lying face down and the wrists had been tied together at the front of the body with plastic cable ties. The body had been wrapped in black plastic refuse sacks, and there were coils of a heavy black plastic coated cable encircling the body. The cable was most evident in the region of the knees and the neck and shoulders. It is probable that originally the body had been totally wrapped in polythene refuse sacks, but in some regions of the body, these had been ripped away exposing the clothed remains below. At the time of examination, the lower leg region was still concealed by partially opened black polythene sacks. The left foot was present, contained soft tissue and was clothed in a sock. The right foot was missing, with the distal ends of the left fibula and tibia exposed. The upper part of the body from the neck to the pelvis was skeletonised and bone was clean and bleached white.

Based on intelligence, the black plastic refuse sack around the head had been recently torn open when the body was discovered, to reveal the back of the head and brown hair. The black plastic covering the torso had been torn open at a much earlier time to reveal the ribs and the vertebrae, which were all skeletonised, and the upper exposed bone surfaces exhibited weathering. This was manifested as a bleached appearance, and some bone had a light-green discolouration, presumably due to algal or other microbiological colonisation. The lower central part of the back was covered with a degraded elasticated textile, which was later identified as a lumbar support. The right scapula was separated from the main articulated skeleton and was an isolated find several metres away. The disarticulated right scapula and missing right foot were consistent with scavenger activity and dispersion of the human remains. A full list of missing skeletal elements was confirmed at the post-mortem; it was evident that the bones of the arms (left and right humeri) as well as the left scapula and clavicles (left and right) and the elements of the right foot (contained within sock and shoe) were all missing. This slightly atypical scavenging pattern was a result of the position of the body (face down), the way it was trussed (wrists tied at front and therefore under the body) and the effect of the elaborate use of electrical cable to contain the body package. This resulted in the shoulders being presumably the most easily accessible to scavengers. Although it cannot be demonstrated, the scavenger species in question is almost certainly the red fox (*Vulpes vulpes*). The pelvic region was skeletonised, with the exposed lumbar vertebrae and *os coxae* exhibiting bleaching and green discolouration, consistent with weathering. A pair of elastic-waisted trousers was on the lower limbs with the waistband coming to the top of the femur, with only the left femoral head being exposed. The thighs were hidden by a combination of clothing, wrappings, vegetation and loose soil, which was confirmed as earthworm upcasts.

After the post-mortem examination, the investigative team recommended that the wider area had to be searched using a human remains detection dog to look for missing elements. This search concentrated along the heavily vegetated area along the road/field margins, which is consistent with the activity routes of the red fox (i.e. keeping to 'cover' rather than unnecessarily crossing open ground) and as a result, all the remaining skeletal elements were recovered. There was the additional advantage that this search revealed other personal effects belonging to the victim, discarded (perhaps at a subsequent time) close to but not at the same location as the body.

A large piece of heavy black plastic sheeting to the west of the body was examined by the forensic archaeologist/anthropologist and a forensic botanist, specifically with respect to colonisation by moss, retardation of plant growth underneath and root penetration. At this stage of the investigation, the team would have been in a position to produce a biological profile for the skeletonised remains, and there was a good chance that the mitochondrial DNA of the victim would be recoverable. It was critical from an investigative perspective to develop an estimate of how long the body had been at the dump site. Given that principal entomological activity around the corpse had ceased, it was decided that vegetational response to the corpse would provide the best estimate. The interpretation by the forensic botanist, with respect to penetration of green plant shoots through the body and associated covering, was critical in narrowing down time scale and hence the number of missing persons potentially concerned.[3] A forensic botanist was present on the scene prior to disturbance and removal of the remains, and worked in conjunction with the forensic archaeologist. Within the plastic sheet was a rodent nest that had utilised textile thread, as well as vegetation for bedding material. This again emphasises that while the principal interest as investigators is the victim and the circumstances of deposition, the deposition site will become modified by a host of natural biological processes, including plant colonisation and growth, animal feeding (mammalian scavenging, insect activity), but also non-feeding use of the deposition site, that has to be investigated too.

The lower legs were wrapped in black plastic refuse sacks as stated above. During the examination of the plastic refuse sacks wrapping, a wallet was recovered, which was lying on the ground surface, but

3 The forensic botanical interpretation enabled a much more focused approach to the missing person profiles, which when used in conjunction with the biological profile generated through physical anthropological analysis enabled a positive identification to be confirmed by DNA.

beneath the plastic. The wallet was examined at the scene and found to be empty. The plastic refuse sacks covering the lower legs had already been partially torn open. On opening up the plastic refuse sacks, the presence of a plastic cable tie around the region of the ankles was revealed. Further plastic cable ties were also located around the lower limbs further up the body in the region of the knees and hips, and a jacket was knotted around the thighs. The lower body garment was a dark-coloured tracksuit bottom with elasticated waist and ankles. The waistband was around the region of the upper thighs. Whilst these were in a position with the waistband lower than the waist, it is not possible to categorically state whether this was due to how the perpetrator left the body, or due to bloating during the decomposition of the body. The lower limbs were bound together by a polyester jacket tied by its sleeves. The jacket had a zip front and empty fly puparia were found in the folds. The front of the jacket revealed a zip pocket that was turned out. It also exhibited red staining, which was most probably of fungal origin.[4] The jacket was largely of polyester construction with a nylon liner. Under the jacket and trousers, surviving pubic hair was observed in the groin region and an elasticated waistband from cotton underwear that had completely decayed.

The *os coxae* were entirely skeletonised and their orientation confirmed that the body had been lying face down. After the removal of sacrum, left and right *os coxae*, the skeletal elements of the hands were revealed and a fingernail was recovered. The orientation of the bones of the hands suggested that they had decayed *in situ* and their association with looped cable ties suggested that the hands had been bound at the wrists in front of the body. In the region of the lower torso, the remains of two medically-related textile items were recovered. The first was the elasticated lumbar support, the fabric of which consisted of a heavily elasticated cotton textile, which had degraded, leaving a structure dominated by the elastic element, polyester stitching and the manufacturer's label. Also recovered was an aorto-bifemoral bypass graft and its associated sutures. Unsurprisingly, this surgical textile had not degraded.

The upper body clothing was missing. This had been a cotton shirt that was only represented at the scene by the blue polyester interlock stitching and the polyester manufacturer's labels. The presence of these labels recovered in association with the upper body (at the post-mortem examination) is indicative of it being clothed in a garment whose main fabric has not survived (i.e. 100% cotton).

29.3.2 Body Wrappings and Preservation of Materials

The body had been bound using cable ties (at the wrists, ankles, knees and thighs). The wrists had been bound in front of the body with the hands in front of the pelvic region. Evidence of a decorative loose upholstery cover (throw) was recovered during the post-mortem examination, with the label found inside the plastic refuse sack that contained the head. This, in conjunction with yarn from an interlocking seam that was recovered with the body, would imply that the clothed body was wrapped in the throw. This had then been wrapped by the black plastic refuse sacks and with thick black electrical cable looped around the body, with interlacing down the front of the body and held with additional cable ties.

This case study illustrates the differential preservation of elements of the body and associated textiles and materials. The preservation of some materials such as textiles have been well documented elsewhere (Janaway 2008), but it is critical that CSI teams understand the principles of differential preservation and the condition materials are likely to occur in a range of different depositional environments.

Material response to exposure to environmental conditions in this case was variable (Table 29.1). Cotton is a natural textile predominantly comprised of cellulosic fibres. It is therefore no surprise

4 One of the principal problems with the time pressures and finance of active casework is that if the question is not pertinent to addressing the primary concerns of the investigation, there is no capacity to assess all material fully.

Table 29.1 Summary of materials preservation.

Material	Items	Condition/Degradation
Cotton	Fabric of shirt	Complete loss of cotton fabric
Leather	Wallet	Leather stiffer due to loss of leather lubricants but otherwise no significant degradation
Polyester	Fabric of jacket Manufacturers labels (shirt, lumbar support)	No significant degradation
Polyethylene	Refuse sacks	No significant degradation
Polyvinyl chloride	Industrial polymer insulated cable	No significant degradation
Nylon	Jacket lining Cable ties	No significant degradation
Elastane	Lumbar support (cotton/elastane fabric) Elasticated waistband of underwear, trousers	The elastane elements of these compound fabrics survived well
Dacron or expanded polytetrafluoro-ethylene (ePTFE)	Aortic Bifemoral Bypass and associated sutures	No significant degradation. Graft and associated monofilament sutures are selected not to break down *in vivo*, so are highly resistant to decay after death

that the cotton fabric was completely degraded, leaving polyester interlock stitching and the polyester manufacturer's labels.

Leather is manufactured from animal skin, which has been chemically treated to inhibit degradation. In addition, various colours, finishes and waterproofing treatments may be added. The leather wallet at the scene was stiff but did not show significant degradation.

The industrial polymer insulated cable that had been used to tie up the body is designed to withstand soil burial, and thus was intact and unaffected by the proximity of the decomposing body and environmental exposure. Historically, in the early 20th century, electrical cables were rubber insulated, with the addition of lead sheathing to provide greater protection. More recently, natural rubber has been replaced by synthetic rubber insulation. For low temperature cables the most common material is polyvinyl chloride (PVC), which is highly durable but can become brittle if the plasticiser is leached out, or if subjected to strong UV radiation. In this case, the length of exposure (only 35 months) and the lack of strong sunlight (combination of northern England, UK, and shade from vegetation) resulted in a similar integrity and flexibility of the cable as from new.

Refuse sacks (i.e. black plastic rubbish bags and bin liners) are made of polyethylene of different thicknesses. Most bags are made of Low Density Polyethylene (LPDE), with the stronger ones being of either Linear Low Density Polyethylene (LLDPE) or High Density Polyethylene (HDPE). They are commonly sold in rolls of between 10 up to 100 bags, separated by perforations that allow them to be individually detached from the roll. They are sold in different thicknesses from ultra-light (80 gauge, ca. 20 mu) up to 1,000 gauge (250 mu), which are sometimes referred to as rubble sacks. Clearly, the thinner sacks will have a tendency to tear more easily. In this instance, there was no significant degradation of the polythene.

Cable ties (also known as zip ties) are constructed with ratchet teeth and pawl to fasten bundles of cables together. They are commonly available from hardware or motorists shops and thus have often been used (as in this case) to tie wrists, ankles, etc. together. Most are made of nylon and, as such, are highly resistant to chemical, biological, or UV degradation under a range of depositional and post-depositional conditions. In this case, like the industrial insulated cable, there was no significant degradation over the 35 months.

29.3.3 Summary of Scene Examination

The degree of skeletonisation and weathering (bleaching and discolouration of the bone) was consistent with some of the wrappings having been open for a considerable length of time. There was good evidence that the body had been laid in a prone position and decomposed *in situ* due to the articulation and orientation of the bulk of the skeletal elements. The surviving soft tissue (on the left upper leg and left foot) was consistent with differential preservation due to relatively intact clothing and wrappings covering these areas of the body, that is, the knotted jacket and footwear. The clothing exhibited differential preservation due to different fabric compositions. The missing skeletal elements (right foot, left scapula, both clavicles and both humeri) were consistent with dispersal due to animal scavenging. With the extensive network of the heavy black cable, the arms (left and right humeri) and the foot were perhaps the easiest to access by scavengers. In other circumstances, the distal elements (e.g. hands, forearms) would also have been targeted by scavengers, but in this case these were shielded by the body. Based on field observations, there was no evidence of deliberate concealment of the body by partial or full burial. Whilst there was some soil overlying the sides of the black plastic refuse sacks, this is consistent with natural post-depositional processes. The body was lying parallel with the slope and immediately adjacent to the trunk of the ash tree. Whilst it is possible that the body was rolled down the slope, coming to rest at the bottom, it is also possible that it was dragged or carried there.

29.4 Conclusion

With the case study above, we can return to the questions posed at the start of this chapter:

- *Are these human bones?* In this case, this was clearly the case, and this was concluded at the scene and confirmed during the post-mortem examination of all the recovered material.
- *Do the remains represent one person?* Although most of the skeleton was articulated in anatomical position, formally all the skeletal elements were identified at the post-mortem examination, and it was confirmed that this was a single individual.
- *Who is this person?* This question is critical to the investigative team, but it was hindered by the fact that, although the body was dumped adjacent to a quiet rural (unclassified) road, the dump-site was less than five minutes travel time by car to part of the major motorway network of the north of England, UK. As a result, less than an hour by car at average speeds would reach a number of cities and, therefore, the remains could potentially be from a large number of victims. The biological profile indicated an elderly male, but to make progress it was important to address the issue of time scale. Positive identification was made by DNA analysis.
- *How long has the person been dead/been present there?* Clearly, these should be two questions – how long has this person been dead, and how long have they been at the deposition site. In this case, where the remains were fully skeletonised and bulk of entomological activity had ceased, the approach was to consider the dump-site as an ecosystem and examine the plant response, including retardation, regrowth and colonisation. This would only address the issue of time scale at the dump-site, although the pattern of skeletal articulation (only affected by scavenging activity)

implies that the bulk of decomposition had taken place at the deposition site, implying a relatively close time between death and deposition.[5]

- *When did this happen?* It is generally important to address questions of seasonality, especially in consideration of aspects such as vegetation growth. For this to be taken into account, it is critical as part of the scene processing that someone, who is suitably qualified in ecology, can make a pre-disturbance survey of plant growth. This needs to be done in conjunction with the team (ideally the forensic archaeologist/anthropologist and SOCOs) as the body and other evidence is recovered. This involves a high degree of integration of forensic archaeology, forensic anthropology and forensic botany.
- *How did the body arrive at this location?* There was no direct physical evidence regarding transport to the site, although the dump-site location at the edge of a relatively quiet rural road strongly implied the use of a motor vehicle. The manner in trussing the body, by using the industrial electrical cable in a manner similar to string on a parcel, indicates some thought regarding the physical containment and movement of the body. The cable held the concealing plastic and textile wrappings in place, while giving the perpetrator something to grip onto when moving the body.
- *Has there been any third-party involvement or foul play?* In this case, it would be hard to postulate that the deceased had wrapped himself at the deposition site. Although in the case of bodies with less elaborate wrappings bindings found in woodland and adjacent to walls or in outbuildings, it is important to consider the possibility that these are the undiscovered remains of a rough sleeper/accident victim rather than a deliberately dumped body. And it is this aspect which requires the attention of the forensic archaeologist with careful recording of the body coverings, vegetation, etc. Were those branches used to conceal a body? Or were they the remains of some kind of sleeping shelter?
- *What are the manner and cause of death?* Strictly speaking, under the legal system of England and Wales, UK, this is the remit of the Home Office appointed forensic pathologist.[6] However, it is critical that scene recording considers taphonomic aspects that might have an implication regarding, for instance, the determination of ante-mortem bone fracture patterns as opposed to post-mortem patterns caused by loading of the body, for example, by overlying rocks.
- *Are all the remains present or are some of them missing and require further search?* By the end of the post-mortem examination, there was a target list of missing skeletal elements. Given the most likely scavenging pattern and the distribution of dense undergrowth along the road/field margins, it was agreed that a human remains detection dog operating on a free search would be the most effective way to recover the missing remains.

To summarise this case study, accessing site formation processes and taphonomic transformations at crime scenes often requires specific knowledge. For example, the spatial relationship between different types of physical evidence has to be documented in such a manner that it will allow the reconstruction of the pre-depositional, depositional and post-depositional processes that took place at the crime scene. Additionally, it is important to analyse and interpret the encountered taphonomic transformations (e.g. human taphonomy, textile degradation, ecological changes) in their context and association. Information that has not been localised, documented and retrieved or sampled at the crime scene will be lost forever. All this shows that the procedures to examine a crime scene, and their sequence, are of extreme importance and should be established prior to accessing any crime scene in close collaboration between the scientists and police forces.

5 This is not always the instance. In another historic case from northern England, UK, partially mummified remains were found in an outdoor location where they had clearly only been recently dumped after a considerable period of storage in a roof space or building cavity, as indicated by the presence of glass fibre insulation fibres.

6 For more information, see: https://www.gov.uk/forensic-pathology-role-within-the-home-office (Accessed 7 August 2015).

Acknowledgements

We thank Mike Groen for his constructive comments to this paper, as well as our two reviewers.

References

Gardner, R.M. (2012) *Practical Crime Scene Processing and Investigation.* CRC Press: Boca Raton.

Gardner, R.M. and Bevel, T. (2009) *Practical Crime Scene Analysis and Reconstruction.* CRC Press: Boca Raton.

Janaway, R.C. (2008) The decomposition of materials associated with buried cadavers. In: Tibbett, M. and Carter, D.O. (eds), *Soil Analysis in Forensic Taphonomy: Chemical and biological effects of buried human remain.* CRC Press: Boca Raton, pp. 153–202.

Janaway, R.C. (2015) Forensic archaeology in the United Kingdom and quality assurance. In: Groen, W.J.M., Marquez-Grant, N. and Janaway, R.C. (eds), *Forensic Archaeology: A global perspective.* Wiley-Blackwell: Chichester, UK, pp. 197–206.

30

Saponified Brains of the Spanish Civil War

Fernando Serrulla, Francisco Etxeberría, Lourdes Herrasti, José Luis Cascallana and Julio Del Olmo

30.1 Introduction: the Spanish Civil War (1936–1939)

Social and political instability characterised Spain during the first third of the 20th century. On 18 July 1936, the General of the Spanish army, Francisco Franco, lead a military coup. From the next day onwards Franco's civil followers (*falangistas* and other supporters) began to kill and arrest people during 3 years of civil war and 35 years of a hard dictatorship. During the Spanish Civil War (1936–1939), approximately 1 million people died. More than 130,000 people died in the first months of this war, mostly through repression, and not by fighting in the war itself. Many of them had become victims of enforced disappearance, suffered physical and psychological torture and were eventually killed following unlawful confinement or simply executed after summary trials. This was a careful strategy designed by the perpetrators of the military coup to spread terror, and to cause chaos and instability to their enemies at the beginning of the fighting (Maestre 2010). The dead bodies were found either along roadsides or buried in mass graves throughout the whole of the Spanish territory (Preston *et al.* 2011). The families of the disappeared were unable to go through the natural grieving process since they did not know with any certainty whether their missing relatives were alive or not. Even today, almost 80 years after the war, there are families still searching for their missing relatives in mass graves.

In 2000, one of the above-mentioned relatives attempted a search for his grandfather in Priaranza del Bierzo (León, Spain). He used scientific archaeological procedures during the excavation of the grave and identified the skeletal remains that were recovered with DNA analysis (Silva and Macías 2003). This example was followed by many others and triggered further exhumations throughout Spain. The majority of exhumations have taken place in the autonomous region of Castilla-León, which is the region in which the mass graves of 'La Pedraja' (Burgos) and 'Villabasta de Valdavia' (Palencia) were found.

This chapter describes the mass grave of La Pedraja and the scientific analysis of the many preserved saponified brains found in this context.

30.2 Two Mass Graves

La Pedraja is a pass located some 30 km east of Burgos, very near (<10 km) to the well-known archaeological site of Atapuerca. Based on historical documents, it was estimated that more than 200 people were buried in the mass grave of La Pedraja. The first stage of the excavation was undertaken by the Aranzadi Science Society in 2010. This mass grave included the remains of 104 people. The 'Pedraja'

Taphonomy of Human Remains: Forensic Analysis of the Dead and the Depositional Environment, First Edition.
Edited by Eline M.J. Schotsmans, Nicholas Márquez-Grant and Shari L. Forbes.

mass grave was a trench 24 m long and 2.5 m wide, where several groups of victims were buried between July and November 1936. Ground altitude at this location is 1,150 m above sea level. The clay-type soil of the mass grave did not allow drainage of rain water. As most of the victims were killed in the same place and buried immediately afterwards, many personal effects were found associated with the human remains, such as glasses, dentures, clothes, and also bullets and cartridge cases. As in many other Spanish Civil War burials, the dead bodies were covered with lime (e.g. Congram *et al.* 2014; Schotsmans *et al.* 2017).

The bones were in very poor condition with only the occipital bone of the crania preserved. Some of the individuals appeared to have a well-preserved brain mass. These brains were about one-sixth of the normal size (Figure 30.1). In total, 45 preserved brains and one preserved heart were recovered in this mass grave (Serrulla *et al.* 2015).

Another six cadavers were exhumed (2012) in Villabasta de Valdavia, a meadow positioned 120 km from La Pedraja. This area is a valley 900 m above sea level where runoff water accumulates in winter. Meteorological conditions here are very similar to those found on the hill of La Pedraja. The bodies were buried at a depth of 60 cm. The burial site consisted of two parts; the first one lay just below the water stream, and included two skeletons. The second compartment, 5 m further, contained another four individuals. According to the villagers, the area tended to be flooded most of the year. As expected, there was considerable poor bone preservation, but the physical structure of the bones was better than those found in the mass grave La Pedraja. Personal effects as those seen in the mass grave La Pedraja were found very close to the bodies, in addition to fragments of bullets. Five preserved reduced brains were recovered. No other preserved organs were observed.

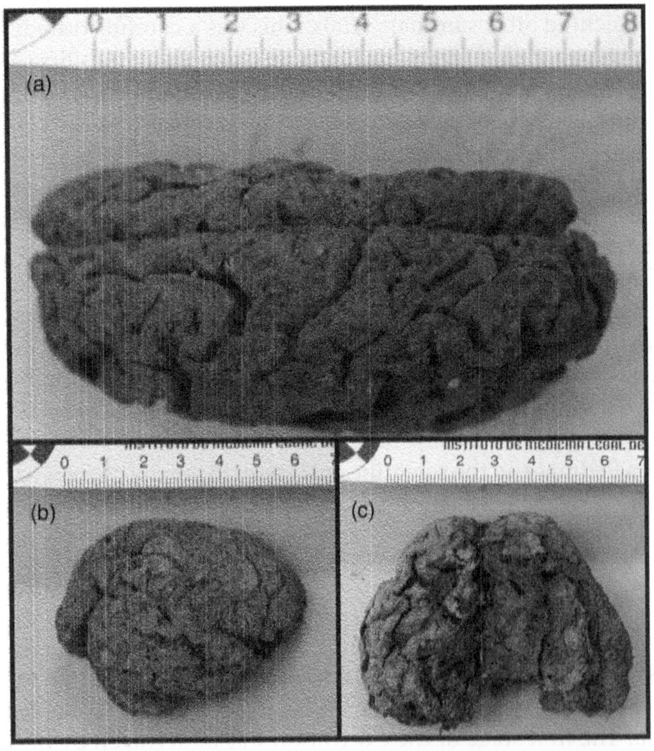

Figure 30.1 Gross morphology of saponified brains found in mass grave 'La Pedraja': (a) brain 25; (b) brain 104; (c) brain 11.

30.3 Methods and Materials

The brain collection, composed of a total of 50 saponified brains, is the largest and best preserved of its type in the world within archaeological and historical contexts. In order to understand the brain preservation and undertake forensic analysis, a team of scientists participated in the study of the brains. Several technical methods and tests were performed, but because of being buried for 77 years, many of the tests failed.

In brief, the following methods were applied. A total of 50 dried brains were morphologically inspected, photographed and examined by conventional X-ray and Computed Tomography (CT) scans. To optimise CT images of brain tissues, parameters of a 'lung' window were used. Stereolithography from CT images was achieved in order to model the brains. For further studies, the most well-preserved brains were selected from the mass grave La Pedraja (brains 11, 25 and 104) and Villabasta de Valdavia (brain 2). A Magnetic Resonance Imaging (MRI) scan was carried out on two of the four selected brains with prior to tissue rehydration. To rehydrate the brains, two different methods were employed: brains 11 and 2 were rehydrated by immersing them in the classical alcohol solution described by Ruffer (1909, 1921) and modified by Prats (Prats-Muñoz *et al.* 2012). Brains 25 and 104 were rehydrated with the glycerol water solution described by Eklektos (2006). After tissue rehydration, the entire brains were fixed in 10% buffered formalin for 2 weeks, coronally sectioned and the cassettes obtained were processed in an automatic tissue processor for dehydration, alcohol cleaning and infiltration with paraffin wax. Blocks were cut into serial 3–5 μm sections. Slides were stained routinely with haematoxylin and eosin (H and E) to demonstrate overall tissue structure, Prussian blue to demonstrate blood rests, Bielschowsky silver stain to show neurons and axons and Sevier Munger silver technique to show myelin in the nervous system. Standard immunohistochemical procedures were performed using antibodies directed against the following antigens: glial fibrillary acid protein (GFAP) for glial cells; CD 31 for endothelial cells and factor VIII for blood-clotting. For transmission electron microscopy (TEM) studies, cross-section samples of the rehydrated cerebellum and cerebral hemispheres were prepared in the conventional way.

To extract and sequence mitochondrial DNA from the brain tissue, ancient DNA techniques were applied (Knapp *et al.* 2012).

Because particular soil types could accelerate the adipocere formation, including sand and silty sand (Forbes *et al.* 2005b), 10 soil samples were collected from each mass grave. The soil samples were dried and sieved and a qualitative chemical analysis was performed on a modern conventional gas chromatograph. Atomic mass spectrometry methodology was used to accomplish the elemental analysis of the soil. Furthermore, the soil samples were characterised by X-ray powder diffraction analysis.

30.4 Results: Taphonomic Factors and Brain Analysis

The factors that are considered to have aided the unique preservation of the brains are outlined below.

30.4.1 Weather Conditions

The weather in the autumn of 1936 was similar in both La Pedraja and Villabasta de Valdavia, being cold and wet. According to the Atapuerca's meteorological observatory, records indicate the rainfall in October 1936 was up to 61 litres/m^2 and the lowest temperature was -8°C.

30.4.2 Soil Composition

Analysis of soil samples from La Pedraja showed a medium level of calcium concentrations fluctuating between 111 to 1,556 mg/kg. The pH of the soil was surprisingly acidic for a clay soil, ranging from 4.7 to 5.6. The amount of natural organic matter, less than 7.6%, was assumed to be very low. The mineral portion of the samples had the features of clay soils as the chemical components were SiO_2 (60%), Al_2O_3 (22%), Fe_2O_3 (7%) and K_2O (4.5%). Furthermore, there were traces (<1%) of several oxides such as Ti, P, Ba, Zr, Ca, S, Rb, Mn, Cu, Zn, Sr and Y. The presence of lime was identified in one of the sections of the mass grave of La Pedraja. Conversely, pH values in samples collected from Villabasta de Valdavia were slightly alkaline (>7.0) and the proportion of total calcium was a little higher at 1,500 mg/kg.

30.4.3 Gross Findings

Gross morphology of the brains was similar in both mass graves. The surface displayed a spongy granulated texture with a dark brown discoloration, being brittle, dry, hard, cracked and fragile to the touch. The weight of the brains was reduced 30 times. The medium size of the brains before rehydration ranged from 6 to 8 cm long and 4 to 6 cm wide. A few brains were fragmented. Soil and variable amounts of vegetable roots were attached to superficial cerebral parenchyma, particularly in the brains collected from Villabasta de Valdavia. Gross anatomy of the brains was easily recognised after careful superficial water cleaning (Figure 30.2). Partial deformation of one cerebral hemisphere was found in almost every brain. The cerebral *gyri* were condensed, and the *sulci* and deep main features were distended. Brain stem and spinal cord were missing in all cases. After coronal sectioning, the cut surfaces showed no grossly identifiable anatomical landmarks. Interestingly, a patchy subarachnoid haemorrhage over the parieto-temporal surface of the left hemisphere was detected in brain 11 (Figure 30.3a).

30.4.4 Radiological Studies

Brain radiographs showed multiple lead shot remains inside the cerebral parenchyma. These metal-density rounded spots were observed in 10 brains of the mass grave La Pedraja. They were of different sizes, suggesting home-made ammunition. None of the brains from Villabasta de Valdavia showed signs of shot in the X-ray examination. The brain images provided by CT and MRI scans did not allow to distinguish between white and gray matter, as the whole cerebral parenchyma showed a homogenous amorphous substance.

30.4.5 Chemical and Toxicological Studies

Qualitative analysis of the brains disclosed the presence of the saturated fatty acids, which are considered to be the components of adipocere (Forbes *et al.* 2005a,b).The saturated fatty acids found were myristic, palmitic and stearic acids. Other unsaturated fatty acids were also occasionally detected in the adipocere, including linoleic, lauric, ricinoleic, capric, lignoceric, caprilic, heptadecanoic, pentadecanoic, nonadecanoic and eicosanoic acids. Toxicological analysis of the brain samples did not reveal illicit drugs.

30.4.6 Genetic Study

Successive attempts to extract DNA from the brain samples failed.

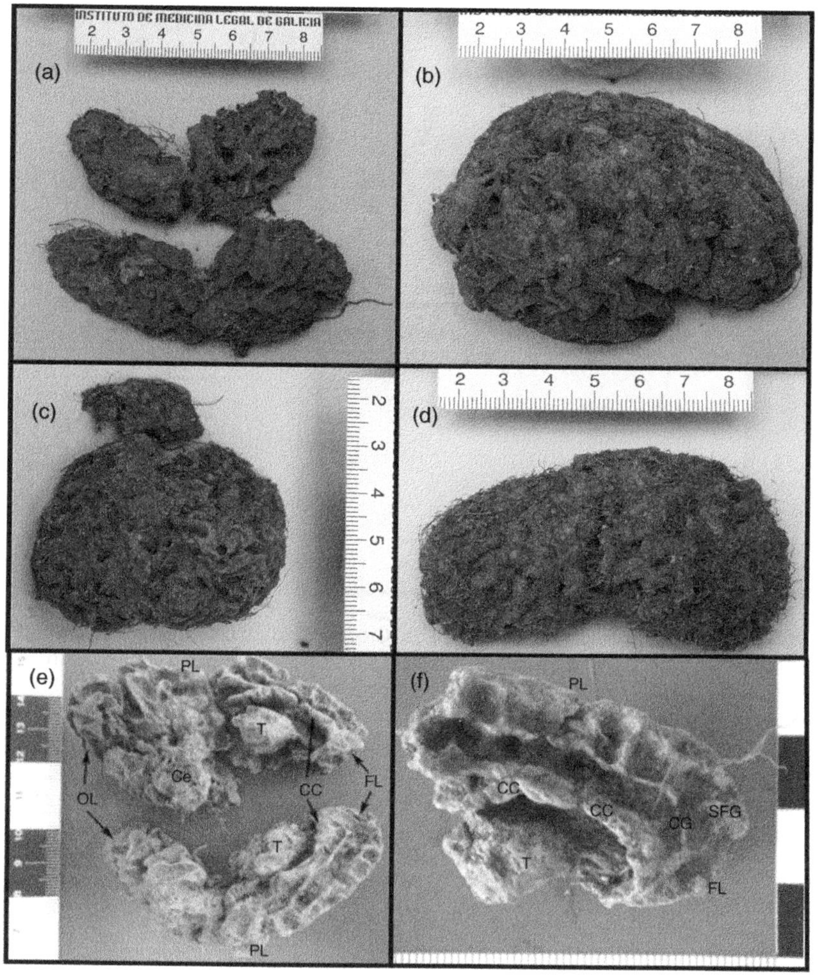

Figure 30.2 Gross morphology of saponified brains found in mass grave 'Villabasta de Valdavia'. Lateral view of (a) brain 2; (b) brain; (c) brain 4; and (d) brain 6. (e) Medial view of brain 2 after rehydration and superficial cleaning; and (f) higher magnification. Some vegetable roots remained attached to cerebral parenchyma. FL: Frontal lobe. PL: Parietal lobe. OC: Occipital lobe. Ce: Cerebellum. T: Thalamus. CC: Corpus callosum. CG: Cingulate gyrus. SFG: Superior frontal gyrus.

30.4.7 Microscopic Features

Due to its state of degradation, the histological specimens had no affinity with most of the stains, therefore white matter could not be discriminated from grey matter. Only Prussian blue dye retained its staining properties.

Extensive hemosiderin deposits were found in the parietal surface and nearby cerebral parenchyma of brain 11, a probe of intracranial ante-mortem haemorrhage (Figure 30.3b). Nearly all brain sections displayed fungi spores due to contamination. Moreover, small vegetable roots or stems were present throughout in the examined slices. The specific immunohistochemical staining showed the presence of very small blood vessels as they were positively lined with both the endothelial cell marker CD31 and factor VIII. At the ultrastructural level, the cerebral parenchyma was represented mainly

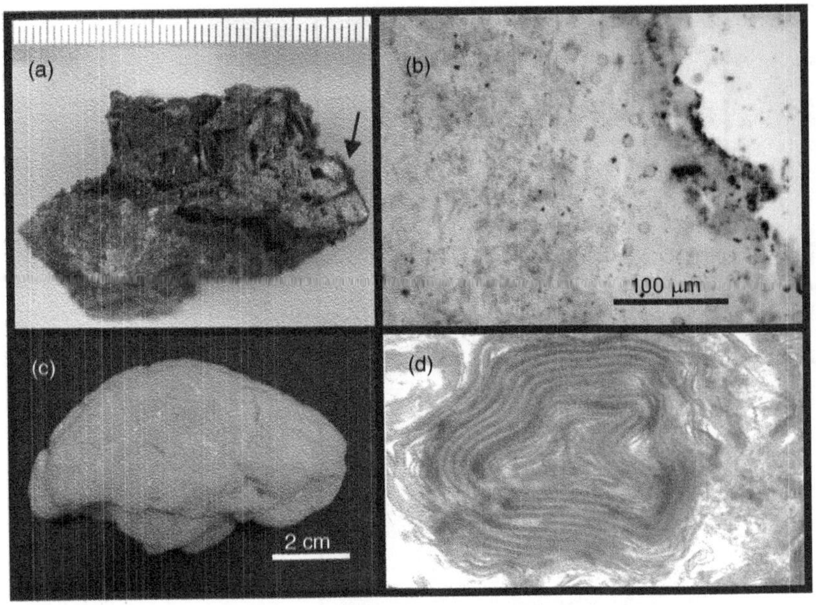

Figure 30.3 (a,b): Intracranial haemorrhage on parietal lobule of brain 11. (a) Gross grey-dark coloured subarachnoid thickening on parietal lobe (arrow). (b) Intraparenchymal dark deposits of hemosiderin in a specimen stained with Perl's stain (Prussian blue); round microorganisms with affinity for neutral red counterstain can also be observed. (c) Plastic scale model of brain 25 after stereolithography composition from CT scans. (d) Electron micrograph of brain 104 showing imperfect concentric arrangement of myelin lamellae and disintegration of central axoplasm.

by clusters of amorphous myelin debris and lipids, which occasionally presented several myelin layers disposed in a concentric organisation around a collapsed axoplasm (Figure 30.3d). No nerve cells, axons or synapsis were found.

30.4.8 Modelling of the Brains

Because environmental factors such as moisture, gram-positive bacteria and fungal growth might cause irreversible breakdown of the stored brains, 3D plastic models of the best preserved saponified brains were developed. A 3D printer generated the brain models using stereolithography files (DICOM format) from CT scans (Figure 30.3c). We modelled 28 brains from individuals from both mass graves.

30.5 Discussion and Conclusion

The major focus in this study was to determine the mechanism of preservation of the brains and what factors have been decisive in this single taphonomic phenomenon. The alluvial earth around the dead bodies was well-defined as an acid clay soil that in 1936 became broadly waterlogged. As established in chemical analysis, the whole brain fat was saponified into adipocere (Chapter 2).

Some authors – under experimental conditions – describe stimulating factors of adipocere formation such as moisture, mild alkalinity, anaerobic surroundings and warm temperature. On the contrary, cold temperature, excessive alkalinity (lime) and aerobic conditions are factors that inhibit adipocere formation (Forbes *et al.* 2005a, b). However, most published cases of preserved brains came across saponified brains in very different circumstances, sometimes in opposite contexts. Often, the mechanism of brain preservation is explained as 'saponification', while sometimes brains can be preserved in an extremely dry environment (Gerstzen 1995; Karlik *et al.* 2007). Furthermore, most of these studies did not execute chemical analysis of the brains, so the mechanism of preservation could have been severe cases of dehydration.

In this context, the authors agree with O'Connor *et al.* (2011) that only the case reported by Papageorgopoulou (2010) could be associated to the presence of adipocere. Therefore, it is necessary to take into consideration that not all published cases of preserved brains have been preserved by saponification. According to these and other authors (Eklektos 2006; Prats-Muñoz *et al.* 2012; Tkocz *et al.* 1979), most cases of saponified brains were found in conditions of high moisture and anaerobic environment. These factors are similar to what we noticed in our experience as forensic pathologists: almost all dead bodies recovered from water appeared to be partially saponified after several weeks of submergence. So the main question remains: what could be the main factor responsible for the development of adipocere? Maybe the microbiology of the bodies and the composition of the soil include the answer.

High moisture and an anaerobic environment, two key factors in brain adipocere formation, could provide the optimal growing conditions for different bacteria. These microorganisms, still not very well identified, can play an essential role in adipocere formation. Experiments have proved the requirement for an abundance of gram-positive bacteria during the early post-mortem period to assist in lipolysing the triglycerides into free fatty acids (Ueland *et al.* 2014). Extensive hydrolysis is enhanced by the presence of sufficient bacterial populations, anaerobic environment and moisture (Yan *et al.* 2001). Moisture is essential for the survival of the bacteria and also for the hydrolysis process (Mohan Kumar *et al.* 2009).

Pfeiffer *et al.* (1998) reported that bacteria found in soil, where adipocere was present, included gram-negative *Pseudomonas*, *Serratia*, *Alcaligenes* and *Enterobacter* and gram-positive *Bacillus*, *Nocardia* and *Cellulomonas*. According to the authors, gram-negative bacteria are believed to be responsible for the formation of adipocere, although this opinion is not shared by other researchers (e.g. Mohan Kumar *et al.* 2009; O'Brien and Kuehner 2007). In any case, it is assumed that bacteria present in the body and/or in the soil play a role in the process of saponification. In the saponified brains dating from the Spanish Civil War, it is assumed that chemical and microbiological changes were involved.

In summary, the mechanisms of adipocere formation are still not completely understood. Although it is not possible to explain exactly what happened to these brains, the authors suggest that the preservation of brain through adipocere formation is the result of primary and secondary factors. The primary factors are the essential factors. They include the presence of adipose tissue, a specific microbiological charge, high moisture and an anaerobic environment. Without primary factors, adipocere cannot be formed. Secondary factors are not necessary for adipocere formation, but the total amount of adipocere is stimulated by it. Secondary factors consist of physical and chemical elements which affect primary factors. Amongst the secondary factors are:

1) Temperature range is determined by the metabolism of the microbiota involved; most cases of saponified brain are observed in cold temperatures. The influence of temperature in enzymatic reactions such as hydrolysis of fats is also well known. On the other hand, cold temperatures reduce the progress of putrefaction;
2) Presence or absence of cations as Sodium (Na^+) and Calcium (Ca^{2+}). These and others cations are necessary to the formation of salts of fatty acids, which are chemical elements that form adipocere;
3) Acid or alkaline soil. Most cases of saponified brains have been preserved in acid soil, but there are cases in alkaline soils too. The pH of the soil affects enzymatic reactions. Probably the microbiological charge in acid soil produces more hydrolysis of the fats or esters.

A last question remains: why were the brains preserved, whereas the bones were in a very poor condition? As most of the victims were reported to be shot dead, severe haemorrhage and exsanguination should be the cause of death. Possibly little blood remained inside the head when the dead bodies were buried. It is well known that the progress of putrefaction occurs mainly throughout blood vessels, but in a brain without blood and in cold temperatures, the decomposition of the brain could have been delayed. In these circumstances the presence of high moisture, anaerobic conditions and a tissue (the brain) with a high proportion of fat (60%) (Tower 1994) represent the primary essential factors for the production of adipocere. The skulls formed a barrier and lead to preservation of the brains in the mass graves.

Acknowledgements

We would like to thank Veronica García Gordo and Yessica Medeiros for their indispensable contribution, which is widely recognised. We also thank Herminia and Miguel for being there. Special gratitude also goes to the full team of the *Aranzadi Science Society* who worked from dawn to dusk in the exhumation of the mass grave at La Pedraja. This study is a part of the doctoral thesis of the first author (FS) at the University of Granada (Spain).

References

Congram, D., Flavel, A. and Maeyama, K. (2014) Ignorance is not bliss: evidence of human rights violations from civil war Spain. *Annals of Anthropological Practice*, **38**: 43–64.

Eklektos, N., Dayal, M.R. and Manger, P.R. (2006) A forensic case study of a naturally mummified brain from the bushveld of South Africa. *Journal of Forensic Science*, **51**: 498–503.

Forbes, S.L., Stuart, B.H. and Dent, B.B. (2005a) The effect of the burial environment on adipocere formation. *Forensic Science International*, **154**: 24–34.

Forbes, S.L., Dent, B.B. and Stuart, B.H. (2005b) The effect of soil type on adipocere formation. *Forensic Science International*, **154**: 35–43.

Gerszten, P.C. and Martinez, A.J. (1995) The neuropathology of South American mummies. *Neurosurgery*, **36**: 756–761.

Karlik, S.J., Bartha, R., Kennedy, K. and Chhem, R. (2007) MRI and multinuclear MR spectroscopy of 3,200-year-old Egyptian mummy brain. *American Journal of Roentgenology*, **189**: W105–110.

Knapp, M., Clarke, A.C., Horsburgh, K. and Matisoo-Smith, E.A. (2012) Setting the stage – building and working in an ancient DNA laboratory. *Annals of Anatomy-Anatomischer Anzeiger*, **194**: 3–6.

Maestre, F.E. (2010) *Violencia roja y azul: España, 1936–1950.* Crítica: Barcelona.

Mohan Kumar, T.S., Monteiro, F.N., Bhagavath, P. and Bakkannavar, S.M. (2009) Early adipocere formation: a case report and review of literature. *Journal of Forensic and Legal Medicine*, **16**: 475–477.

O'Brien, T.G. and Kuehner, A.C. (2007) Waxing grave about adipocere: soft tissue change in an aquatic context. *Journal of Forensic Science*, **52**: 294–301.

O'Connor, S., Al, E., Al-Sabah, S., Anwar, D., Bergström, E. *et al.* (2011) Exceptional preservation of a prehistoric human brain from Heslington, Yorkshire, UK. *Journal of Archaeological Science*, **38**: 1641–1654.

Papageorgopoulou, C., Rentsch, K., Raghavan, M., Hofmann, M.I., Colacicco, G. *et al.*, (2010) Preservation of cell structures in a medieval infant brain: a paleohistological, paleogenetic, radiological and physico-chemical study. *NeuroImage*, **50**: 893–901.

Pfeiffer, S., Milne, S. and Stevenson, R.M. (1998) The natural decomposition of adipocere. *Journal of Forensic Science*, **43**: 368–370.

Prats-Muñoz, G., Malgosa, A., Armentano, N., Galtes, I., Esteban, J. *et al*. (2012) A paleoneurohistological study of 3,000-year-old mummified brain tissue from the Mediterranean Bronze Age. *Pathobiology: Journal of Immunopathology, Molecular and Cellular Biology*, **79**: 239–246.

Preston, P., Muñoz, C.M. and Nacarino, E.V. (2011) *El holocausto español: odio y exterminio en la Guerra Civil y después*. Debate: Barcelona.

Ruffer, M.A. (1909) Preliminary note on the histology of Egyptian mummies. *British Medical Journal*, **1**: 1005.

Ruffer, M.A. (1921) *Studies in the Palaeopathology of Egypt*. University of Chicago Press: Chicago.

Schotsmans, E.M.J., García-Rubio, A., Edwards, H.G.M., Munshi, T., Wilson, A.S. and Rios, L. (2017) Lime burials from the Spanish Civil War (1936–1939). *Journal of Forensic Sciences*.

Serrulla, F., Etxeberria, F. and Herrasti, L. (2015) Corazón conservado 70 años por saponificación. *Revista Española de Medicina Legal*, **41**: 43–44.

Silva, E. and Macías, S. (2003) *Las fosas de Franco: los republicanos que el dictador dejó en las cunetas*. Temas de hoy: Barcelona.

Tkocz, I., Bytzer, P. and Bierring, F. (1979) Preserved brains in medieval skulls. *American Journal of Physical Anthropology*, **51**: 197–202.

Tower, D.B., Thouret, M.-A., Fourcroy, A.-F., Vauquelin, L.N., Couerbe, J.-P. and Frémy, E. (1994). *Brain Chemistry and the French Connection, 1791–1841: An account of the chemical analyses of the human brain by Thouret (1791), Fourcroy (1793), Vauquelin (1811), Couerbe (1834), and Frémy (1841). A second sourcebook in the history of neurochemistry*. Raven Press: New York.

Ueland, M., Breton, H.A. and Forbes, S.L. (2014) Bacterial populations associated with early-stage adipocere formation in lacustrine waters. *International Journal of Legal Medicine*, **128**: 379–387.

Yan, F., McNally, R., Kontanis, E.J. and Sadik, O.A. (2001) Preliminary quantitative investigation of post-mortem adipocere formation. *Journal of Forensic Science*, **46**: 609–614.

31

Analysis and Interpretation of Burned Human Remains from a Homicide

Anne Coulombeix and Yves Schuliar

31.1 Introduction

This chapter presents a French criminal court case that required assistance of anthropologists and fire scene experts of the French Forensic Science Institute of the French National Gendarmerie/Institut de Recherche Criminelle de la Gendarmerie Nationale (IRCGN). The case involved the disappearance of five members of a French family and the subsequent investigation of discovered skeletal remains. Forensic experts reconstructed a fire scene in order to compare the suspect's statement with observations and evidence noticed at the scene (Baccard *et al.* 2004). This case study highlights the crucial role of forensic anthropologists and their contribution to criminal investigation with regard to reconstructing the sequence of events leading to death and interpretation of taphonomic processes.

31.2 Background to the Case

In April 2003, a couple and their three children were reported missing in Haute-Savoie, a department in the Rhône-Alpes region of eastern France. The prosecutor launched a criminal investigation and five months later a suspect was interrogated. Almost immediately, the suspect testified that all five individuals had been killed and set on fire. Based on the suspect's statements, investigators from the IRCGN were able to locate the crime scene, which was located in the Alps at an altitude of 1,300 m. It was situated in a pine forest, close to a road and a mountain stream (Figure 31.1). During that period, heavy rainfall had caused significant flooding across the region. Therefore, five months after burning the bodies, the outlines of the fire had been erased and could not be measured accurately. Other important information such as soil discolouration or evidence of fuel was also lacking. The human remains, deposited at the surface, were scattered, caused by various taphonomic agents, such as abundant rainfall, soil erosion and animal scavenging. Despite the complex nature of the crime scene and its partial destruction, several experts collected contextual evidence.

Taphonomy of Human Remains: Forensic Analysis of the Dead and the Depositional Environment, First Edition.
Edited by Eline M.J. Schotsmans, Nicholas Márquez-Grant and Shari L. Forbes.

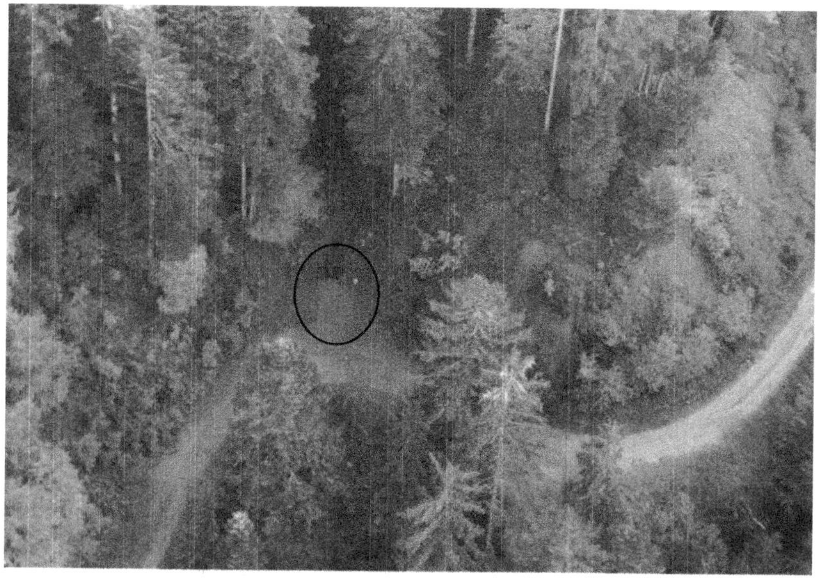

Figure 31.1 Aerial view of the location of the pyre (Haute-Savoie, French Alps).

31.3 Physical Evidence Recovered at the Crime Scene

Five months after the crime, the human remains were scattered and traces of the fire had disappeared. Only isolated bone fragments could be detected (n = 196) (Table 31.1). Detailed information regarding their position and orientation was recorded before recovery. Sediment and soil from the crime scene was subsequently sieved, resulting in the recovery of teeth, human nails, hair, jewels, faunal remains, burned wood and metal fragments from a mattress. Of the initial estimated weight of the complete five human bodies (280 kg), only 10% was recovered, represented exclusively by bones. Based on the analysis of the bones, the total weight of the collected bones and differences in size and age of the skeletal elements, a minimum number of three individuals could be identified (Baccard *et al.* 2004).

Two types of taphonomic modifications were noticed on the bones. The first type was linked to the burning process and the second type was caused by animal activity. Many bone and dental remains showed signs of burning, with heat-induced colour changes from yellow-brown to calcined white, while 24% of the bones showed almost no signs of burning (Figure 31.2). Those colour changes enabled the reconstruction of details of the combustion process through assessment of burn intensity and variability (Schmidt and Symes 2008; Thompson 2004) (Chapter 21). The majority of the bones showed a yellow-brown and black colour, indicating that the temperatures on those bones ranged from between 200°C and 500°C. About 20% of the bones had a blueish grey to white colour, which indicates temperatures between 500°C to 800°C.

The second category of taphonomic damage observed on the human remains was caused by animal scavenging (Chapter 16). The crime scene was clearly affected by scavenging behaviour, resulting in scattered human remains and the disappeareance of many bones. Scavenger inflicted bone modifications were also noticed on the bones, represented mostly by bite marks consisting of pits, punctures, scores and furrows (Figure 31.3). They were likely caused by medium-size carnivores (Binford 1981). The faunal remains recovered during sieving of sediments and soil from the crime scene were not taxonomically identified, nor was a study conducted on the scavenging marks observed on the human remains.

Table 31.1 Overview of skeletal remains disovered at the crime scene.

	Skeletal remains	*n*
JUVENILE	Femur	2
	Vertebrae	2
	Teeth	4
	Pelvis	1
	Radius	1
	Unfused epiphyses	1
	Spongious fragments	4
	TOTAL	**15**
	Skeletal remains	*n*
ADULT	Upper limbs	16
	Lower limbs	14
	Cranium	50
	Teeth	19
	Vertebrae	26
	Ribs	2
	Pelvis	5
	Scapulae	1
	Long bone shaft fragments	21
	Spongious fragments	16
	Non identifiable remains	11
	TOTAL	**181**

31.4 Additional Experiments

Because of doubts of certain elements in the suspect's statement and a lack of crucial information regarding the conditions of the fire, the orientation of the bodies, the utilised fuel and possible accelerants, it was necessary to set up experiments with pig carcasses. The aim was to create comparative data and to evaluate the impact of various taphonomic processes on the human remains. The results of the experiments were compared to the results of the analysis of the remaining skeletal remains collected at the crime scene (Baccard *et al.* 2004).

According to the suspect, the five bodies were piled up on a pyre with wood and 40 to 60 litres of fuel (diesel and petrol) was poured over the individuals. The fire was lit in the second half of the night, lasting for two to five hours. The suspect stated that he did not intervene in the burning process, either to maintain the fire or to rearrange the bodies. At the end of the night, once the fire cooled down, he collected the human remains and placed them in a carpet. The following night, he returned to the crime scene and repeated the process, using 10 litres of methylated spirit (ethanol). The fire lasted for two hours, after which the suspect scattered the remains around.

Two sets of experiments (A and B) using pig carcasses were conducted at the presumed location of the original crime scene in order to compare the results with the suspect's statement.

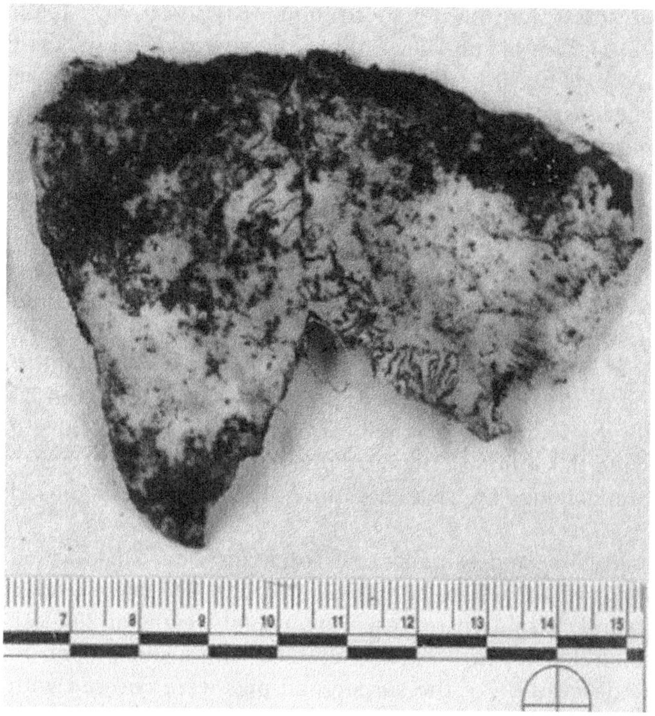

Figure 31.2 Parietal and occipital cranial bones were almost not affected by the fire.

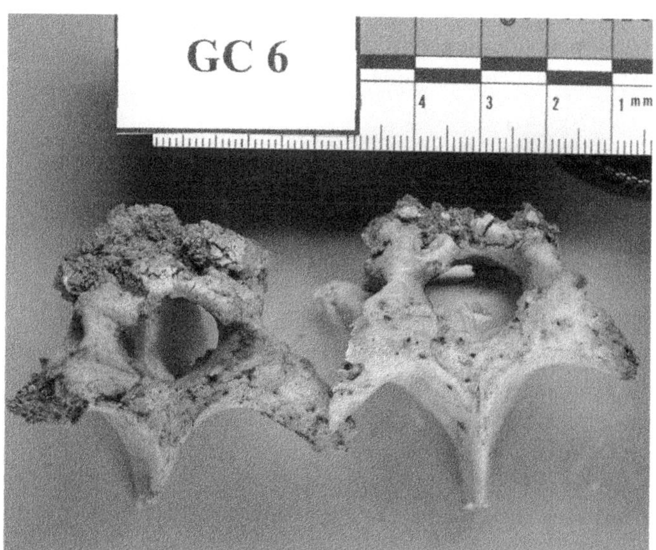

Figure 31.3 Gnawing damage on two thoracic vertebrae caused by a scavenger.

Pigs (*Sus scrofa*) have often been utilised in taphonomic experiments because they have a comparable skin structure, fat-muscle ration, body-mass and physiology to humans (France *et al.* 1992; Rodriguez and Bass 1985; Schoenly *et al.* 1991). Pigs of similar weight to the victims were selected to carry out two different experiments, two pigs of 70 kg for experiment A and five pigs with a similar weight to the family members for experiment B. The following data were collected during the experiments: external temperature, hygrometry, atmospheric pressure, wind speed, fire temperature and fire duration.

For experiment A, two separate fires were created with a 70 kg pig on each of them (pyre A1 and A2). A pyre of 180 cm wide and 80 cm high was made of 220 kg of wood piled up, similar to ritual cremations in India or Nepal. Petrol and diesel was poured over the wood as a accelerant. The two pigs were placed supine on the wood. They were not dressed, so that damage on their bodies could be observed. The fire lasted for a period of six hours, which resulted in the disappearance of most of the wood. Three distinct phases of fire could be identified. The first phase (0–30 min) was quick and immediate, associated with the burning of the petrol. The second phase began after about 30 minutes and lasted for 3 hours. In this phase the temperature remained constant (between 600 and 900°C) and contributed to extensive damage to the animals. The third phase consisted of a decrease in temperature. The fire burned in a less homogeneous way, which required the bodies to be moved in order to destroy them further.

A second experiment (B1) consisted of 5 pigs (2 big and 3 smaller ones) on a 3 m wide, 3 m long and 1 m high pyre of 880 kg wood. This quantity was estimated to be sufficient to complete the intended destruction of the five bodies (i.e. 2 adults and 3 children representing a total weight of 280 kg). In order to take into account the influence of clothes, each pig was dressed with a shirt, a pair of trousers and a sports jacket. Following the description of the suspect, all pigs were covered with sheets and a blanket. Clothes, a carpet and parts of furniture (i.e. chairs and a couch) were also added to the fire, followed by 60 litres of petrol poured on top. This experimental fire lasted for seven hours. The remains of the pigs were seriously damaged, representing 18% of their initial weight. The skeletal remains showed heat-induced colour changes from yellow-brown to calcined white. Afterwards, based on the suspect's statement, bone and tooth fragments were collected and burned again with 10 litres of ethanol. This 'secondary' fire only had a limited impact on the remains, reducing the weight by another 10%. Because ethanol is not a very good accelerant, the fire only lasted an hour.

31.5 Discussion

Direct comparison between experimental burning of pigs with burning of human bodies has limitations. Fatal fire models in the USA have shown that it is not only the head and limbs that are crucially different between pigs and humans but also the soft tissue, underlying subcutaneous fat, muscles, tendons and bones, which results in different responses to fire (Pope and Whitney 2015). Moreover, in this situation, it was difficult to recreate the crime scene in an exact way, because two fires are never exactly alike (in this case, not exactly the same weather conditions, the use of a different species of wood, exact size, duration of exposure, etc.) (Dehaan 2008).

Overall, the main aim of the experiments was to reproduce conditions of the fire in order to obtain similar remains to the skeletal remains found at the crime scene. The experiment revealed that it had been necessary to use an important quantity of wood to obtain similar skeletal remains. Clearly, the proportion of wood and petrol indicated by the suspect was not sufficient to burn five bodies and their artefacts. Furthermore, the quantity of wood required to build a fire, to almost totally destroy five individuals, would have been immense and would have required well-organised logistics.

Although some bones clearly reached temperatures between 500°C and 800°C, many bones were not burned or burned at low temperatures. These observations by the fire scene experts and anthropologists were exclusively based on the skeletal remains still present at the crime scene, five months after the crime took place.

All the above elements support the hypothesis that the five bodies were neither completely burned nor completely destroyed. Therefore, it is very likely that the fire had not destroyed the bodies to a great extent. The absence of soft tissue on the bones was likely the result of the normal decomposition process and animal scavenging. Additionally, the majority of the human remains had disappeared because of animal activity and rainfall on the slope. All these factors resulted in the recovery of only 196 human remains representing 5 individuals. Finally, in addition to the anthropological analysis, DNA analyses confirmed the identity of three of the five victims (Baccard *et al.* 2004).

31.6 Conclusion

Special care is required during the recovery of burned human remains, complicated by the fragile nature of such remains and the complex contexts in which they might occur. Methods of recovery can affect the degree of fragmentation. Distinguishing small burned human bone or tooth fragments from charred pieces of building materials or other items, such as furniture, can be challenging, even for trained anthropologists. Application of traditional archaeological methods by police officers is highly advised in order to locate important pieces of evidence and prevent the loss of significant contextual evidence. Therefore it is recommended to ask a forensic (archaeo-) anthropologist to be the coordinator of an interdisciplinary team during the investigation of a fire scene. Not only can the forensic anthropologist help with the analysis and interpretation of the burned bones, he/she can also aid with the reconstruction of the taphonomic processes. This case study highlights how collaboration between different specialists can contribute to a criminal investigation.

Acknowledgements

The authors would like to thank the fire scene experts for their collaboration on this case. We also wish to thank Aurore Val and Antony Colombo for their comments to the text.

References

Baccard, E., Calisti, C., Grevin, G. and Touron, P. (2004) *Rapport d'examen technique multidisciplinaire.* IRCGN: Paris.

Binford, L.R. (1981) *Bones: Ancient men and modern myths.* Academic Press: New York.

Dehaan, J.D. (2008) Fire and bodies. In: Schmidt, C.W. and Symes, S.A. (eds.), *The Analysis of Burned Human Remains.* London: Academic Press, pp. 1–16.

France, D.L., Griffin, T.J., Swanburg, J.G., Lindemann, J.W., Davenport, G.C. *et al.* (1992) A multidisciplinary approach to the detection of clandestine graves. *Journal of Forensic Sciences*, **37**: 1445–1458.

Pope, E.J. and Whitney, M. (2015) *Burning Models: Human versus pig in taphonomic fatal fire modeling.* Proceedings of the 67th Annual Meeting of the American Academy of Forensic Sciences, Orlando, p. 105.

Rodriguez, W.C. and Bass, W.M. (1985) Decomposition of buried bodies and methods that may aid in their location. *Journal of Forensic Sciences*, **30**: 836–852.

Schmidt, C.W. and Symes, S.A. (eds) (2008) *The Analysis of Burned Human Remains*. Academic Press: London.

Schoenly, K., Griest, K. and Rhine, S. (1991) An experimental field protocol for investigation of postmortem interval using multidisciplinary indicators. *Journal of Forensic Sciences*, **36**: 1395–1415.

Thompson, T.J.U. (2004) Recent advances in the study of burned bone and their implications for forensic anthropology. *Forensic Science International*, **146**: S203–S205.

32

A Soldier's Story: Forensic Anthropology and Blast Injury

Marie Christine Dussault, Martin Brown and Richard Osgood

32.1 Introduction

With the advent of the centenary of the Great War (1914–1918), many more inspiring stories are told by relatives of those who fought, as well as by other witnesses. Amongst these accounts, particularly those of the missing, are some that have been concluded through the application of physical anthropology and archaeology to aid in the identification of individuals. This includes finding the remains and the description and interpretation of the sequence of events of the individual's last moments nearly 100 years later.

The case presented is one such case, describing the anthropological contribution to the identification of Private Alan James Mather, an Australian who lost his life in Belgium. The anthropological examination of the remains permitted an explanation of what had happened to Pte Mather, particularly the circumstances of how he had lost his life.

32.2 Background and Case History

The body of Pte 1983 A.J. Mather was found in July 2008. His remains were uncovered during the archaeological investigation of a section of a German front line trench east of St Yvon, Ploegsteert, Belgium. The excavation formed part of The Plugstreet Project, a conflict landscape investigation led by No-Man's-Land, an archaeological group that includes both professional and amateur archaeologists and historians. The Project was conceived in 2005 following the investigation of training trenches on the British Army's Salisbury Plain Training Area (Osgood and Brown 2009). These trenches were associated with Australian troops of the Third Division (3 Div), part of the Australian and New Zealand Army Corps (ANZAC). From the training grounds of that time, men of 3 Div were deployed to Belgium where they formed the right flank of the attack on Messines on 7 June 1917. As part of this attack, 19 mines, which had been tunnelled out under the German line, were detonated, and the Allied attackers stormed the enemy positions with remarkable success (Passingham 2004). Mather was one of the men killed during this assault and, as his body received no known grave at the time, his name appears on the Menin Gate Memorial to the Missing in Ieper (Ypres). During archaeological excavation of the trench, the body was found lying on its left side, in a slightly crouched position with arms and legs flexed. The body lay at a slight angle against the collapsed rear wall of the German trench. It appeared that the trench wall had collapsed, due either to the shock wave from the mine some 500 m to the south or the barrage that followed it to batter the defences before the Allied assault.

Taphonomy of Human Remains: Forensic Analysis of the Dead and the Depositional Environment, First Edition.
Edited by Eline M.J. Schotsmans, Nicholas Márquez-Grant and Shari L. Forbes.

His body was covered with a deposit very similar to the surrounding soils that formed the sides and parapets of the trench and this is considered to be earth cast up by shell bursts. No other associated remains were found. It is unknown whether the burst that buried Mather was an Allied shell falling short or part of the German fire on the attack.

Following the discovery of the human remains, a careful excavation led by an experienced forensic archaeologist was undertaken (Osgood and Brown 2009), with the final recovery supervised by the Belgium Army as recipient of the remains. As artefacts were lifted, they were placed within a chain of evidence and passed up to the team's conservation laboratory where they were cleaned, stabilised, recorded and packed (Osgood and Brown 2009). During this phase of operations, the fallen soldier gained a limited identity: elements of his equipment, including a rifle, entrenching tool and webbing, indicated that he had been a member of the British Imperial forces; insignia then provided his particular formation. Remnants of his clothing such as webbing, khaki collars and corduroy trousers were identified as consistent with post-1915 British infantry issue. Shoulder titles and badges all showed the man to be a member of the Australian military forces. Meanwhile, deeply personal artefacts, like his toothbrush, proved to have an emotional effect for those involved. The artefacts found with the remains were in good condition, for example the brand name of the toothbrush could be read (France Flexadent) and two ampoules full of iodine were recovered.

His equipment told an important tale. From historical research it is known that only two Australian units were in this particular part of the battlefield and of those only 3 Div was involved in combat, indicated by the 150 rounds of ammunition, Mills grenades and fixed bayonet. Careful consideration of the Order of Battle, showed that the extreme right flank was occupied by the 33rd Battalion (33rd Bn) during the attack, which indicated that this man was a member of that formation (Osgood and Brown 2009). Despite the attack being a success, the 33rd Bn still bore many casualties, with some 50 of those having no known grave. These missing men included soldiers who could not be recovered following the blast, those who had been given battlefield burial and men lost in the fog of war, like Mather. Nevertheless, the Commonwealth War Graves Commission (CWGC) holds records of each and all of these men, including age, date and place of death, often including the address and details of their families. Meanwhile, the Australian National Archives retain the service records of all enlisted men and these include further details, including place of birth and enlistment, medical and dental records and height and weight. It soon became apparent that many of the men in the 33rd Bn were recruited in New South Wales because of a 1916 recruiting drive. Many, but not all, were New South Wales born and bred, but others were incomers from other parts of the world.

32.3 Condition of the Remains and Inventory

The skeletal remains of Pte Mather were examined on 9 February 2010 at the Commonwealth War Graves Commission in Ypres, Belgium. The biological profile was conducted using established anthropological methods to estimate the age, sex and stature of the remains (Buikstra and Ubelaker 1997). Working jointly with a team from The Plugstreet Project, the CWGC under direction from the Australian Ministry of Defence, established two work objectives. First, the biological profile was undertaken with the purpose of aiding in the joint efforts to identify the skeletal remains with the aim of informing any living relatives. This was to be accomplished by comparing the results to a list of missing persons, and with subsequent DNA analysis undertaken by the Australian Ministry of Defence. The second objective was to carry out a trauma analysis to establish the peri-mortem circumstances of the individual's death, in combination with the archaeological and historical records.

The remains were kept in a small coffin and sealed in bags according to general anatomical order. The remains themselves had some adhered soil, which was removed and the bones cleaned. The

Figure 32.1 Inventory of the remains.

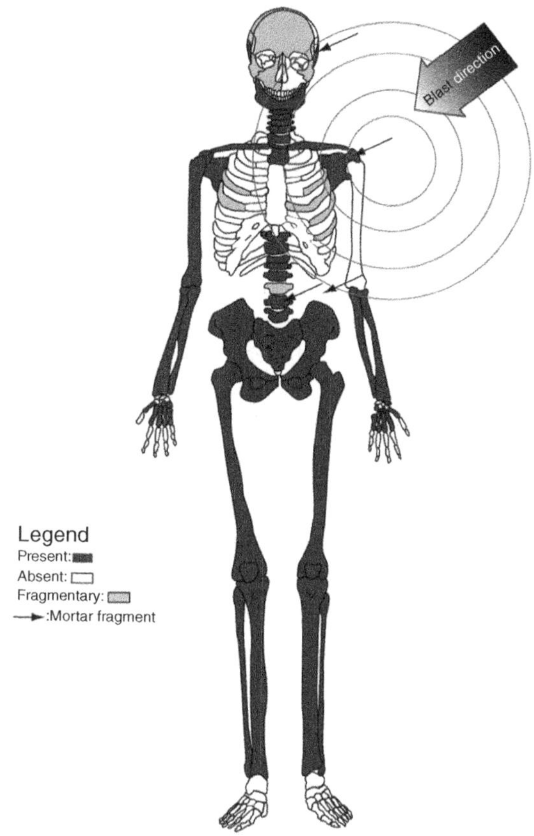

skeleton was nearly complete and the condition of the remains was excellent, with good preservation of the cortical bone. The bones were first laid out in anatomical order on a mortuary table.

An inventory of the remains was made to assess completeness and determine the minimum number of individuals. The cranial bones were fragmentary but mostly present. The cranial vault was reconstructed. Some bones of the face were missing including the sphenoid, palatine, vomer, ethmoid and most of the maxillae. A small portion of the right maxilla was recovered. The mandible was complete but had experienced significant post-mortem tooth loss. As a result, only the first and second left molars, with fillings, remained.

The left and right ribs were very fragmentary and thus a specific rib number could not be identified. The sternum was missing. The left humerus was also absent and was not recovered during the excavation. Most of the hand bones were present, with the exception of some of the right carpal bones. There was also a supernumerary lumbar vertebra, which articulated well with the other lumbar vertebra and the sacrum. Nearly all the foot bones were missing, with the exception of a proximal phalanx. The inventory is illustrated in Figure 32.1.

32.4 Analysis Results

32.4.1 Biological Profile

Estimation of sex was made using morphological and metric methods commonly used in physical anthropology. The bones used were the pelvis and skull. The sciatic notch was narrow and the subpubic angle was narrow. These indicate that the remains were male. In the skull, the nuchal crest of the occipital bone was very prominent, the mastoid process was large and the gonial angle of the mandible flared. These three morphological traits also indicate that the remains were male (Bass 2005).

Measurements were taken from the femoral head and the humeral head. These involve measuring the diameter of the head, in the vertical plane, using callipers. The humeral head measured 51.1 mm and the femoral head measured 49.7 mm. Both these measurements indicate that the remains were male (Bass 2005).

The age of the skeleton was established using assessment of epiphyseal fusion of certain post-cranial elements and the morphological changes of the pubic symphyses, the auricular surface and sternal rib ends. All long bones were fused, indicating that the remains represent an adult individual. Fusion of the hyoid bone was noted. It was fused completely with the sutures obliterated. This particular bone is known to fuse in the late stages of life, particularly the third decade (Scheuer and Black 2004), indicating that the remains represent an individual over the age of 30. In the clavicle, the sternal medial epiphyses were also fused, again indicating an individual over the age of 30 (Bass 2005; Scheuer and Black 2004).

By examining the pubic symphysis using comparative casts (Bass 2005; Buikstra and Ubelaker 1997) and the auricular surfaces using the methods of Bass (2005) and Buikstra and Ubelaker (1997) the age, in both cases, was estimated to be between 30 to 35 years of age. Sternal rib ends of the left ribs (those which could be identified as being ribs number 3 to 5) were also compared using casts and the age from these estimated as 32–40 years.

Using the Fordisc 3.0 method, the estimated stature was calculated from multiple long bone measurements for accuracy (Jantz and Ousley 2005). Using the maximum length of the femur (47.6 cm) and condylar-malleolus length of the tibia (37.9 cm), the stature was estimated as being 165.7 to 178.2 cm (95% prediction interval).

Overall, the skeleton exhibited very robust and well-developed muscle markings. This was evident in the upper body, especially in the clavicles and the right upper arm. The individual was estimated to be a male between 30 and 40 years of age, measuring between 165.7 and 178.2 cm.

32.4.2 Pathology

The skeleton exhibited a number of pathological conditions. In the vertebral column, Schmorl's nodes were observed in the first, third, fourth and fifth vertebra lumbar vertebrae. These were also seen in the thoracic vertebrae with the fourth through to twelfth vertebrae affected. The posterior spinous processes of the vertebrae were also angled to the right, in the majority of the spinal column.

Also noted was extensive osteophytic lipping of the vertebral bodies, indicating the presence of osteoarthritis. Osteoarthritis in the form of osteophytic lipping and pitting was also observed in the acetabulum of the pelvis, bilaterally.

The right femur was bowed anteriorly. In both the femoral heads, a flattening was observed. Cribra orbitalia was present in the left eye socket, exhibited by woven bone.

32.4.3 Trauma

The left and right ribs were extensively fragmented. Examination of the fracture edges showed no evidence of healing, and were broken in an oblique manner, indicating that they had been sustained peri-mortem. The fragments were mostly left fragments and all of these had peri-mortem fractures. The fragments, which could be assigned to specific ribs, showed that trauma was prevalent in the mid-thorax region. This trauma was also seen bilaterally.

The left humerus and sternum (body) were absent; however, the manubrium and both clavicles were present and intact. Multiple metallic fragments were located on the left temporal bone, the left scapula and in the associated matrix. Cranial fragments from the vault were examined and peri-mortem fractures were identified on the left side of the vault, fragmenting the vault into large pieces. No other instances of peri-mortem or ante-mortem trauma were observed.

32.5 Discussion

This case is an example of the potential of blast injury trauma analysis in historical contexts. The forensic anthropologist's knowledge of the appearance of trauma caused by explosives can be very useful in analysing the context of such cases, in conjunction with site data and historical information. This is also applicable to modern forensic cases. It is widely known in the medical literature that fragmenting explosives, such as mortar shells used during World War I and subsequently, cause fragmentation of the human skeleton through various mechanisms such as the blast wave, fragment impact and blast wind causing displacement of bodies and surrounding objects (Covey 2002; Hr *et al.* 2009). The four patterns of injury, from primary to quaternary blast injury, are well documented in the medical literature, but have very rarely been researched from a forensic anthropology perspective (Dussault *et al.* 2014). The first pattern of blast related injury affects the fluid and air-filled organs, such as the bowels and the lungs. The blast wave passing through causes both an increase and decrease in pressure, injuring the organs (Figure 32.2).

The second pattern of blast injury relates to fragmentation injuries. This includes fragments from the casing of explosive munitions and can cause lacerations of soft tissues and fracturing of bone. The third pattern of blast injury occurs when there is crushing of the body, either by the movement of the body or of objects into the body. This is caused by the blast wind, moving the body or objects themselves. The quaternary (or fourth) pattern encompasses the injuries, which are not included in the previous three and are often related to burn trauma. In forensic anthropological cases, familiarity with the consequences of the second and third patterns of injuries is crucial.

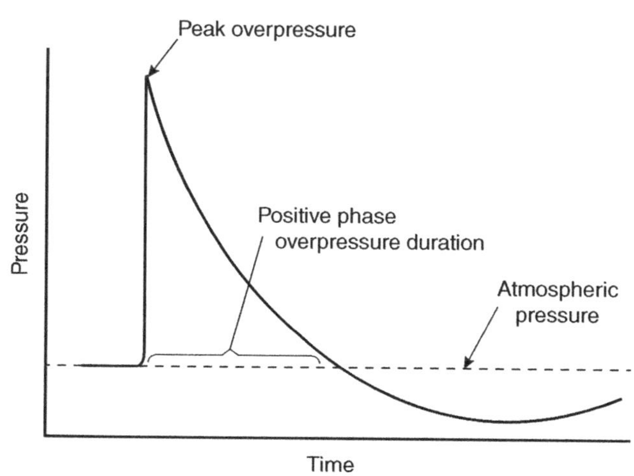

Figure 32.2 Positive and negative pressure phases (adapted from Horrocks and Brett 2000).

Based on the known historical case background, the group of soldiers was under fire from shells during the night of 7 June 1917. The trauma indicates that the man was hit by shellfire from the left, injuring his upper left arm and severely fracturing his ribs. No other nearby skeletal elements, such as the clavicle and scapula, which are in close proximity, were noted to have any damage. Shell fragments were found embedded in his left temporal and left scapula, confirmed by the archaeologists and military history specialists. The fragmented portions of the skull and the ribs were examined and gunshot injuries were ruled out. In blast injuries, large fragments and less fragmentation are noted compared to gunshot wounds. In the skull reconstruction, no entrance wounds were located and no radiating fractures were observed.

Analysing the skeletal trauma and physical evidence found during the excavation strongly points to a situation whereby the soldier was hit by shellfire from the left. During the reconstruction of the skeleton and the examination of the overall pattern of trauma, it was determined that the shell and its fragments would have passed through the upper portion of his arm, through the left side of his chest and exited on the right side of his torso. This was supported by the extensive fragmentation of the ribs in the mid-thorax region. Additionally, metallic fragments were embedded in bones from the left side only. During excavation he was found *in-situ*, covered in dirt that would have been thrown up during the attack and which buried him at a shallow depth. His uniform was also partially intact, apart from the torso area, where no remnants of buttons were found, as would have been expected. This evidence points to the fact that he was hit by shell fragments and was subsequently buried by the resulting cast-off.

The injuries seen in the skeletal remains can be interpreted as secondary and tertiary blast injuries, with fragments of the shell casing embedded in the shoulder girdle and skull as well as potential crush injuries, particularly in the torso from the cast-off, which buried him.

A second important aspect of the case is the appearance of very large muscle markers and pathology, particularly in the spine. The individual's spine exhibited extensive Schmorl's nodes as well as angulation of the spinous processes. Schmorl's nodes occur when there is an extrusion of the centre of the vertebral disk, often due to back trauma or congenital defects. Previously undertaken studies link the presence of Schmorl's nodes in military populations to an increased prevalence and associates these with trauma, probable in this case (Burke 2012). Prominent muscle markings, such as those seen in the shoulder girdles, were also noticed and could indicate physically taxing work, developing large muscles in the arms. The presence of extensive osteophytic activity in the spine was also noted, and combined with the Schmorl's nodes and large muscle attachments, could be linked to occupational stress markers, potentially indicating previous involvement in a very physical occupation (Villotte *et al.* 2010).

The anthropological examination estimated that the individual was male, aged between 30 to 40 years and measured between 165.7 and 178.2 cm. He exhibited extensive osteophytic changes in the spine, with Schmorl's nodes and displaced posterior processes. Both these aspects of the examination aided in answering the first objective set out by the requesting parties and contributed in the identification by confirming the results of stable isotope and DNA analysis.

Reconstruction of the skull and post-cranial skeleton and trauma analysis determined that the individual had been killed by fragments of a German mortar shell hitting him from the left and slightly behind, resulting in extensive fragmentation of the torso, left arm and cranial vault, with fragments embedded in the bones. This corroborates the historical accounts of the events of that day as well as the archaeological evidence.

32.6 Conclusion

In collaboration with archaeologists, the anthropologist can contribute to the analysis of human remains from conflict contexts in order to aid identification. In this case, the anthropological analysis was consistent with the DNA identification of Pte Mather. The examination determined that from the skeletal remains, the individual was a 30- to 40-year-old male, with a stature of between 165.7 and 178.2 cm. Additionally, pathology and muscle markers on the body indicated that he had potentially held an occupation involving physical labour.

Upon return of the DNA results and identification of Pte Mather, more aspects of his life were revealed to the team. Pte Mather was an Australian man who was 37 years old, measured 170 cm and had previously worked as a grazier on a farm in New South Wales, Australia. This is consistent with the anthropological results. Combined with historical evidence from the conflict in Belgium, it was confirmed that indeed he had been killed by shellfire on the night of 7 June 1917.

Through the application of knowledge about the mechanisms of blast injury, forensic anthropology can contribute to contextual evidence in excavations and create a developed profile of the individual whose remains are to be identified, corroborated by the extensive historical documentation of conflict. It is important to understand the mechanisms of blast, the variations with different munitions and the differences to gunshot wounds. This is likely to be particularly relevant in future, as the use of explosive munitions becomes the most prevalent mode of defence in both regular and irregular conflict.

References

Bass, W.M. (2005) *Human Osteology: A laboratory and field manual*. Missouri Archaeological Society: Columbia.

Buikstra, J.E. and Ubelaker, D.H. (1997) *Standards for Data Collection from Human Skeletal Remains*. Arkansas Archaeological Survey: Fayetville.

Burke, K.L. (2012) Schmorl's nodes in an American military population: frequency, formation, and etiology. *Journal of Forensic Sciences*, **57**: 571–577.

Covey, D.C. (2002) Blast and fragment injuries of the musculoskeletal system. *Journal of Bone and Joint Surgery*, **84**: 1221–1234.

Dussault, M.C., Smith, M. and Osselton, D. (2014) Blast injury and the human skeleton: an important emerging aspect of conflict-related trauma. *Journal of Forensic Sciences*, **59**: 606–612.

Horrocks, C. and Brett, S. (2000) Blast injury. *Current Anaesthesia and Critical Care*, **11**: 113–119.

Hr, C., Jb, H. and La, Y. (2009) Injuries from explosions: physics, biophysics, pathology, and required research focus. *The Journal of Trauma*, **66**: 1468–77.

Jantz, R. and Ousley, S. (2005) *FORDISC 3.1. Computerized Forensic Discriminant Functions*. The University of Tennessee: Tennessee.

Osgood, R. and Brown, M. (2009) *Digging up Plugstreet: The archaeology of a Great War battlefield*. Haynes: Sparkford.

Passingham, I. (2004) *Pillars of Fire: The battle of Messines Ridge, June 1917*. Pbk. ed. Sutton Pub: Stroud.

Scheuer, L. and Black, S. (2004) *The Juvenile Skeleton*. Academic Press: San Diego.

Villotte, S., Castex, D., Couallier, V., Dutour, O., Knüsel, C.J. and Henry-Gambier, D. (2010) Enthesopathies as occupational stress markers: evidence from the upper limb. *American Journal of Physical Anthropology*, **142**: 224–234.

33

Decomposition in an Unusual Environment: Body Sealed in Concrete

Maria Cristina de Mendonça

33.1 Introduction

This case study presents a case of burial in concrete, selected as an interesting example of how concrete influences preservation, sealing the body and thus preserving it from environmental conditions, which in this particular case were extreme. The case is anonymised due to the fact that it was performed under the scope of a human rights violation in a conflicted area, so specific details are limited.

33.2 Case Report

The body of a child was found inside a large plastic cylindrical container, filled with concrete, and located in an open space next to an abandoned building in a sandy desert-like area of the northern hemisphere. Weather conditions in this a region are extreme: a large thermal range (very high day temperatures – average high is 35°C, record high being 45.2°C, and low night temperatures – with lows of 0°C, the record low being −32°C), as well as a very low relative humidity. Nevertheless, the body was well preserved in such conditions during two months post-mortem, due to the fact that it was sealed with concrete inside the thick plastic walls of a container. In other forensic cases performed in the same region, bodies left in surface deposition during a similar post-mortem interval, were always found completely mummified, sometimes skeletonised.

The body was identified as a 7-year-old girl who had been reported missing about two months before, in a town close to the site. During that time, no traces were found by investigators from the local police. The discovery came when a man who was rummaging around, found several identical waste containers filled with trash, and tried to remove them. While doing so, he noticed that one particular container was much heavier, so he turned it on its side in order to roll it away. When the side of the container touched the ground the top opened, the plastic sidewall cracked and the man realised that the contents had also cracked. From the plastic sidewall crack, a dark smelly fluid began to leak out and part of a child's foot was visible through the opening. The police were notified and when they arrived at the site, they discovered that the content of the container was a block of concrete, which had to be arduously broken up with a chisel to release a child's body. A forensic investigation was requested and followed accordingly.

The container was 72 cm in height, with a large opening of 45 cm in diameter at the top. The body of the deceased was estimated as 1.20 m tall and was completely naked except for earrings in both ears. The body had been placed upside down in a foetal position inside the container, with the head at the

Taphonomy of Human Remains: Forensic Analysis of the Dead and the Depositional Environment, First Edition.
Edited by Eline M.J. Schotsmans, Nicholas Márquez-Grant and Shari L. Forbes.

bottom and both feet at the top. The condition of the soft tissues was slightly greenish and beginning to decompose, with slippage of the skin and hair, mostly because they had adhered to the concrete. A few maggots were present, as well as vegetal matter stuck inside the skin folds.

A full autopsy was performed. External wounds were perfectly perceptible, as well as internal trauma. Ancillary investigation including genetic and toxicological analysis was undertaken. The cause of death was absolutely clear and violence was evident by blunt trauma to the head perpetrated by a blunt instrument that impacted the scalp by way of several blunt force injuries. Fingerprints, forensic odontology and DNA comparison ascertained identification. Consequently, it became a perfectly straightforward post-mortem examination. The interesting issue in this case is based upon the most unusual environment in which the body had been kept, as far as the interpretation of circumstantial data was concerned. This is discussed below.

33.3 Discussion and Conclusion

The characteristics of the wounds to the head, which were the cause of death, were clearly a result of numerous blunt force injuries. The child was undoubtedly killed outside the container before being placed in it. Placing a dead 1.20 m tall body inside a 72 cm height container would require that no *rigor mortis* be present, allowing the body to be folded into a foetal position. Therefore, it is estimated that this would have happened either during the first few hours after death, before *rigor mortis* set in, or later, when *rigor mortis* had passed and decomposition began (after 36 hours, at the most). The presence of a few maggots on the body points to the second hypothesis.

Maggots and some vegetal matter indicate that the body had been kept out for some time in the open, before entering the container. The greenish discoloration and slippage of soft tissues constituted an obvious sign of decomposition, which according to the hot climate registered in this particular location, can appear in few hours.

Hence it would appear that the victim was killed and left exposed to the environmental conditions for a short while, either naked or dressed. Afterwards the undressed body was placed inside the container, which was then filled with fluid concrete. At the moment the concrete, involving the entire body, filled the container and solidified, decomposition apparently stopped.

It is hypothesised that, as long as the container was hermetically sealed, tissue conditions could endure for an indefinite period, despite the most extreme hot temperatures in sandy desert-like areas, for example, in this particular case, or in other extreme environments where degrading conditions may exist. Depending on the stage of decomposition of the body when it is sealed, forensic investigation will not be compromised, except for the accurate estimation of post-mortem interval.

This case was performed under the scope of a human rights case, therefore no other circumstantial details, nor photographs, are allowed to be disclosed. Nevertheless, it shows that concrete appears, at least in this case, to slow down decomposition of soft tissues in a significant way. If it had not been for such an unusual burial environment, it may be expected that two months after death, in the same climatological circumstances, the body of this little girl would have been completely skeletonised.

34

A Case Study from Los Angeles: Baby in Concrete

Chelsea Parham and Elissa Fleak

34.1 Introduction

In October of 2011, the Los Angeles Police Department (LAPD) informed the Los Angeles County Department of Medical Examiner – Coroner about the discovery of an infant encased in concrete. The case description and examinations that follow are based on the case notes and reports by the Los Angeles County Department of Medical Examiner – Coroner (2011).

34.2 Background to the Case

The baby, a Caucasian male, was believed to have died the previous year (late 2010); at the time of death, the infant was approximately six to eight weeks of age. The parents, who were living in a hotel, had a history of methamphetamine abuse and stated to Police that they were uncertain of how the baby had passed away. The mother reported that she only noticed her son was unresponsive when she attempted to breastfeed. The father suggested that, while co-sleeping, he may have accidently suffocated the child. He also stated that it was possible he strangled the infant in a state of confusion, whilst under the influence of drugs. Neither parent reported the death, and for three days they drove around with the deceased baby in the backseat of the car.

By mutual consent, the parents agreed to place the body in a 121 litres (32-gallon) plastic container and take it to their rented storage space at a facility. The father prepared a mixture of concrete, covered the infant with it and poured household products over it, in an attempt to hide the foul odour that was becoming apparent. However, the smell continued to fill the storage unit and after eight months the parents decided to move the container to the Angeles National Forest where they buried it.

Three months later, the mother was arrested on drug charges. She informed the father that she was planning to disclose information to the police about the death of their baby. The father decided that, with the help of a friend, he would move the tub containing the concrete and infant to another place. However, the friend contacted the police and led them to the location of the burial.

The scene was in a remote area of the Angeles National Forest. The edge of the road was large enough for a vehicle to park. From there, a slope led approximately 10 feet down to a dry streambed, with the clandestine graveside between the hillside and a scrub oak. The tree shaded the container which had a single corner exposed. A thick opaque plastic appeared to be wrapped around the tub. The soil on top of the container had some sprouted seedlings of poison oak, which were beginning to grow. Illegal dumping of household waste was noticed in the surrounding area and photographed; but did not appear to be in connection with the case.

Taphonomy of Human Remains: Forensic Analysis of the Dead and the Depositional Environment, First Edition.
Edited by Eline M.J. Schotsmans, Nicholas Márquez-Grant and Shari L. Forbes.

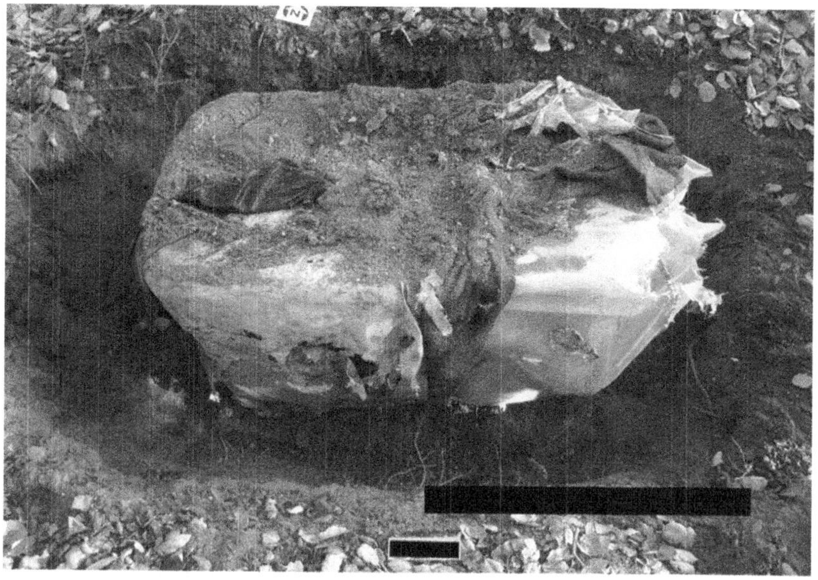

Figure 34.1 The container containing the infant encased in concrete (Source : Reprinted with permission of the Los Angeles County Department of Medical Examiner – Coroner).

Due to the difficult location and the remains being buried, the Special Operations Response Team within the Coroner's office was requested for the recovery. The thick plastic wrap and storage container, still holding the baby and concrete, were fully recovered (Figure 34.1) and brought back to the Forensic Science Centre for examination.

The grey tub was secured with a lid and wrapped, not only in the plastic, but also a fleece blanket and a fitted sheet. Once the lid was removed, a white, crystalline substance and bleach-like smell was noticed and identified as a combination of concrete and household cleaning products.

The container was approximately half full of concrete (Quikrete® Fast-Setting Concrete Mix) and portions of a blanket-like material could be seen. After X-rays were taken of the block to identify the positioning of the infant, the container was inverted to assist in the careful removal of the content. The presence of the blanket created natural fault lines, which assisted in the separation of the concrete into pieces. The top section of concrete was removed to show the infant's body wrapped in additional blankets and at least one towel. These coverings created a barrier to stop the concrete from coming into contact with the baby (Figure 34.2).

34.3 External Examination

Once the infant was unwrapped from the blankets and towel, a disposable diaper and cotton bodysuit was noticed. The bodysuit however, was only covering the arms and the front was left open – the infant's legs were not within the garment. The baby was laid in the supine position inside the container and confirmed to be a boy.

Upon removal from the concrete and the clothes, the body appeared to have normal development and had been well nourished. There was no evidence to suggest any significant ante-mortem trauma externally. Signs of post-mortem trauma were the collapse of the chest cavity and flattening of the nose tip (Figure 34.3).

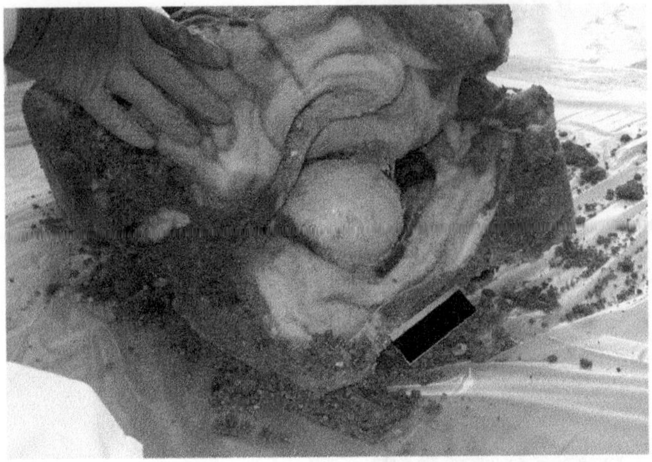

Figure 34.2 Image of the concrete block with fleece blanket and the infant's cranium being exposed (Source : Reprinted with permission of the Los Angeles County Department of Medical Examiner - Coroner).

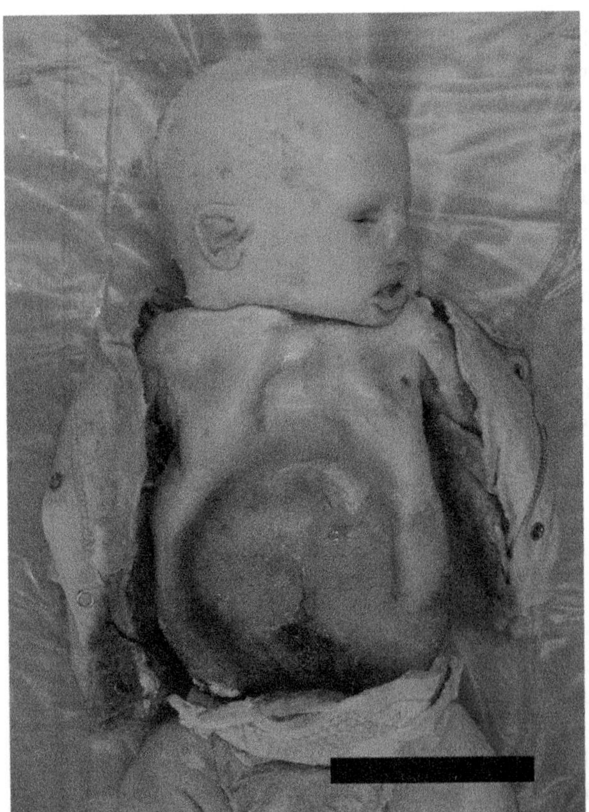

Figure 34.3 The baby was well preserved after about 11 months in concrete (Source : Reprinted with permission of the Los Angeles County Department of Medical Examiner – Coroner).

The skin, relatively intact and preserved, had a slight shade of yellow with mild white crusting on several lower portions of the body. The toes had a pink-orange tint, while the lower abdomen and genital region showed brown and black discolouration. The back, buttocks, posterior thighs and neck were a mild grey hue. There was a mark noted underneath the chin that was faintly brown. Also, the fingers were noticed to have a grey-black tint.

The skin that was exposed (i.e. not covered by the diaper or bodysuit) was firm to the touch. Some of the areas felt rubber-like and had a waxy texture. The portions that were covered by the diaper were soft and when pressed, remained fixed in indentation. The skin also looked as though it was waterlogged, though the body was not exposed to any outside fluids.

The hair of the head, eyebrows and eyelids was absent. Also absent were the toenails and the left thumbnail. The hands, found clenched, still had fingernails and the right thumbnail.

The infant's body, after the completion of an external examination, was issued a Y-shaped incision autopsy and cranial inspection.

34.4 Internal Examination

It was apparent by the softening and discolouration of the internal soft tissues, that the infant's body was moderate to severely decomposed. The organs in the neck and chest regions were well preserved compared to the counterparts in the abdomen. The tongue and oral cavity were well preserved and identifiable. The larynx and hyoid bone were intact with no fractures or signs of ante- or peri-mortem trauma. The oesophagus was identifiable through its course with normal features and colours.

The chest cavity had sunken in but it appeared that there were no true rib fractures. Both lungs were collapsed and grey in colour, but normally formed. The heart had also collapsed but did not appear to have signs of trauma. The aorta however, was unable to be identified below the diaphragm.

The liver was of a black-brown colour and the gallbladder appeared to be collapsed. Only a small portion of what possibly could have been splenic tissue was collected and appeared in normal condition. The kidneys and adrenal glands were dramatically different on each side. A portion of the right kidney and the entire gland were easily identifiable, while the left pair were unable to be documented due to the breakdown of tissues; the pancreas and stomach were also unidentifiable in the region. Overall, the left upper abdominal quadrant was soft, almost clay-like in composition and of grey-black colour. It was believed that this material was composed of the organs in that section that were unable to be examined.

The majority of the gastrointestinal tract was recognisable, including the small bowel and colon; the appendix however, was not seen. The bladder and prostate were identified and intact. Decomposition of the genitalia did not allow for the documentation of the testes and the lymph nodes in that region were also deteriorated.

When the scalp was opened, a large amount of yellow-grey liquid was released. The cranial sutures were not fused and connective tissue was absent. This caused partial collapse of the cranial bones at the crown and frontal portion, but no evidence of fractures. The *dura mater* at the crown had become a transparent, yellow gelatinous material, yet the lateral areas had *dura mater* of the usual opaque, white appearance; all of which was still intact with no damage.

Once further examined, the brain appeared with a normal convolutional pattern on the surface with a white-grey colour. However, at the point of removal, it became a liquid-like consistency and degenerated. The spinal cord, whilst identifiable, was not dissected or removed.

During the autopsy, samples of the liver, thymus and lungs were taken for examination under the microscope. Tissue from the liver and brain was collected for toxicology. Blood, bile, urine or stomach contents were unable to be obtained due to the stage of decomposition of the infant's body.

34.5 Discussion

Based on the statements given at the time of the arrest, the first period of the infant's encasement in concrete was spent located in an un-airconditioned and unventilated storage unit as indicated to the police by the father. This had an outer average temperature of 17°C over a time period of approximately eight months.

For the three following months, the concrete tub with baby was buried in the Angeles National Forest with an average temperature of 25°C, no precipitation and 14% mean humidity. The differences between these locations' data are due to seasonal and environmental (urban versus rural) changes, and an elevation difference of 402 m, with a distance of roughly 16 km (10 miles) between the locations.

The timescale indicated that the baby passed away about 11 months ago. However, the baby's outer appearance suggested a shorter post-mortem interval. This is often noticed in case studies with concrete (Chapter 33) and in the experimental literature (Gibelli, 2013; Phillips 2012).

The skin was firm to the touch in all areas except for the region that was covered by the diaper and skin slippage was not present. It is hypothesised that the concrete block and the blankets surrounding the body, created a microclimate that provided a mechanism for preservation. This was supported by an experiment carried out by Parham (2014), who investigated whether a barrier to concrete altered decomposition rates in porcine samples. Pig trotters covered with cotton cloth were buried in concrete for three months. After three months, the porcine samples were preserved superficially, with a waterlogged appearance of the skin that was soft to the touch. The inner portions of the trotters had begun to decompose and were in the earliest stages of putrefaction. While the results of Parham's experiment (2014) are similar to the characteristics that were observed in the infant, one has to keep in mind that experiments with pig trotters are not the same as an entire carcass with internal organs and its bacterial community, responsible for putrefaction. On the other hand, a new-born's gut does not contain many microorganisms yet, which leads to a reduced putrefaction (Janaway 1996).

Most of the moisture could have been absorbed and drawn away from the baby's body by the blankets and surrounding concrete. The diaper however, being tight around the waist, perhaps kept the moisture closer to that area and thus caused the change in consistency and colour of the skin.

Regarding the hair and nails, it is possible that the infant was born with a sparse amount of hair or had insufficient life to develop, whereas nails should have been existent on all digits given the normal and understood parameters of development. The only nails that had survived post-mortem were the nails of both hands except for the left thumb. The clenched fists possibly protected the nails from deterioration. Whether the loss of both hair and toenails was caused by the alkalinity of the concrete or the use of household cleaning products to cover the smell, was not determined. One of the most noticeable effects of the concrete on the baby's body was the collapsed chest cavity; not only identified externally by the concaved appearance, but also internally by the crumpled lungs and heart. The infant did not display signs of suffocation from co-sleeping or the possible strangulation that the father had suggested. If more concrete had been used on top of the deceased, additional damage may have been observed and perhaps altered the decomposition superficially and within the body.

The organs of the abdomen were severely decomposed. This is often noticed in concrete cases (e.g. Gibelli 2013) and due to the gut bacteria. While young babies do not have the same amount of gut microorganisms as observed in adults (Janaway 1996), clearly there were enough gut bacteria to initiate putrefaction.

34.6 Conclusion

While the infant had been deceased for nearly a year at the time of discovery, the body was still easily recognisable as an individual. The outer appearance did not show any ante- or peri-mortem trauma intentionally inflicted and was intact. As for the inner cavities, severe decomposition was seen in the lower portion of the torso, while the rest was well preserved. This could have been caused by a variety of factors, including the encasement in concrete. Had the baby been buried without concrete, it is possible that the remains would never have been found or only partially recovered.

The cause of death was determined by the medical examiner by means of the toxicology report that the baby had most likely died from the intake of methamphetamine, received through breast milk or by parental administration. Due to the parents' attempt to conceal the body, the mode of death was deemed homicide.

References

County of Los Angeles, Department of Medical Examiner – Coroner (2011) Autopsy Report (Case No. Redacted – John Doe). Los Angeles, California.

County of Los Angeles, Department of Medical Examiner – Coroner (2011) Case Notes (Case No. Redacted – John Doe). Los Angeles, California.

County of Los Angeles, Department of Medical Examiner – Coroner (2011) Investigator's Narrative (Case No. Redacted – John Doe). Los Angeles, California.

County of Los Angeles, Department of Medical Examiner – Coroner (2011) Laboratory Analysis Summary Report (Case No. Redacted – John Doe). Los Angeles, California.

County of Los Angeles, Department of Medical Examiner – Coroner (2011) Medical Report (Case No. Redacted – John Doe). Los Angeles, California.

County of Los Angeles, Department of Medical Examiner – Coroner (2011) Microscopic Report (Case No. Redacted – John Doe). Los Angeles, California.

Gibelli, D., Di Giancamillo, A., Taborelli, A., Porta, D., Andreola, S. *et al.* (2013) Burial of piglet carcasses in cement. *The American Journal of Forensic Medicine and Pathology*, **34**: 43–49.

Janaway, R.C. (1996) The decay of buried human remains and their associated materials. In: Hunter, J., Riverts, C. and Martin. A, (eds). *Studies in Crime: An introduction to forensic archaeology*. Routledge: London, pp. 58–85.

Parham, C. (2014) *Taphonomic Changes to Wrapped and Unwrapped Porcine Samples within Concrete*. MSc Dissertation, Cranfield University: Cranfield.

Phillips, G. (2012) *Decomposition Rates of Rats and Pigs when Concealed within Concrete: The 'Piggy Hoffa' experiments*. MSc Dissertation, University of Nebraska: Kearney.

Part V

Past, Present and Future Considerations

35

History and Development of the First Anthropology Research Facility, Knoxville, Tennessee

Giovanna M. Vidoli, Dawnie W. Steadman, Joanne B. Devlin and Lee Meadows Jantz

35.1 Introduction

The Anthropology Research Facility (ARF) at the University of Tennessee (UT), Knoxville, USA, is the first, and the most famous, human decomposition facility in the world. Although it is often referred to by its moniker 'The Body Farm', first coined by the author Patricia Cornwell in 1994, the nickname does not thoroughly capture the magnitude of research or the extensive training conducted at the ARF, nor does it convey the respectful treatment of the donors by the researchers and staff. The ARF is one of the many resources managed by the Forensic Anthropology Center (FAC), which also includes a vibrant Body Donation Program, the William M. Bass Donated Skeletal Collection, the McCormick Skeletal Collection, a Forensic Skeletal Collection and the William M. Bass Forensic Anthropology Building. The mission of the FAC is to lead research that advances the field of forensic anthropology, provide consulting services to law enforcement agencies, medical examiners and attorneys, and train students and professionals in the forensic sciences.

In this chapter, past and current research in human decomposition and taphonomy is highlighted, including its contribution to innovative studies between decomposition facilities, university departments and government agencies. This chapter begins with the history of the ARF and an overview of all the interlocking operations that are necessary for a functioning and successful human decomposition research facility. Additionally, the contributions of decomposition facilities to research and training, and to a growing body of knowledge regarding human decomposition, skeletal anatomy and grave detection, are discussed.

35.2 History of the ARF

In 1971, the Department of Anthropology at the UT hired Dr William M. Bass to lead the department. He became the primary forensic anthropology consultant to law enforcement and medical examiners throughout Tennessee and the southeast. Despite his extensive archaeological and anthropological experience and expertise, Bass soon became aware of how little was known about human decomposition and that limited our understanding of estimating the post-mortem interval (PMI). The case that notoriously ignited his determination to rectify the problem was that of Colonel William Shy, where Bass notably says 'I got the age, sex, race, height and weight right but I was off on the time of death by 113 years!' (Nashville Banner, 9 January 1978). He initially estimated that the individual had been

Taphonomy of Human Remains: Forensic Analysis of the Dead and the Depositional Environment, First Edition.
Edited by Eline M.J. Schotsmans, Nicholas Márquez-Grant and Shari L. Forbes.

deceased for 6 to 12 months before other evidence indicated that the deceased was embalmed during the Civil War (1861–1865). Bass recognised that PMI estimates could only improve by empirical study in a controlled environment.

In 1980, Bass approached the UT Administration and proposed a human decomposition research facility. He was granted a parcel of wooded and secluded land behind the UT Medical Center, approximately 6 km from the main University campus, and initiated the first systematic study of human decomposition in a natural outdoor laboratory. To obtain human subjects for his research, Bass began a formal body donation programme in 1981. Once decomposed and cleaned, the skeletons of each donor were accessioned into the William M. Bass Donated Skeletal Collection. To manage the growing resources, Bass established the FAC in 1987, as a research centre in the Department of Anthropology.

The initial ARF was approximately half an acre; however, early decomposition studies took place on a 4.9 m^2 (16 square feet) concrete pad completely surrounded by a chain link fence (Figure 35.1). At the time, the surrounding wooded area was isolated and therefore was not enclosed by a privacy fence, but soon after the decomposition studies were initiated, the Medical Center began expanding their parking lot towards the ARF boundaries. Due to this expansion, there was increased public awareness of the facility, and a group called Solutions to Issues of Concerned Knoxvillians (SICK) was established to protest against the human decomposition facility. The concerns and public protestations were short-lived once a privacy fence and a chain link fence topped with razor wire were erected around the ARF boundaries to prevent public curiosity and animal intrusions. Since then, about three decades later, there have been no other public outcries and the ARF has become a source of pride and recognition in the community.

Unfortunately, not all proposed decomposition facilities in the USA have enjoyed the same public support as the ARF. Recently, Carson-Newman University in Jefferson County, Tennessee (50 km from UT) had planned to establish a decomposition research facility but was met with objections, and eventually a lawsuit, from the surrounding community members who were concerned about contamination of their well-water and surrounding soils. While the City Council ultimately approved the facility, public opposition was strong. Efforts to establish the Carson-Newman research facility, which

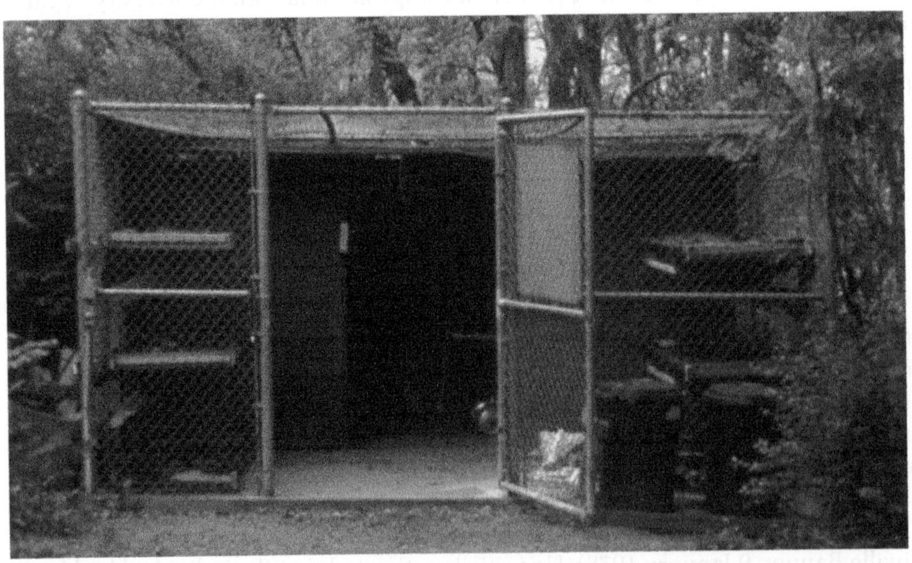

Figure 35.1 Image of the original ARF, a 4.9 m square concrete block surrounded by chain link fence.

Table 35.1 List of human decomposition facilities in the USA.

Decomposition Facility	Location	Year Founded[a)]	Size
ARF	Knoxville, TN	1980	Approx. 3 acres
Forensic Anthropology Research Facility	Texas State University San Marcos, TX	2008	26 acres
Southeast Texas Applied Forensic Science Facility	Sam Houston State University Huntsville, TX	2009	9 acres
Forensic Investigative Research Station	Colorado Mesa University, CO	2013	30 acres
Forensic Osteology Research Station	Western Carolina University Cullowhee, NC	2006	12×15 m^2
Complex for Forensic Anthropology Research	Southern Illinois University Carbondale, IL	2012	0.33 acre

a) First year human donors accepted for decomposition studies

would focus on the environmental effect of human and animal decomposition on soil, air and water, was indefinitely suspended in 2014. The research at Carson-Newman would have added greatly to a valuable body of literature that examines the effect of large-scale cattle decomposition on surrounding soils, leachate and ground water (Hawkins *et al.* 2012; Schwartz *et al.* 2013; Yuan *et al.* 2013) and previous research examining the effect of human and pig decomposition on the soil environment (Damann 2010; Damann *et al.* 2012; Schwartz *et al.* 2013; Van Belle *et al.* 2009).

By the late 1980s, Bass realised that the small space limited to a concrete pad would not suffice for decomposition studies, as it lacked the realism of the body–ground interface. Bass was granted an additional 2 to 3 acres from the UT Medical Center and the additional land expanded the potential for greater research opportunities. Throughout the 1990s, this area was sufficient to support a growing academic programme and the number of annual body donations to the FAC. In 1999, the FAC began a partnership with the Federal Bureau of Investigation (FBI) to deliver annual training to agents. The week-long training focuses on decomposition processes and the systematic recovery of scattered and buried human remains. Additionally, in 2001, the FAC began a relationship with the Law Enforcement Innovation Center (LEIC) to provide a week-long course in surface recoveries and burial excavations for the National Forensic Academy. These commitments, as well as expanded research agendas and increasing numbers of body donations, necessitated more space. In 2004, the ARF had expanded to approximately 1.5 acres and in 2013, the ARF expanded again to its present size of just over 2 acres.

While the ARF is not physically the largest decomposition facility in the USA (Table 35.1), it continues to be a leader in research into PMI studies and actualistic training programmes. Ironically, when Dr Bass founded the ARF, he expected the research to be a finite endeavour, though it is now clear that the resources provided by the ARF and other facilities create limitless opportunities for novel research. Furthermore, with additional decomposition facilities across the USA, and the potential in other countries, collaborative and comparative research is expanding our understanding of decomposition in different environments.

35.3 Daily Operations of the FAC

The Body Donation Program is the heart and soul of the FAC and is the basis for all research and training conducted at the research centre. The Body Donation Program began in 1981, and was initially promoted by the Tennessee State Medical Examiner, Dr Jerry Francisco. In that first year, the programme received four donated bodies and one the following year. Figure 35.2 demonstrates the trend in body donations since its inception in 1981. Though the number of donations grew steadily during its second decade, a dramatic increase occurred in the early 2000s. This is likely due to the increase of forensic television shows that included storylines about 'the Body Farm' and decomposition in general. Due to this extremely high interest in the FAC, it is no longer possible to accommodate all interested donors and, in 2012, the FAC began to record the number of individuals who were declined (Figure 35.2). Over the last few years, the number of body donations that are not accepted is nearly twice the number that is accepted. Potential donors are now declined if the Anthropology Research Facility is at capacity, if the individual has certain communicable diseases, including HIV, hepatitis, tuberculosis or Methicillin-resistant *Staphylococcus aureus* (MRSA), or if the individual is unidentified. In the beginning of the programme, unidentified remains from the medical examiner's office were accepted at the ARF for research. However, that policy has since changed and only identified remains donated by the individual, or their family (legal next of kin), are accepted.

The FAC currently has over 4,000 pre-registered individuals who have arranged to donate their body to the FAC. As part of the donation process, individuals complete a questionnaire that gathers information on their medical and personal histories including age, sex, ancestry, stature, weight, medical histories, residence histories, occupations and parity. With this life history documentation, the research potential of the Body Donation Program is unparalleled in forensic science, and also serves

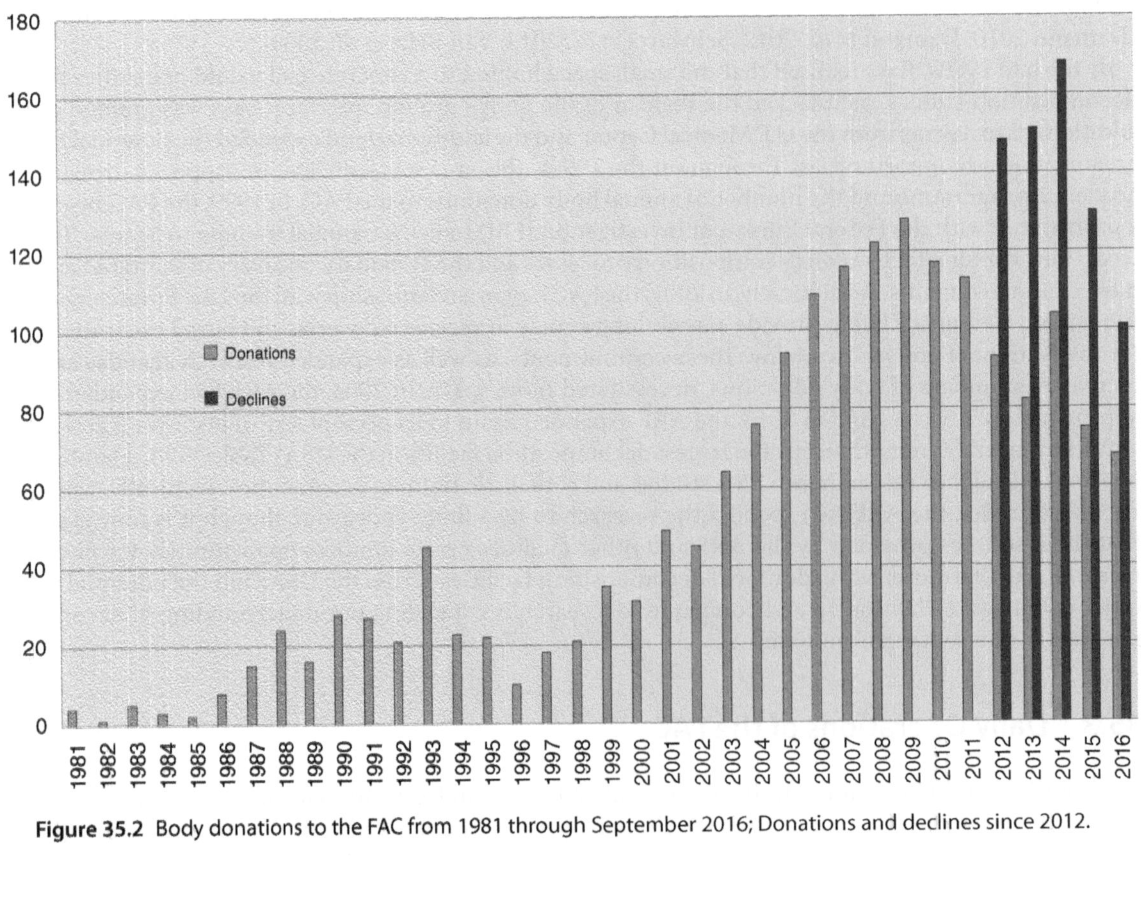

Figure 35.2 Body donations to the FAC from 1981 through September 2016; Donations and declines since 2012.

research partners in clinical medicine, biomechanics, physics, biology, chemistry, serology, immunology and genetics. In addition to research on donated bodies, a large subset of FAC pre-donors have agreed to participate in research involving living human subjects, including written surveys, genetics, biometrics and medical research.

At the time of death, the donor is either transported to the FAC with arrangements made by the family or, if the individual is within a 160 km radius (100 miles), they are transported by FAC staff. Upon arrival at the FAC, a process called 'Intake' is conducted, which includes collection of biological samples, including blood, fingernails and hair. Additional data collected during Intake include cadaver stature and weight, full body and facial (direct and lateral) photographs, presence and location of scars and tattoos, and whether the individual was an organ donor or autopsied. Additionally, mesh bags are placed around the hands and feet to protect the loss of small bones during the decomposition process. Though personal anonymity is maintained, these data and information are available to researchers and can be used in conjunction with ante-mortem data, decomposition data and skeletal data.

Once Intake is complete, the donor is placed at the ARF, for research and training during decomposition. If the donor is not part of an active research project, they are placed prone and covered with a black plastic sheet. The objective of placing them in this manner is to minimise loss of teeth and smaller bones and to quicken the decomposition process as insects, particularly maggots, are more active when protected from direct sunlight and other elements. Unless the donor is utilised for research, the objective of accelerating decomposition is to allow skeletal recovery and placement of another donor. Donors not placed on the surface are placed in shallow graves for research and training in burial excavation techniques.

In 2011, the FAC established a daily decomposition photo database. This database contains daily photographs of each donor placed at the Facility until decomposition ceases. These photographs are also available for research and include the date and ambient temperature at time of photograph. Once the donor has decomposed and is skeletonised, the remains are recovered from the ARF as part of training for law enforcement, young professionals or UT undergraduates. The skeletal remains are recovered using archaeological methods and this training allows participants to practice appropriate methods for documenting and mapping the position of the skeletal remains.

After the skeletal remains are recovered, they are brought to the Bass Forensic Anthropology Building where undergraduate volunteers clean the remains. Once they are cleaned, the skeletons are accessioned into the William M. Bass Donated Skeletal Collection. The accessioning process consists of inventorying, labelling, measuring and packaging the human skeletal remains. The Bass Collection consists predominantly of older white males but donations of females and individuals of other self-reported racial groups are increasing. Additionally, the Bass Collection includes unpulverised cremated remains and foetal remains. The cremated remains are often from donors who have a disease preventing normal body donation, while the foetal remains are family donations. As of publication, there are 40 foetal skeletons and 67 cremations. The long-term availability of donor skeletons and cremated remains is one of the major differences between the Body Donation Program and other scientific body donation programmes, such as medical schools, where the bodies are utilised for only a few months or years. There are currently over 1,700 skeletons available for onsite research and teaching, making it the largest documented skeletal collection of contemporary Americans. Space for the Bass Donated Skeletal Collection is becoming more limited as the collection continues to grow and research interest increases. The Bass Collection grows at a rate of about 100 donations a year and spatial availability for long-term curation and research is an important consideration for decomposition research facilities that maintain skeletal collections. Each December, the FAC senior staff estimate the number of donations required to meet the anticipated training and research needs for the following year. This strategy has been effective for maintaining the number of donations that meet FAC research and training needs, yet do not overwhelm spatial constraints.

The Bass Collection contributes to a wide variety of research topics in biological anthropology. In addition to methodological studies designed to create and validate new methods of skeletal identification, the Bass Collection is a crucial component of ongoing research, examining secular change in craniofacial morphology and long bone length that has greatly expanded understanding of biological responses to environmental change (Jantz 2001; Jantz and Jantz 1999; Jantz and Meadows Jantz 2000; Wescott and Jantz 2005). The Bass Collection is also utilised for the development of new orthopaedic devices and a variety of health studies that shed light on contemporary diseases, such as diabetes, obesity, chronic heart disease and cancer. Several large-scale studies have focused on the effects of diabetes and obesity on the skeleton and discovering skeletal markers of these diseases for the purposes of identification (May 2014; Moore 2008; Moore and Schaefer 2011). These studies include the use of CT scans, X-rays, DEXA scans, micro-CT, isotopes, genetics, protein assays and bone histology. Additionally, as skeletal collections with different demographics at other decomposition facilities grow, the possibilities for comparative research will increase, further strengthening identification methods in forensic anthropology.

35.4 Research at the ARF

Since its inception, the ARF has led research on human decomposition. The initial studies focused on the variables that affect decomposition and burial location (i.e. Bass 1984; Mann *et al.* 1990; Rodriguez 1982; Rodriguez and Bass 1983, 1985; Vass 1991; Vass *et al.* 1992; Watkins 1983). These studies increased understanding of the complexity and unpredictability of decomposition and the many variables that affect calculating the PMI (Vass 2011). Later studies, many conducted as Master's theses, examined the effect of water (O'Brien 1994; O'Brien and Kuehner 2007), clothing (Cahoon 1992; Miller RA 2002), sun and shade areas (Srnka 2003), fabric and plastic body coverings (Dautartas 2009) and indoor versus outdoor locations (Ritchie 2005; Tomlinson 2003) on rates of decomposition. These studies added greatly to the understanding of the factors that affect human decomposition and the difficulty in estimating an accurate PMI. Additionally, they paved the way for projects that examined by-products of decomposition, including decay odour (Love 2001; Vass *et al.* 2004), post-mortem tooth loss (McKeown and Bennett 1995), and the effect of decomposition on soil ecology (Damann 2010; Damann *et al.* 2012). Additionally, there are hourly and daily climatic data for the ARF from the Biosystems Engineering and Soil Science Department at the UT, allowing integration of environmental data into research questions. The Biosystems Engineering and Soil Science Department collects climate data throughout various locations in Tennessee, including just north of the ARF on the west side of the main UT-Knoxville campus. According to their data, which is accessible from the Biosystems Engineering and Soil Science Department website, the average daily high temperatures from 2012 to 2014 were 23.8°C, daily lows were 11.1°C, relative humidity was 67.7% and average annual rainfall was 90.3 cm. These data are consistent with those reported by Damann (2010) between 2003 and 2007.

Although the ARF is geographically small, decomposition processes are not homogenous throughout the facility and mummification and adipocere formation varies across the ARF landscape. These decomposition patterns may be a result of raccoon scavenging (Jeong *et al.* 2014) or the effect of decomposition by-products on the soil environment. Damann tested the soils inside and outside of the ARF for moisture and organic content, soil pH, total nitrogen and carbon content and lipid-bound phosphorous, to examine how the soil had been affected by 30 years of decomposition at the ARF (Damann 2010; Damann *et al.* 2012). Overall, he found increased soil pH and increased levels of total nitrogen, soil-extractable phosphorous and soil moisture content within the ARF (consistent with high-quality nutrients) compared with a control area outside of the ARF. As a result of this information, the FAC now regularly tests local soils before placement of donors for research projects.

Researchers at Southeast Texas Applied Forensic Science Facility (STAFS) at Sam Houston University also compared the soil chemistry below and around decomposing human bodies to control samples, in order to map the spatial extent of the cadaver decomposition islands (Aitkenhead-Peterson *et al.* 2012). They found significant downslope movement of grave soil chemistry, although this study needs to be replicated with a larger sample size. Although soil samples at the ARF were not taken decades ago, with the onset of research, areas throughout the ARF will continue to be tested to record how the soil environment continues to change, and if there is any relationship between soil ecology and decomposition. A forthcoming project will further examine the factors affecting decomposition trends across the ARF.

The early studies highlighted the need for human decomposition facilities in different environments and the need to replicate decomposition studies in discrete ecosystems. The Forensic Anthropology Research Facility (FARF) at Texas State University, San Marcos, has examined the regional factors that affect decomposition in central Texas (Parks 2011; Sears 2013; Suckling 2011; Wescott *et al.* 2013), including the effect of clothing (Phalen 2013) and autopsy (Bates 2014) on decomposition in Texas. Additionally, while rodent scavenging is common at the ARF (Jeong *et al.* 2014; Klippel and Synstelein 2007), studies at Texas State and Sam Houston have shown different scavenging patterns, including vultures (Reeves 2009; Spradley *et al.* 2012) and bobcat (Rippley *et al.* 2012), as well as the effect of the red fire ant on fly activity and, therefore, PMI estimation (Lindgren *et al.* 2011). Additional studies at the facilities in Colorado and Illinois will hopefully expand our understanding of decomposition in more arid environments than Tennessee or Texas.

Although other institutions, mostly outside the USA where human decomposition facilities have yet to be established, are utilising non-human models to examine decomposition in different environments (Adlam and Simmons 2007; Bachmann and Simmons 2010; Komar and Beattie 1998; Simmons *et al.* 2010a, 2010b; Wilson *et al.* 2007) as proxies for human decomposition, systematic testing of the decomposition differences and similarities between humans and non-humans has never been done. A National Institute of Justice (NIJ)-sponsored research project at the ARF is the first to critically and quantitatively evaluate the validity of using non-human animals as proxies for humans in decomposition research (Dautartas *et al.* 2015). Three trials of human, pig and rabbit subjects will assess similarities and differences in decomposition patterns and rates, insect behaviour and scavenger behaviour. Additionally, soil samples will be taken to test differences in microbial patterns among the three species. The results from this study will provide guidelines for when and how pigs and other non-human animals can be utilised as a proxy for human decomposition in forensic contexts.

While the first studies focused on macroscopic changes of decomposition and added greatly in our understanding of decomposition, recent studies are incorporating new technology and microscopic techniques. Current research partners for such endeavours are at Oak Ridge National Laboratories (ORNL), the UT Space Institute and a number of agencies under the Department of Defense. One example is a mass grave project that will determine which remote sensing technologies are effective in detecting mass graves of varying size over time (Corcoran and Mundorff 2014; Corcoran and White 2013). Four mass graves containing one, three and six individuals and one control grave were placed to test a variety of remote sensing technologies over a three-year period. The purpose is to assess how long certain remote sensing technologies, such as LiDAR and thermal sensing, are useful in detecting mass graves. While earlier studies at the ARF using ground penetrating radar have provided information on its utility to detect burials throughout the decomposition process (Miller, M.L. 2002; Miller *et al.* 2002), new technological advances in remote sensing allow more distant (aerial) and more sensitive data to locate graves. This current work has resulted in a research and development agreement with the USA federal government that allows the FAC to participate with federal laboratories to test sensitive equipment. For additional testing, the government requested a second grave with 25 human subjects to be placed at the ARF. Several research projects are also being conducted on these mass grave projects, including research on plant and soil isotopes, DNA contamination within the grave and soil microbes within and around the mass graves over time. The FAC will organise an international field school at the end of each project to provide anthropologists and human rights workers from conflict and post-conflict countries with training on mass grave excavation techniques.

The FAC works with a number of laboratories and private companies to develop and test other new types of technologies. For instance, the FAC is working with ORNL and their product development partners to test classified and commercially available iris and fingerprint scanners. The purpose is not only to analyse the sensitivity and accuracy of the scanners, but also to determine the post-mortem duration in which the scanners can provide accurate information. This has immediate field implications for military personnel in identifying fallen US personnel and adversaries.

Current research at the FARF and the STAFS is examining the changing bacterial community structures and soil chemistry during decomposition to aid in PMI estimation (Benbow *et al.* 2014; Lynne *et al.* 2014; Singh *et al.* 2014). These projects will allow researchers to test soils to determine if decomposition has occurred there, even if the body is no longer present, as well as the use of soil microbes to quantitatively assess the PMI. The FAC also works with researchers in the UT Department of Biosystems Engineering and Soil Science to examine the relationships within soil microbial communities when human bodies decompose, as well as how soil isotopic values change during decomposition (Cobaugh 2013). Additionally, a current project at the ARF is examining the persistence of DNA in the soil under a decomposing body (Emmons 2014). These projects highlight the growth and expansion of human decomposition research beyond gross macroscopic changes, in order to further understand how the whole environment, from soil ecology to microbes, is affected by and affects decomposition.

Interest in human decomposition has also expanded into the realm of cultural anthropology, with studies that examine attitudes of individuals who work at the ARF towards death (Compton 2012) and why people donate their bodies to the human decomposition facilities (Martinez 2013). These studies demonstrate that human decomposition facilities can contribute to all aspects of anthropology and can foster open dialogues about the ethics and policies surrounding body donation and human decomposition facilities.

The FAC resources are available to UT faculty and students as well as external researchers upon request. The FAC has established a formal review process of research requests. Researchers send their requests to the FAC Director who then forms a review panel comprised of FAC staff and the appropriate anthropology faculty. Research requests are evaluated based on scientific merit, efforts to minimise the loss of bone tissue and whether the FAC can reasonably facilitate the research. Research requests allow tracking of current research, provide transparency in the selection process and offer feedback to researchers. The research request forms and a list of current publications and presentations using FAC resources can be found on the FAC website.

35.5 Training Opportunities at the ARF

In addition to research, the ARF has offered many opportunities for training and continues to broaden its sphere of influence through its training programmes. Daily operations of a decomposition facility, body donation programme and skeletal collection require tremendous planning, foresight and organisation. The FAC staff must track research, plan for future research, manage ante- and post-mortem databases, curate multiple skeletal collections, manage volunteers and interns and deliver training and outreach services. These operations would not be possible without the aid of graduate assistants, undergraduate volunteers and interns, allowing a mutually beneficial relationship between the FAC and students. The FAC engages well over 70 undergraduate students each semester in the archaeological recovery of remains from ARF and the processing of those skeletal remains. Students receive valuable crime scene training at the ARF, including mapping and photo documentation of skeletal remains. The process of skeletal recoveries and cleaning and labelling skeletal remains provides undergraduates with training in crime scene processing, maceration techniques and laboratory practices. The graduate students receive unique training in working with a body donation programme and mentoring undergraduate students in field recoveries, in addition to countless research opportunities at the ARF and Bass Collection. Training at the FAC includes younger individuals and in 2014, the FAC began an after-school internship programme for local high school students to introduce them to forensic anthropology and research methods in the forensic sciences. Their internship culminates in a presentation of their research project to their parents, teachers and local community members.

Additionally, since 2006, short courses at the ARF have brought students and professionals from around the world to UT to be trained in grave identification, burial excavation, surface recovery and documentation processes. The FAC currently offers approximately ten short courses a year that target law enforcement and research communities. Additionally, agency-specific short courses can be provided to school groups and law enforcement agencies. Short courses are typically three to five days long and the staff consist of experts from UT and around the world. The field-based courses stress the complexities of excavations and recoveries, allowing law enforcement to gain appreciation for what forensic anthropologists can add to crime scene investigation. As a result, these courses also function to guide law enforcement on whom to call when faced with skeletal remains. The ARF and other human decomposition facilities are unique in that burial excavation and field recovery courses allow classroom lectures to also have a field component, where different stages of decomposition, the effect of scavenging on remains, differential decomposition in burials from the same depositional events and features of recent and older clandestine graves can all be demonstrated. Laboratory-based short courses focus on osteology, methods in biological profile, pathology and trauma and advanced subjects such as histology, commingling and taphonomy. The Bass Collection offers extensive examples of pathologies, surgical interventions, taphonomic changes and human variation to provide the course participants with many illustrations of skeletal response to intrinsic and extrinsic factors.

The short courses, and volunteer and internship opportunities at the ARF and the FAC allow the continual training and education of future forensic anthropologists, crime scene investigators, medical examiners and other professionals who work with human remains. Additionally, these training opportunities serve as valuable examples of the importance of human decomposition facilities for outreach and education.

35.6 Conclusion

The ARF has been instrumental in decomposition studies over the past 35 years and has made a tremendous impact on forensic investigations. Not only did the ARF undertake and generate the first systematic research into post-mortem changes, but it also inspired the establishment of other decomposition facilities. Its influence is also tangible in investigations, as outcomes of work completed at the ARF often impact casework conducted on behalf of the medicolegal community. While no one case has ultimately been solved solely because of research conducted at the facility, numerous cases have been influenced by what the facility has contributed to our understanding of the PMI. Research in human decomposition continues to grow in fields outside of anthropology, providing a more holistic understanding of human decomposition and its effect on the micro-environment and PMI estimation. Additionally, the expansion of human decomposition research to cultural anthropology demonstrates a growing interest in the decisions surrounding body donation, and shows promise for additional discourses about attitudes towards death and body donation.

While the ARF, the Bass Skeletal Collection and the FAC would not have been possible without the body donation programme and the donors, daily operations would not be possible without the aid of graduate assistants, undergraduate volunteers and interns. The future of human decomposition facilities is bright as forensic anthropologists continue to reach beyond disciplinary boundaries and collaborate with scientists in other scientific fields, to further discover and quantify variables affecting human decay and the PMI.

References

Adlam, R.E. and Simmons, T. (2007) The effect of repeated physical disturbance on soft tissue decomposition – are taphonomic studies an accurate reflection of decomposition? *Journal of Forensic Sciences*, **52**: 1007–1014.

Aitkenhead-Peterson, J., Owings, C., Alexander, M., Larison, N. and Bytheway, J.A. (2012) Mapping the lateral extent of human cadaver decomposition with soil chemistry. *Forensic Science International*, **216**: 127–134.

Bachmann, J. and Simmons, T. (2010) The influence of preburial insect access on the decomposition rate. *Journal of Forensic Sciences*, **55**: 893–900.

Bass, W.M. (1984) Time interval since death: a difficult decision. In: Rathbun, T.A. and Buikstra, J.E. (eds), *Human Identification: Case studies in forensic anthropology*. Charles C. Thomas: Springfield, pp. 136–147.

Bates, L. (2014) *Comparison of Decomposition Rates between Autopsied and Non-Autopsied Human Remains in Central Texas.* MA thesis, Texas State University: San Marcos, TX.

Benbow, M.E., Pechal, J., Singh, B., Tomberlin, J.K., Tarone, A.M. *et al.* (2014) *Initial Assessment of the Structure and Function of the Postmortem Human Microbiome: Forensic applications.* Paper presented at the American Academy of Forensic Sciences, Seattle, WA.

Cahoon, S. (1992) *Effects of Clothing on Human Decomposition and Deterioration of Associated Yarns.* MA thesis, University of Tennessee: Knoxville, TN.

Cobaugh, K.L. (2013) *Soil Microbial Community Succession during Cadaver Decomposition.* MS thesis, University of Tennessee: Knoxville, TN.

Compton, K. (2012) *(Re)conceptualizing Death: Examining attitudes toward death at the Anthropological Research Facility.* MA thesis, University of Tennessee: Knoxville, TN.

Corcoran, K. and Mundorff, A. (2014) *A Multidisciplinary Data Fusion Based Approach to Remote Human Grave Detection.* Paper presented at the American Academy of Forensic Sciences, Seattle, WA.

Corcoran, K. and White, D. (2013) *Fusion of Remotely Sensed Data for Human Grave Detection.* Paper presented at the CaGIS/ASPRS Specialty Conference on Imaging and Mapping for Disaster Management.

Damann, F.E. (2010) *Human Decomposition Ecology at the University of Tennessee Anthropology Research Facility.* PhD thesis, University of Tennessee: Knoxville, TN.

Damann, F.E., Tanittaisong, A. and Carter, D.O. (2012) Potential carcass enrichment of the University of Tennessee Anthropology Research Facility: a baseline survey of edaphic features. *Forensic Science International*, **222**: 4–10.

Dautartas, A.M. (2009) *The Effect of Various Coverings on the Rate of Human Decomposition.* MA thesis, University of Tennessee: Knoxville, TN.

Dautartas, A.M., Meadows Jantz, L., Vidoli, G.M. and Steadman, D.W. (2015) *A Multidisciplinary Validation Study of Non-Human Animal Models for Forensic Decomposition Research: A time series approach.* Paper presented at the American Academy of Forensic Sciences, Orlando, FL.

Emmons, A. (2014) *The Preservation and Persistence of Human DNA in Soil during Cadaver Decomposition.* MA thesis, University of Tennessee: Knoxville, TN.

Hawkins, S., Menn, F., Cobaugh, K. and DeBruyn, J. (2012) *Leachate Analysis from an Organic Burial Pit Containing Euthanized Large Animals.* Paper presented at the ASA, CSSA and SSSA International Annual Meeting, Cincinnati, OH.

Jantz, L.M. and Jantz, R.L. (1999) Secular change in long bone length and proportion in the United States, 1800–1970. *American Journal of Physical Anthropology*, **110**: 57–67.

Jantz, R.L. (2001) Cranial change in Americans: 1850–1975. *Journal of Forensic Sciences*, **46**: 784–787.

Jantz. R.L. and Meadows Jantz, L. (2000) Secular change in craniofacial morphology. *American Journal of Human Biology*, **12**: 327–338.

Jeong, Y., Synstelien, J.A., Smith, J. and Jantz, L.M. (2014) *Raccoon Scavenging at the Anthropological Research Facility at the University of Tennessee.* Paper presented at the American Academy of Forensic Sciences, Seattle, WA.

Klippel, W.E. and Synstelien, J.A. (2007) Rodents as taphonomic agents: bone gnawing by brown rats and gray squirrels. *Journal of Forensic Sciences*, **52**: 765–773.

Komar, D. and Beattie, O. (1998) Postmortem insect activity may mimic perimortem sexual assault clothing patterns. *Journal of Forensic Sciences*, **43**: 792–796.

Lindgren, N.K., Bucheli, S.R., Archambeault, A.D. and Bytheway, J.A. (2011) Exclusion of forensically important flies due to burying behavior by the red imported fire ant (*Solenopsis invicta*) in southeast Texas. *Forensic Science International*, **204**: E1–E3.

Love, J.C. (2001) *Evaluation of Decay Odor as a Time Since Death Indicator.* PhD thesis, University of Tennessee: Knoxville, TN.

Lynne, A., Haarmann, D., Hyde, E.R., Petrosino, J.F., Zhang, X. *et al.* (2014) *The Living Dead: An investigation into the internal microbiome of human decomposition.* Paper presented at the American Academy of Forensic Sciences, Seattle, WA.

Mann, R.W., Bass, W.M. and Meadows, L. (1990) Time since death and decomposition of the human body: variables and observations in case and experimental field studies. *Journal of Forensic Sciences*, **35**: 103–111.

Martinez, H.M. (2013) *I Don't Need It, You Can Have It: Motivations for whole body donation.* MA thesis, Texas State University: San Marcos, TX.

May, S.E. (2014) *An Investigation of Diabetes Mellitus in Postmortem Human Remains.* PhD thesis, University of Tennessee: Knoxville, TN.

McKeown, A.H. and Bennett, J.L. (1995) A preliminary investigation of postmortem tooth loss. *Journal of Forensic Sciences*, **40**: 755–757.

Miller, M.L. (2002) *Coupling Ground Penetrating Radar Applications with Continually Changing Decomposing Human Targets: An effort to enhance search strategies of buried human remains.* MA thesis, University of Tennessee: Knoxville, TN.

Miller, M.L., Freeland, R.S. and Koppenjan, S. (2002) *Searching for Concealed Human Remains using GPR Imaging of Decomposition.* Paper presented at the 9th International Conference on Ground Penetrating Radar, Santa Barbara, CA.

Miller, R.A. (2002) *The Affects of Clothing on Human Decomposition: Implications for estimating Time Since Death.* MA thesis, University of Tennessee: Knoxville, TN.

Moore, M.K. (2008) *Body Mass Estimation from the Human Skeleton.* PhD thesis, University of Tennessee: Knoxville, TN.

Moore, M.K. and Schaefer, E. (2011) A comprehensive regression tree to estimate body weight from the skeleton. *Journal of Forensic Sciences*, **56**: 1115–1122.

O'Brien, T.G. (1994) *Human Soft-tissue Decomposition in an Aquatic Environment and its Transformation into Adipocere.* MA thesis, University of Tennesse: Knoxville, TN.

O'Brien, T.G. and Kuehner, A.C. (2007) Waxing grave about adipocere: soft tissue change in an aquatic context. *Journal of Forensic Sciences*, **52**: 294–301.

Parks, C.L. (2011) A study of the human decomposition sequence in Central Texas. *Journal of Forensic Sciences*, **56**: 19–22.

Phalen, K. (2013) *The Effects of Clothing on Human Decomposition.* MA thesis, Texas State University, San Marcos, TX.

Reeves, N.M. (2009) Taphonomic effects of vulture scavenging. *Journal of Forensic Sciences*, **54**: 523–528.

Rippley, A., Larison, N.C., Moss, K.E., Kelly, J.D. and Bytheway, J.A. (2012) Scavenging behavior of *Lynx rufus* on human remains during the winter months of Southeast Texas. *Journal of Forensic Sciences*, **57**: 699–705.

Ritchie, G.T. (2005) *A Comparison of Human Decomposition in an Indoor and an Outdoor Environment.* MA thesis, University of Tennessee, Knoxville, TN.

Rodriguez, W.C. (1982) *Insect Activity and its Relationship to Decay Rates of Human Cadavers in East Tennessee.* PhD thesis, University of Tennessee, Knoxville, TN.

Rodriguez, W.C. and Bass, W.M. (1983) Insect activity and its relationship to decay-rates of human cadavers in East Tennessee. *Journal of Forensic Sciences*, **28**: 423–432.

Rodriguez, W.C. and Bass, W.M. (1985) Decomposition of buried bodies and methods that may aid in their location. *Journal of Forensic Sciences*, **30**: 836–852.

Schwarz, M., Bonhotal, J., Bischoff, K. and Ebel, Jr., J. (2013) Fate of barbiturates and non-steroidal anti-inflammatory drugs during carcass composting. *Trends in Animal and Veterinary Sciences Journal*, **4**: 1–12.

Sears, A.M. (2013) *Decomposition in Central Texas and Validity of a Universal Postmortem Interval Formula.* MA thesis, Texas State University, San Marcos, TX.

Simmons, T., Adlam, R.E. and Moffatt, C. (2010a) Debugging decomposition data-comparative taphonomic studies and the influence of insects and carcass size on decomposition rate. *Journal of Forensic Sciences*, **55**: 8–13.

Simmons, T., Cross, P.A., Adlam, R.E. and Moffatt, C. (2010b) The influence of insects on decomposition rate in buried and surface remains. *Journal of Forensic Sciences*, **55**: 889–892.

Singh, B., Crippen, T.L., Tarone, A.M., Pechal, J., Benbow, M.E. *et al.* (2014) *Utility of Bacteria Associated with Human Cadavers in Estimation of Postmortem Interval (PMI).* Paper presented at the American Academy of Forensic Sciences, Seattle, WA.

Spradley, M.K., Hamilton, M.D. and Giordano, A. (2012) Spatial patterning of vulture scavenged human remains. *Forensic Science International*, **219**: 57–63.

Srnka, C.F. (2003) *The Effects of Sun and Shade on the Early Stages of Human Decomposition.* MA thesis, University of Tennessee, Knoxville, TN.

Suckling, J.K. (2011) *A Longitudinal Study on the Outdoor Human Decomposition Sequence in Central Texas.* MA thesis, Texas State University, San Marcos, TX.

Tomlinson, K.D. (2003) *Death as a Process: Human decomposition in an insect-restricted environment.* MA thesis, University of Tennessee, Knoxville, TN.

Van Belle, L.E., Carter, D.O. and Forbes, S.L. (2009) Measurement of ninhydrin reactive nitrogen influx into gravesoil during above-ground and below-ground carcass (*Sus domesticus*) decomposition. *Forensic Science International*, **193**: 37–41.

Vass, A.A. (1991) *Time Since Death Determinations of Human Cadavers utilizing Soil Solution.* PhD thesis, University of Tennessee, Knoxville, TN.

Vass, A.A. (2011) The elusive universal post-mortem interval formula. *Forensic Science International*, **204**: 34–40.

Vass, A.A., Bass, M., Wolt, J.D., Foss, J.E. and Ammons, J.T. (1992) Time since death determinations of human cadavers using soil solution. *Journal of Forensic Sciences*, **37**: 1236–1253.

Vass, A.A., Smith, R.R., Thompson, C.V., Burnett, M.N., Wolf, D.A. *et al.* (2004) Decompositional odor analysis database. *Journal of Forensic Sciences*, **49**: 760–769.

Watkins, L.L. (1983) *Late Postmortem Changes in Three Human Bodies in Knox County, Tennessee.* MA thesis, University of Tennessee, Knoxville, TN.

Wescott, D. and Jantz, R.J. (2005) Assessing craniofacial secular change in american blacks and whites using geometric morphometry. In: Slice, D.E. (ed.), *Modern Morphometrics in Physical Anthropology.* Kluwer Academic/Plenum Publishers: New York, pp. 231–245.

Wescott, D.J., Hamilton, M.D., Spradley, M.K., Mavroudas, S., Sears, A.M. *et al.* (2013) *Regional Factors in Central Texas affecting Postmortem Decomposition.* Paper presented at the American Academy of Forensic Sciences, Washington, DC.

Wilson, A.S., Janaway, R.C., Holland, A.D., Dodson, J.I., Baran, E. *et al.* (2007) Modelling the buried human body environment in upland climes using three contrasting field sites. *Forensic Science International*, **169**: 6–18.

Yuan, Q., Snow, D.D. and Bartelt-Hunt, S.L. (2013) Potential water quality impacts originating from land burial of cattle carcasses. *Science of the Total Environment*, **456**: 246–253.

36

Crime Scene Investigation, Archaeology and Taphonomy: Reconstructing Activities at Crime Scenes

W.J. Mike Groen and Charles E.H. Berger

36.1 Introduction

Archaeologists make use of analytical reasoning when reconstructing the past from excavated material finds and features, or the material record. They aim to reason backwards, from the observed material record in the present to the human activities that caused it in the past. This perception of physical evidence as a proxy for past (human) activity is not unique for archaeology; it is also encountered in forensic science, for example during the investigation of a crime scene[1] (i.e. the Crime Scene Investigation practice, or CSI practice). This similarity between archaeology and CSI practice has also been noted in scene of crime textbooks (Gardner 2012; Gardner and Bevel 2009; Houck and Siegel 2010; Houck *et al.* 2012). However, archaeology and CSI practice apply dissimilar lines of reasoning when analysing and interpreting past (human) activity. For example, in archaeology, the interpretation of the archaeological record starts before the actual excavation and is supported by a theoretical framework and background knowledge. Archaeological research methodologies are research question driven and integrate GIS[2] and database features with archaeological field procedures. Scenes of crime officers (SOCOs) traditionally focus on collecting physical evidence from crime scenes as completely and systematically as they can (the investigative phase), trusting that the issues of analysis and interpretation regarding the crime, or events leading to the deposition of a body, can be postponed until the results from the forensic laboratory arrive (the evaluative phase).[3] Each CSI is perceived as a unique and isolated event that is often performed under time pressure; the physical (trace) evidence is in danger of degrading or disappearing altogether and the culprit must be found before more crimes are committed. The SOCOs' decisions on what physical evidence should be collected are generally

1 For the sake of simplicity, the term 'crime scene' is used in this chapter to refer to any scene upon which crime scene investigation (CSI) is performed.

2 GIS (Geographic Information System) is a tool specially developed to integrate, analyse and display different types of spatial information, including databases, within one analytical framework, and is therefore perfectly suited to identify, analyse and predict (quantitatively and qualitatively) the spatial distribution of physical evidence.

3 During the investigative phase, the SOCOs (and some forensic scientists) collect evidence relevant to the case and utilise, generally speaking, abductive reasoning to offer possible explanations for their findings. During the evaluative phase, forensic scientists use inductive reasoning (based on the Bayesian paradigm) to evaluate the evidential value of the examination results, using a pair of propositions.

Taphonomy of Human Remains: Forensic Analysis of the Dead and the Depositional Environment, First Edition.
Edited by Eline M.J. Schotsmans, Nicholas Márquez-Grant and Shari L. Forbes.

based on their knowledge and past experience, not on solid scientific grounds. The collection of evidence can also be guided by information gained from the work of the detectives on the case. This can greatly improve efficiency, but can also carry the risk of confirmation bias in the collection of physical evidence.

Most forensic scientists who work at a forensic laboratory do not examine crime scenes and, if they do, will only examine one type of physical evidence at a crime scene (e.g. blood spatter); their methods of investigation are therefore laboratory-based and focus mainly on analysing and interpreting the collected physical evidence itself. Most forensic scientists tend to work within a narrow forensic discipline and generally do not (or are not allowed to) combine their results with the results obtained from other forensic disciplines. This is, generally speaking, the prosecution's job, or that of the police. SOCOs and forensic scientists rarely receive feedback from magistrates concerning the consequences of their reports.

Even though the archaeological paradigm[4] has already been integrated in forensic science in the discipline of forensic archaeology (e.g. Dupras *et al.* 2011; Groen *et al.* 2015; Hunter *et al.* 2013), this paradigm is largely unknown to most SOCOs and forensic scientists. The knowledge that a more traditional archaeological discipline, i.e. bioarchaeology/human osteoarchaeology (e.g. Buikstra and Beck 2009; Duday 2006; Larsen 2015), is methodologically closely similar to a medico-legal investigation, also seems to be lacking. This is unfortunate as understanding past (human) activity – a phenomenon that is not observable directly, but only through the (absence of the) material record it has produced – has been a key issue in the archaeological discourse since the 19th century. Questions such as: 'How is it possible to convert contemporary observations of the results of past activity into meaningful statements concerning the past?' and 'How is it possible to infer and test hypotheses concerning past activities, utilising only contemporary observations?' have already been critically addressed. An outcome of the archaeological discourse was that archaeological research methodology differs from the research methodology used in the classical experimental sciences.[5] The latter focuses strongly on the testing of hypotheses in a controlled laboratory setting and the identification of (deterministic) laws and (statistical) regularities in the natural world. The status of archaeological reconstructions about past human activities is also debated;[6] are such reconstructions scientific and objective, or mainly the result of a hermeneutic process? When compared to archaeology, CSI practice also seems to lack an interpretative framework for physical evidence collected at crime scenes. This is despite the fact that criminalistics has an interpretative framework (Evett 2015) that could be extended for application in CSI. The fact that every crime scene is the result of a mix of human and non-human (taphonomic) processes, and that it is essential to develop ways to link the observations obtained during the CSI (i.e. the empirical data), with inferences about the (human) activities that have created the observed results in the first place, is – from an archaeological point of view – not fully acknowledged. Finally, a distinction between an investigative phase and a follow-up evaluative phase, as encountered in forensic science and CSI practice, is alien to archaeology, because it does not operate within the judicial context.

In this chapter the authors explore the applicability of the archaeological paradigm in the CSI practice – as related to major crimes (e.g. murder, manslaughter, arson), the perception of physical

4 A paradigm or scientific framework integrates (epistemological and ontological) assumptions, methodology and research objectives of a scientific discipline (e.g. Scotland 2012).

5 This observation is not unique to archaeology. It is also valid in, for example, geology, planetary science, palaeontology and evolutionary biology (Cleland 2011; Jeffares 2008). All these sciences explain contemporary observable phenomena in terms of their past causes (see also Houck and Siegel 2010).

6 This debate involved questions concerning the ontological and epistemological nature of the collected material record (e.g. Alberti *et al.* 2013; Chapman and Wylie 2015; Lucas 2012; Sullivan 1978; Wylie 2002). Ontology is a branch of philosophy that focuses on the nature of reality. Epistemology is concerned with the nature of scientific knowledge itself and questions such as how we know that something is true.

evidence, site formation processes and taphonomic transformations (e.g. decay, degradation, corrosion). This chapter starts with a discussion on the fundamentals of CSI, after which it focuses on the archaeological paradigm as relevant to the CSI practice. In Section 3, the archaeological perception of physical evidence as assemblages, with emphasis on the archaeological site formation processes, is discussed. The chapter ends with a conclusion summarising the value of integrating the archaeological and criminalistic frameworks in the CSI practice.

36.2 CSI Fundamentals

As all forensic science begins at a crime scene, the CSI forms an integral part of this science. The crime scene is the location from where most physical (trace) evidence will be collected. Forensic science is, generally speaking, using comparison as a method of examination. The comparative method aims to provide evidence to support one of at least two mutually exclusive hypotheses (pair of propositions). Such hypotheses could, for example, concern who left the material at the crime scene. Crime scene traces with unknown origin are compared with material collected from a known person, for example an accused (i.e. a reference sample).

Rule 401 of the US Federal Rules of Evidence[7] states that: 'Evidence is relevant if:

a) it has any tendency to make a fact more or less probable than it would be without the evidence; and
b) the fact is of consequence in determining the action'.

Those 'facts' include when the crime was committed, how the crime was committed, who was involved and sometimes why the crime was committed. Physical evidence can be anything from a massive object to microscopic trace evidence (e.g. fibres, latent human biological traces) and can be transferred during the criminal activity.[8] Such transfer can be primary or direct (i.e. from a source to a target), or secondary or indirect (i.e. from a source to a target via an intermediary object). Tertiary, quaternary, etc. transfers are also possible. To observe the trace in the present, it does not only need to have been transferred, but it also needs to have persisted and been recovered. Finally, contact can also transform traces or wipe them out entirely, or the once present traces can degrade and disappear with time.

Physical evidence can be either classified as coming from a class of sources, or individualised as coming from one specific source. For prediction of the forensic value of physical evidence, an 'evidentiary triangle' is used to predict what type of physical evidence could be linked to the victim, the suspect and the crime. SOCOs are, generally speaking, most interested in the physical evidence that can be linked to all three, because this physical evidence could potentially lead to the (unknown) offender.

Questions, inferences and conclusions based on the examination can be at the source level or at the activity level (Cook *et al.* 1998a; Evett *et al.* 2000).[9] The evidentiary value will depend on the context of the case (i.e. the relationships between the suspect, the victim and the location where the crime was committed), and the hypotheses[10] used to evaluate this evidence. Forensic laboratories will also

7 For more information, see: https://www.law.cornell.edu/rules/fre/rule_401 (accessed 10 October 2016).
8 This transfer is often related to Locard's Exchange Principle (Locard 1920, 1930), simplistically translated as 'every contact leaves a trace'. Of importance is that Locard merely stated that this transfer could take place, there is no guarantee.
9 Within criminalistics, three hierarchical levels of hypotheses are defined: (1) the source level (source of the trace); (2) the activity level (activity or actor that led to the transfer of the trace); and (3) the offence level (crime during which the trace was transferred).
10 A forensic hypothesis is a translation of a relevant question into some realistically possible answers. A hypothesis that does well at explaining the observed results could be integrated into a scenario (see footnote 11).

use likelihood ratios (LR) when reporting their conclusions using mutually exclusive hypotheses to evaluate the evidence (ENFSI 2015). An LR is the probability of the evidence under hypothesis A, divided by the probability of the evidence under hypothesis B. The probabilistic conclusions consider the probability of the evidence and not the probability of the hypotheses themselves (Cook *et al.* 1998a, 1998b; Evett *et al.* 2000; Robertson *et al.* 2016), because the prior odds of the hypotheses are considered to be the task of the court. However, during the CSI (the investigative phase of the case), the SOCO can consider the prior odds of the hypotheses of interest to optimise the chances of collecting the most relevant physical evidence. In the Bayesian paradigm, finding the truth is probabilistic and all probabilities are conditional; the conclusions can change if the hypotheses or the contextual information change.

A crime scene is, technically speaking, the 'location where an illegal act occurred; for purposes of the CSI' (Houck *et al.* 2012). CSI practice is generally considered a technical police activity and demands three elements of the investigator: a general understanding of the CSI practice and forensic science, experience in dealing with – and processing of – crime scenes and the ability and willingness to be impartial (Gardner and Bevel 2009). Some SOCOs and forensic scientists also employ a hypothetico-deductive model for the interpretation and decision-making during the CSI. In this model the 'investigator begins with observation of the scene leading to a cycle of hypotheses creation and testing, with other information being supplied only after the initial scene examination and hypotheses creation' (Jamieson 2004). The CSI practice itself consists of a sequence of procedures (Gardner 2012; Gardner and Bevel 2009):

1) securing and protecting the scene to minimise the loss of physical evidence
2) assessing the scene for visible physical evidence or traces (and also for health and safety risks)
3) formulating forensic scenarios[11] (i.e. composite hypotheses) concerning what could have happened at the crime scene
4) non-intrusive preliminary walkthrough, observation and documentation
5) intrusive search (for non-visible traces), collection and documentation of the localised physical evidence
6) (scientific) analysis of the collected evidential material, mostly in a forensic laboratory
7) interpretation of the results of the analysis of physical evidence recovered at the crime scene

The possibility to fall back in the CSI sequence is essential, for example if new physical evidence has been encountered or new questions have been raised. What kind of physical evidence is collected and how it is collected depends for example on the knowledge and experience of the SOCOs (and forensic scientists), the evidentiary value, the limitations of laboratory tests (i.e. false positives and false negatives), the protocols used in forensic laboratories (Gardner 2012; Gardner and Bevel 2009; Houck *et al.* 2012) and the national jurisdictions. Generally speaking, the collected physical evidence should be able to:

- support a forensic scenario or its alternative, or possibly exclude it (e.g. a forensic scenario based on eye-witness statements)
- offer investigative leads to identify the people present at the crime scene during the criminal act (e.g. victim, witness, perpetrator) and, if possible, their interrelationships
- offer preliminary findings regarding the manner of death (natural, accidental, homicide, suicide or undetermined) and the cause of death (disease or injury responsible for the death). The final findings are provided by the coroner or medical examiner

11 A forensic scenario is defined as a combination of forensic hypotheses. Preliminary forensic scenarios are based on the issues in the case, background knowledge, tactical information (e.g. a witness statement) and/or empirical observations at a crime scene. The forensic scenarios that remain after CSI will be based on confirmed or supported forensic hypotheses only.

- establish logical and defensible forensic scenarios regarding what happened at the crime scene, after analysis of physical evidence at the forensic laboratory

It is vital to collect physical evidence in accordance with best practice guidelines, to prevent (cross-) contamination and therefore mistakes, misleading evidence, or loss of evidence. The CSI sequence consequently follows a strict 'chain of custody', to guarantee that all investigative steps have been taken and to avoid rejection of evidence by the court. 'Chain of custody' refers to the chronological documentation (traceability and continuity) of evidence from the crime scene to the court. Crime scene integrity issues are, according to Gardner (2012), addition of new material, destruction of material and movement of material across the scene. SOCOs and forensic scientists should also be aware that perpetrators could manipulate physical evidence to conceal crimes or postpone detection (Beauregard and Bouchard 2010; Beauregard and Martineau 2014).

36.3 The Archaeological Paradigm

Archaeology, as an academic discipline, applies theories and methodologies derived from the humanities (e.g. history), the social sciences (e.g. economics, sociology and cultural anthropology) and the natural sciences (e.g. biology, earth sciences and taphonomy). We define theory as an intellectual framework used to interpret the archaeological record and methodology as 'the procedures and approaches used to carry out a piece of archaeological research, whether it is an excavation, survey, artefact study, or any other kind of analysis' (Darvill 2002). Archaeological excavation and research is data- and theory-driven and there are different theoretical frameworks within archaeology.[12] The primary goal of archaeology is the study and reconstruction of past human activities and the effect of these activities on the natural processes, through the systematic recovery, analysis and interpretation of the archaeological record. Archaeologists agree that the retrieved archaeological record is not only affected by past site formation processes, but also by the methods used during the process of recovery, mostly upon excavation. To recognise patterns in the archaeological record, background knowledge of past activities (e.g. databases and models) is used. Archaeologists only interpret the archaeological record in its context and association (e.g. *in situ*). Because this record is mainly caused by past human activity, they use anthropogenic models to explain the archaeological record as the result of this human activity. In summary, although archaeology and CSI practice are sometimes perceived as similar, the archaeological framework differs greatly from the one used during the CSI practice. The authors believe that archaeological insights should be incorporated into the CSI practice, especially if the goal of the CSI is to interpret at the level of human activities. The most important insights are addressed below.

36.3.1 Theory-Driven Research

In archaeology, data analysis and data interpretation are inter-dependent rather than independent (Carver 1990; Gibbon 1989; Hodder 1986, 1992; Wylie 1992, 2011). Collection, analysis and interpretation of physical evidence therefore go hand-in-hand. Today's archaeologists agree that collection, analysis and interpretation of the material record are affected by theoretical and methodological aspects and the socio-cultural background of the observer. All observations of physical entities are observer-dependent and constructed in the context of their research. Every archaeologist acknowledges that it is impossible to collect the entire archaeological record. And even if full collection was

12 This is not surprising since archaeologists study a wide range of past human activities, ranging from the production of ceramics to funerary symbolism, requiring different explanatory theories and models. For more information on archaeological theory, see for example Bentley *et al.* 2009 or Johnson 2010.

possible, the archaeologist would still face the dilemma of how much of the collected material record should be stored, examined, analysed, interpreted and published. Hence, data collection and sampling is always subject to a selection process and interpretation driven. An archaeological excavation is always theory-driven (in the vocabulary of the SOCO: 'scenario-driven'); its field methodology is designed to answer specific research questions.

36.3.2 Use of Empirical Databases

Archaeologists use quantitative and qualitative empirical databases containing (site transcendent) information acquired from past archaeological excavations and successive research of the excavated material record (i.e. background knowledge). Most of these databases are GIS-related and link spatial find and feature locations, as mapped during the process of excavation, with databases containing information on these finds and features (i.e. attribute tables). Furthermore, archaeological databases are used during different stages of research. During the preliminary desktop research or desk-based assessment (DBA), archaeologists use GIS-related databases to predict where archaeological sites are located (e.g. Banning 2002), to predict which finds and features can expect to be encountered during the forthcoming excavation in order to form hypotheses, and to develop a valid and reliable field methodology. During the process of excavation, a relational GIS database forms an integral part of the excavation recording strategy to provide an up-to-date view of the excavated finds and features and their spatial relationships (e.g. Smith and Levy 2014), to help detect possible omissions in field documentation and to test hypotheses. After excavation, GIS-related databases are used as analytical tools to analyse and reconstruct the excavated material record, to test and/or adjust hypotheses, and to help structure the archaeological record for analysis and publication (e.g. tables, graphs, layouts, plans). Archaeological databases are constantly updated with new information obtained from excavations and subsequent research to ensure that they are up-to-date to inform preliminary desktop research in subsequent cases.

36.3.3 Assemblages and Site Formation Processes

As mentioned above, archaeologists do not have direct access to materialised past human activity; they only have access to what remains of this activity in the present. No matter how refined the archaeological theory and methodology, the physical evidence of past activities will always remain a – possibly incomplete – combination of residues of these activities (e.g. Bailey 2007). This is due to site formation processes, or events that have created and subsequently affected the archaeological site, for example taphonomic transformations. The physical evidence of past activities should therefore be seen as resulting from a combination of events, forming – in archaeological terms – an assemblage, or a combination of finds and features *in situ* and in a defined space (e.g. Lucas 2012).[13] The concepts of assemblages and site formation processes will be discussed more extensively further on in this chapter.

36.3.4 Anthropogenic Models

An archaeological record is dynamic, it is the result of spatio-temporal human (and non-human) activities and processes. Anthropogenic models help to interpret past human activities using generalisations made from descriptions of past and/or ongoing human practice. In other words, these models of behaviour seek spatio-temporal regularities that occur within the archaeological record and link

13 Assemblage has an additional meaning in archaeology; it can also refer to a specific (typological) set of artefacts found at one or more archaeological site(s), for example flints (i.e. flint assemblages) or pottery (i.e. pottery assemblage). This second meaning falls outside the scope of this chapter.

these regularities – while acknowledging the importance of site formation processes and taphonomic transformations – to human activity.[14] This is done by creating hypotheses that are testable by means of the archaeological record. The models used can be based on inductive reasoning (evidence based), deductive reasoning (theory-based exclusion) or abductive reasoning (e.g. by linking the localised material record to hypotheses, to find a new explanation), depending on the archaeological questions that need to be answered. For example, archaeologists often integrate abductive interpretation of the results of an archaeological excavation, with deductive interpretations, as obtained from archaeological experimental studies. Predictive models tell where more physical evidence is expected, based on what has been found so far and knowledge concerning the human activity that caused the physical evidence. Anthropogenic models (together with other types of background knowledge) can also be used during predictive modelling, since they also have (some) predictive power (e.g. Verhagen and Whitley 2012). New archaeological excavations will undoubtedly expose new archaeological records, finding the current anthropogenic models somewhat deficient. The continuing feedback corrections from the archaeological record will result in updated models, allowing the development of new hypotheses that again will be tested by new archaeological records.

Archaeological reconstructions of the past are thus based on background knowledge, anthropogenic models and/or actualistic experiments, which re-enact the predicted human activity. They can provide scientifically-tested models concerning which human activity caused which type of assemblage. In view of the above, archaeological research design covers a sequence of steps to ensure that archaeological research is organised, efficient, reliable and valid. Each step in this sequence (after Swartz 1967), although distinct, might have to be revisited:

1) *Preliminary desktop research*: formulation of problem, accessing background knowledge, formulating preliminary questions, forming of hypotheses, development of excavation methodology
2) *Field survey*: limited testing of hypotheses, updating of hypotheses, limited collection of archaeological record
3) *Final desktop research*: formulation of final research questions, finalising of research hypotheses, finalising excavation methodology
4) *Excavation*: collection of archaeological record during fieldwork and data processing
5) *Data analysis*: site formation analysis, placing of the archaeological assemblages in a spatial and sequential (i.e. spatio-temporal) framework through classification and contextual association, partly during the fieldwork
6) *Interpretation*: study of the archaeological record (e.g. how were certain finds and features made and used), testing of hypotheses, use of anthropogenic models for site-specific socio-cultural reconstruction, partly during the fieldwork
7) *Integration*: post-excavation synthesis of the interpreted parts of the archaeological record, reconstruction of past site-specific ways of life by means of anthropogenic models and background knowledge
8) *Comparison*: identification of cultural (dis)similarities with previous archaeological studies, further testing of hypotheses, evaluation of research methodology
9) *Abstraction*: formulation of (new) ideas about the past, updating of background knowledge, consolidation or revision of general laws, development of new research questions

---

14 For example, in archaeology, middle-range theories (e.g. Binford 1977, 1981; Schiffer 1976) are developed to link the excavated archaeological record to the behaviours of past people that caused this record. These theories are, generally speaking, developed by engaging in contemporary experiments (actualistic studies) and ethno-archaeological observations concerning the object or process to be studied in order to find regularities in the observed outcomes and to produce general analogies for interpretation of the archaeological record.

36.4 Assessing Archaeological Assemblages and Site Formation Processes

An archaeological site can be seen as an accumulation of materialised patterns of past human (and non-human) activities, often with an unknown timeframe. As mentioned, materialised patterns of past physical activity can be interpreted as assemblages, or combinations of finds and features *in situ* and in a defined space. Assemblages therefore also refer to a process (sequence of activities) and can thus be seen as proxy witnesses. Assemblages can also be used for dating purposes, by means of their internal configuration and their relations to the environments where they have been found *in situ*. Archaeologists have developed terminology to sequence the finds and features in assemblages through relative and absolute chronologies. The absolute chronology is described in calendar years. The relative terminology is subdivided into terms for events that precede other events, events that follow other events and events that occur more or less simultaneously. It is important to keep in mind that every excavation disperses the assemblages as once present during the fieldwork, to re-assemble the disconnected parts (i.e. different types of finds and features encountered) again into whole new assemblages (i.e. the recovered and analysed material record). If the process of excavation and reconnection is not performed correctly, the evidentiary value of an assemblage could be lost. Or worse, will result in misleading evidence. Archaeological discourse has also shown that to be able to understand the importance of an archaeological find or feature in an assemblage, the spatial relations and contextual associations of all finds and features in the assemblage have to be spatially known in 3D space, *in situ*. Archaeological mapping furthermore enables the archaeologist to easily and quickly oversee the whole archaeological site, the localised archaeological record and the different assemblages present in this record. Mapping is thus also a reconstruction tool, especially if the analysis and interpretation of the excavated material record is performed within a GIS application (e.g. Bianchini *et al.* 2015).

Additionally, physical evidence of past human activities can be understood as a sequence of formative and retrieval processes (Clarke 1973; DeBoer 1983; Lucas 2012; Schiffer 1972, 1976, 1983, 1996). This sequence can be sub-divided into:

1) the full range of human activity in the past, or the 'pre-depositional activities'
2) the pre-depositional activities that have been materialised and deposited, or the 'depositional assemblages'
3) remains of the depositional assemblages that have survived into the present, or the 'post-depositional assemblages'
4) remains of the post-depositional assemblages that are recognised and recorded during the investigation, or the 'localised assemblages'
5) remains of the localised assemblages that are recovered/sampled, or the 'sampled assemblages'
6) remains of the sampled assemblages that are analysed and interpreted, or the 'analysed assemblages'
7) remains of the analysed assemblages that are reported, or the 'reported assemblages'

Each of the above-mentioned steps results, generally speaking, in a progressive loss of physical evidence as one goes forward in time, resulting in a progressively smaller material record (Figure 36.1).

The relationship between a localised assemblage and a reported assemblage is therefore not the same as the relationship between a depositional assemblage and a reported assemblage. To comprehend the transformations between the depositional assemblages and the post-depositional assemblages, one needs to understand the site-specific formation processes that have created and preserved the archaeological site and the evidentiary value of its material record. Additionally, taphonomic transformations have (or could have) distorted, masked and/or deleted a part of the once available

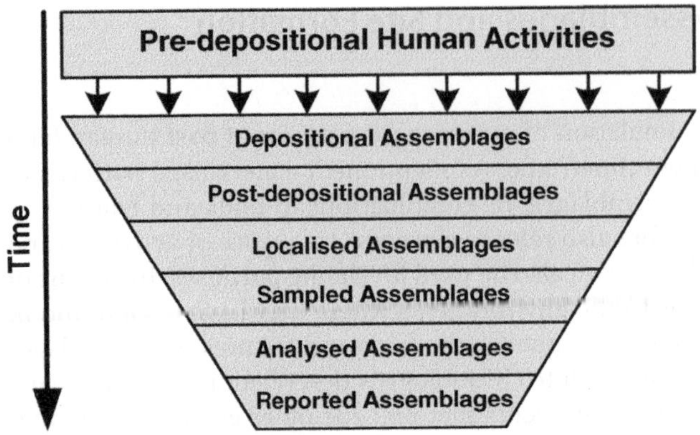

Figure 36.1 A schematic representation of archaeological formative and retrieval processes.

depositional assemblages. Since site formation processes and taphonomic transformations are not only reductive but also additive, they can also introduce new patterns into the localised assemblages. Since all site formation processes and taphonomic transformations have spatial and temporal components, they also can be used for predicting absolute or relative timing (sequence) of events and human activity. In summary, the excavated archaeological assemblages are always transformed due to past human and non-human processes and therefore only partly represent the originally deposited finds and features within these assemblages. The interpretation of an archaeological find or feature also requires considering its spatio-temporal location within an assemblage.

36.5 The CSI Practice, an Archaeological and Criminalistic Perspective

From the archaeological point of view, today's CSI is, in practice, unable to test hypotheses concerning past human (criminal) activity. For example, since forensic databases and their functionalities are not integrated into CSI recording methodologies, SOCOs (and forensic scientists that attend crime scenes) are unable to objectively learn from patterns encountered during past casework. Localised physical evidence cannot be regarded as an objective 'snapshot' of the past that is able to 'speak for itself', but should be seen as the result of past (human) action, site formation processes and taphonomic transformations. The process of interpretation is further determined by the research methodology and the theoretical framework used to interpret the evidence. Since collected physical evidence on its own is 'silent', the development and use of anthropogenic models to help interpret the localised evidence at activity level should, from an archaeological point of view, be promoted during the CSI. Archaeologists aim to chronologically order human activity, which is also beneficial during the CSI. An example is the case of a body with questions related to time of death, post-mortem interval (PMI) or time since deposition. The information can also be used to:

- create background knowledge
- develop research driven strategies to predict where certain types of physical evidence could be encountered (predictive modelling) and what could be their evidentiary value
- predict why certain types of physical evidence are, or could be, no longer present

Accessing background knowledge at a crime scene could inform SOCOs of where physical evidence is expected, support certain hypotheses and scenarios or suggest new ones and predict what form this evidence could have. This should mostly take place during the CSI and not later, after all physical evidence has been collected for analysis in a forensic laboratory. However, accessing background knowledge to guide investigations could also cause contextual bias, or 'the psychological principle that the desires and expectations with which people approach the task of observation measurably affect their perceptions and interpretations of what they observe' (Saks *et al.* 2003). SOCOs and forensic scientists performing CSI should therefore obtain all the information needed for crime scene assessment and the development of the CSI research methodology and hypotheses, but not more than that because of the risks of contextual bias (Champod 2014; Ditrich 2015; Kassin *et al.* 2013; Ribaux *et al.* 2010a; Saks *et al.* 2003; Stoel *et al.* 2014). It is also important to integrate the objectives of research and development (R&D) projects, such that resulting findings can be applied in CSI practice to maximise retrieval and interpretative potential. For example, performing an experimental study to comprehend how people are strangled in order to maximise the recovery of DNA traces associated with strangling by means of analogical reasoning.

In summary, looking at lessons learned from archaeology, the CSI practice should start before the actual CSI and should not end with submitting a CSI report. Figure 36.2 visualises the proposed integration of the CSI practice with the discussed archaeological research design to formulate a theoretical and methodological framework, which makes the CSI objectives and procedures explicit. Each step in the nine-step sequence will be discussed separately.

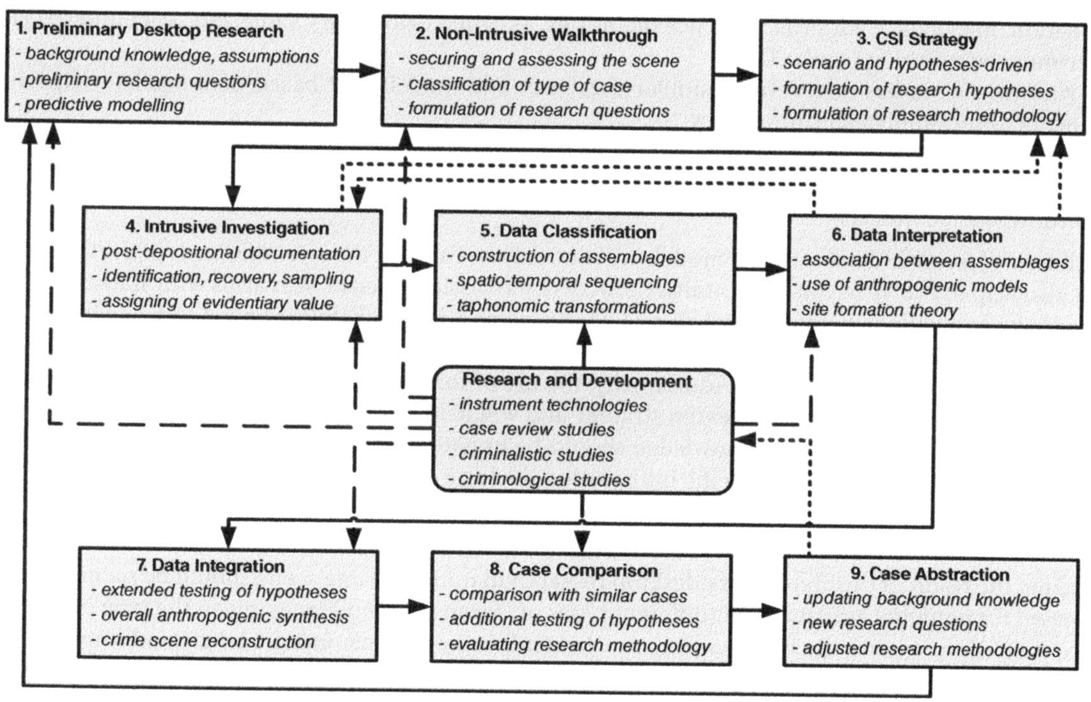

Figure 36.2 Archaeological framework and the CSI practice. The solid lines relate to the proposed CSI sequence. The dashed lines relate to the proposed R&D. The dotted lines represent feedback.

36.5.1 Step 1. Preliminary Desktop Research

Desktop research is the backbone of an archaeological excavation. By accessing information acquired from previous excavations and subsequent research, archaeologists are able to express (to some extent) an expectation of what the excavation results will be and are therefore also able to develop specific research methods that will enable them to answer specific research questions and to test hypotheses. Although a typical investigation of a crime scene does not have as much preparation time as an archaeological excavation, integrating desktop research with the CSI practice would strongly benefit the CSI. To be able to do this, the (already available) forensic background knowledge and experience would have to be combined in forensic databases and models. For example, crime-specific models could be developed by studying the location and distribution of forensic assemblages, as resulting from different types of criminal activities. Although no two crimes are the same, crimes of the same type can share enough characteristics to form patterns, to help predict where the most useful crime-related traces can be found and which hypotheses should be considered. The use of forensic databases and models would not only provide an empirical link between a specific human activity and the material outcome of this activity, but would also enable – as a diagnostic tool – the SOCOs and forensic scientists to assign an evidentiary value to a forensic assemblage, given the hypotheses used. Additionally, three types of R&D studies could provide valuable background knowledge for the recognition of physical evidence at the crime scene, the interpretation and the assignment of evidentiary value:

- case review studies used to develop databases and models that for specific types of crime hold information on evidence patterns, evidence quantities, assigned evidentiary value, etc., encountered at crime scenes during regular CSI
- criminalistic studies that develop similar databases and models, but based on actualistic experiments using simulated crime scenes
- criminological studies that develop databases and models related to certain types of crime and acquired from the study of human (criminal) pre-depositional and depositional activities (i.e. the anthropogenic models)

The use of forensic databases and models will not only strengthen the scientific basis of the CSI, but will also help to evolve beyond the intuitive process by assessing forensic scenarios with statistical aid (predictive modelling), before the intrusive CSI. Knowing what probabilities need to be assigned to outcomes and which research questions should be asked, given a certain type of forensic scenario, will improve the investigative process. Additionally, the use of forensic databases and models during the CSI will aid the development of a search strategy and will help to generate hypotheses at the activity level. The available background knowledge should be updated before performing an intrusive CSI, preferably after obtaining case-specific information during a police briefing.

36.5.2 Step 2. Non-Intrusive Walkthrough

Keeping the result of the preliminary desktop research in mind, a crime scene should be secured and assessed for potential availability of (different types of) forensic assemblages, given the type of crime encountered, to update the background knowledge. In other words, using background knowledge would enable the SOCOs and forensic scientists to identify forensic assemblages that could provide evidence for past (human) activities at the crime scene. To be able to do this, a crime scene should preferably be mapped in 3D with the aid of a 3D-scanner, a total station[15] and/or photogrammetry, and investigated by means of visual aid and non-intrusive CSI equipment (e.g. a forensic light

15 A total station is an electronic device which integrates the functions of a theodolite (vertical measurement) and a distance meter (horizontal measurement). In archaeology, total stations are mainly used to record – in a database format – surveys and excavations (e.g. the spatial *in situ* locations of the localised finds and features). The recorded data is used to produce archaeological site plans, for example within a GIS (see footnote 2).

source) to obtain an overview of the crime scene and to answer specific questions. For example, what type of crime, if any, occurred? What is the nature and extent of the crime scene? What type of formation processes (human and non-human) could have been responsible for the creation and subsequent modification of the encountered forensic assemblages? Which materials or remains from the scene could have been transferred from the scene to the perpetrator, or *vice versa*? The non-intrusive walkthrough will help the SOCOs (and forensic scientists attending the crime scene) to update their background knowledge. It will also help them to develop a CSI strategy and to specify the questions to be answered during and after the CSI. Non-intrusive search methods are preferred over intrusive ones, which will be discussed in Step 4.

36.5.3 Step 3. CSI Strategy

The above makes clear that CSI practice should be scenario-driven and centred on the forensic assemblages, site formation processes and taphonomic transformations encountered during the non-intrusive walkthrough. The CSI research methodology should take into the account the available background knowledge to optimise the allocation of search efforts. The methodology used should be able to detect background analogies, 'smoking guns'[16] and 'downstream effects',[17] given certain hypotheses.

While for evaluative work in the forensic laboratory, inductive reasoning based on the Bayesian paradigm should be used, a crude deductive reasoning can be applied during the CSI. To quote Jeffares (2008):

> Take multiple observations of evidence: $[o^a, o^b, o^c]$. Now take two hypotheses, H_1 and H_2. If H_1 accounts for $[o^a + o^b]$ but is incompatible with $[o^c]$ and H_2 accounts for all three observations $[o^a + o^b + o^c]$, then $[o^c]$ is the 'smoking gun' that discriminates between two hypotheses about a historical event. This single downstream effect not only supports one hypothesis, it works against the alternative hypothesis.

In other words, looking for a 'smoking gun' or a 'downstream effect' could help the SOCOs to discriminate between hypotheses. However, it should be kept in mind that excluding one hypothesis does not demonstrate the other to be true when there are more than two hypotheses.

The research methodology should also focus on the reconstruction of the situation prior to the investigated (criminal) event, on the reconstruction of the encountered crime scene formation processes and on the assignment of (preliminary) evidentiary value to the encountered assemblages, given the hypotheses used. The research methodology should be adjusted if unexpected (physical) evidence is encountered, or if the hypotheses used are falsified. Finally, if one wishes to use data and information acquired from individual crime scenes to improve background knowledge, it is necessary to ensure that all crime scenes are routinely and consistently recorded, preferably digitally. Digital recording will not only improve precision, it will also improve the 'chain of custody'.

36.5.4 Step 4. Intrusive Investigation

Generally speaking, a crime scene – like an archaeological site – will (and can) be only processed once. The CSI search strategy and type of search (e.g. lane, grid, trail or spiral) should depend on the

16 A 'smoking gun' is a trace (or traces) 'that unambiguously discriminates one hypothesis from among a set of currently available hypotheses as providing "the best explanation" of the traces thus far observed' (Cleland 2002).

17 The 'downstream effect' stands for the dispersal of traces or remains that have resulted from different past activities. Different activities will produce different assemblages and therefore produce different 'downstream effects' (Jeffares 2008).

type of crime scene, terrain and light conditions, logistics and time available, manpower and experience present, type and size of the physical evidence being searched for, and the forensic scenarios and hypotheses used. Each SOCO and forensic scientist should be briefed about the search strategy before the search. Archaeological principles (e.g. principle of superposition, principle of original horizontality, principle of lateral continuity) should be used to sequence the physical evidence found, something that is recognised in CSI textbooks (Gardner 2012; Gardner and Bevel 2009; Houck and Siegel 2010; Houck *et al.* 2012). The search should start with areas most likely to contain relevant evidence (i.e. the point of entry or exit, paths suspected of having been used by the perpetrator, points of contact between the perpetrator, the victim and the crime scene). Physical evidence collection strategies should be based on background knowledge and should address relevant, case-specific hypotheses. However, physical evidence that is in danger of being destroyed by natural or human activity should be collected first, even if the evidentiary value of this evidence seems low at the time. It is widely acknowledged that all steps in the investigation should be documented in such a way that it will be possible to reconstruct all actions and decisions made during the CSI, for example for the purposes of the court. From an archaeological point of view, crime scene documentation should not only consist of photographs (and film) and written documentation (e.g. forms and notes), but should also include (3D) mapping. An evidentiary item should never be moved before it has been mapped *in situ* (i.e. in an assemblage), ideally using a 3D-scan, a total station and/or photogrammetry. If this is not available, traditional archaeological mapping techniques (i.e. rectangular measurements, triangulation or baseline measurements) could be used. If an item is moved before recording, it should never be put back in place to be mapped. Sketches should only be used as an additional mnemonic device, since a sketch is unreliable as a mapping method, not linked to a database, and above all, already an interpretation of the encountered situation. A GIS application should preferably be used to link the locations of the mapped physical evidence to an attribute table containing (quantitative and qualitative) information on this evidence.

36.5.5 Step 5. Data Classification

From an archaeological point of view, *in situ* examination of the localised physical evidence should start during the CSI, by reconstructing and sequencing the localised (crime-related) assemblages and by analysing the site formation processes and taphonomic transformations encountered. Presumptive testing (e.g. for blood and semen) will offer an additional possibility to find spatio-temporal sequences in the localised forensic assemblages. This sequencing will not only help to take the passing of time into account, but also to look for post-depositional changes that could have transformed the localised assemblages.

36.5.6 Step 6. Data Interpretation

In archaeology, data interpretation begins during the process of excavation, mainly with the aid of (3D) site plans. If a GIS application is used, the site plans can be linked to evidentiary logs. The site plans show, among other things, the spatial locations of all localised assemblages. Site plans should also be integrated with CSI practices. For example, site plans in combination with scene of crime formation processes will help the SOCOs (and forensic scientists) to infer from the localised assemblages, the once deposited assemblages, by accounting for the taphonomic transformations that occurred on the site. Thinking in terms of assemblages helps to comprehend how physical evidence was originally deposited; it enables reasoning backwards from the localised assemblages (taking into account the probability of recovery) to the post-depositional assemblages (e.g. probability of persistence), to the depositional assemblages (e.g. probability of transfer), to the (human) activities that took place. In this process, the probabilities of transfer, persistence and recovery of physical evidence are applied and updated. All these probabilities are (together with context) key factors in activity level interpretation in forensic science. By accessing forensic assemblages at the crime scene, hypotheses could also be supported or falsified during the CSI, since the statistical data to inform the assignment of LRs could be derived from the forensic databases containing background data. Technological innovations (e.g. lab-on-a-chip) will speed up this process and therefore offer new possibilities to support a hypothesis or its alternative, not only in the laboratory, but also at the crime scene.

It is also necessary to use anthropogenic models to improve CSI practice. It is perfectly fine to analyse and compare forensic evidence without the use of anthropogenic models at the source level, but for interpretation at the activity level the anthropogenic models are necessary. Forensic anthropogenic models should be used to generate hypotheses and to investigate the support of localised assemblages for one or the other hypothesis. The use of such models could also improve how CSI strategies cope with incomplete assemblages, by identifying the (causal) processes underlying these assemblages.

36.5.7 Step 7. Data Integration

In archaeology, the process of data integration takes place post-excavation and combines separate analyses and interpretations of different types of assemblages into one overall synthesis. Archaeologists use the data integration predominantly to reconstruct the way of living and the environment at and near the excavated site. In other words, archaeologists combine remaining hypotheses into a consistent and causal explanation. GIS visualisations clarify the spatial layout of assemblages, inform whether an interpretation is plausible and clarify whether evidence could have been missed due to site formation processes and taphonomic transformations. In this manner the GIS possibilities are fully exploited, producing queries, analysing the spatial distribution of evidence and presenting the results of all these operations in images, graphs or databases. These methods could also improve CSI practice.

The integration of all observations, hypotheses and background knowledge will attempt to offer a better reconstruction than the separate items of evidence can alone. When considering the integrated reconstruction, some items of evidence will turn out not to be relevant or even misleading. After the analysis of evidence in the laboratory, the resulting evidence can also be integrated into the interpretation of the localised assemblage to further aid the reconstruction of what took place at the crime scene. Using the Bayesian framework to interpret the physical evidence will not only provide a methodology for weaving together different strands of reasoning, it will also force the SOCOs and forensic scientists to be explicit about their strands of reasoning.

36.5.8 Step 8. Case Comparison

In archaeology the interpretation and synthesis of an excavation are always compared to other excavations, to test new hypotheses and to evaluate the excavation methodology employed. Although case comparison is not regarded today as part of the CSI practice, a comparison between similar types of crime scenes would be very beneficial to the final interpretation of the crime scene examined. The analysed forensic assemblages and their evidentiary value, given the used hypotheses, could be compared to analysed assemblages from earlier forensic cases. The comparison could lead to new hypotheses, new ideas about taphonomic transformations and an evaluation of the CSI strategy, for example whether it was adequate for localising the relevant physical evidence. This is especially important when the evidence gathered was not enough to establish a solid forensic scenario. For example, because not enough physical evidence was localised or sampled, or perhaps because the evidence sampled was of too low evidentiary value. After case comparison, a CSI report, from an archaeological point of view, is ready to be submitted.

Additionally, case comparison will aid an intelligence-led framework of policing, since the 'newly collected forensic case data will feed crime intelligence in order to fully use their informative potential' (Ribaux *et al.* 2010a). Securing forensic evidence at crime scenes should therefore also be seen as a tool for providing crime intelligence (Ribaux *et al.* 2010a, 2010b).

36.5.9 Step 9. Case Abstraction

In archaeology, abstraction is the final research step. Abstraction enables the archaeologist to formulate new ideas about the past, to update the existing background knowledge and to develop new research questions and hypotheses that will be answered or tested by new excavations and/or laboratory research. Case abstraction therefore offers much needed feedback for future preliminary desktop research. CSI casework should not be an end in itself; it should also be used to generate new (anthropogenic) models and to update the existing (GIS-related) forensic databases to improve their predictive value.

36.6 Conclusion

At first glance, archaeology and CSI practice appear similar; both disciplines use the remaining physical evidence resulting from previous human activity to reconstruct human activity while taking taphonomic changes into account. However, archaeology and CSI practice use dissimilar lines of reasoning to reach their conclusions, a difference that is explained by the dissimilar historical paths both disciplines took to evolve. It is believed that archaeology, as a scientific discipline, offers opportunities to evaluate and develop the CSI practice. Archaeology is all about past human interaction, between humans and their environments and between humans themselves. Additionally, archaeology, like CSI practice, is seldom able to offer certainty; it cannot test new interpretations of the remote past by performing controlled experiments. However, archaeological research can weigh new interpretations by means of anthropogenic models and other types of background knowledge, and test hypotheses – upon which the new interpretations are based – by means of actualistic experimental studies and the excavated archaeological record, in order to support a particular hypothesis or its alternatives.

This chapter presents an archaeological, criminalistic and criminological framework for evidential reasoning in CSI that is based on forensic background knowledge (e.g. databases and models), experimental studies, anthropocentric theories (e.g. criminological studies), mutually exclusive hypotheses and the physical evidence (i.e. empirical input) recovered at a crime scene. From an archaeological point of view, CSI practice can only develop scientifically if it is broadened beyond the traditional boundaries of a technical investigation. If every CSI is considered as a single and isolated event – as it is in current practice – then it will not be able to learn from the past. If CSI practice is re-defined as a circular scientific process, it will not only be able to generate new forensic knowledge (e.g. forensic intelligence) and new ways to look for physical evidence, but it will also be able to improve future CSI by means of case abstraction. Additionally, the adoption of GIS-based recording strategies will not only help to develop new ways of CSI evidence documentation, analysis, interpretation and visualisation, but it will also offer better accuracy and save time. The introduction of crime scene formation models and the concept of forensic assemblages will aid SOCOs and forensic scientists to localise physical evidence that is capable of discriminating between hypotheses through linking the localised evidence to human activities that took place before, during and after the crime committed. This can be done largely directly at the crime scene and not only afterwards at the forensic laboratory. The above offers a framework to consider where to look for certain types of physical evidence, what could be its evidentiary value, and for explaining why certain types of physical evidence were not recovered. Additionally, without proper knowledge of site formation processes, SOCOs and forensic scientists might lack the theoretical understanding needed to formulate appropriate hypotheses, might fail to recognise and therefore recover relevant evidence and might not be able to link the localised evidence to relevant hypotheses.

Introducing the archaeological paradigm into the CSI process will undoubtedly bring with it new challenges. For example, national laws could obstruct central storage and use of case-specific information. Additional challenges and questions are, for example:

- How can the already available forensic background knowledge best be accessed, unified and stored?
- How can databases and models be accessed during the CSI, especially to check how reasonable the assumptions are and to develop mutually exclusive hypotheses?
- How can we test that the technical methods used to recover decomposing or degraded physical evidence are suitable in the first place?
- How should we deal with the risk of contextual bias at crime scenes, especially when accessing police information to aid forensic investigation?

Despite all these challenges, integrating the archaeological framework with CSI practice will not only help to improve CSI, it will also help the SOCOs and forensic scientists to access the information needed for answering questions at the activity level. Furthermore, it will help the CSI practice to benefit from lessons learned in archaeology during the last 200 years.

Acknowledgements

The authors would like to express their gratitude to Marcel van Beest, Dennis Boon, Jurrien Bijhold, Gerda Edelman, Paul van den Hoven, Roosje de Leeuwe, Gerard Stor, Matthijs Zuidberg (Netherlands Forensic Institute), Nicholas Márquez-Grant (Cranfield University, UK) and Rob Janaway (University of Bradford, UK) for their helpful and constructive comments on the earlier versions of this chapter that greatly contributed to its final version. The final manuscript has also benefitted from useful suggestions provided by Eline Schotsmans and Christopher Knüsel (University of Bordeaux, France).

References

Alberti, B., Jones, A.M. and Pollard, J. (2013) *Archaeology after Interpretation: Returning materials to archaeological theory*. Left Coast Press: Walnut Creek.

Bailey, G.N. (2007) Time perspectives, palimpsests and archaeology of time. *Journal of Anthropological Archaeology*, **26**: 198–223.

Banning, E.B. (2002) Archaeological survey as optimal search. In: Burenhult, G. and Arvidsson, J. (eds), *Archaeological Informatics. Pushing the envelope, computer applications and quantitative methods in archaeology*, Proceedings of the 29th Annual CAA Conference, Gotland, April 2001. Archeopress: Oxford, pp. 341–350.

Beauregard, E. and Bouchard, M. (2010) Cleaning up your act: forensic awareness as a detection avoidance strategy. *Journal of Criminal Justice*, **38**: 1160–1166.

Beauregard, E. and Martineau, M. (2014) No body, no crime? The role of forensic awareness in avoiding police detection in cases of sexual homicide. *Journal of Criminal Justice*, **42**: 213–220.

Bentley, R.A., Maschner, H.D.G. and Chippindale, C. (2009) *Handbook of Archaeological Theories*. AltaMira Press: Plymouth.

Bianchini, C., Borgogni, F. and Ippolito, A. (2015) Advantages and disadvantages of digital approach in archaeological fieldwork. In: Giligny, F., Djindjian, F., Costa, L., Moscati, P. and Robert, S. (eds), *CAA2014, 21st Century Archaeology. Concepts, Methods and Tools.* Proceedings of the 42nd Annual CAA Conference, Paris, April 2014, Archeopress: Oxford, pp. 95–105.

Binford, L.R. (1977) General introduction. In: Binford, L.R. (ed.), *For Theory Building in Archaeology: Essays on faunal remains, aquatic resources, spatial analysis and systematic modelling*. Academic Press: New York, pp. 1–10.

Binford, L.R. (1981) Behavioural archaeology and the 'Pompeii premise'. *Journal of Anthropological Research*, **37**: 195–208.

Buikstra, J.E. and Beck, L.A. (2009) *Bioarchaeology: The contextual analysis of human remains*. Left Coast Press: San Diego.

Carver, M. (1990) Digging for data: archaeological approaches to data definition, acquisition and analysis. In: Francovich, R. and Manacorda, D. (eds), *Lo scavo archeologico. Della diagnosi all'edizione.* All'Insegna del Giglio SAS: Florence, pp. 45–120.

Chapman, R. and Wylie, A. (eds) (2015) *Material Evidence: Learning from archaeological practice.* Routledge: New York.

Champod, C. (2014) Research focused mainly on bias will paralyse forensic science. *Science and Justice*, **54**: 107–109.

Clarke, D.L. (1973) Archaeology: the loss of innocence. *Antiquity*, **47**: 6–18.

Cleland, C.E. (2002) Methodological and epistemic differences between historical science and experimental science. *Philosophy of Science*, **69**: 474–496.

Cleland, C.E. (2011). Prediction and explanation in historical natural sciences. *The British Journal for the Philosophy of Science*, **62**: 551–582.

Cook, R., Evett. I.W., Jackson, G., Jones, P.J. and Lambert, J.A. (1998a) A hierarchy of propositions: deciding which level to address in casework. *Science and Justice*, **38**: 231–239.

Cook, R., Evett, I.W., Jackson, G., Jones, P.J. and Lambert, J.A. (1998b) A model for case assessment and interpretation. *Science and Justice*, **38**: 151–156.

Darvill, T. (2002) *The Concise Oxford Dictionary of Archaeology.* Oxford University Press: Oxford.

DeBoer, W.R. (1983) The archaeological record as preserved death assemblage. In: Moore, J.A. and Keene, A.S. (eds), *Archaeological Hammers and Theories.* Academic Press: New York, pp. 19–36.

Ditrich, H. (2015) Cognitive fallacies and criminal investigations. *Science and Justice*, **55**: 155–159.

Duday, H. (2006) Archaeothanatology or the archaeology of death. In: Gowland, R. and Knüsel, C. (eds), *Social Archaeology of Funerary Remains*. Oxbow Books: Oxford, pp. 30–56.

Dupras, T.L., Schultz, J.J., Wheeler, S.M. and Williams, L.J. (2011) *Forensic Recovery of Human Remains: Archaeological approaches*. CRC Press: Boca Raton.

ENFSI (European Network of Forensic Science Institutes) (2015) *ENFSI Guideline for Evaluative Reporting in Forensic Science: Strengthening the evaluation of forensic results across Europe (STEOFRAE)*. Available at: https://www.unil.ch/esc/files/live/sites/esc/files/Fichiers%202015/ENFSI%20Guideline%20Evaluative%20Reporting (accessed 15 September 2015).

Evett, I.W. (2015) The logical foundations of forensic science: towards reliable knowledge. *Philosophical Transactions B*, **370**: article ID 20140263.

Evett, I.W., Jackson, G. and Lambert, J.A. (2000) More on the hierarchy of propositions: exploring the distinction between explanations and propositions. *Science and Justice*, **40**: 3–10.

Gardner, R.M. (2012) *Practical Crime Scene Processing and Investigation*. CRC Press: Boca Raton.

Gardner, R.M. and Bevel, T. (2009) *Practical Crime Scene Analysis and Reconstruction.* CRC Press: Boca Raton.

Gennard, D. (2012) *Forensic Entomology: An introduction*. Wiley-Blackwell: Oxford.

Gibbon, G. (1989) *Explanation in Archaeology*. Blackwell: Oxford.

Groen, W.J.M., Márquez-Grant, N. and Janaway, R.C. (2015) *Forensic Archaeology. A global perspective.* Wiley-Blackwell: Oxford.

Hodder, I. (1986) *Reading the Past: Current approaches to interpretation in archaeology*. Cambridge University Press: Cambridge.

Hodder, I. (1992) *Theory and Practice in Archaeology*. Routledge: London.

Houck, M.M. and Siegel, J.A. (2010) *Fundamentals of Forensic Science*. Academic Press: Burlington.

Houck, M.M., Crispino, F. and McAdam, T. (2012) *The Science of Crime Scenes*. Academic Press: Oxford.

Hunter, J., Simpson, B. and Sturdy Colls, C. (2013) *Forensic Approaches to Buried Remains*. Wiley-Backwell: Oxford.

Jamieson, A (2004) A rational approach to the principles and practice of crime scene investigation: I. Principles. *Science and Justice*, **44**: 3–7.

Jeffares, B. (2008) Testing times: regularities in the historical sciences. *Studies in History and Philosophy of Biological and Biomedical Sciences*, **39**: 469–475.

Johnson, M. (2010) Archaeological Theory: An introduction. Wiley-Blackwell: Oxford.

Kassin, S.M., Dror, I.E. and Kukucka, J. (2013) The forensic confirmation bias: problems, perspective and proposed solutions. *Journal of Applied Research Memory and Cognition*, **2**: 42–52.

Larsen, C.S. (2015) *Bioarchaeology: Interpreting behaviour from the human skeleton*. Cambridge University Press: Cambridge.

Locard, E. (1920) *L'enquête criminelle et les méthodes scientifiques*. Ernest Flammarion: Paris.

Locard, E. (1930) The analysis of dust and traces. *American Journal of Police Science*, **1**: 279–298 and 401–418.

Lucas, G. (2012) *Understanding the Archaeological Record*. Cambridge University Press: Cambridge.

Ribaux, O., Baylon, A., Roux, C., Delémont, O., Lock, E. *et al.* (2010a) Intelligence-led crime scene processing. I: Forensic intelligence. *Forensic Science International*, **195**: 10–16.

Ribaux, O., Baylon, A., Lock, E., Delémont, O., Roux, C *et al.* (2010b) Intelligence-led crime scene processing. Part II: intelligence and crime scene examination. *Forensic Science International*, **199**: 63–71.

Robertson, B., Vignaux, G.A. and Berger C.E.H. (2016) *Interpreting Evidence: Evaluating forensic science in the courtroom*. 2nd edition. Wiley: Chichester.

Saks, M.J., Risinger, D.M., Rosenthal, R. and Thompson, W.C. (2003) Context effects in forensic science: A review and application of the science of science to crime laboratory practice in the United States. *Science and Justice*, **43**: 77–90.

Schiffer, M.B. (1972) Archaeological context and systemic context. *American Antiquity*, **37**: 156–165.

Schiffer, M.B. (1976) *Behavioural Archaeology*. Academic Press: New York.

Schiffer, M.B. (1983) Toward the identification of formation process. *American Antiquity*, **48**: 675–706.

Schiffer, M.B. (1996) *Formation Processes of the Archaeological Record*. University of Utah Press: Salt Lake City.

Scotland, J. (2012) Exploring the philosophical underpinnings of research: relating ontology and epistemology to the methodology and methods of the scientific, interpretative, and critical research paradigms. *English Language Teaching*, **5**: 9–16.

Smith, N.G. and Levy, T.E. (2014) ArchField in Jordan: real-time GIS data recording for archaeological excavation. *Near Eastern Archaeology*, **77**: 166–170.

Stoel, R.D., Berger, C.E.H., Kerkhoff, W., Matthijssen, E.J.A.T. and Dror, I.E. (2014) Minimizing contextual bias in forensic casework. In: Strom, K.J. and Hickman, M.J. (eds), *Forensic Science and the Administration of Justice: Critical issues and directions*. SAGE Publications: Thousand Oaks, pp. 67–86.

Sullivan, A.P. (1978) Inference and evidence in archaeology: a discussion of the conceptual problems. *Advances in Archaeological Method and Theory*, **1**: 183–222.

Swartz, B.K. Jr,, (1967) A logical sequence of archaeological objectives. *American Antiquity*, **32**: 487–497.
Verhagen, P. and Whitley, T.G. (2012) Integrating archaeological theory and predictive modelling: a live report from the scene. *Journal of Archaeological Method and Theory*, **19**: 49–100.
Wylie, A. (1992) 'On heavily decomposing red herrings': scientific method in archaeology and the ladening of evidence with theory. In: Embree, L. (ed.), *Metaarchaeology: Reflections by archaeologists and philosophers*. Kluwer: Boston, pp. 296–288.
Wylie, A. (2002) *Thinking from Things: Essays in the philosophy of archaeology*. University of California Press: Berkley, CA.
Wylie, A. (2011) Critical distance: stabilizing evidential claims in archaeology. In: Dawid, P., Twining, W. and Vasilaki, M. (eds), *Evidence, Inference and Enquiry*. Oxford University Press: Oxford, pp. 371–394.

Index

Note: Page numbers appearing in **bold** indicate tables, page numbers in *italic* indicate figures.

a

Taphonomy of Human Remains: Forensic Analysis of the Dead and the Depositional Environment, First Edition.
Edited by Eline M.J. Schotsmans, Nicholas Márquez-Grant and Shari L. Forbes.

r